LUMBAR SPINAL STENOSIS

Lumbar Spinal Stenosis

Gunnar B.J. Andersson, M.D., Ph.D.
Professor and Associate Chairman
Department of Orthopaedic Surgery
Rush Medical College
Senior Attending Surgeon
Rush–Presbyterian–St. Luke's Medical Center
Chicago, Illinois

Thomas W. McNeill, M.D.
Associate Professor
Department of Orthopaedic Surgery
Rush Medical College
Senior Attending Surgeon
Rush–Presbyterian–St. Luke's Medical Center
Chicago, Illinois

Forewords by
Alf L. Nachemson, M.D.
Henry La Rocca, M.D.

Mosby Year Book

St. Louis   Baltimore   Boston   Chicago   London   Philadelphia   Sydney   Toronto

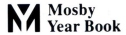
**Mosby
Year Book**

Dedicated to Publishing Excellence

Sponsoring Editor: James D. Ryan
Assistant Editor: Joyce-Rachel John
Associate Managing Editor, Manuscript Services: Deborah Thorp
Production Supervisor: Carol A. Reynolds

Mosby–Year Book, Inc.
11830 Westline Industrial Drive
St. Louis, MO 63146

1 2 3 4 5 6 7 8 9 0 CL CL MB 96 95 94 93 92

Library of Congress Cataloging-in-Publication Data
Lumbar spinal stenosis / [edited by] Gunnar B.J. Andersson, Thomas W.
  McNeill.
      p. cm.
    Includes bibliographical references and index.
    ISBN 0-8016-0090-1
    1. Spinal canal—Stenosis. 2. Spinal canal—Stenosis—Surgery.
3. Lumbar vertebrae—Surgery. I. Andersson, Gunnar, 1942– .
II. McNeill, Thomas W., 1936– .
    [DNLM: 1. Spinal Stenosis.   WE 750 L95662]
RD771.S74L86 1991
617.3'75—dc20   91-35006
DNLM/DLC   CIP
for Library of Congress

AMJAD ALI, M.D.
Associate Professor of Diagnostic Radiology and Nuclear
  Medicine
Rush Medical College
Associate Attending Physician
Rush–Presbyterian–St. Luke's Medical Center
Chicago, Illinois

GUNNAR B.J. ANDERSSON, M.D., PH.D.
Professor and Associate Chairman
Department of Orthopaedic Surgery
Rush–Presbyterian–St. Luke's Medical Center
Chicago, Illinois

CHARLES N. APRILL, III, M.D.
Spine Radiologist
Diagnostic Conservative Management, Inc.
New Orleans, Louisiana

SCOTT D. BODEN, M.D.
Assistant Professor Orthopaedic Surgery
The George Washington University School of Medicine
Washington, D.C.

RUSSELL BODIN, R.T.
Diagnostic Conservative Management, Inc.
New Orleans, Louisiana

MICHAEL BONFIGLIO, M.D.
Professor Emeritus
Orthopaedic Surgery
Department of Orthopaedics
University of Iowa Hospital
Iowa City, Iowa

NEIL I. CHAFETZ, M.D.
Rothman-Chafetz Medical Group
Torrance, California

JEN-YUH CHEN, M.D.
Biomechanics Laboratory II
Department of Biomedical Engineering
University of Iowa
Iowa City, Iowa

HENRY V. CROCK, A.O., M.D., F.R.C.S., F.R.A.C.S.
Consultant Spinal Surgeon
Senior Lecturer/Honorary Consultant
Royal Postgraduate Medical School
Cromwell Hospital
London, England

GIACOMO A. DELARIA, M.D.
Head, Division of Cardiac Surgery
Scripps Clinic and Research Foundation
La Jolla, California

CHARLES C. EDWARDS, M.D.
Professor of Orthopaedic Surgery
University of Maryland
Director, Spine Surgery Program
University of Maryland Hospital
Baltimore, Maryland

ERNEST W. FORDHAM, M.D.
Professor and Associate Chairman
Department of Diagnostic Radiology/Nuclear Medicine
Rush–Presbyterian–St. Luke's Medical Center
Chicago, Illinois

JOHN W. FRYMOYER, M.D.
Professor of Orthopaedics
Director, McClure Musculoskeletal Research Center
Department of Orthopaedics and Rehabilitation
University of Vermont
Orthopaedic Surgeon
Medical Center Hospital of Vermont
Burlington, Vermont

VIJAY K. GOEL, PH.D.
Professor and Chairman
Department of Biomedical Engineering
University of Iowa
Iowa City, Iowa

EDWARD J. GOLDBERG, M.D.
Department of Orthopaedics
Rush–Presbyterian–St. Luke's Medical Center
Chicago, Illinois

DIETER GROB, M.D.
Schulthess Klinik
Department of Orthopaedics
Zürich, Switzerland

LEON GROBLER, M.D.
Assistant Professor
Department of Orthopaedics
University of Vermont
Burlington, Vermont
Director of Surgical Services
Spine Institute of New England
Williston, Vermont

J. GWON, M.D.
Biomechanics Laboratory II
Department of Biomedical Engineering
University of Iowa
Iowa City, Iowa

SCOTT HALDEMAN, D.C., M.D., PH.D.
Associate Clinical Professor
Department of Neurology
University of California at Irvine
Irvine, California

KIM W. HAMMERBERG, M.D.
Assistant Professor
Section of Spinal Surgery
Department of Orthopaedic Surgery
Rush Medical College
Rush–Presbyterian–St. Luke's Medical Center
Chicago, Illinois

J. HAN, M.S.
Biomechanics Laboratory II
Department of Biomedical Engineering
University of Iowa
Iowa City, Iowa

TOMMY HANSSON, M.D., PH.D.
Professor and Chairman
Department of Orthopaedics I
Sahlgren Hospital
Göteborg, Sweden

MARK B. KABINS, M.D.
Spine Fellow
Department of Orthopaedic Surgery
University of California at Davis
Sacramento, California

TONY KIM, M.D.
Clinical Instructor
Neuroradiology Fellow
Department of Radiology
The University of Chicago
Chicago, Illinois

JOHN P. KOSTUIK, M.D., F.R.C.S.C.
Professor of Orthopedics
Director, Spine Service
Department of Orthopaedic Surgery
Johns Hopkins University
Baltimore, Maryland

TAO-HONG LIM, PH.D.
Biomechanics Laboratory II
Department of Biomedical Engineering
University of Iowa
Iowa City, Iowa

JEFFREY R. McCONNELL, M.D.
Division of Orthopaedic Surgery
University of Maryland Hospital
Baltimore, Maryland

THOMAS W. McNEILL, M.D.
Associate Professor
Department of Orthopedics Surgery
Rush Medical College
Senior Attending Surgeon
Rush–Presbyterian–St. Luke's Medical Center
Chicago, Illinois

KJELL OLMARKER, M.D., PH.D.
Department of Orthopaedics
Sahlgren Hospital
Göteborg University
Göteborg, Sweden

MALCOLM H. POPE, PH.D., DR. MED. SCI.
McClure Professor of Musculoskeletal Research
Director of Orthopaedic Research
University of Vermont
Vermont Rehabilitation Engineering Center
Burlington, Vermont

RICHARD W. PORTER, M.D., F.R.C.S., F.R.C.S.E.
Professor of Orthopaedics
Department of Orthopaedics
University Medical Buildings
Fosterhill, Aberdeen, Scotland

RUTH G. RAMSEY, M.D.
Professor of Radiology
Head, Section of Neuroradiology
The University of Chicago
Chicago, Illinois

WOLFGANG RAUSCHNING, M.D., PH.D.
Research Professor
Swedish Medical Research Council
Department of Orthopaedic Surgery
University Hospital
Uppsala, Sweden

JORDAN D. ROSENBLUM, M.D.
Instructor, Department of Radiology
The University of Chicago
Chicago, Illinois

ANDREW ROSENSON, M.D.
Department of Diagnostic Radiology/Nuclear Medicine
Rush–Presbyterian–St. Luke's Medical Center
Chicago, Illinois

STEPHEN L.G. ROTHMAN, M.D.
Consultant Radiologist
Spinal Injury Service
Rancho Los Amigas Hospital
Rothman-Chafetz Medical Group
Torrance, California

BJÖRN RYDEVIK, M.D., PH.D.
Associate Professor Orthopaedic Surgery
University of Göteborg
Associate Professor
Department of Orthopaedics
Sahlgren Hospital
Göteborg, Sweden

NILS SCHÖNSTRÖM, M.D., PH.D.
Department of Orthopaedics
Kalmar Hospital
Kalmar, Sweden

KEISUKE TAKAHASHI, M.D., PH.D.
Department of Orthopaedics
Kanzawa University School of Medicine
Kanzawa, Japan

HENK VERBIEST, M.D., PH.D.
Professor of Neurosurgery
Emeritus Chairman
Department of Neurosurgery
Utrecht University
Utrecht, The Netherlands

SUNJAY VERMA, M.D.
Clinical Instructor
Department of Radiology
The University of Chicago
Chicago, Illinois

BARRIE VERNON-ROBERTS, M.D.
George Richard Marks Professor and Head
Department of Pathology
University of Adelaide
Head, Division of Tissue Pathology
Institute of Medical and Veterinary Science
Adelaide, South Australia

ROBERT G. WATKINS, M.D.
Kerlan Jobe Orthopaedic Clinic
Inglewood, California

JAMES N. WEINSTEIN, D.O.
Professor, Department of Orthopaedics
Director, Spine Diagnostic and Treatment Center
University of Iowa Hospitals and Clinics
Iowa City, Iowa

SAM W. WIESEL, M.D.
Professor and Chairman
Department of Orthopaedic Surgery
Georgetown University Hospital
Washington, D.C.

LEON L. WILTSE, M.D.
Clinical Professor of Orthopaedic Surgery (Honorary)
University of California at Irvine
Irvine, California
Active Medical Staff
Memorial Medical Center at Long Beach
Wiltse Spine Institute
Long Beach, California

FOREWORD

The accurate diagnosis of spinal stenosis has long been a matter of controversy. This book certainly attempts to tackle that problem by a multidisciplinary and multidimensional approach. There is little doubt that this entity will be of increasing interest for spinologists over the next decade.

Our population aged 60 years or older will increase by 10% to 20% in the industrialized nations until the year 2010. In the future there will be more attention to this problem than ever before; the aging population will for various reasons have an increased demand on mobility and they will have the desire to add life to their "golden years," not just years to a handicapped life. In this context, a comprehensive review of the various aspects of spinal stenosis is urgently needed. What is also urgently needed, however, is a much better knowledge of the natural history of the patient with the clinical syndrome. It has been demonstrated by Johnsson and collaborators from Malmö, Sweden, that even with both clinical and radiological signs of spinal stenosis the natural history over at least four years is far from a picture of relentless deterioration. The condition of a majority of patients remains the same; some improve and only a few deteriorate.

The specificity and sensitivity of the various diagnostic tests need to be better investigated, and some studies in the literature already demonstrate that even though the sensitivity of our various radiologic tests such as CT, MR, and myelography is 80% to 90%, the specificity is less good.

The reader should be aware, also, of the increasing number of complications reported in the recent literature from the rather extensive surgery that is sometimes contemplated for aged patients. Not infrequently, less than satisfying results have been published. It is therefore mandatory that this text be reviewed with a critical eye. Everyone with experience in the field of spinal stenosis surgery can, after a few years of observation, identify his happiest and most thankful patient as well as less happy ones and even serious catastrophes. It is hoped that this comprehensive update will help us to avoid the mistakes of the past, to operate on fewer patients with less morbidity, and to successfully treat the majority with a more conservative approach.

ALF L. NACHEMSON, M.D., PH.D.
Professor and Chairman
Department of Orthopaedics
Göteborg University
Göteborg, Sweden

FOREWORD

Over the years, I have had several opportunities to work with Drs. Andersson and McNeill on a variety of projects focused on the organization and dissemination of information concerning the spine. A new opportunity was granted when I received an invitation to compose this foreword to their current educational effort, physically represented by this volume. Knowing well the quality of their work and the import of their separate and joint contributions to the field, I was eager to respond.

In producing this text, Drs. Andersson and McNeill have considered the broad range of topics that must be mastered before a comprehensive understanding of spinal stenosis can be had. On one level, stenosis is a pathoanatomic phenomenon in which the several spaces inside the bony spine are reduced in their dimensions. Yet, while appreciating the morphometric abnormality that is essential to the stenotic state, of even greater import is the effect that stenosis exerts on the contents of those spaces. This effect alone determines if and when stenosis transcends being merely an anatomical variation to become a clinical problem. In the degenerative sequence that can occur *pari passu* with normal aging, quite remarkable space constriction may arise with no attendant symptoms or findings. Further, all spinal traumatologists must admit that alarming degrees of canal constriction can result from the acute intrusion of fracture fragments in the patient who remains clinically intact.

While the ultimate determining factor in clinically significant stenosis is probably not yet known, crucially important new studies of the vascular anatomy of the neural elements have revised outmoded concepts. Coupling these with the elegant recent work of the pathophysiology of compressed neural structures inside the spine establishes that arterial insufficiency and venous stasis not only impair neural function, but they also contribute to demyelination and fiber death. Moreover, chronic intraneural edema sets the stage for intraneural fibrosis. Such anatomical changes create both local functional abnormalities in the affected nerves and more remote (and pernicious) disruptions in the spinal cord.

With this fundamental knowledge, exploration of the diverse etiologies of spinal stenosis permits recognition of the mode of insult that is common to them all, thus unifying a host of unrelated disorders. Practical matters, including the clinical assessment of the problem with all manner of contemporary technology, can now flow logically from such basic data.

Given a clinically significant case, the next unsolved issue in spinal stenosis is the choice of appropriate therapy. Once adequate conservative treatment has proved wanting, a surgical decision to decompress that which is compressed would seem automatic. How much decompression is required, however, remains a matter of opinion. Concerns about destabilizing the spine by removing what must be taken away are not yet resolved satisfactorily in the current literature. Even so, because bony resection must often be generous, a compelling case can be made for deploying internal fixation to regain the stability that has been deliberately sacrificed. Of course, since no internal fixation device can withstand the forces applied to it indefinitely, fusion must occur in order to obtain the desired outcome. Which fusion techniques are most reliable is not solidly established, but considering spinal biomechanics following extensive resection, efforts to minimize the risk of fusion failure become imperative.

All of these issues are admirably addressed herein, and the first truly comprehensive treatise on the subject has been launched.

HENRY LA ROCCA, M.D.
Clinical Professor of Orthopaedic Surgery
Tulane University Medical School
New Orleans, Louisiana

PREFACE

From the beginning, spinal stenosis has been a controversial topic. While there was always agreement that pressure of nervous tissue could cause pain, this was typically associated only with fractures, deformity, and herniated discs. The controversy was understandable, since earlier diagnostic techniques had poor sensitivity and did not provide cross-sectional images. Unfortunately, even at present, spinal stenosis is not a clear concept. It remains an entity that is poorly understood, with poorly described clinical features and confusing terminology and classification. Although discussed in all contemporary books on back pain, there is a lack of comprehensive text detailing all aspects of spinal stenosis. This is becoming even more noticeable as we begin to understand the problem better, as new diagnostic techniques emerge, and as we apply new surgical approaches to solve the problem. Against that background it is unfortunate that information is still scattered between disciplines and, thus, is difficult to access. This book is an attempt to remedy this situation.

When deciding on the content of the book, we had a number of goals:

- To describe spinal stenosis clinically, morphologically, physiologically, and pathologically. This required introductory basic science chapters.
- To detail the multiple etiologies while acknowledging that degenerative changes are responsible for the majority of problems.
- To review current diagnostic techniques and attempt to advise on the different choices.
- To present a management philosophy, including nonoperative and operative treatment alternatives, and to discuss the surgical techniques and their consequences.
- To alert the reader, in a clear fashion, to the diversity of thought in treatment choices.
- To make the reader aware of possible complications arising from treatment and the management of such complications.

We also wanted to make sure that the book was contemporary and provided expert opinion. This required asking a large number of outstanding scientists and clinicians to devote their time to this effort. We are grateful to our contributors who worked so diligently and provided such excellence. We are also grateful to our editors, James Ryan and Joyce-Rachel John, for their understanding and unfailing support. Our families have been remarkable in their understanding and support. They have allowed books, papers, and phone calls to interfere with our family lives and accepted that we have spent long hours away from home. We are deeply grateful.

Many people contributed to this book by devoting their particular skills. Judith Weik provided illustrations of superb quality. Dorothy Bell provided excellent secretarial support. Margaret Hickey, Suzanne Buckner, Mary Jo Przybylowicz, and Glenda Sinkora helped in many aspects of the effort. Finally, we wish to thank the FAX machines around the world, without whose presence we would not have been finished on time.

GUNNAR B.J. ANDERSSON, M.D., PH.D.
THOMAS W. McNEILL, M.D.

CONTENTS

Spinal Stenosis: The Concept

Henk Verbiest, M.D., Ph.D., Hon. F.R.C.S., Eng.

I accepted the editors' invitation to participate in this book as a charming challenge. My charge was to present my personal experience with stenosis of the lumbar spinal canal. This is a rare opportunity to present an inside story in a medium in which, it seems, only the outside stories determine the scientific values of the community.

My inside story of spinal stenosis is unique. During the past 56 years, I have published scientific papers on various subjects. However, stenosis has been the only subject that has kept me fascinated from my first stenosis paper in 1949 to the present. This is because stenosis has many faces that are, in the end, human faces.

THE EARLY DAYS

The first period of my story encompasses the years from 1949 to the early 1960s. This was a personal period of solitude in which I mobilized my mental and physical efforts.

The discovery of developmental stenosis was not simply the result of thought. The thought followed the physical efforts of removing very thickened laminae, leaving me with blisters on my hands and confusion. The confusion arose from not having found any abnormality in the vertebral canal to explain the partial or complete caudographic block that had been one of my surgical indications. I discussed this quandary with my neurosurgical colleagues, some of whom had had similar experiences. They were unable to provide an explanation or additional information or to suggest appropriate steps to investigate this phenomenon. After some thought, I then

decided to approach the problem systematically. I would make exact clinical and surgical reports of future cases using a fixed protocol. By this approach I hoped to detect common properties among these cases.

My first three cases had thickened laminae and a complete caudographic block in common. The next step in my protocol was to "inspect the vertebral canal thoroughly." This provided me with a striking example of the psychological difference between "looking" and "seeing." I suddenly became aware of the narrowness of the vertebral canal in the area of the thickened laminae. There is no doubt that narrow spinal canals have existed before. Thickened laminae as a cause of neurologic problems have, in fact, been reported by a few authors since 1900.[2, 19, 21] The authors "saw," however, the thickened laminae but not the narrow canal as the culprit.

In two of my three cases the thickened laminae involved one vertebra and in the third case two vertebrae. In one of the cases the dural sac dilated after laminectomy. The other two required additional decompression of the dural sac. In all three patients the signs and symptoms disappeared following the decompression. This, I believed, confirmed the reality of the thesis that the narrow vertebral canal was the cause of the symptoms. It was also encouraging good luck since in later years complete cure did not always follow decompressive surgery.

My first paper (1949) was published in a commemorative volume in memory of my teacher, Professor Clovis Vincent.[25] Unfortunately, this volume is no longer available (although several hundred copies may exist in a Paris depot). It was in this paper that I baptized the narrowing of the bony vertebral canal as "stenosis" since the passage of contrast medium was impeded. This paper included measurements of the spinal canal (which had been done from the beginning) and made the distinction between absolute and relative stenosis. The clinical picture presented mentioned walking disturbance.

My earliest work also included morphologic measurements, namely of the interpedicular distances of the lumbar vertebral canal, based on anteroposterior (AP) radiographs of 100 Dutch volunteers who were symptom-free.[25, 26] The interpedicular distance of my first three patients fell within the range of normals established by this study. It was by deduction that I concluded that the abnormal narrowing was in the sagittal diameter and was caused by thickened laminae and articular processes.

In 1950 I published my first stenosis paper in the *Nederlands Tijdschrift Voor Geneeskunde*.[26] I now had a detailed analysis of a total of five cases and was therefore able to present a more thorough description of the clinical and morphologic picture of lumbar spinal stenosis. The clinical symptoms described were disturbances of walking or standing which included pain, paresthesias, and loss of power or sensation, or both. The walking disturbance was called "intermittent claudication" and was considered to be pathognomonic of stenosis of the lumbar vertebral canal. Three of the five patients had intermittent claudication, the pathophysiology of which was unknown, as was the source of its variation in causative signs and symptoms among patients. Hypothetical causes for the intermittent claudication and the variation among patients were advanced. The possibility of increased local pressure on the nerve roots by the wall of the vertebral canal during upright posture or an increased gradient of spinal fluid above and below the area of stenosis were considered. The absence of symptoms of intermittent claudication in some patients with stenosis was thought to be due to differences in tolerance of the caudal nerve roots to pressure and wear and tear caused by standing and walking.

The morphologic properties of stenosis as seen in radiographs, frontal tomograms, and caudograms were also described. The plain radiographs and tomograms may reveal a great height of the laminae obliterating the interlaminar space. There may be an acute angle between the inferior articular processes which may reach to the midline and obliterate the interlaminar space. Contrast studies (caudograms) reveal a block to the passage of contrast medium. The block is greater posteriorly than anteriorly as a consequence of the hypertrophic laminae or facets,

or both. The "toothed" appearance of extradural compression is present. Since the pathologic changes often consist of thickening of the laminae and hypertrophy of the articular processes, laminectomy alone often is insufficient. The medial portion of the articular processes may need to be removed also.

In the years 1948 and 1949 the frequency of surgery for stenosis vs. herniated disc was 5 vs. 159 in our department.

In an English translation of this early work, I coined the term *developmental* in order to distinguish it from congenital (existing at birth) described by Sarpyener in 1945 and 1947.[22, 23] In none of our patients were symptoms of stenosis present before adult life. I meant to infer by this terminology that I believed that in my cases the stenosis was not fully developed at birth, but rather was due to thickening

UNIVERSITY CLINIC OF NEUROLOGY, UTRECHT

UNUSUAL FORMS OF COMPRESSION OF THE CAUDA EQUINA

REPORT OF TWO CASES OF LUMBO-SACRAL EXTRADURAL CYSTS AND OF ONE CASE OF ‹KNOTTING› OF A CAUDAL NERVE ROOT

BY

Dr. H. VERBIEST
Chief of the Neurosurgical Department

PAPER READ AT THE MEETING OF THE LUSO-SPANISH SOCIETY AND THE BRITISH SOCIETY OF NEUROLOGICAL SURGEONS, MADRID, APRIL, 26, 1951

1953

VALENCIA

FIG 1–1.
Predestined oblivion of a paper through external measures.[27] For explanation, see text.

of the laminae and articular processes caused by abnormal postnatal bone growth. Unfortunately, ambiguity persisted as dictionary definitions of *developmental* varied. Confusion persists to this day with some authors using developmental stenosis as a synonym for congenital stenosis.[1] Fortunately, a clearer definition of *developmental* vs. *congenital* is now given by *Churchill's Medical Dictionary* (1989): "In current use developmental is often preferred to congenital because the former refers to the total span of development, whether embryonic, fetal or postnatal. Congenital implies that the condition originated prenatally and was present at birth." It is remarkable to me that there exists no equivalent in German, Dutch, or French for the English term *developmental*.

My English paper (which now included nine cases) was rejected repeatedly by editorial boards of important English and American neurosurgical and neurologic journals. The reasons given for rejection varied from disbelief to irrelevant comments about spinal fluid protein variability among the patients treated. This caused me great concern and mental stress, since because of language barriers my views remained unnoticed outside of my country. The breakthrough came 4 years later when the English version of my paper was published (1954). It was ironic to me, a neurosurgeon, that the paper was not published by a neurosurgical or neurologic journal, but rather by the British volume of the *Journal of Bone and Joint Surgery*.[29] It is regrettable that 4 years were lost.

During the period of time that I was working on getting the English version of my paper accepted, two others were published. In a paper given at the combined meetings of the British, Spanish, and Portuguese Neurosurgical Societies in Madrid on April 26, 1951, I described "knotted" caudal nerve roots in a case of stenosis. This paper was published in Valencia in 1953[27] for distribution to the members of the societies (Figs 1–1 and 1–2). The publisher did not list his name, and the distribution was limited. No wonder that this condition was rediscovered 17 years later under the name "redundant" caudal nerve root.[5] The second paper dealing with stenosis was published in the *Nederlands Tijdschrift Voor Geneeskunde*.[28] This paper attempted to give a fundamental classification of vertebral disorders (stenosis) based on three basic categories. These categories were derived from the capacity of the vertebral canal, the condition of the motion segment, and the condition of the hard tissues of the spine.

BASIC STUDIES

Since I had hypothesized, but not proved, that developmental stenosis was the result of excessively small sagittal diameters, it was necessary to measure midsagittal diameters (MSDs) in our stenotic patients and compare them with those of a normal population. The MSD was chosen because it is the only measurement with constant reference markers and thus liable to comparative investigation.

Unfortunately, there were no published data with reference to MSDs that I was able to find in the literature. I needed to find a way to generate these figures myself. I requested the aid of Dr. J. J. A.

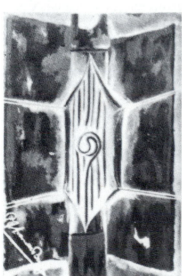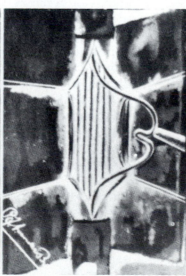

FIG 1–2.
Left, illustration showing knotted caudal nerve root. *Right*, illustration showing abnormal length of the same caudal nerve root after disentanglement of the knot through perineurolysis. This drawing appeared in the paper whose title page is pictured in Fig 1–1.

Huizinga who was later to become professor of physical anthropology in our faculty. By a happy coincidence, Dr. Huizinga had been charged with the identification of the ancient skeletal remains of a person who was buried in a common grave.* This gave us access to 50 Dutch lumbar spines for measurements. He found that the minimal MSDs in these spines were: L1, 14 mm; L2, 13 mm; L3, 12 mm; L4, 11 mm; and L5, 12 mm. Since there was a very high frequency of MSDs of 11 mm at L4, it was felt that measurements of this magnitude were not sufficiently small to produce symptoms of stenosis (called in this instance "absolute stenosis"). Absolute stenosis was thought to probably occur in spines with MSDs of 10 mm or less.

International acceptance of the concept of stenosis was very slow indeed. The first independent English-language papers appeared in the United States in 1961 and 1962. They were presented by Elihu Friedman,[10] an orthopaedic surgeon, and Joe Epstein, a neurosurgeon, and colleagues.[9] Meanwhile, during the period from 1955 to 1961 we quietly continued our studies which were reasonably well received in Europe and well received in the Netherlands. It was in 1955 that I received the Winkler Medal (given once every 4 years for neurologic research) from the Dutch Neurologic Society. This came at a time when I was beginning to have doubts about stenosis and the honor provided needed encouragement to continue my investigations.

THE TURNING POINT

My 19 years of taciturnity on the subject of stenosis came to an end in 1974 with an invitation from Harry Farfan to participate in the founding of the International Society for the Study of the Lumbar Spine. I decided to give a talk on the pathomorphology of developmental stenosis based upon measurements. The planning of this paper led to new insights and a future strategy.

We had developed a measurement device, the "stenosimeter,"[30] which allowed us to safely make intraoperative measurements of the stenotic area in 97 cases. Intraoperative measurements could not be

Johan van Oldebarnevelt was, along with William of Orange, a founder of the Dutch Republic. He, unfortunately, fell into disgrace with William of Orange's son who had him beheaded and buried in a common grave. The present-day Dutch government has restored the reputation of van Oldebarnevelt and placed his remains in a mausoleum.

safely done by the method that Dr. Huizinga used on the skeletal remains. The clinical measurements could only be done in the interlaminar space. This yielded additional insight. The ratio of MSD measurements from the cephalad border and the caudad border is normally less than 1. In some stenosing vertebrae, this ratio may be reversed. It was also noted that the stenosis may occur only at the cephalad or caudad border of the so-called stenosing arch. In stenotic areas there may be discontinuities where the measurements are normal. Prior to computed tomography (CT) scanning, these discontinuities were a source of surgical error. It was in this presentation[32] that the concept of foraminal stenosis was introduced.

NEUROGENIC INTERMITTENT CLAUDICATION

I was asked to write chapters on neurogenic intermittent claudication (NICL) for the *Handbook of Clinical Neurology* and in a monograph.[33, 34] This required additional focus and exploration of fields that had not received attention in the neurologic literature to date. Further, it required the establishment of criteria for the diagnosis of NICL.[31] One of my difficulties was that the syndrome was often more impressive to the physician than to the patient. NICL becomes, however, not manifest during clinical examination. It remains the patient's private experience. He is not capable of recognizing the particularities of NICL and usually verbalizes this complaint in terms of declining vitality or early fatigue. Charcot encountered similar difficulty, having described vascular intermittent claudication in 1858.[3] Charcot complained 29 years later (1887) that he had not encountered even a single physician who had seen this disturbance.[4] He asked, "Is there a more impressive syndrome than this one?"

Failing intellectual capacity for self-analysis by the patient and failure by the physician to ask the correct questions results in masked NICL. I needed to exactly define the fundamental properties of NICL in the most simple and clear manner so that the pertinent questions could be adapted for the anamnestic low back patient protocol. The questions about walking were:

1. How long can you walk? (My patients are unsure about distances.)

2. What causes you to stop walking? (This should not consist of an exaggeration of resting [pre-walking] signs and symptoms but rather of a new disturbance.)

3. What causes you to stop walking? (Was it pain, parasthesias, loss of power, backache, urinary incontinence. Were one or both legs involved? What is the relationship to the symptoms at rest?)

4. After a short rest can you resume walking?

5. How long does the rest need to be?

This detailed analysis resulted in some unexpected findings[39] such as the spread of symptoms present at rest to a larger area during walking. The most frequent symptom associated with NICL was loss of power. Pain or sensory deficit was half as frequently given as the cause to stop walking. A curious phenomenon was the suppression while walking of resting (permanent) leg pains in about one half of the patients who were experiencing resting leg pains, while 17 of 22 patients without resting leg pains experienced them when walking!

NICL was present in 72% of 195 patients. NICL was found with MSDs in the range between 4 and 10 mm which was no different from the MSDs found in the patients who did not experience NICL. This indicates that both the narrowness of the vertebral canal and the individual tolerance of the nerve roots to compression were determinants of NICL.

Two theories as to the cause of NICL were debated by various authors. Some supported the thesis that NICL was caused by pressure on the nerve roots and others supported the idea that NICL was a result of nerve root ischemia. These theories were based upon findings in acute experiments. In my view, the differences in individual tolerance of nerve roots to chronic stenotic compression might result in nerve roots that remain intact, nerve roots developing permanent neural deficit, and nerve roots that develop subclinical changes which only become manifest during additional stenotic compression while standing or walking and produce NICL.[39, 42, 43] I based this view upon Gilliatt and Wilson's findings,[12, 13] that subclinical changes in a nerve may become symptomatic through additional proximal compression of the nerve. In a few of our cases it appeared that symptoms (NICL) persisted because one cephalad stenotic segment had not been decompressed.[33, 34] Reoperation with decompression of the additional stenotic level caused the remaining NICL to disappear.[37] In any case, NICL appears to be caused by additional compression (ischemia) of already subclinically "injured" nerve

roots. The clinical relevance of this conclusion appears to be that one cannot be sure of the "symptomatic level" in NICL, the exception being isolated neuroforaminal stenosis producing NICL.

DISC HERNIATIONS

Our material revealed a high incidence of disc herniations at L3–4 and higher levels[33, 34, 39, 42] and a higher frequency of multiple disc herniations in stenotic patients. In our patients a disc herniation at L1–2 was always associated with developmental stenosis, which may be outside of the area of herniation, causing the stenosis to remain unidentified. These findings bear a remarkable resemblance to those seen in achondroplasia[42] and raise some interesting questions.

RADIOGRAPHIC MEASUREMENT
OF THE SPINAL CANAL

In the years 1974 to 1976, Gargano et al.[11] and Jacobson et al.[16, 17] introduced Takahashi's method[24] of axial transverse tomography for examining the stenotic lumbar canal. This method became obsolete in the same year (1976) with the introduction of body CT scans which produced much better images. In 1979, I published the measurement of MSDs using CT.[38] It was now possible to determine when the decompression can be confined to the caudad portion of the lamina,[42, 43] thus, limiting the surgery to the areas affected.

Radiographic (CT) analysis in cases of degenerative spondylolisthesis and traumatic deformity of the spinal canal causing NICL were often associated with stenosis in neighboring portions of the canal.[33, 34, 38] The identification of this more extensive stenosis is important. A decision as to whether or not treatment must consist of reducing the deformity by means of instrumentation or limiting the decompression to the area of deformity will be dependent upon these findings.

Radiologists often give attention to the bony structures surrounding the vertebral canal and neglect the structural properties of the canal itself. Gestalt psychology explains that for recognition of a pattern a background is needed. Further, if the background is also a pattern, then the subject cannot perceive both patterns at the same time.[40] Therefore, radiologists and spinal surgeons should be trained to first examine in CT scans the pattern of the bony walls of the vertebral canal with the lumen of the canal as background followed by evaluating the pattern of the lumen of the vertebral canal.

MEASUREMENTS BY OTHER AUTHORS

Investigators who are interested in measurements may become confused in their interpretation of the data. For example, physical anthropologists, who do not know the medical history of the original "owner" of the spine, may be tempted to exceed the limits of statistical information. Huizinga found the smallest MSDs in the region of L3–4. He called this a region of "physiologic stenosis" suggesting that the developmental stenosis might be an exaggeration of the physiologic stenosis.[15] Our measurements showed that developmental stenosis most often occurred at L5, although it may be confined to the upper lumbar levels.[33, 34]

Eisenstein accepted MSDs of 11 to 13 mm as being stenotic.[6, 7] Our measurements showed that these measurements were not a cause of neural problems in the absence of other factors. So-called relative stenosis is not a pathologic condition. This relative stenosis is prone to a pathologic condition. Minor degenerative changes may produce absolute stenosis.

Postacchini et al. measured MSDs of skeletal lumbar vertebrae from the caudal portion of the laminar junction overlying the caudad border of the vertebral body. This method did not take into account the MSDs of the caudad border of the laminae where they overroof the intervertebral discs.[43]

CLINICAL STENOSIS

Clinical stenosis can only be analyzed through measurements in patients with clinical disturbances. Even then, the interpretation of the findings may be erroneous.

The neural arch is the cause of symptomatic stenosis when the MSD is too small. In cases of interpedicular distances that are too small, a growth dis-

turbance of the vertebral body must be inferred. Thus, measurements may indicate the site of abnormal bone growth.

Different morphologic types of stenosis may produce the same reduction in cross-sectional area of the theca and be equally symptomatic. Therefore, patients with MSDs that are too small, interpedicular distances that are too narrow, or concentric narrowing of the vertebral canal (achondroplasia) may all benefit from decompressive laminectomy.

CLINICAL RADIOGRAPHY

Plain radiographic examination may reveal that stenosis is present. When there is an acute angle between the inferior articular processes on the AP view, there is a significant chance of stenosis at that level. This is especially true if the interlaminar space is occluded by the articular processes. The examination of the plain radiographs for signs of stenosis is especially important since, for economic reasons, CT scans are usually limited to L3 to S1. Clinically important stenosis may be present above these levels.[8,42] Sagittal magnetic resonance imaging (MRI), particularly the T2-weighted images, may give an idea of the fluid content of the dural theca but do not visualize the bony structures well. Myelography of the entire lumbar spine remains the safest method for the diagnosis and localization of stenosis.[33, 34, 42]

LINGUISTICS AND CLASSIFICATION

This topic concerns the role of linguistics in nomenclature and classification.[35, 36, 41–43] As editor in chief of *Neuro-Orthopaedics*, it frequently happens that I must call the attention of authors to their use of linguistically dubious or ambiguous terminology. Often they agree with my objections but insist on using the inadequate term because it is now in general use. They are afraid that using a better term may not carry the intended meaning to the linguistically preconditioned reader.

The term *lumbar stenosis* is now canonized by tacit convention. Medical circles like vague old Latin or Greek expressions. Molière ridiculed this trend in the 17th century but it remains to this day.

A study of the etymology of stenosis[36] revealed that in the classical period it was used to indicate small orifices (Aristotle: small esophagus; Galen: small veins). Stenosis disappeared from the medical vocabulary until the 19th century when it came into use to indicate a small channel or orifice which impedes the transport of gases, liquids, or solid matter. The word *stenosis* was also briefly used to indicate a reduced capacity of the cranial cavity.

The basic disturbance in lumbar stenosis is not in the transport of some physiologic matter, but rather a narrowing that produces constriction of fixed living tissue.[35, 36, 42, 43] I therefore distinguish between "transport stenosis" and "compressive stenosis."

Shortly after the introduction of the word *stenosis* to describe narrowing of the lumbar spinal canal, it was employed in a classification system.[1] At that time, the authors felt obliged to give a definition also. The result was a failing consensus for the use of the term *stenosis*. Some authors use it to indicate a vertebral canal that is too narrow or intervertebral foramina that are too narrow. Others apply it to small lateral recesses, which in reality are portions of a canal and not channels. Some authors have gone so far as to invent illusionary walls for the "lateral recess."[18, 43] The term *lateral stenosis* has become very popular. This term is applied not only to narrowing of an intervertebral foramen due to bone growth changes but to all sorts of degenerative changes of the intervertebral foramen which may impinge on the nerve roots. Many of these changes were described in earlier years.[14] Now they wear a new garment and are called "lateral stenosis."

In later years, I have regretted having introduced the term *stenosis* of the lumbar spinal canal. I chose this term because the flow of contrast medium was obstructed in these narrow lumbar canals. It would have been better if I had used the term *narrow vertebral canal*. This can easily be translated into all languages and is easily understood.

Some authors consider congenital and developmental stenosis to be identical. This is not our intention. Sarpyener's papers on congenital stenosis called attention to a condition of vertebral canal narrowing which was present at birth and was part of a larger malformation.[22, 23] We have had experience with congenital stenosis that became manifest in adulthood. These were dysraphic states or errors of segmentation[32, 33, 35, 42, 43] which were surely present at birth. The stenosis in these patients was not due to bony hypertrophy as in developmental stenosis. Developmental stenosis exists in achondroplasia. In this instance, the stenosis is not the disease per se but the symptom of a disease characterized by a generalized growth disturbance.[42]

CONCLUSIONS

I hope that, in the future, the adjective *idiopathic* can be removed from the term *developmental stenosis*. Many differing causes are now coming to light, making the term *idiopathic* inappropriate. Possibly, the term *osteoblastic stenosis* will be substituted for developmental stenosis, should the osteogenic importance be confirmed. CT scans should provide quantification of the progressive thickening of the bone and be applied to longitudinal follow-up studies which need to last for 10 years or longer.

The neurophysiologic aspects of NICL should be explored in the laboratory using a treadmill, electromyelograms, NCVs, etc.

I have enjoyed the opportunity to present this short review of my life story as it pertains to developmental stenosis. I understand that the reader may agree or disagree with my theories, but, in any case, this story demonstrates that those interested in stenosis of the vertebral canal will encounter various intriguing fields of research that ought to keep him or her busy for a lifetime.

REFERENCES

1. Arnoldi CC, Brodsky AE, Cauchoix J, et al: Lumbar spinal stenosis and nerve root entrapment syndromes. *Clin Orthop* 1976; 115:4–5.
2. Bailey P, Casamajor L: Osteoarthritis of the spine as a cause of compression of the spinal cord and its roots. *J Nerv Ment Dis* 1911; 38:588–609.
3. Charcot JM: Sur la claudication intermittente. *C R Soc Biol (Paris)* 1858; 225–238.
4. Charcot JM: Lecons du Mardi à la Salpétrière. Policlinique 1887–1888. Paris, Aux Bureaux du Progrès Médical et Louis Bataille 1892; 1:44.
5. Cressman NR, et al: Serpentine myelographic defect caused by redundant nerve root. Case report. *J Neurosurg* 1968; 28:391–393.
6. Eisenstein SM: The morphometry and pathological anatomy of the lumbar spine in South African Negroes and Caucasians with special reference to spinal stenosis. *J Bone Joint Surg [Br]* 1977; 59:173–180.
7. Eisenstein SM: Lumbar vertebral morphometry for computerized tomography in spinal stenosis. *Spine* 1983; 8:187–191.
8. Elsberg CA, Dyke CG: The diagnosis and localization of tumors of the spinal cord by means of measurements made in x-ray films of the vertebrae and the correlation of the clinical and the x-ray findings. *Bull Neurol Inst NY* 1934; 3:359–394.
9. Epstein J, Epstein BS, Lavine LS: Nerve root compression associated with narrowing of the lumbar spinal canal. *J Neurol Neurosurg Psychiatry* 1962; 25:165–170.
10. Friedman E: Narrowing of the spinal canal due to

thickening of the laminae, a cause of back pain and sciatica. *Clin Orthop* 1961; 21:190–197.

11. Gargano FP, Jacobson RE, Rosomoff H: Transverse axial tomography of the spine. *Neuroradiology* 1974; 6:254–258.

12. Gilliatt RW, Wilson TG: A pneumatic tourniquet test in the carpal tunnel syndrome. *Lancet* 1933; 2:595–597.

13. Gilliatt RW, Wilson TG: Ischemic sensory loss in patients with peripheral nerve lesions. *J Neurol Neurosurg Psychiatry* 1954; 17:104–114.

14. Hadley MD: *Anatomo-Roentgenographic Studies of the Spine.* Springfield, Ill, Charles C Thomas, Publisher, 1964.

15. Huizinga J, Heiden JA, Vander Vinken PJJG: The human vertebral canal. A biometric study. *Proc R Neth Acad Sci* 1952; C55:23–33.

16. Jacobson R, Gargano FP, Rosomoff H: Transverse axial tomography of the spine. Part I. Axial anatomy of the normal lumbar spine. *J Neurosurg* 1975; 42:406–411.

17. Jacobson R, Gargano FP, Rosomoff H: Transverse axial tomography of the spine. Part II. The stenotic spinal canal. *J Neurosurg* 1975; 42:412–419.

18. Kirkaldy-Willis WH: Lumbar spinal stenosis (editorial comment). *Clin Orthop* 1976; 115:2–3.

19. Parker HL, Adson AW: Compression of the spinal cord and its roots by hypertrophic arthritis. *Surg Gynecol Obstet* 1925; 41:1–14.

20. Postacchini F, Ripani M, Carpano S: Morphometry of the lumbar vertebrae. *Clin Orthop* 1983; 172:296–303.

21. Sachs B, Fraenkel J: Progressive ankylotic rigidity of the spine (spondylose rhizomélique). *J Nerv Ment Dis* 1900; 27:1–15.

22. Sarpyener MA: Congenital stricture of the spinal canal. *J Bone Joint Surg [Br]* 1945; 27:70–79.

23. Sarpyener MA: Spina bifids aperta and congenital constricture of the spinal canal. *J Bone Joint Surg [Br]* 1947; 29:817–821.

24. Takahashi S: *An Atlas of Axial Transverse Tomography and Its Clinical Application.* New York, Springer-Verlag, 1969.

25. Verbiest H: Sur certaines formes rares de compression de la queue de cheval. Les sténoses osseuses du canal vertébral, in *Hommage à Clovis Vincent.* Paris, Maloine, 1949.

26. Verbiest H: Primare stenose van het lumbale wervelkanaal bij volwassenen. Een nieuw ziektebeeld. *Ned Tijdschr Geneeskd* 1950; 94:2415–2433.

27. Verbiest H: Unusual compression of the cauda equina. Report of two cases of lumbo-sacral extradural cysts and of one case of "knotting" of a caudal nerve root, in *Libro de Communicationes of the Combined Meeting of the Luso-Spanish Neurosurgical Society and the British Society of Neurological Surgeons.* Madrid, April 26, 1951. Valencia, 1953.

28. Verbiest H: Moderne overwegingen over compression medullae. *Ned Tijdschr Geneeskd* 1954; 98:2972–2982.

29. Verbiest H: A radicular syndrome from developmental narrowing of the lumbar vertebral canal. *J Bone Joint Surg [Br]* 1954; 36:230–237.

30. Verbiest H: Further experiences on the pathological influence of a developmental narrowness of the bony lumbar vertebral canal. *J Bone Joint Surg [Br]* 1955; 37:576–583.

31. Verbiest H: Neurogenic intermittent claudication in cases of absolute and relative stenosis of the lumbar vertebral canal, (ASLC and RSLC), in cases with narrow intervertebral foramina and in cases with both entities. *Clin Neurosurg* 1973; 20:204–214.

32. Verbiest H: Pathomorphological aspects of developmental lumbar stenosis. *Orthop Clin North Am* 1975; 6:177–196.

33. Verbiest H: Neurogenic intermittent claudication. Lesions of the spinal cord and cauda equina, stenosis of the vertebral canal, narrowing of intervertebral foramina and entrapment of peripheral nerves, in Vinken PJ, Bruyn GW (eds): *Handbook of Clinical Neurology,* vol 20, pt 2. New York, North Holland/American Elsevier, 1976, pp 611–807.

34. Verbiest H: *Neurogenic Intermittent Claudication. With Special Reference to Stenosis of the Lumbar Vertebral Canal.* New York, North Holland/American Elsevier, 1976.

35. Verbiest H: Fallacies of the present definition, nomenclature and classification of the stenoses of the lumbar vertebral canal. *Spine* 1976; 1:217–225.

36. Verbiest H: *Neurogenic Intermittent Claudication. With Special Reference to Stenosis of the Lumbar Vertebral Canal.* New York, North Holland/American Elsevier, 1976, pp 199–205.

37. Verbiest H: Results of treatment of idiopathic developmental stenosis of the lumbar vertebral canal. A review of twenty seven years experience. *J Bone Joint Surg [Br]* 1977; 59:181–188.

38. Verbiest H: The significance and principles of computerized tomography in idiopathic developmental stenosis of the bony lumbar vertebral canal. *Spine* 1979; 4:369–378.

39. Verbiest H: Stenosis of the lumbar vertebral canal and sciatica. *Neurosurg Rev* 1980; 3:75–89.

40. Verbiest H: Words, images, knowledge and reality. Reflections from the neurosurgical perspective. Fourth European lecture. By invitation from the European Association of Neurosurgical Societies. *Acta Neurochir* 1983; 69:163–193.

41. Verbiest H: Introduction, in Hopp E (ed): *Spinal Stenosis. State of the Art Review,* vol 1. Philadelphia, Hanley & Belfus, 1987, pp 361–367.

42. Verbiest H: Lumbar spine stenosis, in Youmans JR (ed): *Neurological Surgery,* Philadelphia, WB Saunders Co, 1990, pp 2805–2855.

43. Verbiest H: Lumbar spinal stenosis, in Weinstein JN, Wiesel S (eds): *The Lumbar Spine.* Philadelphia, WB Saunders Co, 1990, pp 546–589.

2

Definition and Classification of Lumbar Spinal Stenosis

Gunnar B. J. Andersson, M.D., Ph.D.
Thomas W. McNeill, M.D.

Few things should be easier than providing a definition of a disease. Once a disease entity has been described, a name is elected, and the process is completed. Problems arise, however, when there are several alternative bases for definition, and when trying to achieve general acceptance of a definition. In reality, there are few items creating as much controversy as definitions. This is particularly true when the boundaries of what is to be defined are uncertain. Yet, definition and classification are necessary for meaningful communication between physicians, as well as between physicians and insurance companies, lawyers, and other parties in the health care process. Further, patients should know the name of their disease, and the name should, if at all possible, be meaningful to them. As will be evidenced in this chapter and throughout the book, definition and classification of spinal stenosis is controversial and, to a degree, arbitrary. It is not our purpose to present a new definition or a new classification system or even advocate one of those in current use. Rather, we review common definitions of, and classification systems for spinal stenosis, and fold them into an organizational structure.

DEFINITIONS

The most frequently used definition of spinal stenosis was published by a group of more than 20 orthopaedic surgeons and neurosurgeons in 1976.[2]

They defined stenosis as "any type of narrowing of the spinal canal, nerve root canals, or intervertebral foramina." The narrowing could be local, segmental, or generalized. It could be caused by bone, soft tissue, or combinations thereof. It might involve the vertebral canal or the dural sac, or both. This definition, while simple and logical, does not define what constitutes a narrowing—and thus is arbitrary and qualitative. It is also not helpful in defining the character of the stenotic lesion, or its cause. To that purpose, a classification system was developed.

Verbiest[18] has criticized the definition, suggesting instead the following: "...stenosis is an abnormal narrowness of cavities, tubular organs, orifices, or valves capable of producing disease through its influence upon its contents." His definition allows (as does the "Arnoldi" definition), but does not provide, quantification in terms of cross-sectional areas or diameters. Verbiest further divides stenosis into two subclasses: transport stenosis and compressive stenosis. Transport stenosis is related to fluids and gases and manifests itself distal to the narrowing, causing no local damage. Compressive stenosis, on the other hand, involves the compression of fixed living matter. Symptomatic compressive stenosis causes damage to the content in the narrowed area and distal effects are caused by the local damage. Lumbar spinal stenosis is clearly a form of compressive stenosis by this definition. Verbiest also distinguishes between "stenosis of the bony vertebral canal and stenosis produced by ligamentous or cartilaginous portions or parts of the walls of the vertebral canal."[18] Compression of the nervous content, according to Verbiest,[19] takes place between opposite aspects of the wall of the vertebral canal. This view is shared by Kirkaldy-Willis who defined stenotic compression as "squeezing of the spinal cord or nerve roots of the cauda equina between opposed parts of the wall of the vertebral canal. Similarly stenotic compression of a spinal nerve or nerve root may occur in the intervertebral canal."[8]

The nerve root canal as defined by Kirkaldy-Willis and McIvor "starts in the spinal canal at the point where the nerve root sheath comes off the dural sac and ends where the nerve root emerges from the intervertebral foramen."[9] The point where the nerve sheath comes off the dural sac is located well inside the vertebral canal, which includes the lateral recess. Since the recess is part of the spinal canal, it is not part of the intervertebral or nerve root canal. This anatomic observation supports the view of Verbiest: "the narrow lateral recess is part of the vertebral canal giving access to the intervertebral foramen."[18] The medial opening of this foramen is called by him the "ostium internum."[18]

Others have specifically addressed the fact that in clinical practice stenosis is only important when the neural structures which are housed inside the vertebral canal are influenced by a narrowing.[14] The relationship between the sizes of the dural sac and the vertebral canal is uncertain, but when the bony vertebral canal is below a certain size, the dural sac is always affected.

Normally there is ample space in the spinal canal, the nerve root canals, and the intervertebral foramina. When congenital narrowing is present the available space is smaller, but rarely is the narrowing so severe that the neural structures are affected in childhood (see Chapter 12). In most cases of stenosis, the narrowing occurs because of enlargement of the different structures which combine to form the walls of the canal. At the level of the pedicle the walls are essentially made up of bone, while at disc level the walls are made up of disc tissue anteriorly, facet joints and ligamentum flavum laterally, and laminar structures posteriorly (Fig 2–1). Enlargement of any of these structures, such as bulging or herniation of the disc, thickening or buckling of the ligamentum flavum, and degenerative changes of the facet joints can all contribute to narrowing of the canal (Fig 2–2).

CLASSIFICATION

The purpose of classification is to arrange entities (or objects) on the basis of similarities and differences. At least four different classes of classification can be used for lumbar spinal stenosis: (1) classification based on etiology, (2) classification based on morphology, (3) classification based on clinical presentation, and (4) classification based on pathoanatomic considerations. These classes of classification are not competing, but complementary.

Arnoldi et al.[2] presented the most accepted etiologic classification in 1976 (Table 2–1). It divides ste-

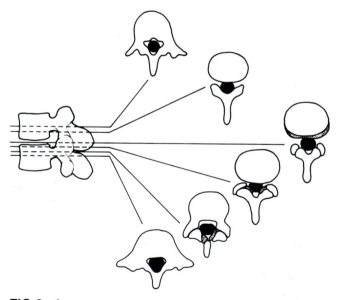

FIG 2–1.
Tracings of CT scan cuts from different levels of a spinal motion segment illustrating what constitutes the walls of the canal. (Adapted from Schönström NSR, Bolender N-F, Spengler DM: *Spine* 1985; 10:43–48.)

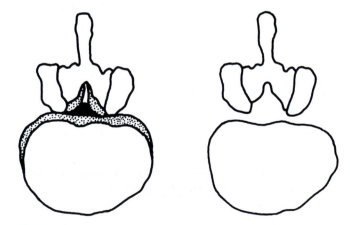

FIG 2–2.
The importance of the soft tissues to the size of the vertebral canal at disc level. (Adapted from Schönström NSR, Bolender N-F, Spengler DM: *Spine* 1985; 10:43–48.)

TABLE 2–1.

Classification of Spinal Stenosis.*

I. Congenital-developmental stenosis
  a. Idiopathic (hereditary)
  b. Achondroplastic
II. Acquired stenosis
  a. Degenerative
  b. Combined congenital and degenerative stenosis
  c. Spondylolytic/spondoylolisthetic
  d. Iatrogenic
    i. Post laminectomy
    ii. Post fusion
    iii. Post chemonucleolysis
  e. Posttraumatic
  f. Metabolic
    i. Paget's disease
    ii. Fluorosis

*Modified from Arnoldi CG, Brodsky AE, Cauchoix J, et al: *Clin Orthop* 1976;115-4–5. Used by permission.

nosis into two congenital-developmental groups, and six acquired groups. This classification is all-inclusive from an etiologic perspective, but does not provide information about where the narrowing is located. To that purpose, they also suggested distinguishing between stenosis in the central portion of the vertebral canal (also referred to as central stenosis) and in the peripheral portion, lateral recesses, and nerve root canals. Peripheral has been replaced by lateral, but definitions of what constitutes the lateral recess and nerve root canal remain controversial (Table 2–2). Verbiest suggests that earlier proposed definitions create confusion, and defines the term *narrow lateral recess* as "the part of the vertebral canal giving access to the intervertebral foramen."[18] He further suggests that "if the narrow lateral recess is continuous with a narrowed lateral wing of a trefoil canal, the combination of both will be called the narrow lateral gutter."[18] The usefulness of an anatomic classification is obvious when considering surgical decompression.

We have used a simple system to describe the

anatomic location of a lateral stenosis.[1] As illustrated in Figure 2–3, the anatomy is divided into three zones based on the relationship to the pedicle. Zone 1 is the lateral recess and is the area under the articular process medial to the pedicle. It is also referred to as the subarticular zone.[10] Zone 2 is the portion of the nerve root canal which is immediately distal to (below) the pedicle, while zone 3 is the area lateral to the pedicle. Zone 2 is sometimes referred to as foraminal, while zone 3 is termed extraforaminal.[10]

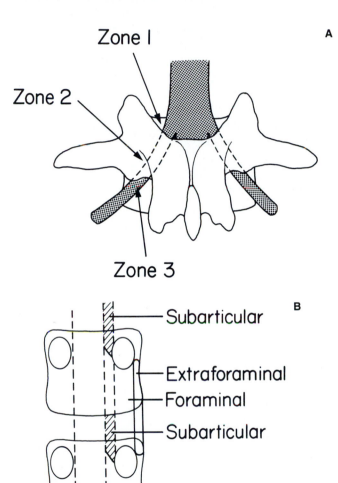

FIG 2–3.
A, the lateral zones in AP perspective. (Adapted from Andersson GBJ, McNeill TW: *Lumbar Spine Syndromes.* Vienna, Springer-Verlag, 1989.) **B,** The lateral zones in AP perspective with the posterior elements removed. (Adapted from McCulloch JA: Microsurgical spinal laminectomies, in Frymoyer JW (ed): *The Adult Spine: Principles and Practice.* New York, Raven Press, 1991, pp 1821–1831.)

TABLE 2–2.

The Pathway of the Lumbar Nerve Root*

Anatomic Zone		Synonyms
Entrance zone		Lateral recess Subarticular zone Ostium internum
Midzone	Intervertabral or nerve root canal	Pedicle level
Exit zone		External exit Ostium externum
Far lateral zone		

*Modified from van Akkerweeken PF: *Lateral Stenosis of the Lumbar Spine* (thesis). University of Utrecht, Netherlands, 1989.

Vertebral Canal Stenosis (Central Stenosis)

Admitting that it is impossible to develop an all-inclusive binary or ternary taxonomy of the stenoses of the vertebral canal, Verbiest[18] suggests a pathomorphologic classification for the bony portions of the vertebral canal (Table 2–3). He argues that there is no place for acquired stenosis in a taxonomy of vertebral stenotic disease and that instead the name of the underlying disease should be used. Congenital stenosis by Verbiest's definition includes only stenosis existing before or at birth. This is different from the Arnoldi classification in which idiopathic and achondroplastic stenoses were also included (see Table 2–1). By Verbiest's classification they would be developmental stenoses, i.e., the result of a growth disturbance of the vertebral arches that continues until adult age. Achondroplasia, discussed in Chapter 12, is the most frequent form of developmental stenosis.

Lateral Stenosis

Van Akkerweeken has particularly addressed the definition and subclassification of lateral lumbar stenosis, proposing the following: "Lateral lumbar stenosis is defined as an abnormal narrowing of the pathway of the lumbar nerve root, the dorsal root ganglion and/or the spinal nerve. This pathway begins at the point where the nerve root sheath takes off from the dura and ends at the area lateral to the pedicle."[16]

To classify lateral stenosis, he proposed the following five classifications:

1. Classification based on etiology.
   a. Congenital: spinal dysrhaphism, failure of segmentation.
   b. Developmental: uncommon variation in shape, size, or orientation of the articular processes.
   c. Degeneration: degenerative spondylolisthesis, osteophyte formation, and loss of disc height with telescoping facets; intraforaminal disc protrusion.
   d. Trauma: burst fracture of the vertebral body leading to a narrow lateral recess; fracture of the superior articular process with dislocation.
   e. Tumor: metastases in the pedicle and posterior aspect of the vertebral body.
2. Classification based on localization of abnormal narrowing.
   a. Ostium internum or entrance zone (lateral recess).
   b. Pedicle zone or midzone.
   c. Ostium externum or exit zone.
   d. "Far lateral" zone (strictly speaking, no narrowing).
3. Classification based on clinical presentation.
   a. Pain present at rest: atypical leg pain or nerve root compression.
   b. Pain only upon walking: neurogenic intermittent claudication.
   c. Negative Lasègue's sign, etc.: atypical leg pain.
   d. Positive Lasègue's sign, etc.: nerve root compression.
   e. Impaired nerve root function present at rest: radiculopathy.
   f. Impaired nerve root function only upon walking: neurogenic intermittent claudication.
   g. Any combination of the above.
4. Classification based on the pathoanatomy of the narrowness (one factor or a combination of factors).
   a. Ligaments.
      (1) Ligamentum flavum: hypertrophy, calcification, ossification.
      (2) Ligamentum longitudinale posterius: calcification.
   b. Disc.
      (1) "Bulging" annulus in the case of severe degeneration.
      (2) Severe loss of disc height.
      (3) Protrusion.
   c. Facet joint.
      (1) Synovitis with synovial hypertrophy and effusion.
   d. Bone.
      (1) Articular process: osteophyte formation, uncommon shape and orientation.
      (2) Vertebral body: osteophyte formation posteriorly or laterally.

TABLE 2–3.

Taxonomy for Stenosis of the Bony Portions of the Vertebral Canal

I. Congenital
II. Developmental
  A. Through inborn errors of skeletal bone growth
  B. Idiopathic developmental stenosis
    1. In the presence of bony hypertrophy of structures of the vertebral arch
    2. In the absence of bony hypertrophy of structures of the vertebral arch (rare)

*Modified from Verbiest H: Lumbar spinal stenosis: Morphology, classification and long-term results, in Weinstein J, Wiesel S (eds): *The Lumbar Spine.* Philadelphia, WB Saunders Co, 1990, pp 546–589.

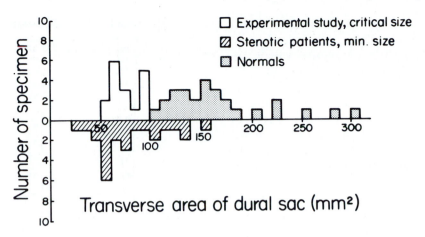

FIG 2–4.
Histogram of measurement of the transverse area of the dural sac. (Adapted from Schönström N: *The Narrow Lumbar Spinal Canal and the Size of the Cauda Equina in Man* (thesis). University of Goteborg, Sweden, 1988.)

(3) Lamina: hypertrophy, spondylolysis with granulation tissue.
5. Classification based on pathobiomechanics of the lumbar motion segment as a whole.
   a. Fixed rotational deformity.
   b. Segmental hypermobility ("dynamic stenosis").

Measurements

We have already mentioned the problem of defining what size of the vertebral canal constitutes stenosis. In this respect stenosis has been divided into absolute—where there is no reserve capacity—and relative—where there is limited reserve space and, for example, a small disc bulge is sufficient to cause symptoms.[17] In absolute stenosis the midsagittal diameter (MSD) is 10 mm or less, while in relative stenosis it is 10 to 13 mm. Patients with MSD of 10 mm or less may be asymptomatic, however. The probable reason for this is that the cross-sectional area of the vertebral canal is sufficient to accommodate the nerve roots inside the dural sac. Schönström[13] found that the transverse area of the dural sac on computed tomography (CT) scans was the best measure of a central (vertebral canal) stenosis. The critical size, below which there is not enough space for an uncompressed cauda equina, was found to be 120 mm[2] in a clinical study.[14] Experimentally, Schönström[13] determined that the critical size is probably less and suggested an interval between 50 and 100 mm[2] (Fig 2–4). These data compare well with the transverse area of the nervous tissue of the cauda equina in man, which has been reported by Hasue et al.[4] The suggestion of an interval indicates that individual differences exist, perhaps owing to differences in geometry, the size of the nerve roots, and the response of the nerve roots to compression. Changes in posture and load cause changes in the available space for the nerve roots. Thus, it has been found that both flexion-extension and axial loading can change the transverse area of the vertebral canal.[11, 13, 15, 21] Schönström[13] found changes in the magnitude of 40 to 50 mm[2], and argues that these dynamic changes may explain the intermittent symptoms of spinal stenosis.

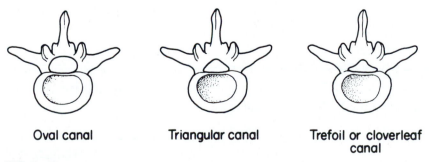

Oval canal   Triangular canal   Trefoil or cloverleaf canal

FIG 2–5.
Main types of spinal canals. (Adapted from Weinstein PR, Ehm G, Wilson CB: *Lumbar Spondylosis.* St Louis, Mosby–Year Book, 1977.

The shape of the lumbar vertebral canal is also important. As discussed in Chapter 3, there is considerable individual variation. Triangular canals are the most common (Fig 2–5), but in 15% of the population a trefoil shape occurs at L5, and in a few percent less at L4. Trefoil canals often have smaller MSDs but it is particularly in the lateral recesses where the nerve roots are at risk because of the shape of the canal. Oval canals are more uncommon, but of course are advantageous from a geometric perspective.

The normal variation in MSD is significant. Huizinga et al.[6] measured MSDs in 51 Dutch skeletons and found the lowest value to range from 14 mm at the L1 level to 11 mm at the L4 level. The anteroposterior (AP) and interpedicular diameters were generally not related and stenosis generally occurred in the AP diameter.

Eisenstein[3] measured the lumbar spinal canal in 485 skeletons of blacks and whites. Little difference was found between men and women in the AP and transverse diameters of the canal. The AP diameter alone was found to be the essential parameter in assessing spinal stenosis. He found the lowest normal limits of this diameter to be 10 mm in blacks and 12 mm in whites and the smallest diameters were found at the L2, L3, and L4 levels. The transverse (interpedicular) diameter increased steadily from L1 to the L5 vertebra. The lower limit of normality was 17 mm. This confirms previous observations by Haworth and Keillor[5] (Fig 2–6).

Postacchini et al.,[12] in a morphometric study of 121 skeletons (63 Italian and 58 Indian), found the mean dimensions to be significantly greater in the Italian skeletons. The lowest normal AP diameter was 12.6 mm in the Italian skeletons and 11.5 mm in the Indian series. Midsagittal diameters of less than 11 mm were almost always found in the L4 and L5 vertebrae.

Other Definitions

With reference to the symptoms occurring in spinal stenosis, an additional term, *neurogenic intermittent claudication*, should also be defined. Verbiest has defined neurogenic intermittent claudication by two primary criteria:

1. Neural disturbances impede the continuation of walking.
2. Walking can be resumed after 10 to 20 minutes of rest.

Currently, the two most accepted theories for neurogenic intermittent claudication, also referred to as pseudoclaudication, are:

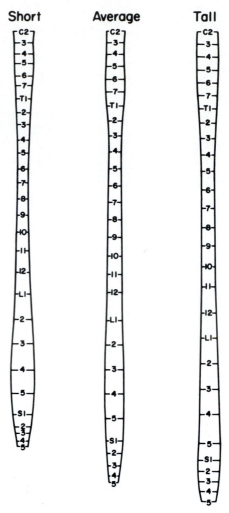

FIG 2–6.
Average spinal canal width (transverse diameters) in adults of different heights, illustrating the shape of the canal in the lumbar area. (Adapted from Haworth JB, Keillor GW: *Radiology* 1962; 79:109.)

1. Increased lordosis during standing and walking reduces the size of the vertebral canal.
2. The necessary increase in blood supply to the nerve roots and spinal ganglia needed during walking is inhibited by a vascular constriction caused by stenosis.

Although both of these causes are dynamic in nature, the specific cause of the symptoms in individual patients remains obscure.

SUMMARY

Spinal stenosis can most easily be defined as a narrowing of the vertebral canal, lateral recesses, and vertebral foramina. Based on location, it can be divided into vertebral canal (central) or lateral stenosis. It can have different etiologies, can present in different anatomic variations, and does not always result in clinical symptoms. Clearly there need be a mismatch between the available space and its contents for symptomatic stenosis to occur. Measurements, therefore, are not always conclusive. Because of significant interindividual differences and the difficulty in measuring dynamic changes within the canal, clinical correlation with measurements is always necessary.

REFERENCES

1. Andersson GBJ, McNeill TW: *Lumbar Spine Syndromes.* Vienna, Springer-Verlag, 1989.
2. Arnoldi CC; Brodsky AE, Cauchoix J, et al: Lumbar spinal stenosis and nerve root entrapment syndromes: Definition and classification. *Clin Orthop* 1976; 115:4–5.
3. Eisenstein S: The morphometry and pathological anatomy of the lumbar spine in South African Negroes and Caucasoids with special reference to spinal stenosis. *J Bone Joint Surg [Br]* 1977; 59B:173.
4. Hasue M, Kikukchi S, Sukuyama Y, et al: Anatomic study of the interrelation between lumbosacral nerve roots and their surrounding tissues. *Spine* 1983; 8:50–58.
5. Haworth JB, Keillor GW: *Radiology* 1962; 79:109.
6. Huizinga J, Hejden JA, Von den Vinken PJJG: The human lumbar vertebral canal: A biometric study. *Proc K Ned Akad Wet* 1952; 55:22.
7. Johnsson K-E: *Lumbar Spinal Stenosis (thesis).* University of Lund, Sweden, 1987.
8. Kirkaldy-Willis WH: *Managing Low Back Pain.* New York, Churchill-Livingston, Inc, 1984.
9. Kirkaldy-Willis WH, McIvor GWD: Editorial comment. Lumbar spinal stenosis. *Clin Orthop* 1976; 115:2–3.
10. McCulloch JA: Microsurgical spinal laminotomies, in Frymoyer JW (ed): *The Adult Spine: Principles and Practice.* New York, Raven Press, 1991, pp 1821–1831.
11. Penning L, Wilmink JT: Biomechanics of lumbosacral dural sac. A study of flexion-extension myelography. *Spine* 1981; 6:398–408.
12. Postacchini F, Ripain M, Carpano M: Morphometry of the lumbar vertebrae. *Clin Orthop* 1983; 172:296.
13. Schönström N: *The Narrow Lumbar Spinal Canal and the Size of the Cauda Equina in Man.* (thesis). University of Goteborg, Sweden, 1988.
14. Schönström NSR, Bolender N-F, Spengler DM: The pathomorphology of spinal stenosis as seen on CT scans of the lumbar spine. *Spine* 1985; 10:43–48.
15. Sortland O, Magnaes B, Hauge T: Functional myelography with metrizamide in the diagnosis of lumbar spinal stenosis. *Acta Radiol Suppl (Stockh)* 1977; 355:42–54.
16. Van Akkerweeken PF: *Lateral Stenosis of the Lumbar Spine* (thesis). University of Utrecht, Netherlands, 1989.
17. Verbiest H: Further experiences on the pathological influence of a developmental narrowness of the bony lumbar vertebral canal. *J Bone Joint Surg [Br]* 1955; 37:476–583.
18. Verbiest H: Fallacies of the present definition, nomenclature and classification of the stenoses of the lumbar vertebral canal. *Spine* 1976; 1:217–225.
19. Verbiest H: Lumbar spinal stenosis: Morphology, classification and long-term results, in Weinstein J, Wiesel S (eds): *The Lumbar Spine.* Philadelphia, WB Saunders Co., 1990, pp 546–589.
20. Weinstein PR, Ehni G, Wilson CB: *Lumbar Spondylosis.* St Louis, Mosby-Year Book, Inc. 1977.
21. Wilmink JT, Penning L: Influence of spinal posture on abnormalities demonstrated by lumbar myelography. *AJNR* 1983; 4:656–658.

SECTION I

Basic

3

Pathoanatomy of Lumbar Spinal Stenosis: A Pictorial Outline

Wolfgang Rauschning, M.D., Ph.D.

This chapter provides a brief pictorial outline of some typical pathoanatomic features of degenerative lumbar spinal stenosis. Rather than attempt to describe structural changes in the text, I have used figures and their legends to explain important pathoanatomic changes associated with degeneration (Figs 3–1 through 3–7). The figures have been selected from numerous recorded images and, as such, provide a structural description of degenerative lumbar spinal stenosis. In my opinion, pictures are more easily memorized than paragraphs of text. Further, the sheer complexity and interindividual variation of the changes defy any attempt to describe them verbally.

The human spine is extremely complex, both with respect to its supporting structures and the spinal neural elements and blood vessels. In addition, various portions of the spine are highly dissimilar. A systematic descriptive account of all morphologic features would exceed the scope of this chapter which is aimed at an understanding of basic anatomic facts of clinical importance. Throughout, I have used the nomenclature proposed by the glossary of spinal terminology as published by the American Academy of Orthopaedic Surgeons, with two exceptions. I use the term *spinous process* instead of spine and I sometimes use the term *spinal canal* instead of vertebral canal, which is the correct anatomic term, but is not as well established clinically.

METHODOLOGIC CONSIDERATIONS

Conventional dissection, by definition, entails the destruction of layers of tissue which inevitably leads to distortion of topographic relationships. Conventional histologic examinations necessitate fixation and decalcification which leads to shrinkage and deformation of important neurovascular relationships. The images in this chapter are cryosectional surface images from frozen cadaveric spines. Since the whole torso or sections of the spine were frozen in situ, the relationship of the spinal soft tissues to the vertebrae is "frozen" both in neutral positions and in typical and clinically significant functional positions. The spine segments were also radiographed and examined with a computed tomography (CT) scanner in the axial, sagittal, and coronal planes.

The specimens were sectioned on a heavy-duty sledge cryomicrotome using a surface cryoplaning technique which I developed in 1977. Photographs of the leading surface of the block taken at submillimeter cutting height intervals render undistorted color images in which structures can be recognized by their natural colors and texture. More important, the spatial relationships are preserved in every specimen.

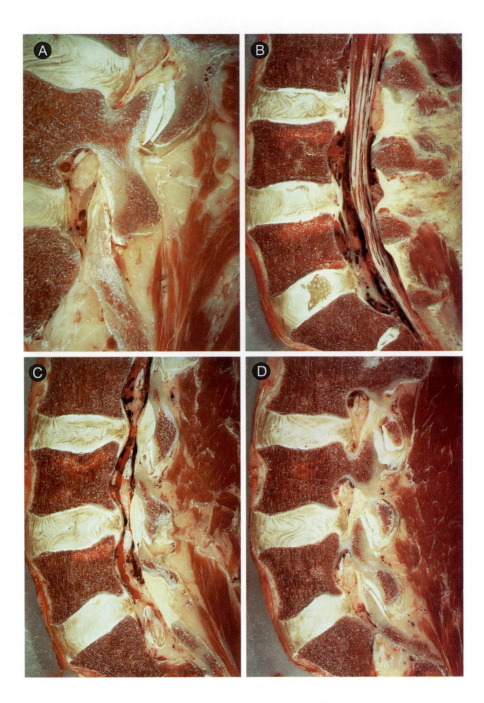

FIG 3–1.

A, normal L4 and L5 foramina and facet joints in a specimen from a 42-year-old man. The specimen had been frozen with the spine in the neutral position. At L4–5 the boundaries of the foramen are clearly outlined: the upper portion or story is identical with the so-called subpedicular notch (anatomically formed by the incisura vertebralis inferior) and is bounded predominantly by bone—the lower half of the vertebral body anteriorly, the pedicle superiorly, and the bony base of the inferior articular process posteriorly in the entrance zone and the medial portion of the infundibular "pedicle zone" of the root canal. Note that the anatomy varies considerably between the L4–5 foramen (root canal)

and the L5–S1 foramen (root canal). The specimen has been sectioned exactly in the sagittal plane. The disparity of the anatomy is due to the fact that the vertebral canal has wider transverse (medial to lateral) dimensions at L5–S1 than at higher levels. The L4 and L5 nerves are thus located in the midpedicle zone and the infundibular entrance zone, respectively. Although seemingly patent on lateral radiograms, the lower portion of the L4–5 foramen is virtually obliterated by the physiologic bulge of the disc and the insertion of the outer annular fibers into the shallow groove at the superior aspect of the pedicle below (anatomically the incisura vertebralis superior). In the midpedicle and lateral

VERTEBRAL COLUMN VS. SPINE

For didactic reasons, it is useful to distinguish between the vertebral column and the spine. The *vertebral column* is a multisegmented mobile structure of bone, discs, and ligaments with several physiologic curvatures in the sagittal plane. It provides stability and support to the trunk, head, and upper extremities and, at the same time, allows mobility. The pattern of motion varies greatly in the various regions of the spine. The most mobile portions are the cervical spine and the mid and lower lumbar spine. Every spinal motion segment has a typical range and pattern of motion which is determined by the geometry of bony and articular surfaces as well as by the state of the discs, and the location and mechanical properties of ligaments and joint capsules. Mobility is controlled by the muscles attaching to the vertebral column, and influenced by their mass and fiber composition as well as their orientation in space.

The term *spine* encompasses more than just the musculoskeletal elements of the vertebral column. Its architecture forms osseoligamentous spaces which accommodate, protect, and transmit vital and delicate neurovascular structures. These spaces are the *vertebral canal* and the two *intervertebral foramina* or *root canals* at each spinal level. The root canal morphology varies significantly from one vertebral level to the next and there is also a wide and significant range of interindividual variations with respect to canal size and configuration.

The pathologic anatomy of the stenotic spinal canal as described by Verbiest (see Bibliography) conceives lumbar spinal stenosis as a developmental narrowing of the central spinal canal. According to Verbiest, stenosis indicates a pathologic condition which compresses the contents of the spinal canal in contrast to a narrow spinal canal in which the neural structures are encroached upon but not compressed.

---

portion of the foramen (root canal) the ligamentum flavum inserts into the anterior aspect of the superior articular process way down to the top of the pedicle. Both the annulus and the ligamentum flavum, which forms the facet joint capsule, narrow the lower (retrodiscal) portion of the foramen to a narrow slit. The nerve structures are invariably located in the upper subpedicular part of the foramen, surrounded by sparse veins and the vertebral artery located anterior to the nerve. At both L4−5 and L5−S1, by far the most voluminous constituent of the "root" is the dorsal root ganglion which, owing to its rich intrinsic vasculature, has a dark-yellow coloration which distinguishes it from the light-yellow ventral or motor roots which lie snugly at the anterior aspect of the ganglion.

B−D, anatomy in a specimen from a 62-year-old woman. Radiographs showed very short pedicles which results in constitutionally reduced dimensions of both the (central) spinal (vertebral) canal and of the foramina and lateral conduits of the spine. In the midline the thecal sac (dura and arachnoid membrane) have the shape of a narrow tube in which the roots of the cauda equina and accompanying blood vessels are firmly constricted. The dura is surrounded by large layers of epidural veins which probably are engorged since the cadaver was frozen in the supine position. All discs have normal height and bulge posteriorly into the vertebral canal, most pronounced at L3−4. This disc shows signs of disintegration of the normal architecture of the fiber arrangement of the annulus fibrosus with broken lamellae and fissures extending from the intermediate and medial layers of the annulus fibrosus and replacing the nucleus pulposus (cf. the L5−S1 disc with a macroscopically normal nucleus pulposus). Following the disc margins from **B** to **D** it becomes apparent that the "bulge" of the disc is in fact circumferential. Posteriorly in the midline the narrow bands of cortical laminar bone are connected by the much wider bands of the interlaminar ligamenta flava. Note the buckling of the ligamentum flavum at L4−5. At L5−S1 the ligamentum flavum is very thin; more laterally it increases in thickness **(C).** The decreased anteroposterior dimensions of this spine not only cause a reduction of the sagittal diameter (and volume) of the spinal canal within the confines of the medial borders of the pedicles but also pronounced decrease of the sagittal dimensions of the spinal canal between the dura and the pedicles **(C).** Note that the spinal canal is segmentally encroached upon at the levels of the motion segment which is bounded by the disc annulus anteriorly and the ligamentum flavum−joint capsule posteriorly which both form an hourglass-shaped hiatus at each intervertebral level. The root sleeves pass through this hiatus at each level, bounded by soft tissue and not in contact with bone at any level. By contrast, the vertebral canal is wide at the level of the bony ring (vertebral body-pedicle-lamina), to a large degree owing to the marked concavity of the posterior wall of the vertebral bodies **(B,C). D** shows the foramina at L3−4, L4−5, and L5−S1. Note that owing to the wider transverse dimensions of the lower lumbar spine, three different medial-to-lateral levels of the foramina are displayed in one section. The inverted teardrop shape of the foramen with complete obliteration of the retrodiscal portion is best seen at L4−5. (From Rauschning W: Normal anatomy of the vertebral canal and the lumbar neural structures, in Postacchini F (ed): *Lumbar Spinal Stenosis.* Heidelberg, Springer-Verlag, 1989, pp 21−48. Used by permission.)

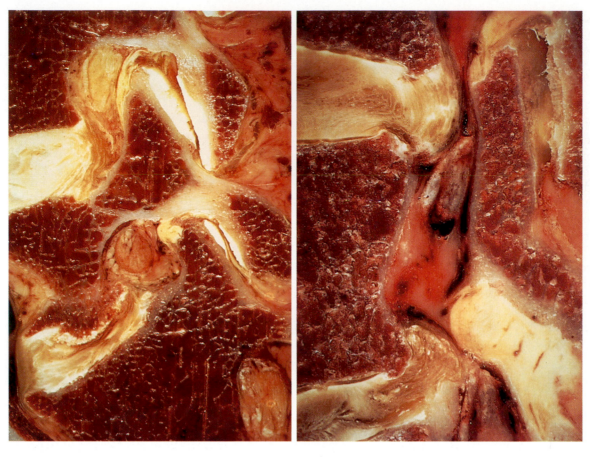

FIG 3–2.

Sagittal section of a spine which had been frozen in extension in situ in the intact cadaver by supporting the lumbar lordosis with a towel. No axial loading was applied. By freezing of the spine before removal of the specimen the undistorted soft tissue–bone relationships are maintained. The extension induces a sagittal rotation of L4 posteriorly on L5 whereas there is less motion at L5–S1. The oblique orientation of the joints to the coronal plane induces a slight posterior translation of L4 on L5 and the tip of the inferior articular process rests on the pars interarticularis of L5. From inferiorly the pars is pinched by the superior articular process of S1. The joint capsule is stretched and compressed. Owing to the combination of translation (retrolisthesis) and sagittal rotation, the joint space opens superiorly in a wedge-shaped fashion. Loose areolar tissue and a meniscoid synovial tag protrudes into the joint space, probably because of negative pressure. The ligamentum flavum joint capsule attaches broadly to the anterior surface of the superior articular process which rotates into the foramen from posteriorly, encroaching upon the subpedicular notch, pushing the ganglion anteriorly against the unyielding bone, and compressing and flattening the dorsal surface of the root ganglion. As in Figure 3–1,A, ventral roots lie anterior to the ganglion. (From Rauschning W: Normal anatomy of the vertebral canal and the lumbar neural structures, in Postacchini F (ed): *Lumbar Spinal Stenosis*. Heidelberg, Springer-Verlag, 1989, pp 21–48. Used by permission.)

FIG 3–3.

Sagittal section through a spine with degenerated discs at L4–5 and L5–S1 immediately medial to the pedicles. The intact cadaver was frozen with the lumbar spine in extension (lordosis) and a rotatory force applied by twisting the pelvis against the trunk. Note the gross disruption of the intervertebral discs. A cleft in the lower portion of the annulus of the L4–5 disc along the apophyseal ring detaches the annulus with the exception of the outer "capsular" layer of the annulus. At L5–S1 this outer annular layer tracks or dissects superiorly by detaching the periosteum of the vertebral body. The rotation of L5 in relation to L4 causes the L5 lamina to move anteriorly toward the L4–5 disc which is pulled posteriorly by the posteriorly moving L4 body. The L5 root sheath is caught between the disc and the lamina. The rotational position is evident from the gaping of the L4–5 facet joint which displays a vacuum phenomenon. At the L5–S1 level the S1 root sleeve passes between the disc and the thick infolding ligamentum flavum. (From Rauschning W: Normal anatomy of the vertebral canal and the lumbar neural structures, in Postacchini F (ed): *Lumbar Spinal Stenosis*. Heidelberg, Springer-Verlag, 1989, pp 21–48. Used by permission.)

NORMAL ANATOMY

The lumbar vertebral canal can be divided into a central portion, two lateral portions, and a posterior portion corresponding to the interlaminar corner. The central portion represents the central vertebral canal; each lateral portion constitutes the nerve root canal or radicular canal.

The central portion of the spinal canal is roundish and occupied by the dural tube. Stenosis of the central portion of the vertebral canal has often been called *central spinal stenosis,* in contrast to lateral spinal stenosis or nerve root canal stenosis. This terminology implies that in central spinal stenosis the nerve root canals may not be stenotic. However, this is not the case because stenosis of the central portion is consistently associated with stenosis of the lateral corners of the vertebral canal. To avoid the misconception that only the central portion may be stenotic, I prefer the term *stenosis of the spinal canal* or *spinal canal stenosis* to central spinal stenosis.

The nerve root canal is the tubular structure in which the nerve root runs from the lateral aspect of the dural sac to the entrance into the intervertebral foramen. This canal consists of two parts: the proximal—subarticular or intervertebral—,and the distal, corresponding to the lateral recess, i.e., the lateral corner of the vertebral foramen at the level of the pedicles. The proximal part is bounded anteriorly by the intervertebral disc and posterolaterally by the anterior part of the superior articular process which is covered by the ligamentum flavum, which at these levels merges with the articular capsule of the facet joint. The distal part begins at the level of the superior end plate and ends at the entrance of the intervertebral foramen. The nerve root canal does not have a medial wall; it can be considered to consist of the lateral aspect of the dural sac. The nerve root canal may be stenotic in the absence of any significant narrowing of the central spinal canal. This condition should be called *isolated nerve root canal stenosis.*

The intervertebral foramen, or neural foramen, which is more of an osseofibrous canal than a real foramen, is formed by two adjacent vertebrae and the intervertebral disc. The entrance and the exit of the foramen correspond to the medial and lateral aspect of the pedicle. Many authors include the neuroforamen in the nerve root canal and consider the intervertebral foramen to be its most distal portion. In my opinion, there are valid reasons to separate the neural foramen from the nerve root canal and thus

to identify stenosis of the intervertebral foramen as a separate entity. Nerve root canal stenosis is common, either isolated or associated with stenosis of the central portion of the spinal canal, whereas compression of the nerve root within the intervertebral foramen is extremely rare.

An example of developmental stenosis is found in specimens with short pedicles. In such specimens, the dorsal walls of the vertebral bodies display a marked concavity which commonly is further accentuated by prominent vertebral end plates. The intervertebral discs physiologically bulge into the spinal canal, i.e., a bulging disc is not a pathologic finding as such.

DYNAMIC NEUROVASCULAR COMPRESSION

The sagittal dimensions of the spinal canal increase in flexion and decrease in extension. In flexion, the laminae of the adjacent vertebrae move apart and the interlaminar space widens. This results in lengthening and thinning of the ligamentum flavum. At the same time, the posterior portion of the annulus fibrosus is also stretched. These changes increase the sagittal dimensions of the spinal canal. In extension, on the other hand, the ligamenta flava shorten, become thicker, and buckle into the vertebral canal, and the annulus fibrosus bulges posteriorly. This results in a decrease in the sagittal dimensions of the canal at the intervertebral level.

If the vertebral canal has a large reserve space for the nervous structures, the decrease in size caused by extension of the spine is of no pathologic consequence (see Chapter 7). If the reserve space is limited or the spinal nerve roots or dural sac is already somewhat compressed owing to spinal stenosis, then further narrowing caused by extension will increase the compression of the nervous structures. Changes in the size and shape of the vertebral canal occurring in flexion and extension, and particularly those caused by the ligamenta flava, involve primarily the central area of the vertebral canal and thus the dural sac and its contents. The dural sac is constricted at the intervertebral level, and there is often associated dilatation at the midvertebral level. Such dynamic changes can also occur in the nerve root canal, but are less marked than in the central spinal canal. In the root canal, they are caused by bulging of the posterolateral region of the disc into the subartic-

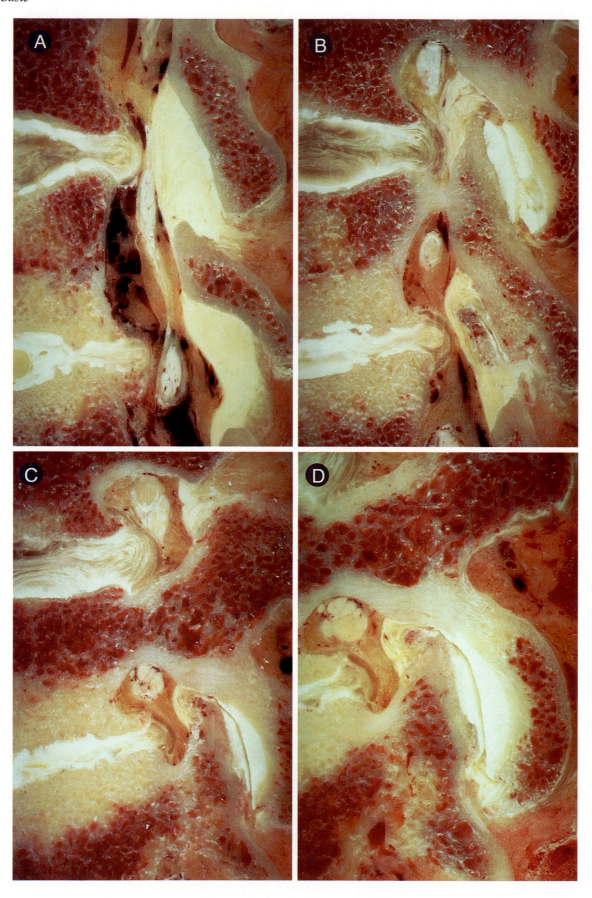

ular portion of the nerve root canal and by buckling of the anterior capsule of the facet joint, with its covering ligamentum flavum, caused by a downward sliding of the inferior articular process during extension of the spine.

Rotation will also affect the subarticular portion of the nerve root canal. When one vertebra rotates in relation to its neighbor, there is a posterior displacement of the lateral portion of the proximal vertebra and a marked posterior protrusion of the disc on the side toward which torsion occurs. On that side, the nerve root canal decreases in width, which can cause compression of the nerve root, particularly if the canal is narrow or stenotic.

In summary, the dimensions and volume of the lumbar spinal canal vary considerably as a function of flexion, extension, and rotation of the motion segment. Dynamic variations in flexion and extension are mainly caused by changes in the degree of bulging of the intervertebral disc and in the thickness and buckling of the ligamentum flavum. Rotation mainly affects the nerve root canals which narrow as a result of both changes in the soft tissue volume and vertebral displacement.

The vertebral canal and foramina (root canals) contain the spinal cord and the lumbosacral roots of the cauda equina which are contained and ensheathed by the thecal sac, a tubular structure which is continuous at the foramen magnum level with the thecae of the skull. Thus, the dura mater spinalis is continuous with the dura mater of the skull (pachy-

meninx). The thecal sac is completely lined internally by the arachnoid membrane (leptomeninx), and is filled with cerebrospinal fluid (CSF) in which the spinal cord, the roots of the cauda equina, and some free subarachnoid blood vessels float freely. The neural thecal envelopes are attached to the vertebral column at the level of the neuroforamina where a variable number of cauda equina roots converge toward a strut-shaped infundibular expansion of the thecal sac. The free intrathecal roots become ensheathed by the meninges. The arachnoid membrane terminates at the medial border of the nerve root ganglion, while the dura is contiguous with the capsule of the ganglion and the perineurium of the segmental spinal nerves.

While the intrathecal neural elements are mobile, the thecal sac is segmentally attached to the vertebral column by several important ligaments and membranes, some of which are commonly known as the Hofmann ligaments. The thecal sac does not expand appreciably when intrathecal pressure rises because the dura is moderately elastic. It offers minimal resistance to compression, and thus cannot protect the cauda equina roots. The thecal sac is surrounded by epidural fat and epidural veins (see Chapter 8). The epidural veins are somewhat arbitrarily divided into the anterior and posterior internal veins. The former constitute a plexus of veins behind the vertebral bodies; the latter, fewer and smaller, line the inner aspect of the laminae. The contents of the vertebral canal and the root canals

---

FIG 3–4.

Sagittal section through a degenerated lower lumbar spine. At L5–S1 the intervertebral disc is completely resorbed and the cartilaginous end plates have fused completely. A marked subchondral end-plate sclerosis has developed adjacent to the former disc. Posteriorly the hard annulus fibrosus protrudes into the root canal. The dorsal root ganglion is smaller than in Figures 3–1 and 3–2. The total resorption of the disc also entails a severe shortening in the posterior elements as demonstrated here by the axial shortening subluxation of the facet joint. Immediately medial to the pedicle **(A)** the L5 and S1 root sleeves pass through the narrow hiatus between disc and ligamentum flavum. The thickness of the ligamentum flavum reflects a retraction and volume redistribution as a result of the decrease of the intervertebral distance rather than a hypertrophy. In the foramina the relatively small roots are surrounded by fat which is only sparsely interspersed with veins. **B, C,** and **D** show a typical feature of degenerative lumbar spondylosis (defined as a degeneration of the "disc joints"): the lower rim of the vertebral body at the insertion site of the outermost layers of the annulus fibrosus have hypertrophied forming circumferential

ridges or flanges which project posteriorly and sometimes slightly superiorly into the foramina (root canals). The nerve root (root sleeve, ganglion, postganglionic nerve) invariably lie above these spondylosis flanges and at a safe distance from the superior articular process of the vertebra below. Some of the marked "ridging" may be due to resorption of the vertebral body wall above the insertion of the outer annulus fibrosus. The grotesque subluxation and interlocking of the facet joint reflects a stable situation at the L5–S1 level: the reduction of the height of the motion segment causes the tip of the superior articular process of the sacrum to hit the interarticular pars from inferiorly causing arthrosis with osteophyte formation of the tip of the superior articular process. Note that the vertical, probably less loaded articular portion of the joint facet carries macroscopically normal cartilage, whereas the superior tip of the upper articular process erodes into the inferior aspect of the pars interarticularis of L5. (From Rauschning W: Normal anatomy of the vertebral canal and the lumbar neural structures, in Postacchini F (ed): *Lumbar Spinal Stenosis.* Heidelberg, Springer-Verlag, 1989, pp 21–48. Used by permission.)

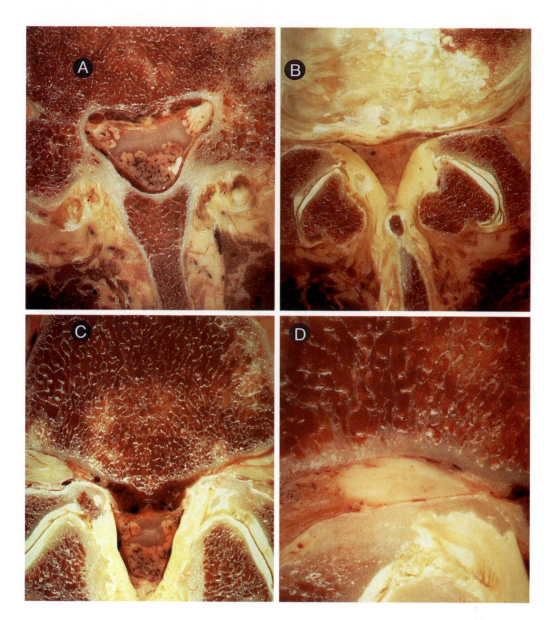

FIG 3–5.

Severe degenerative spinal stenosis at L4–5 which is most pronounced at the level of the intervertebral disc. **A** shows the trefoil configuration of the vertebral canal at the level of the osseous ring (vertebral body-pedicles-lamina). At the *right* of the figure the root sleeve lies in the entrance zone of the foramen, i.e., lateral to the medial border of the pedicle, whereas the root on the *left* snugly follows the medial border of the pedicle. The cauda equina roots are small and layered posteriorly in the thecal sac which contains small amounts of CSF. At the disc level **(B)** the thecal sac is severely compressed. Anteriorly, the circumferential "ballooning" of the disc decreases the sagittal diameter of the canal and also completely obliterates the retrodiscal portion of the root canals. Posterolaterally, the thecal sac is encroached upon by the thick ligamentum flavum causing it to assume a triangular configuration. The roots of the cauda equina are tightly squeezed without any CSF surrounding them. **C** shows the anatomy halfway between the lower end plate and the pedicle and **D** is a close-up showing the relation-

ships of the ganglion and the superior articular process osteophytes. The two ligamenta flava are continuous posteriorly with the thick and degenerated interspinous ligament. The posterior contour of the vertebral body is beveled and V-shaped. From posteriorly, large osteophytes at the insertion of the ligamentum flavum into the superior articular processes cause complete obliteration of the subpedicular notch and of the lateral recess. The ganglia are flattened against the pedicles by the pressure exerted by the protruding disc below. Anteriorly in the vertebral canal the veins are engorged, probably owing to obstruction of the venous drainage. The thecal sac is flattened from the sides, but has a much wider diameter in this less mobile portion of the motion segment, and the thin cauda equina roots are surrounded by CSF. (From Rauschning W: Normal anatomy of the vertebral canal and the lumbar neural structures, in Postacchini F (ed): *Lumbar Spinal Stenosis.* Heidelberg, Springer-Verlag, 1989, pp 21–48. Used by permission.)

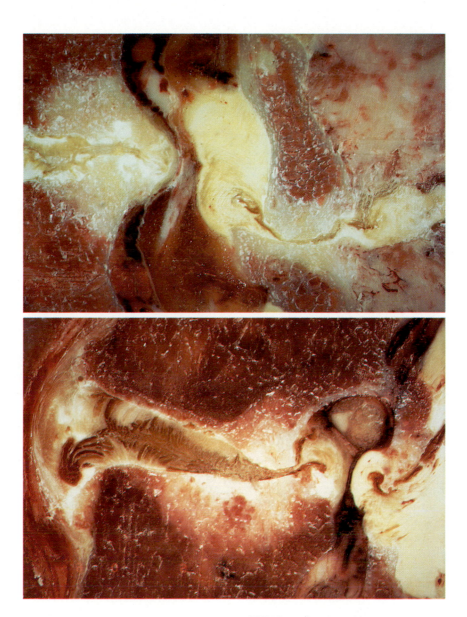

FIG 3–6 (top).
Compression of the L4–5 root sleeve in a specimen with complete disc resorption 2 cm lateral to the midline. The spondylosis changes are more pronounced than those in Figure 3–4. In the posterior disc space marked sclerosis has developed adjacent to the end-plate ridging. Only a dark line remains representing the outer annulus portion of the intervertebral disc. The sclerotic end-plate flanges and intervening hard annulus remnant form a "beak" which markedly projects posteriorly into the spinal canal and abuts the infolding of the redundant ligamentum flavum which "mushrooms" into the spinal canal. Owing to the collapse of the disc height, the laminae are grinding on each other, causing pseudojoints to form which are covered with a thin layer of cartilage. Synovial fluid is contributing to the protrusion of the ligamentum flavum. (From Rauschning W: Normal anatomy of the vertebral canal and the lumbar neural structures, in Postacchini F (ed): *Lumbar Spinal Stenosis.* Heidelberg, Springer-Verlag, 1989, pp 21–48. Used by permission.)

FIG 3–7 (bottom).
Isthmic spondylolisthesis at L4–5. Sagittal section through the medial border of the pedicle. The "beak" formed by the base of the inferior articular process plunges into the interlaminar ligamentum flavum, causing it to project into the foramen. L4 is rotated posteriorly and the disc is severely degenerated and its posterior annulus is partially detached superiorly from the apophyseal rim, allowing the posterior annulus fibrosus to project posteriorly and virtually blocking the canal immediately medial to the pedicle. The extension and rotation of L4 on L5 causes the pedicle to push the ganglion inferiorly against the unyielding annulus. Note the end-plate sclerosis at the areas of contact between the vertebral bodies. (From Rauschning W: Normal anatomy of the vertebral canal and the lumbar neural structures, in Postacchini F (ed): *Lumbar Spinal Stenosis.* Heidelberg, Springer-Verlag, 1989, pp 21–48. Used by permission.)

can be conceived of as a hydraulic system in which the filling and emptying of the epidural veins and sinuses facilitate almost instantaneous variations in the volume of the canals.

DEGENERATIVE CHANGES

With degeneration, a number of changes occur in the spinal motion segment, all of which contribute to the development of spinal stenosis. Because of the reduced disc height, the intervertebral discs tend to bulge into the vertebral canal, and the ligamenta flava thicken and buckle, further reducing available space. Further, the apophyseal joints degenerate and hypertrophy, which contributes to the development of stenosis, as discussed below.

Degenerative changes of the posterior joints consist not only in hypertrophy but also in remodeling of the articular processes which elongate anteromedially and posterolaterally and assume a more transverse orientation. This abnormal orientation is probably due to the abnormal relationship of the facets caused by vertebral slipping. It is possible that the process of remodeling represents a compensation mechanism aimed at limiting vertebral slipping. Degenerative changes of the superior articular processes are responsible for narrowing of the nerve root canals. This narrowing may be slight and may not cause compression of the spinal nerve roots, but may also be significant, producing stenosis of the nerve root canals. When there is significant hypertrophy and outgrowth of the medial border, the central vertebral canal can also be influenced and there can be compression of the thecal sac.

In developmental, degenerative, and combined stenoses, compression of the nervous structures occurs at the intervertebral level, since only this portion of the canal is bordered by anatomic structures that may undergo degenerative changes. At the level of the posterior wall of the vertebral body, the vertebral canal may be narrow, but this narrowing is not severe enough to cause compression of the neural contents.

Figures 3–4 and 3–5 illustrate advanced degenerative lumbar spinal stenosis. At the disc level, the ballooning of the disc itself and the marked thickening of the ligamenta flava in combination with the hypertrophy of the superior articular processes reduces the vertebral canal to a small triangular tube in which the thecal sac and its content is com-

pressed. The subpedicular portion of the foramen is severely encroached upon by osteophytes at the insertion areas of the ligamentum flavum. The nerve roots are compressed from inferiorly by the protruding disc and from posteriorly by large facet joint osteophytes and pinched against the unyielding pedicle.

When degenerative spondylolisthesis occurs, the situation is further complicated. Owing to the integrity of the posterior vertebral arch, the dural sac follows the slipped vertebra and becomes wedged between the intervertebral disc and the posterosuperior end plate of the vertebra below on the one side, and the superior articular processes of the vertebra below and the posterior arch of the slipped vertebra as well as the ligamenta flava on the other side. The pathologic effects of degenerative changes of the articular processes and olisthesis are strictly related to the dimensions of the vertebral canal. If the latter is wide and vertebral slipping slight, compression of the dural tube may not occur. When the spinal canal is of medium size, the dural sac is usually encroached upon laterally, where there is direct contact with the medial border of the facet joints. If the dimensions of the spinal canal are at the lower limits of normal or below these, marked compression of the dural sac and nerve roots occurs even in the presence of only mild degenerative changes of the articular processes or moderate vertebral slipping.

ACKNOWLEDGMENTS

This work has been supported by the Swedish Medical Research Council (project no. B90-17X-07474-05A) and the Research Foundation of the Trygg Hansa Insurance Co., Stockholm.

BIBLIOGRAPHY

American Academy of Orthopaedic Surgeons: *Glossary of Spinal Terminology.* AAOS, Park Ridge, Ill, Document 675-80.

Bergström K, Nyberg G, Pech P, et al: Multiplanar spinal anatomy: Comparison of CT and cryomicrotomy in postmortem specimens. *AJNR* 1983; 4:590–592.

Bose K, Balasubramaniam P: Nerve root canals of the lumbar spine. *Spine* 1984; 9:16.

Breig A: *Adverse Mechanical Tension in the Central Nervous System: An Analysis of Cause and Effect: Relief by Functional Neurosurgery.* New York, John Wiley & Sons, 1978.

Crock HV, Yoshizawa H: *The Blood Supply of the Vertebral*

Column and Spinal Cord in Man. Vienna, Springer Verlag, 1981.

Eisenstein S: The morphometry and pathological anatomy of the lumbar spine in South African Negroes and Caucasoids with specific reference to spinal stenosis. *J Bone Joint Surg [Br]* 1980; 59:73.

Eisenstein S: The trefoil configuration of the lumbar vertebral canal. A study of South African skeletal material. *J Bone Joint Surg [Br]* 1980; 62:73.

Epstein JA, Epstein BS, Levine LS: Nerve root compression associated with narrowing of the lumbar spinal canal. *J Neurol Neurosurg Psychiatry* 1962; 25:165.

Farfan HF: The pathological anatomy of degenerative spondylolisthesis. A cadaver study. *Spine* 1980; 5:412–418.

Hadley LA: Anatomico-roentgenographic studies of the posterior spinal articulations. *AJR* 1961; 86:270–276.

Hofmann M: Die Befestigung der Dura mater im Wirbelkanal. *Arch Anat Physiol (Anat Abtg)* 1898; 403:1898–1911.

Kirkaldy-Willis WH, Wedge JH, Yong-Hing K, et al: Pathology and pathogenesis of lumbar spondylosis and stenosis. *Spine* 1978; 3:319–328.

Lee CK, Rauschning W, Glenn WV: Lumbar lateral spinal canal stenosis. Classification, pathologic anatomy and surgical decompression. *Spine* 1988; 13:313–320.

Lewin T: Osteoarthritis of lumbar synovial joints: A morphologic study. *Acta Orthop Scand Suppl* 1964; 73:1–112.

Lewit K, Sereghy T: Lumbar peridurography with special regard to the anatomy of the lumbar peridural space. *Neuroradiology* 1974; 8:233–240.

Louis R: Topographic relationships of the vertebral column, spinal cord and nerve roots. *Anat Clin* 1978; 1:3–12.

Monajati A, Wayne WS, Rauschning W, et al: The cauda equina: MR imaging considerations. *AJNR* 1987; 8:893–900.

Parke WW, Watanabe R: The intrinsic vasculature of the lumbosacral spinal nerve roots. *Spine* 1985; 6:508.

Postacchini F, Ripani M, Carpano S: Morphometry of the lumbar vertebrae. An anatomic study in two Caucasoid ethnic groups. *Clin Orthop* 1983; 172:296.

Ramsey RH: The anatomy of the ligamenta flava. *Clin Orthop* 1966; 44:129–136.

Rauschning W: Computed tomography and cryomicrotomy of lumbar spine specimens. A new technique for multiplanar anatomic correlation. *Spine* 1983; 8:170–180.

Rauschning W: Detailed sectional anatomy of the spine, in Rothman SLG, Glenn WV (eds): *Multiplanar CT of the Spine.* Baltimore, University Park Press, 1985, pp 33–85.

Rauschning W: Correlative multiplanar computed tomographic anatomy of the normal spine, in Post MJD (ed): *Computed Tomography of the Spine.* Baltimore, Williams & Wilkins Co, 1983, pp 1–57.

Rauschning W: Anatomy of the normal and traumatized spine, in Sances A, Thomas DJ, Ewing CL, et al. (eds): *Mechanics of Head and Spine Trauma.* New York, Aloray, 1986, pp 531–563.

Rauschning W: Normal and pathologic anatomy of the lumbar root canals. *Spine* 1987; 12:1008–1019.

Rauschning W: Detailed anatomy of the lumbar spine, in Cauthen JC (ed): *Lumbar Spine Surgery: Indications, Techniques, Failures and Alternatives,* ed 2. Baltimore, Williams & Wilkins Co, 1988, pp 5–16.

Rauschning W: Pathomorphology of lumbar spinal stenosis, in Postacchini F (ed): *Lumbar Spinal Stenosis.* Heidelberg, Springer-Verlag, 1989, pp 87–99.

Rauschning W: Normal anatomy of the vertebral canal and the lumbar neural structures, in Postacchini F (ed): *Lumbar Spinal Stenosis.* Heidelberg. Springer Verlag, 1989, pp 21–48.

Rauschning W: Imaging anatomy of the lumbar spine (Chapter 6A) in Weinstein JN, Wiesel SW (eds): *The Lumbar Spine.* Orlando, Fla, WB Saunders Co, 1989, pp 23–48.

Rauschning W: Anatomy and pathology of the cervical spine, in Frymoyer J (ed): *The Adult Spine: Principles and Practice.* New York, Raven Press, 1990, pp 907–928, 1465–1486.

Rauschning W, Bergström K: Correlative craniospinal anatomy studied by computed tomography and cryomicrotomy. *J Comput Assist Tomogr* 1982; 7:8–13.

Rauschning W, Genant HJ, Hamberg M, et al: *Clinical and Imaging Anatomy of the Lumbar Spine and Sacrum, Electronic Laser Barcode Atlas.* St Louis, Mosby–Year Book, Inc, 1990.

Reicher MA, Gold RH, Halbach VV, et al: MR imaging of the lumbar spine: Anatomic correlations and the effect of technical variations. *AJR* 1986; 147:891–898.

Schmorl G, Junghanns H: *The Human Spine in Health and Disease,* ed 2. New York, Grune & Stratton, Inc, 1971.

Schneck C: The anatomy of lumbar spondylosis. *Clin Orthop* 1985; 193:20.

Spencer DL, Irwin GS, Miller JAA: Anatomy and significance of fixation of the lumbosacral nerve roots in sciatica. *Spine* 1983; 8:672–679.

van Schajk JPJ, Verbiest H, van Schajk FDJ: The orientation of laminae and facet joints in the lower lumbar spine. *Spine* 1985; 10:59.

Verbiest H: Pathomorphologic aspects of developmental lumbar stenosis. *Orthop Clin North Am* 1975; 6:177–196.

Yong-Hing K, Reilly J, Kirkaldy-Willis WH: The ligamentum flavum. *Spine* 1976; 1:226–234.

4

Posterior Surgical Approaches to the Lumbar Spine

Robert G. Watkins, M.D.

The initial important aspect of the approach to the posterior lumbar spine is to have proper "depth perception thinking." That is, by identifying posterior structures, the surgeon should be able to know the location of anterior structures in relation to the posterior anatomic landmarks. Three-dimensional thinking is important in determining the location of the pedicle and the intervertebral disc in relation to the interlaminar area. While the L5–S1 disc is at the level of the interlaminar area, as one progresses cephalad, the disc space, proportionately, is in a more cephalad position in relation to the interlaminar area. Therefore, exposure of the L3–4 disc requires more removal of the caudal edge of the L3 lamina than would exposure at L5–S1. The disc will be in a more cephalad position compared to the interlaminar area the higher one progresses in the lumbar spine (Fig 4–1).

LEVEL IDENTIFICATION

Three-dimensional thinking is important in identifying levels in surgery. We recommend that at least one intraoperative radiograph be taken to establish the level of the operation in each lumbar spine approach. The spinous process may be large, bulbous, and extend well below the disc or interlaminar space. While this can be used as a general guideline for a large skin incision, it has not been the best landmark for locating a disc or even a fusion level. For a limited exposure, as with a microscopic lumbar

discectomy and facetectomy, two 18-gauge or two 20-gauge spinal needles are placed approximately three fingerbreadths lateral to the spine after appropriate sterile preparation. These are inserted directly vertical and a transtable lateral radiograph is taken. Using the needles relative to the disc space, the surgical approach should be exactly over the disc space itself: not the interlaminar area, not the spinous process, but the disc space itself. This will allow the best visualization of the disc space for a limited-exposure disc excision. For a broader, more extensive exposure, the radiograph is taken after subperiosteal dissection and clearance of one side of the spine. The laminar and interlaminar areas are exposed out to the facet joint, self-retaining retractors are placed, and an instrument such as a Kocher clamp is placed in the interlaminar area. We prefer using the interlaminar area as the key anatomic landmark to identify the spinal level. The interlaminar area is just caudal to the disc space of the motion segment involved. Using the spinous process can be deceptive as is using the lamina. To summarize, for a limited exposure, we use lateral paraspinous needles for the skin incision, followed by a Kocher clamp placed in the interlaminar area of the disc to be exposed. Opening the interlaminar area allows access to the disc space which is just cephalad.

When the transverse process is to be exposed, an 18-gauge needle is inserted dorsally over the proposed pedicle or at the base of the transverse process, which, on the lateral view, would identify a pedicle. The marker establishes the levels to be fused, as a fusion should be from pedicle to pedicle. This is the best marker for a fusion. Using the spi-

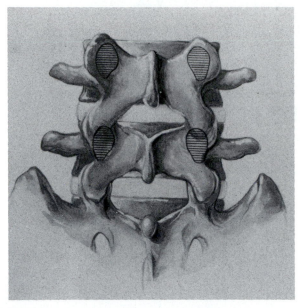

FIG 4–1.
Three-dimensional thinking starts with visualization and palpation of the spinous process and progresses to the anterior column of the spine, the intervertebral disc, the vertebral bodies, and the neurologic structures. The usual posterior approach to the lumbar spine begins with the spinous process. After exposure of the lamina, the facet joint is visualized. Location of the facet joint allows one to distinguish the inferior facet from the superior facet. The base of the superior facet leads to the transverse process. Visualization of the superior facet and the transverse process in the interlaminar area can lead to very specific locations of the pedicle. Dorsally, the critical angle marks the location of the exiting nerve root. The critical angle is the junction of the cephalad edge of the caudal lamina with the base of the superior facet. The exiting nerve root exits immediately under this point. The pedicle is in the cephalad half of the intervertebral body. (From Watkins RG: *Surgical Approaches to the Spine.* New York, Springer-Verlag, 1983, p 157. Used by permission.)

nous process may be quite confusing as the transverse process is very far cephalad to the spinous process of the level to be fused.

THE MIDLINE APPROACH TO THE SPINE

Discussion of specific anatomic structures is best done while presenting the approach. The approach begins with positioning. The ideal position should avoid any abdominal pressure, either from the side or directly anteriorly. We prefer the Andrews frame for the majority of our patients. The hips and the knees are flexed at 90 degrees. Touching the frame are the chest, knees, and chin. There are two well-padded, lateral thigh pads. The abdomen hangs entirely free. In operations involving internal fixation of the lower lumbar spine, positioning the patient with the proper amount of lumbar lordosis is a critical factor. Having the patient with his hips flexed at 90 degrees may not allow sufficient lumbar lordosis. In cases where this is critical we use the four-poster frame, allowing the hips to be extended, which may produce a greater amount of lordosis.

The actual approach begins with a straight midline incision through the dermis only. Epinephrine 20 mL 1-500,000 is injected through the dermal incision into the subcutaneous tissue and the subfascial muscle layer. The "deep" knife extends the incision through to the fascial layer. Self-retaining Gelpi retractors are placed gently. A great deal of care is taken not to crush the subcutaneous fat tissue and every attempt is made to avoid creating an unnecessary dead space in this very important layer.

With the fascia exposed in the midline and the preoperative decision having been made as to whether to do a midline approach or a paraspinous fascial approach, the exposure is extended subfascially by one of these two means.

When the spinous process is to be removed, the electrocautery cuts directly down onto the bone of the spinous process and the fascia is opened in this midline area. The cautery is used to remove as much of the fascial insertion as possible from the bone to allow a better postoperative repair when the spinous process is removed. The surgeon uses two Cobb elevators to sweep the tissue off the tip of the spinous process, exposing the bone alone, and then dissecting over the bulbous tip of the spinous process onto the lamina. All soft tissue is removed as the two Cobb elevators sweep out laterally on the lamina. The assistant follows with the electrocautery and the cell-saver sucker. The lateral dissection ends at the medial portion of the facet joint capsule, and self-retaining retractors are then placed.

A second approach to the spine involves operations in which the spinous process is to be preserved. In these instances the Cobb elevator is used to sweep gently out laterally to the bulbous tip of the spinous process and a paraspinous fascial incision is made just off the bulbous tip of the spinous process. This leaves a medial leaf of lumbodorsal fascia to sew back to. It allows the Cobb elevators to be introduced under this fascial leaf and dissection laterally on the lamina to the medial portion of the facet joint capsule. Exposure of the interlaminar area is carried out with the Cobb elevators and a self-retaining Williams retractor, or similar retractor, is placed. The point of the retractor extends medially, usually just caudal to the spinous process, and the blade exposes the interlaminar area. In cases of lateral recess stenosis, in which an interlaminar operation is to be done, preserving not only the spinous process but most of the laminae, exposure of the interlaminar area is all that is needed. The caudal portion of the lamina is identified above. The caudal edge of the cephalad lamina is then followed around to the medial portion of the inferior facet.

The facet joint is another important landmark that is exposed during the initial stages of the posterior approach (Fig 4–2). After identification of the facet joint, remember that the superior articular process is anterolateral, or volar and lateral, to the infe-

rior articular process. The inferior articular process is the first bone encountered when using a dorsal approach. The facet joint may be markedly distorted in cases of spinal stenosis. A huge, hypertrophic facet joint, with a hypertrophic capsule and a synovial cyst protruding into the interlaminar area, is not an uncommon occurrence. With the same motion as the lamina is cleared, the Cobb elevators are used to sweep the inferior surface of the lamina. With identification of the inferior facet and the facet joint capsule, the next step is to identify the medial articular surface of the superior facet and the pars interarticularis. In order to identify the articular surface of the superior facet, the medial portion of the inferior facet must be osteotomized with a chisel or burred to reveal the glistening dorsal surface of the superior facet. To identify the most caudal superior facet or the pars interarticularis, the caudal portion of the inferior facet may also have to be osteotomized. Care is taken to protect the major portion of the facet capsule. After sweeping over the dorsal surface of the

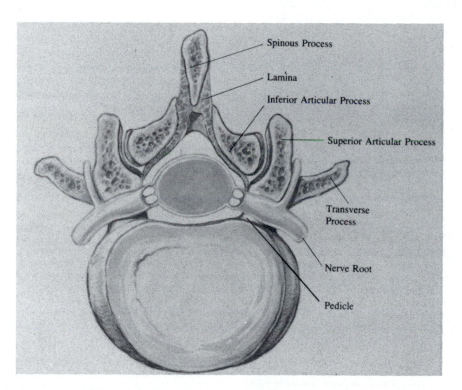

FIG 4–2.
The transverse plane section of the lumbar neuromotion segment emphasizing the orientation of the transverse process, superior articular process, and pedicle as a three-pronged structure. The facet joint is seen as the roof of the lateral recess. The nerve exits below the pedicle at each level. The nerve branches into a dorsal primary ramus that innervates from one to three facet joints at adjoining spinal levels. The ventral primary ramus is responsible for limb function and sensation. (From Watkins RG: *Surgical Approaches to the Spine*. New York, Springer-Verlag, 1983, p 155. Used by permission.)

pars interarticularis with a small Cobb elevator, the cautery is used to clear off the pars interarticularis itself. There are always significant bleeders just lateral to the pars interarticularis. These can be avoided by not extending the dissection lateral to the pars interarticularis.

In cases of total laminectomy, significant foraminotomy, or significant facet arthropathy, we usually take the time to expose the pars interarticularis. This gives us a reasonable idea of the farthest lateral extent of the dissection (Fig 4–3). With the pars interarticularis exposed, the interlaminar area is defined and self-retaining Wiltse retractors are used to hold back the muscle mass. By identifying the facet joints, the location of the transverse process is known. In cases of spinal fusion, the initial stages

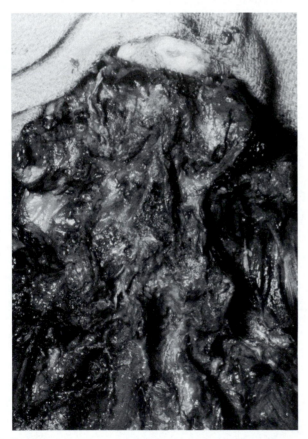

FIG 4–3.
The initial stages of exposure should expose the pars interarticularis. This defines the lateral limits of the bony posterior column and allows the surgeon to leave adequate bone to prevent fracture when cutting the pars interarticularis during the laminectomy. The pars interarticularis is best thought of as the base of the superior facet. (From Watkins RG: *Surgical Approaches to the Spine.* New York, Springer-Verlag, 1983, p 161. Used by permission.)

of the exposure consist of extending the dissection with the Cobb elevators over the facet joint onto the transverse process, initially preserving the capsule. The transverse process extends caudally and laterally from the facet joint. The surgeon dissects over the facet joint capsule, feeling with the Cobb elevators gently. The elevators are then swept down laterally, one cephalad and one caudad until the transverse process, is exposed. Electrocautery, on a low setting, is used to dissect the soft tissue from the dorsal surface of the transverse process. Again, the Wiltse self-retaining retractor provides the best exposure of these areas lateral to the facet joint.

With the transverse process exposed, removal of the facet joint capsule may then be carried out in cases of spinal fusion with exposure of the articular surfaces to allow removal of the lateral portions of articular cartilage and impaction of bone into a portion of the facet joint.

The interlaminar area is bordered by laminae cephalad, and caudad, by the spinous process medially, and laterally by the facet joint. The floor is the ligamentum flavum (Fig 4–4). The ligamentum flavum consists of two layers: the superficial and the deep layer. The deep layer has the typical vertical striations of ligament and is typically thought of as the yellow ligament. The insertion of the ligamentum flavum is approximately 50% cephalad on the undersurface of the cephalad lamina to the edge of the caudal lamina. It blends with the facet joint capsule laterally and then extends out over the nerve root (Fig 4–5) to form a portion of the roof of the intervertebral foramen. The undersurface of the articular facet forms a portion of the lateral recess, and the roof of the entry zone of the foramen. The ligamentum flavum forms a major portion of the soft tissue in the lateral recess (Fig 4–6). There is a cleft in the middle of the ligamentum flavum, creating two leaves, one from the right side and the other from the left. In passing sublaminar wires, the surgeon often takes advantage of this interval beneath the two leaves of ligamentum flavum.

Opening of the ligamentum flavum is done by one of several means. One may cut the lateral edge of the superficial ligament medial to the facet joint with a knife or by electrocautery. Removal of the superficial portion of the ligamentum flavum can then be done from lateral to medial with a curette and pituitaries to expose the deep ligament. The deep portion of the ligamentum flavum may be incised vertically to allow exposure of the epidural space. This

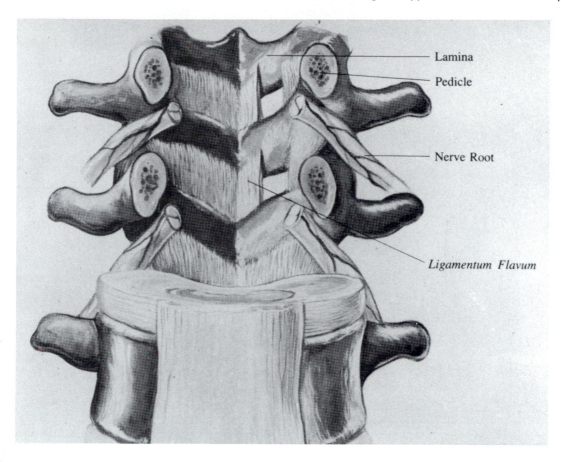

FIG 4–4.
The ligamentum flavum inserts approximately midway under the cephalad lamina and inserts on the cephalad edge of the caudad lamina. This underview of the posterior elements from the intervertebral canal demonstrates the ligamentum flavum and its insertion on the lamina. The ligamentum flavum is the principal stabilizing ligament of the posterior elements. Prediction of spinal stability often depends on the integrity of the posterior soft tissue column, specifically the ligamentum flavum. With a vertical laminar fracture, the principal function of the ligamentum flavum is maintained. By contrast, with a displaced horizontal laminar fracture of the slice variety, the integrity of the ligamentum flavum is disrupted. The ligamentum flavum is thinner in the midline. It can be opened in the midline by passing a Penfield dissector under this midline portion and cutting onto the dissector. The two halves of the ligament can be opened by retracting each laterally. This midline cleft is useful in passing the laminar wires for segmental fixation. (From Watkins RG: *Surgical Approaches to the Spine.* New York, Springer-Verlag, 1983, p 158. Used by permission.)

vertical knife incision is best done by feathering the blade so that the point does not extend deep into the ligamentum flavum, which sometimes is a very thin structure. In this way, an incision can be made at the junction of the middle and lateral thirds of the ligamentum flavum, down to the bluish hue of its undersurface. At this point, the Penfield no. 4 dissector is used to gently penetrate the lower layers of the ligament. The Penfield no. 4 dissector is extended into the epidural space. The dura is identified and the dissector is directed laterally under the lateral leaf of the ligamentum flavum, gently protecting the dura and blood vessels to allow excision of the lateral leaf of the ligamentum flavum with the Kerrison rongeur. At times, with lateral recess stenosis, the nerve root can be severely compressed in the lateral recess and great care should be taken to dissect gently.

After resection of the more medial horizontal portion of the ligamentum flavum, the vertical lateral portion can be excised (carefully protecting the nerve root). Using a Kerrison rongeur angled at 40 degrees, the lateral portion of the ligamentum flavum is removed between the nerve root and the lateral leaf. The ligamentum flavum can also be dissected with a sharp curette starting at the medial and volar surface of the superior facet. It can be detached cephalad by dissection with a curette under

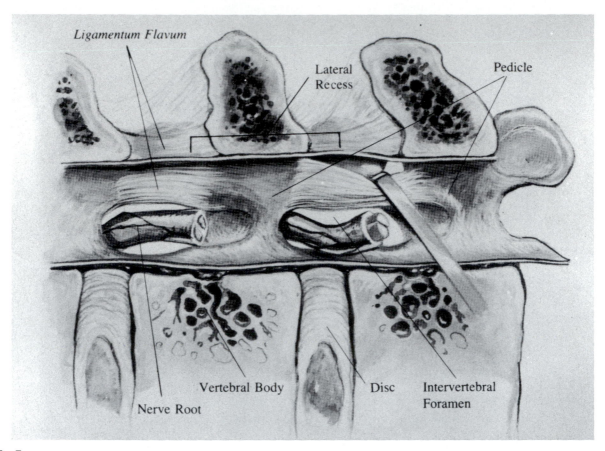

FIG 4–5.
Understanding the intervertebral foramen and the tissues present in the foramen are of critical importance regardless of the exact type of nomenclature used. The interpedicular foramen is the area between the two pedicles. This is lateral to the medial wall of the pedicle. The far lateral intervertebral foramen is the area lateral to the lateral wall of the pedicle. The foramen begins at the medial border of the pedicle and extends laterally from that point. The soft tissues in the intervertebral foramen are important. The floor of the intervertebral foramen in patients with spinal stenosis is frequently annulus of the disc covering a spur and/or herniation. The roof of the intervertebral foramen is the ligamentum flavum and the facet joint capsule. (From Watkins RG: *Surgical Approaches to the Spine.* New York, Springer-Verlag, 1983, p 160. Used by permission.)

the cephalad lamina and by removing the most cephalad attachment of the ligament. The attachment is quite far underneath the lamina and its detachment requires use of the curette completely out of view of the surgeon, who relies on tactile sensation for staying on the undersurface of the lamina. While the caudal portion of the ligamentum flavum which is attached to the cephalad edge of the caudal lamina is easier to detach, it must be remembered that the nerve root exits exactly under this area at a critical angle, where the ligamentum flavum is attached. Therefore, staying directly on the bone of the caudal lamina and base of the superior facet is important in detaching the ligament without injuring the nerve root. Detaching the ligament laterally and caudally and then retracting it medially may allow a better exposure of the root and disc.

THE EPIDURAL SPACE

After opening the ligamentum flavum and entering the epidural space, the pedicle is identified. The key to the anatomy and pathology in the canal is the pedicle (Fig 4–7). In order to understand the intracanal anatomy and pathologic conditions as they are related to clinical symptoms, it is important to understand the concept of individual neuromotion seg-

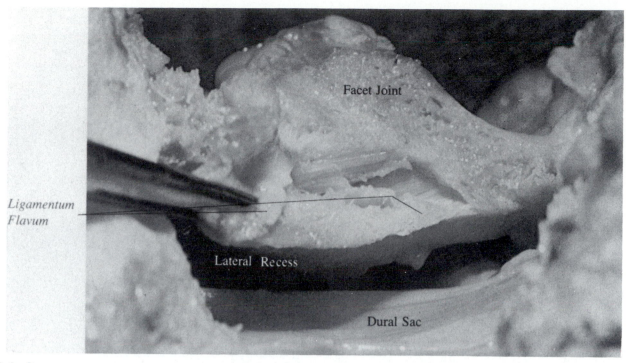

FIG 4–6.
The lateral recess is medial to the wall of the pedicle. Obstruction occurs from the superior facet and ligamentum flavum pressing the nerve root down on the disc or floor of the spinal canal medial to the pedicle. (From Watkins RG: *Surgical Approaches to the Spine.* New York, Springer-Verlag, 1983, p 162. Used by permission.)

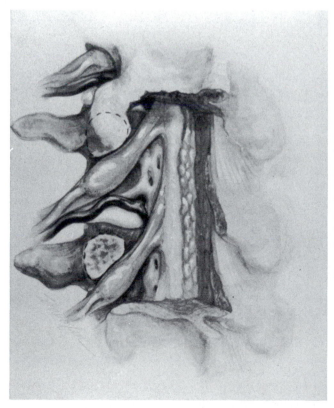

FIG 4–7.
The pedicle is the anatomic key to vertebral canal anatomy and pathology. The disc is immediately cephalad to the pedicle. The traversing nerve root is immediately medial to the pedicle. The exiting nerve root of the segment below is just caudal to the pedicle. The vascular leash exits in the intervertebral foramen caudal to the nerve root, over the caudal intervertebral disc. (From Watkins RG, Collis JS Jr: *Lumbar Discectomy and Laminectomy.* Rockville, Md, Aspen, 1991, p 164. Used by permission.)

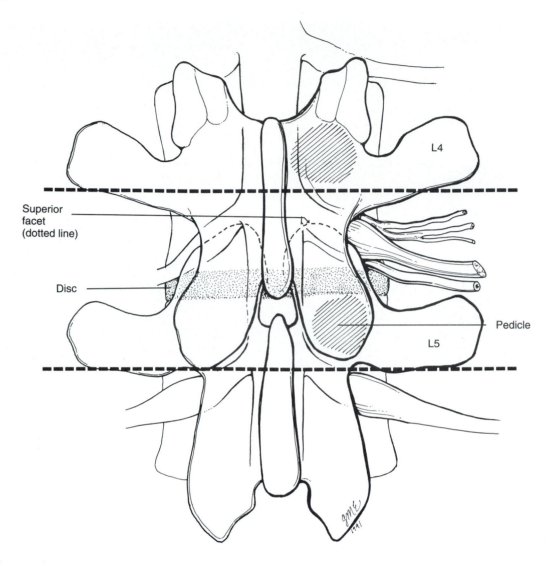

FIG 4–8.

Localization of pathologic entities requires understanding of the concept of a neuromotion segment. A neuromotion segment is defined as the vertebra, disc, ligament, facet joints, nerves, and vessels of one spinal level. A segment begins at the cephalad tip of a superior facet and extends to the caudal pedicle wall of that vertebral body. The terms *exiting* and *traversing nerve root* are important concepts. For example, the traversing nerve root at L4–5 is the fifth nerve. The exiting nerve root at L5–S1 is the fifth nerve. If the patient has a foraminal stenosis at L5–S1, and has S1 symp-

toms, it is not caused by an interpedicular foraminal stenosis at L5–S1. That would affect the L5 root, not the S1 nerve root. A foraminal stenosis at L4–5 should have no direct effect on the L5 nerve root because the exiting nerve root through the intervertebral foramen at L4–5 is the fourth nerve. Therefore, one must not only describe the anatomic abnormalities of the spinal column, such as the location of an area of stenosis, but one must also relate that to the neurologic column and the symptoms produced by these anatomic structures.

ments. Each segment has one pedicle (Fig 4–8). The pedicle itself is immediately anterior to the base of the superior articular facet. The transverse process, the superior facet, and the pedicle form a three-pronged structure with the pedicle projecting anteriorly in the transverse plane, the transverse process projecting laterally in the coronal plane, and the superior articular facet projecting cephalad in the

parasagittal plane. Knowing the location of the pedicle tells you that:

1. The disc space is less than 1 cm cephalad to the pedicle, often appearing immediately cephalad (Fig 4–9).
2. The intervertebral foramen is just caudal to the pedicle. The traversing nerve root of a segment

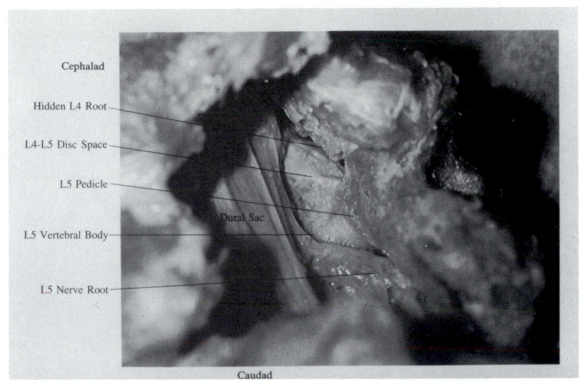

FIG 4–9.
A specimen cleaned of veins shows the relationship of the disc to the pedicle as visualized from a partial hemilaminectomy. The nerve root exits around the pedicle and the disc space is immediately cephalad to the pedicle. (From Watkins RG: *Surgical Approaches to the Spine.* New York, Springer-Verlag, 1983, p 163. Used by permission.)

(i.e., the fifth root at L4–5) becomes the exiting nerve root of the level below (the fifth root at L5–S1) The exiting nerve root traverses around the pedicle to exit caudally in the intervertebral foramen.

3. Immediately dorsal and cephalad to the pedicle is the superior facet. The superior facet of L5 is immediately dorsal and cephalad to the pedicle of L5. The superior facet is the roof of the intervertebral foramen for the exiting nerve root and a portion of the roof for the lateral recess for the traversing nerve root. The superior facet is covered on its undersurface by the facet joint capsule and the ligamentum flavum.

4. Just medial to the pedicle is the traversing nerve root. The key to identifying the traversing nerve root of that neuromotion segment is identification of the pedicle. The base of the pedicle is well vascularized. The tube of the pedicle can be identified by localizing the structures on the dorsal elements. The projection of the tube of the pedicle is found by identifying a point made by a line bisecting the center of the transverse process in the coronal plane and a perpendicular line just medial to the lateral wall of the superior articular facet in the parasagittal plane (Fig 4–10). From this point, the direction of the pedicle may vary from 15 to 25 degrees from the midline angled from lateral to medial (see Fig 4–10). The angle of the pedicle decreases as one progresses cephalad in the lumbar spine and the tube of the pedicle may become elliptic in the upper lumbar spine. Palpation for the pedicle with, for example, a dental tool may produce significant bleeding in this area and should be gentle and just enough to identify the cephalad and caudad border of the pedicle. Often, with significant hypertrophy of the superior facet, the medial border of the superior facet is mistaken for the pedicle and only with more volar palpation is the full lateral extent of the pedicle appreciated. With identification of the pedicle and then the nerve root, the lateral recess is better appreciated.

The lateral recess is bounded cephalad by the tip of the superior facet and caudad by the caudal border of the pedicle. The roof is the superior facet and ligamentum flavum. The floor is the disc and vertebral body medial to the medial wall of the pedicle.

The lateral recess is medial to the medial wall of the pedicle and lateral recess stenosis involves im-

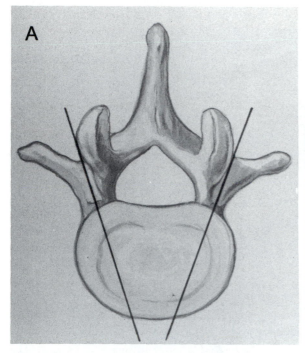

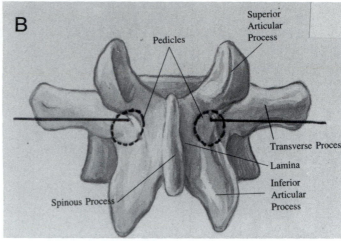

FIG 4–10.
A and **B,** the angle of the pedicle in the transverse plane is angled out from approximately 20 degrees in the lower spine to 10 degrees in the upper lumbar spine. The pedicle is found by the intersection of two lines: the transverse line that bisects the width of the transverse process and the parasagittal line that is just inside the outer border of the superior facet. The projection of the angle of the pedicle for in-sertion of the pedicle screw after location of the point of the intersection of the parasagittal and transverse plane lines allows one to properly angle an interpedicle device down the tube of the pedicle. (From Watkins RG: *Surgical Approaches to the Spine.* New York, Springer-Verlag, 1983, p 156. Used by permission.)

pingement of the traversing nerve root in this area. The intervertebral foramen is divided into the entry zone, which starts at the medial portion of the medial caudal wall of the pedicle, and the interpedicular portion, which is just lateral to the medial wall of the pedicle between the two pedicles, which form the cephalad and caudad borders of the intervertebral foramen. The lateral intervertebral foramen is the portion of the foramen just lateral to the lateral caudal wall of the pedicle.

Identification of the pedicle leads immediately to identification of the traversing nerve root. In spinal stenosis and disc herniation, the traversing nerve root may be tightly adherent to the medial wall of the pedicle. Do not retract the nerve root against a major obstacle. Gentle palpation with the Penfield no. 4 dissector and the microsucker retractor allows one to test the tension in the nerve root medial to the medial wall of the pedicle. It is safer to attempt to gently retract and test for tension in the nerve root more cephalad than the pedicle, at the disc space level, and closer to the shoulder of the nerve root.

If the nerve root is tight, several measures are used to avoid injuring the nerve root by retracting it. The key is to know the anatomy. Knowing the exact location of the pedicle in the canal is the most significant first step in avoiding injury to the nerve. Expose the disc cephalad to the pedicle and slightly lateral to the medial wall of the pedicle. This will involve a partial medial facetectomy. Removing more of the medial portion of the superior facet will permit easy palpation and even visualization of the medial wall of the pedicle. By extending the exposure significantly more cephalad, you will eventually run into the exiting nerve root of the segment above. There is usually a safe area immediately cephalad and lateral to the medial wall of the pedicle.

The first step is to obtain a more lateral exposure until you can easily visualize the medial wall of the pedicle and expose the floor and disc of the canal just cephalad and lateral to the pedicle. The traversing nerve root should not be in this area as it is medial to the medial wall of the pedicle. Next, explore the axilla of the traversing nerve root with the Penfield dissector. This may require removal of more of the caudad lamina. Exploring the axilla may allow you to remove a fragment that will prevent any medial retraction of the nerve root. Bleeding may be encountered in this area as well. Enter the disc space lateral to the nerve root in the safe area. Try to pull out disc material and decompress the nerve root from that area and then gently work under the nerve root, removing disc material from medial to lateral. Extend the exposure cephalad. Remove more of the caudal lamina of the cephalad vertebra and remove enough lamina up to the most cephalad insertion of the ligamentum flavum. This should provide adequate clearance of the cephalad portion of the root. Extend the foraminotomy around the pedicle, removing bone from the "critical angle." The critical angle is the junction of the caudal lamina and the superior facet, under which the nerve root exits. Open this area by following the nerve root around

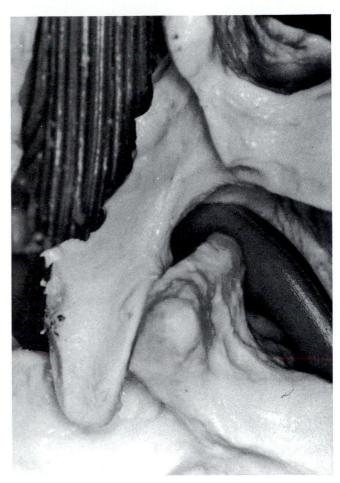

FIG 4–12.
Laminotomy. The transverse process and the inferior facet are shown. The superior facet of a subluxated facet joint projects into the exiting nerve root as it passes through the intervertebral foramen.

the pedicle as it exits, and do an entry zone foraminotomy. Remove the roof of the canal over the nerve as it exits around the pedicle. A foraminotomy of the foramen below may allow better retraction of the nerve root.

After opening the lateral recess, identify the root and the pedicle and follow the root around the pedicle past its medial wall to enter the intervertebral foramen. The cephalad boundary of the intervertebral foramen is the caudal surface of the cephalad pedicle. The caudal boundary is the cephalad portion of the caudad pedicle. The roof of the intervertebral foramen is formed by the superior facet and the pars interarticularis. The floor of the intervertebral foramina is the caudal portion of the vertebral body above and the intervertebral disc space (Fig 4–11).

With rotational deformities of the motion segment, the superior facet may be subluxated anteri-

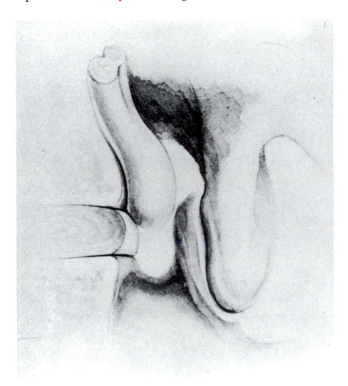

FIG 4–11.
The limits of the intervertebral foramen are: cephalad—the pedicle above; caudad—the pedicle below; the roof is the superior facet and pars from the segment below; and the floor is the caudal portion of the vertebral body above and the intervertebral disc. Distortions in rotation and hypertrophy of the facet joint can produce a narrowing of the intervertebral foramen from two major sources. Firstly, hypertrophy of the tip of the superior facet presses downward and cephalad on the nerve root. Secondly, marginal osteophyte on the back of the body above produces obstruction volar to the nerve root.

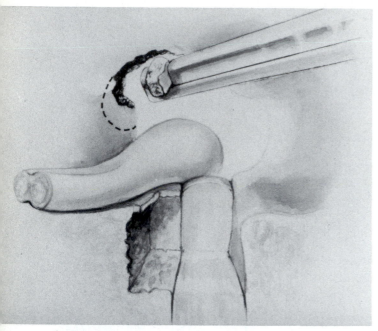

FIG 4–13.
Two types of foraminotomy. A volar bone spur has been removed. The space created by the evacuation of the spur under the nerve root demonstrating relief of the obstruction over the nerve root as well. More common is the undercutting of the roof of the foramen. (From Watkins RG, Collis JS Jr: *Lumbar Discectomy and Laminectomy.* Rockville, Md, Aspen, 1991, p 164. Used by permission.)

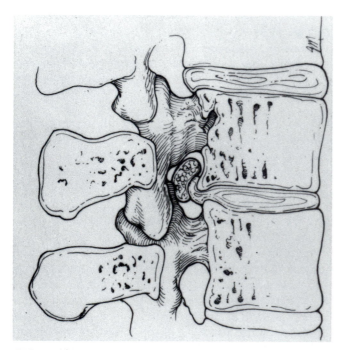

FIG 4–14.
A foraminal disc herniation and bone spur on the back of the body above. This is a left foramen viewed from inside the spinal canal. It shows the volar pressure on the nerve root itself.

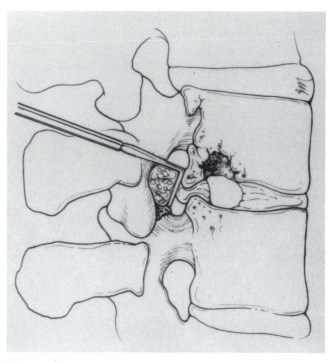

FIG 4–15.
The first step in relieving volar pressure on the nerve root is to burrow under the marginal osteophyte to create room and space for impaction of the osteophyte. The intervertebral disc is entered in order to create the room within the intervertebral disc. The end plate is curetted and burrowed under the spur to produce room for the spur.

orly and downward pressing against the pedicle above and the posterior caudal body of the vertebral body above. Not only the bone of the facet joint but the ligamentum flavum and the facet joint capsule may contribute to a soft tissue stenosis in that area. A vertical subluxation of the tip of the superior facet can pinch the nerve root against the pedicle above. When performing a foraminotomy, one must remove the undersurface of the superior facet to provide an adequate excursion of the entry zone of the foramen (Figs 4–12 and 4–13). At times, a significant bony spur arising from the vertebral body, under the nerve root, in the intervertebral foramen, must be removed. This is best done by opening the intervertebral disc below and curetting under the spur to create a space. The spur can be pushed down into the space created in the inferior surface in the body above (Figs 4–14 through 4–16).

Extraforaminal ligaments may bind the exiting nerve root to the floor of the intervertebral foramen and provide a significant impediment to the excursion of the nerve root. Changes in anatomy due to degenerative disease may allow these structures to become a significant portion of the potential obstruction to the intervertebral foramen.

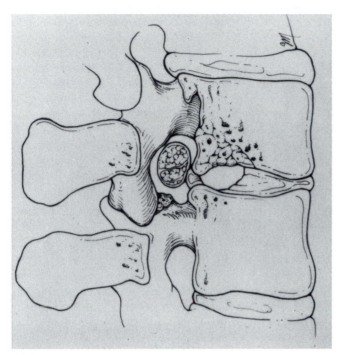

FIG 4–16.
Impaction of the spur into the space to relieve volar pressure under the nerve root.

The vascular leash extends from the central portion of the spinal canal out of the intervertebral foramen, usually caudal to the exiting nerve root. The vascular leash will extend over the intervertebral disc, caudal to the nerve root. There are significant vertically extending veins under the lateral portion of the dura. Obviously, identification of the vascular leash in extensive exposures of the floor of the spinal canal is important. Often these vessels are thick and not easily appreciated as vascular structures. They may mimic the nerve root or a conjoined or accessory nerve root. The key is that the structures coursing on the cephalad edge of the pedicle, over the disc space, are usually vascular, while the nerve root exits in the cephalad portion of the intervertebral foramen, just caudal to the pedicle above. The vessels exit around the cephalad edge of the pedicle and the caudal portion of the intervertebral foramen.

An extensive exposure of the disc, such as that needed for a posterior lumbar interbody fusion, requires that one ligate and transect the vascular leash. Because significant medial retraction of the dura is necessary, cephalad retraction of the exiting nerve root and a full exposure of the disc necessitates that the vascular leash be excised through this area. In standard disc excisions, the vascular leash can be dissected bluntly, from caudad to cephalad, and retracted cephalad to the disc to allow adequate opening of the disc and removal of the significant portion of intradiscal material.

THE PARASPINAL APPROACH TO THE SPINE

The paraspinal approach to the spine may be used to excise a lateral disc herniation, do a foraminotomy from the outside in, expose the transverse process and pedicles for pedicle screw insertion, expose the transverse process and outer portion of the facet for a posterior lateral fusion, or any combination of these.

We prefer a midline skin incision with adequate length to allow lateral retraction of the skin to expose the lumbodorsal fascia and the bulk of the paraspinal muscle mass. A paraspinal fascial incision is made at that point. For lateral exposure of the disc, the paraspinal fascial incision is about two fingerbreadths off the midline. For a more extensive posterior lateral exposure, or, for example, several levels for fusion, we use a curvilinear incision, three fingerbreadths from the midline in its center portion down to one fingerbreadth at the caudad and cephalad extent of the exposure. The paraspinal incision is a muscle-splitting incision. After incising the fascia with the cautery, fingers are used to vertically separate the muscle fibers down to the lateral portion of the facet and the transverse process. There is a tendency to proceed too medially and end up on the lamina. Going directly down in a lateral position puts one onto the transverse process. After muscle spreading and splitting is done with the fingers, the self-retaining Wiltse retractors are inserted and the Cobb elevators used to expose the transverse processes while the assistant on the opposite side of the table uses a cautery on a low setting and a sucker to aid in the exposure of these lateral structures. Exposure of the disc from the lateral approach is carried out by identifying the transverse processes above and below the intertransverse area to be explored. For an L4–5 disc, this is the L4 transverse process and the L5 transverse process. Dissection on the cephalad transverse process proceeds medially to the base of the transverse process, and the superior facet is identified. The pars interarticularis will be more dorsal in the wound, and should be exposed. One approach is to proceed medially on the caudad surface of the transverse process and proceed directly into the intervertebral foramen from this point. We usually go more dorsal, expose the pars interarticularis caudal to this transverse process at the level of the superior facet and better define the borders of the intertransverse area which are the cephalad transverse process cephalad, the caudad transverse process caudad, the intertransverse ligament laterally, the superior facet and the pars medially, and anteriorly, the most lateral portion of the intervertebral disc and vertebral body and the nerve, vessel, and retroperitoneal space structures (Fig 4–17).

The next step is to detach the intertransverse ligament from the cephalad transverse process proceeding immediately along the pars interarticularis and then out on the cephalad portion of the caudal transverse process. The ligament can be dissected free with a curette, gently clamped, and retracted from medial to lateral. Use of the Bovie cautery and magnification at that point is important. We specifically use the bipolar Bovie cautery on the vessels exiting with the nerve root from the spinal canal out

into the intervertebral foramen and intertransverse area. Identify the nerve root by following the caudal surface of the cephalad transverse process medially to the lateral caudal wall of the pedicle. By following the transverse process to the pedicle, the nerve root can be found just caudal to the caudal wall of the pedicle. Therefore, use the transverse process above, and then the pedicle above, to find the exiting nerve root. Identification of the nerve root in an avascular plane, after bipolar cauterization of the vessels, is the key to protecting the nerve root while exposing the intertransverse area. Identify the nerve root as it exits from the canal around the pedicle above to avoid injury. Identification of the nerve root at this point often may reveal the intrusion onto the nerve root by the facet or other obstructing structures. A disc fragment is sometimes seen directly volar to the exiting nerve root and the tension and retractability of the nerve root is gently tested. It

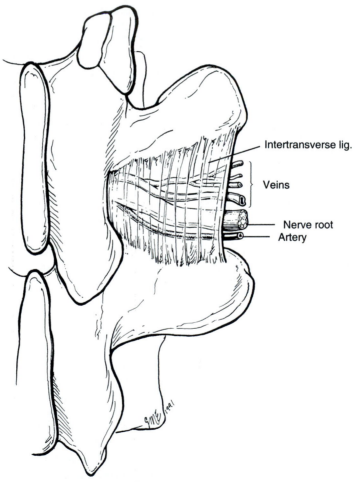

FIG 4–17.
The intertransverse approach. Note the location of the nerve and vascular structures (see text).

may be necessary to use the chisel and Kerrison rongeurs to resect a lateral portion of the superior facet in order to be able to expose this exiting portion of the nerve root. Excision of a portion of the lateral wall of the superior facet does not cause major damage to the facet joint. After exposure of the nerve root, the pathologic conditions may require additional exposure of the pedicle below. By approaching medially to the caudal transverse process to the caudal pedicle, one can identify the intervertebral disc, which is always immediately cephalad to the caudal pedicle. Often the nerve root will course over the disc in this area, but additional exposure above and below the nerve root may add in the foraminotomy or excision of disc material. A large, lateral, volar spur may be removed by identifying the pedicle above the spur on the caudal surface of the vertebral body from above.

The paraspinal approach for fusion is carried out by dissecting directly down on the transverse processes. Insertion of the Wiltse retractor and exposure of the transverse process and outer border of the superior facet is carried out. This is done with the Cobb elevators and the cautery on a low setting. Exposure in this area allows better decortication of the outer border of the superior facet and the transverse process and allows lateral application of the bone graft. The insertion site for the pedicle screws is the point made by a line bisecting the transverse process and a parasagittal line just medial to the lateral wall of the superior facet. Insertion at this point is carried out from lateral to medial. The paraspinal approach provides a better lateral exposure for the lateral to medial orientation of the pedicle screws.

5

The Development of the Vertebral Canal

Richard W. Porter, M.D.

The syndromes of low back disability may be divided into two groups: those of compromise of the neural contents of the vertebral canal, and those in which the source of pain is outside the vertebral canal. The former includes protrusion of the intervertebral disc, root entrapment syndrome from lateral canal stenosis, and neurogenic claudication—spinal stenosis syndromes. This is a significant part of low back pain problems, and hence our understanding of the anatomy of the vertebral canal, its pathology, and its development are essential.

ANATOMY

The term *vertebral canal* refers to that highly complicated space posterior to the vertebral bodies and discs, within the neural arch, which widens and narrows at each vertebral level in both the coronal and sagittal planes. There is regional variation at each vertebral level, differences among populations, and also considerable individual variation within a population.

The vertebral canal is arbitrarily divided into the central canal and the root canal. At the level of the pedicles, the central canal is bounded laterally by the two pedicles, anteriorly by the posterior surface of the vertebral body, and posteriorly by the cranial aspect of the laminae and the medial aspect of the superior apophyseal joints. At the level of the intervertebral discs, the central canal has an artificial lateral boundary which extends from one pedicular level to the next. The central canal contains the cauda equina in its dural envelope.

The root canal is that space lateral to the central canal, in the intervertebral region (Fig 5–1). Anteriorly it is bounded by the posterior surface of the vertebral body above, the posterolateral aspect of the disc, and the posterior surface of the vertebral body below. Superiorly it is bounded by the pedicle of the vertebra above, and inferiorly by the pedicle of the vertebra below. Its posterior relations are the lateral aspect of the lamina, and the superior articulation of the apophyseal joint of the vertebra below. It opens into the central canal medially, and ends laterally at the intervertebral foramen. The root canal at L5 is considerably longer than at other levels because of the broad L5 pedicle.

The lateral recess is that lateral part of the central canal at the pedicular level, anterior to the medial aspect of the superior apophyseal joint.[35] Dome-shaped canals do not have a lateral recess because of the continuous concave posterior surface of this type of canal. Trefoil canals with their "cocked-hat" appearance, however, have a deep lateral recess (Fig 5–2).

In the sagittal plane, the vertebral canal pursues a serpentine course (Fig 5–3). The cranial aspects of the laminae indent the canal posteriorly at the levels of the upper borders of the vertebrae, and posteriorly the canal is indented by the bulging annulus of the intervertebral discs. In the coronal plane, the canal is narrowest at the pedicular levels, widening into each root canal at the level of the discs.

48   *Basic*

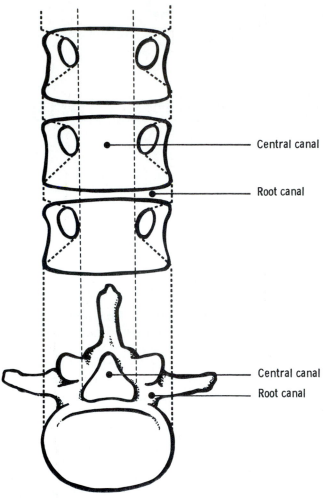

FIG 5–1.
Diagram of the central and root canals in the coronal and transverse planes.

Central canal
Root canal
Central canal
Root canal

The general dimensions of the vertebral canal tend to follow a consistent pattern throughout the lumbar region. When measured in the sagittal plane at the cranial aspect of the laminae, the canal is widest at L1, decreasing toward L4; in dome-shaped canals, it widens again at L5. In trefoil-shaped canals, L5 is equal to or smaller than L4.

There are population differences in the size of the vertebral canal. Spines from the Indian subcontinent are small compared with spines of present-day whites and archaeological Anglo-Saxon and Romano-British spines.[23, 29] Within a population there are also considerable variations in the canal's size, those in the 90th percentile being approximately 50% larger than those in the 10th percentile.[18] Women tend to have slightly wider canals than men in the same population.[6]

THE CLINICAL SIGNIFICANCE OF THE VERTEBRAL CANAL

It might be argued that the size and shape of the vertebral canal has little clinical significance because the epigenetic factors responsible for the canal's development probably ensure that the canal is always matched in size to its contents. An individual with large nerves is likely to have a correspondingly capacious canal.

This concept, however, does not agree with clinical observations. Following the early papers of Sarpyener,[34] Verbiest,[38] and Van Gelderen,[39] others confirmed that a variety of back pain syndromes are related to spinal pathologic conditions in the presence of an already small canal.[9, 12, 25, 26, 30, 32, 41] Edwards and La Rocca[5] showed that 71% of patients with back pain and degenerative change had canal diameters below the mean. Kornberg and Rechtine[14] demonstrated an inverse relationship between the vertebral canal size and the morbidity of disc protrusion. Forsberg and Walloe[11] reported that patients who made a poor recovery from disc surgery had canals that were narrower than those of patients who recovered uneventfully.

We now know that despite the canal's size matching the variable size of the neural contents, there is also a degree of mismatch, and that subjects who have limited space in the vertebral canal are vulnerable to a variety of back pain syndromes when there are added abnormalities. A disc protrusion into a restricted space can produce more troublesome symptoms than a protrusion into a wider canal. The trefoil shape places the nerve root at considerable risk in the presence of a posterolateral protrusion. A far-lateral disc protruding into the root canal, however, quickly involves the root irrespective of the central canal's size.

Similarly, the variable space in the root canal is a significant factor in the development of root entrapment syndrome from lateral canal stenosis. The root can be spared when degenerative change develops in a wide root canal, but be at risk when a similar pathologic change occurs in a small canal (Fig 5–4).

In the presence of segmental instability, the neural contents may not be compromised by dynamic changes when the canal is of adequate size, but stenotic symptoms can arise with segmental deformation if the canal is small.[10] The vertebral canal is un-

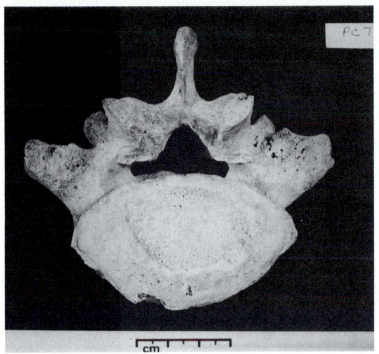

FIG 5–2.
Photograph of a Romano-British L5 vertebra, with a trefoil-shaped central vertebral canal. There is a deep lateral recess.

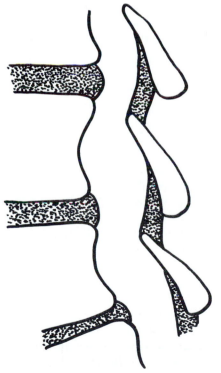

FIG 5–3.
Diagram of a sagittal section of the central vertebral canal, showing its serpentine course. It is indented by the soft tissue of the annulus anteriorly, and posteriorly by the attachment of the ligamentum flavum to the cranial lip of the lamina.

doubtedly a risk factor in many back pain syndromes.

THE SOFT TISSUE COMPONENT OF THE VERTEBRAL CANAL

The cauda equina and nerve roots are generally compromised at the intersegmental region of the vertebral canal. With advancing age, the dura is indented anteriorly at disc level by a bulging degenerate annulus, and the prominent posterior vertebral bars of the vertebrae above and below. Posteriorly, the ligamentum flavum attached to the cranial lip of the lamina also indents the canal (see Fig 5–3). In addition, the fibrous capsule of the apophyseal joints can compromise the canal's contents at the same level. The thickened ligamentum flavum extending laterally around the root canal will add to any bony stenosis. Thus the soft tissue constitutes important boundaries to the central and root canal at the intersegmental level which can have important clinical significance. This does not diminish the relevance of the shape and size of the bony boundaries of the vertebral canal. An individual who has a stenotic bony canal will also have limited space at the

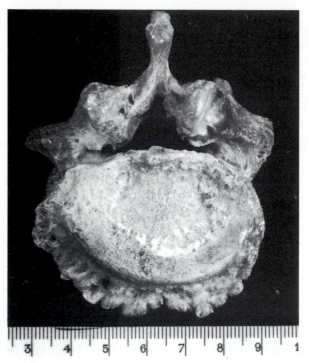

FIG 5–4.
Photograph of an Anglo-Saxon L5 vertebra, showing how degenerative change can further diminish the space in an already small root canal.

intersegmental level, even though much of this boundary is composed of soft tissue, because the soft tissues are attached to bony structures. A canal with large bony diameters provides more adequate space for the soft tissue contents. In addition, at the intersegmental level, the cranial end of the lamina forms an important constriction in central canal stenosis. And the apophyseal joints can similarly constrict both central and root canals. The fact that soft tissues often form the immediate boundary to the canal does not negate the relevance of a small bony canal.

MULTIFACTORIAL ASPECTS OF BACK PAIN SYNDROMES

It is too simplistic to believe that back pain has a single cause. Rather, each syndrome has a multifactorial set of causes. Spinal stenosis and the size and shape of the vertebral canal can never be described as causes of back pain although they are significant

risk factors; they are part of a constellation of factors responsible for the development of symptoms. For example, in symptomatic disc protrusion we tend to concentrate our attention on the protrusion or sequestration because annular damage is generally the acute episode that has precipitated the symptoms. However, in the pathogenesis of the condition, we must consider the strength of the annulus, which is influenced by familial and occupational factors.[27] Age, sex, and diurnal changes have significance,[1] along with the effects of fatigue and the occupational insults that cause annular damage. The relative strength of the bone and disc determines whether failure occurs at the bone or disc level.[21] The integrity of the musculoligamentous complex, muscular strength, and efficient reflex activity also play a part. Biochemical factors and individual differences in the pain mechanism may be important. Roots tethered by dural ligaments,[36] and anomalous roots,[13] can be more readily affected by disc protrusion than freely mobile roots.

One cannot ignore spinal stenosis. The space within the bony canal available to the nerve root which is compromised by a disc is also an important factor, but it is, of course, only one risk factor. It is the balance of factors that produces the symptoms.

THE EARLY DEVELOPMENT OF THE VERTEBRAL CANAL

Archaeological studies have shown that the vertebral canals in small children are remarkably large. It is difficult to obtain archaeological spines from individuals under 4 years of age, but vertebrae at that age have a mean midsagittal diameter 10% wider than the mean midsagittal diameter of adults in the same population.[29] The subsequent reduction in size of the midsagittal diameter is the result of the changing shape of the posterior border of the vertebral body from concave to convex (Fig 5–5). The mean interpedicular diameter at 4 years of age is approximately 85% of the adult size, and it gradually widens with the increasing breadth of the vertebral bodies and the widening pedicles. The upper lumbar vertebrae mature before those in the lower lumbar spine. At maturity approximately 15% of canals are trefoil-shaped at L5,[7] but the trefoil shape has not been seen in specimens of individuals less than 12 years of age.

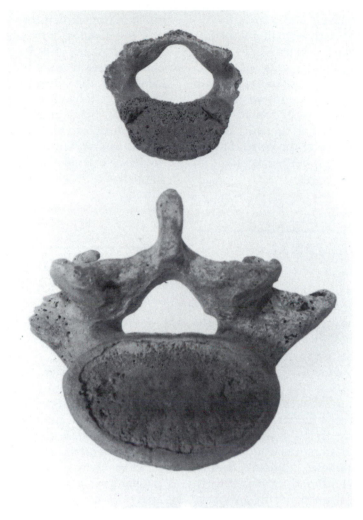

FIG 5–5.
Photograph of two L5 vertebrae from a Romano-British collection. The vertebra above is of an infant, and the vertebra below, an adult. The cross-sectional area of the infant vertebral canal is the same as the adult's. The midsagittal diameter is greater than the adult's because of the concave posterior border of the vertebral body.

FACTORS WHICH INFLUENCE THE DEVELOPMENT OF THE VERTEBRAL CANAL

Anthropometric measurements provide a clue to the development of the vertebral canal. A comparison between the size of the vertebral canal and the length of skeletal long bones showed a useful correlation between the length of the femur and the interpedicular diameter; a tall subject will have a large transverse diameter of the vertebral body, with widely spaced pedicles.[23] There were few useful correlations between the midsagittal diameter of the canal and other bony measurements. The anteroposterior and lateral diameters of the skull had a weak correlation with the midsagittal diameter of the canal, but it seems that this clinically important diameter is largely independent of other skeletal growth. Perhaps this is not surprising, when we know that much of the long bone growth occurs in childhood and adolescence, while the sagittal diameter of the vertebral canal is already mature by 4 years of age.

Clark and co-workers[2] suggested that the size of the vertebral canal may be affected by factors that impair early childhood development. They examined two archaeological populations and found that a malnourished population tended to have shallow vertebral canals. Another study of two archaeological populations[29] compared the canal size with four physiologic stress indicators (cribra orbitalia, porotic hyperostosis, dental hypoplasia, and Harris lines). Dental hypoplasia correlated with a small interpedicular diameter at L1, L2, and L3; Harris lines correlated with a small midsagittal diameter at L1, L3, and L5, a small area at L5, and a more trefoil canal at L4 and L5. There was supportive evidence that an adverse environment in early life is associated with a shallow vertebral canal. No doubt, genetic factors have some influence on the size of the canal, but an adverse early environment is probably important in impairing its growth.

THE TREFOIL CANAL

The trefoil shape occurs in approximately 15% of canals at L5; it is less common at L4 and rare at more proximal levels.[26] It is clinically significant not only because the L5 root is at risk in the shallow lateral recess but also because trefoil-shaped canals tend to have small midsagittal diameters.

The differential growth of the canal's midsagittal and interpedicular diameters makes a hypothesis possible about the trefoil development. The midsagittal diameter matures first, before 4 years of age, and probably much of this diameter is established in utero. The interpedicular diameter, however, continues to mature throughout childhood. Impaired early neuro-osseous development can result in an infant having a small midsagittal diameter, and in the absence of catch-up growth, that subject will be left with a permanently shallow canal. After infancy, however, an improved environment may allow for adequate growth in stature, resulting in a tall individual with broad vertebral bodies, wide pedicles, and a wide interpedicular diameter of the canal. The sagittal diameter remains small, but the interpedicular diameter broadens out to a trefoil shape.

THE CANAL AND ITS CONTENTS

Without a disparity between the canal's size and its contents, it is difficult to explain the body of literature describing the clinical problem of a small vertebral canal. A mismatch can be explained by the differential growth of the cord and canal.

In utero, when the conus is in the sacral canal, the epigenetic influence of the spinal cord on the surrounding structures causes the size of the cord and the canal to be related. Impaired nutrition and impaired neuro-osseous development will result in a small vertebral canal matched to small contents. In infancy, as the conus rises to L2, improved nutrition may arrive too late to benefit the sagittal diameter of the canal, but with improved stature, longer limbs, good muscles, and larger peripheral nerves, the cauda equina will also be relatively large yet with a shallow vertebral canal—a clinically dangerous situation if that canal becomes pathologically compromised.

SPINA BIFIDA OCCULTA

The neural tube develops in a craniocaudal manner and is usually complete at the 26th day after gestation. Failure of closure results in spina bifida overta, and failure of closure of the neural arch, in spina bifida occulta. Spina bifida occulta appears to be not an affection of a single segment, even when there is a deficiency of only one neural arch, but there are subtle changes in the more proximal vertebrae. The midsagittal diameter of the vertebral canal in the vertebrae more proximal to the bifid segment is wider than in unaffected skeletons in the same population.[20, 33] A delay in closure of the neural arch influences at least the two more proximal vertebrae, leaving the canals wider than those of unaffected skeletons.

Spina bifida occulta and overta appear to be related conditions. The parents of children with open spina bifida are four times more likely to have the occult lesion than are other members of the population.[16] Neural tube defects are probably related to periconceptional vitamin deficiency.[15] If vitamin deficiency is also related to the development of the occult lesion and a wider canal proximally, and if, then, in another situation impaired nutrition and development can result in spinal stenosis, there must be two complex interacting environmental factors.

SPONDYLOLISTHESIS

Vertebral displacement in isthmic spondylolisthesis widens the sagittal diameter of the vertebral canal, as the floating lamina is left behind and the

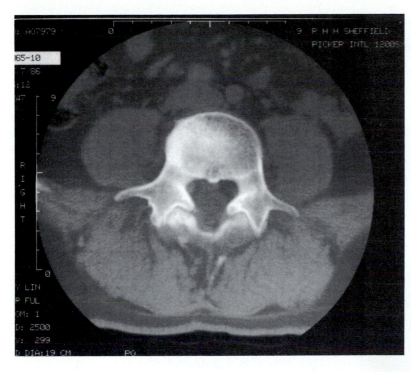

FIG 5–6.
Computed tomography scan of a patient with an isthmic spondylolisthesis at L5, showing the increased sagittal diameter of the central canal; the vertebra is displaced forward, leaving behind the floating lamina.

vertebral body is displaced forward (Fig 5–6); the pars becomes elongated, and the canal dome-shaped. The trefoil configuration is unusual in the presence of spondylolisthesis. Because the canal is so wide it is unusual to find an isthmic spondylolisthesis in patients with a symptomatic disc protrusion or with neurogenic claudication.[24] The L4–5 disc is not uncommonly pathologic above an isthmic defect at L5, but the large vertebral canal protects the cauda equina (Fig 5–7).

Vertebrae with unilateral spondylolysis occur at about one fourth of the incidence of bilateral spondylolysis.[8, 31, 40] The asymmetry of the canal provides some understanding of the changes observed in the bilateral condition, and of the effect of mechanical forces on the plasticity of the growing canal. There is elongation of the pars, horizontal orientation of the lamina, and asymmetry of the inferior apophyseal joints and the posterior elements in vertebrae with unilateral spondylolysis. The combination of these effects produces a rotation of the spinous process away from the side of the lesion, and the inferior facet joint on the side of the defect is placed more dorsally than the superior facet. This produces a unilaterally capacious vertebral canal (Fig 5–8).[28]

If unrestrained shearing forces can alter the shape of a vertebral canal in subjects with unilateral spondylolysis, what might be the effect of other mechanical forces on the vertebral canal? If a pliable tri-

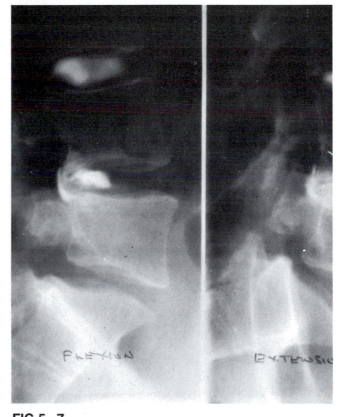

FIG 5–7.
A lateral radiograph of discograms at L3–4 and L4–5 in a patient with an isthmic spondylolisthesis at L5. There is complete disruption of the posterior annulus at L4–5. The patient had back pain only, with no root symptoms or signs.

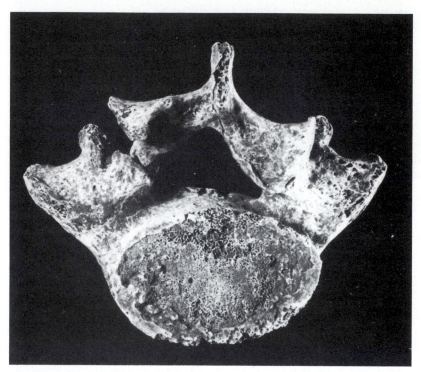

FIG 5–8.
Photograph of an Anglo-Saxon L5 vertebra, with a left-sided unilateral spondylolysis, showing asymmetry of the neural arch and vertebral canal.

angular tube is bent, it will develop a trefoil configuration, which could be a factor in some spines becoming trefoil with the development of the secondary curve of lumbar lordosis.[19] This might explain why the trefoil shape is uncommon in small children.

NEURO-OSSEOUS DEVELOPMENT AND THE IMMUNE SYSTEM

Clark[3] suggested that infantile malnutrition might not only impair the development of the vertebral canal but might also affect the simultaneously developing immune and central nervous systems. If this hypothesis is correct, one might expect the small adult vertebral canal, being a marker of deficient early development, also to be associated with poor function of the adult immune and central nervous systems. The growth curves of the thymus and of the central nervous system are similar to that of neuro-osseous development, and they are likely to be similarly affected by an adverse early environment.

A relationship exits between the size of the vertebral canal and the thymus hormone thymosin α_1.[4] This is compatible with the observation that adults with spinal stenosis attended their physicians in childhood and adulthood with infections more frequently than did subjects with wider canals.[22] There is also some evidence that the academic performance of children with wider vertebral canals at 16 years of age is better than that of their peers with narrower canals; whether this is a reflection of their socioeconomic status or their early neurologic development is not established.

There is growing evidence that subjects with spinal stenosis are at risk of being disadvantaged, not only in developing back pain when the canal is compromised but also in their general health and academic and socioeconomic status. A search for factors which affect spinal development is likely to have wider significance than the investigation of back pain. Growth abnormalities are most likely to occur during the rapid growth phase from the 8th to the 16th intrauterine week, when the crown-rump length increases from 5 to 15 cm.[37] Specific insults to the sensitive enzyme systems at this stage are likely to be more significant than maternal malnutrition to which the fetus is remarkably resistant.[17] A study of such factors in the development of the vertebral canal could be rewarding, with considerable medical, social, and economic consequences.

REFERENCES

1. Adams MA, Dolan P, Hutton WC, et al: Diurnal changes in spinal mechanics and their clinical significance. *J Bone Joint Surg [Br]* 1990; 72:266–270.
2. Clark FA, Panjabi MM, Wetzel FT: Can infant malnutrition cause adult vertebral stenosis? *Spine* 1985; 10:165–170.
3. Clark GA: *Heterochrony, Allometry and Canalisation in the Human Vertebral Column: Examples From Prehistroic Amerindian Populations* (thesis). Massachusetts University Graduate School, 1985, pp 375–381.
4. Clark GA, Hall NR, Aldwin CM, et al: Measures of poor early growth are correlated with lower adult levels of thymosin. *J Hum Biol* 1988; 60:436–451.
5. Edwards WC, La Rocca SH: The developmental segmental sagittal diameter in combined cervical and lumbar spondylolisthesis. *Spine* 1985; 10:42–49.
6. Eisenstein S: Morphometry and pathological anatomy of the lumbar spine in South African Negroes and Caucasoids with specific reference to spinal stenosis. *J Bone Joint Surg [Br]* 1977; 59:173–180.
7. Eisenstein S: The trefoil configuration of the lumbar vertebral canal. *J Bone Joint Surg [Br]* 1980; 62:73–77.
8. Eisenstein SMC: Spondylolisthesis. A skeletal investigation of two population groups. *J Bone Joint Surg [Br]* 1978; 60:488–494.
9. Epstein JA, Epstein BS, Levine I: Nerve root compression associated with narrowing of the lumbar spinal canal. *J Neurol Neurosurg Psychiatry* 1962; 25:165–176.
10. Farfan HF, Gracovetsky S: The nature of instability. *Spine* 1984; 9:714–719.
11. Forsberg L, Walloe A: Ultrasound in sciatica. *Acta Orthop Scand* 1982; 53:393–395.
12. Helivoaara M, Vanharanta H, Korpi J, et al: Herniated lumbar disc syndrome and vertebral canals. *Spine* 1986; 11:433–435.
13. Kadish LJ, Simmons EH: Anomalies of the lumbosacral nerve roots: An anatomical investigation and myeolgraphic study. *J Bone Joint Surg [Br]* 1984; 66:411–416.
14. Kornberg M, Rechtine GR: Quantitative assessment of the fifth lumbar spinal canal by computed tomography in symptomatic L4/L5 disc disease. *Spine* 1985; 10:328–330.
15. Laurence KM, James N, Miller MH, et al: Double-blind randomised controlled trial of folate treatment before conception to prevent recurrence of neural tube defects. *Br Med J* 1981; 282:1509–1511.
16. Lorber J, Levic K: Spina bifida cystica. Incidence of spina bifida occulta in parents and controls. *Arch Dis Child* 1967; 42:171–173.
17. Ounstead M, Ounstead C: On fetal growth rate. *Clin Dev Med* 1973; 46:9.
18. Porter RW: *Measurement of the Lumbar Spinal Canal by Diagnostic Ultrasound* (thesis). University of Edinburgh, 1980.
19. Porter RW. *Management of Back-pain.* Edinburgh, Churchill Livingstone, 1986, p 35.
20. Porter RW: The significance of spina bifida occulta in patients with low back pain. *Clin Anat* 1990; 3:238.
21. Porter RW, Adamas MA, Hutton WL: Physical activity and the strength of the spine. *Spine* 1989; 14:201–203.
22. Porter RW, Drinkall JN, Porter DE, et al: The vertebral canal. Part 2: Health and academic status. *Spine* 1987; 12:907–911.
23. Porter RW, Hibbert C: Relationship between the spinal canal and other skeletal measurements in a Romano-British population. *Ann R Coll Surg Engl* 1981; 63:437.
24. Porter RW, Hibbert CS: Symptoms associated with lysis of the pars·interarticularis. *Spine* 1984; 9:755–758.
25. Porter RW, Hibbert C, Wellman P: Backache and the lumbar spinal canal. *Spine* 1980; 5:99–105.
26. Porter RW, Hibbert C, Wellman P, et al: The shape and the size of the lumbar spinal canal. *Proc Inst Mechanical Engineers* 1980; 51–58.
27. Porter RW, Oakshott GHL: Familial aspects of disc protrusion. *J Orthopaed Rheumatol* 1988; 1:173–178.
28. Porter RW, Park W: Unilateral spondylolisthesis. *J Bone Joint Surg [Br]* 1982; 64:344–348.
29. Porter RW, Pavitt D: The vertebral canal: Nutrition and development, an archaelogical study. *Spine* 1987; 12:901–906.
30. Porter RW, Wicks M, Hibbert C: The size of the lumbar spinal canal in the symptomatology of disc lesions. *J Bone Joint Surg [Br]* 1978; 60:485–487.
31. Roche MB, Rowe GG: The incidence of separated neural arch and coincident bone variations: A survey of 4200 skeletons. *Anat Rec* 1951; 109:233–252.
32. Salibi BS: Neurogenic claudication and stenosis of the lumbar spinal canal. *Surg Neurol* 1976; 5:269–272.
33. Sand PG: *The Human Lumbo-Sacral Vertebral Column: An Osteometric Study* (thesis). University of Oslo, 1970.
34. Sarpyener MA: Congenital stricture of the spinal canal. *J Bone Joint Surg [Br]* 1945; 27:70–79.
35. Schatzker J, Pennal GF: Spinal stenosis, a cause of cauda equina compression. *J Bone Joint Surg [Br]* 1968; 50:606–618.
36. Spencer DL, Irwin GS, Miller JAA: Anatomy and significance of fixation of the lumbo-sacral roots in sciatica. *Spine* 1983; 8:672–679.
37. Thompson D'Arcy W: *Maximum Velocity of Growth at Fourth Month Intra-Uterine Life. Growth and Form,* ed 2. London, Cambridge University Press, 1942.
38. Verbiest H: A radicular syndrome from developmental narrowing of the lumbar vertebral canal. *J Bone Joint Surg [Br]* 1954; 36:230–237.
39. Van Gelderen V: Ein orthotisches (lordotisches) Kauda Syndrom. *Acta Psychiatr Neurol Scand* 1958; 23:57.
40. Willis TA: The lumbo-sacral vertebral column in man, its stability of form and function. *Am J Anat* 1923; 32:95–123.
41. Winston K, Rumbaugh C, Colucci V: The vertebral canals in lumbar disc disease. *Spine* 1984; 9:414–417.

6

The Normal Aging of the Spine: Degeneration and Arthritis

Barrie Vernon-Roberts, M.D.

AGE-RELATED CHANGES OR DEGENERATION?

Potential Importance of the Distinction Between Aging and Pathologic Changes

Changes in the discs, which occur with increasing frequency as adult life progresses, are frequently the subject of discussion, or even dispute, as to whether such changes are a normal part of aging or are the result of truly pathologic processes. This is not unique, but similar to the discussion of some other "disease" processes, such as atheroma of the aorta. While some may consider this distinction not to be helpful, and others may consider that aging itself is a pathologic process, the distinction is potentially important if it can be shown that some detrimental disc changes can be triggered by episodes such as trauma, which are avoidable, or may respond to focused treatment. Similarly, it would be important to identify, and perhaps modify, factors which may accelerate the aging process.

Definition of Degeneration

The 1990 *Concise Oxford Dictionary* defines the adjective *degenerate* as "Having lost the qualities that are normal and desirable or proper to its kind, fallen from former excellence." However, at this stage of our knowledge it is not yet possible to establish, in most instances, whether some or many of the structural differences between young "normal" discs and "abnormal" elderly adult discs are age-related and unavoidable, or pathologic and potentially avoidable. Nevertheless, it is undeniable that alterations in the structure of spinal components, resulting from aging or pathologic changes, are accompanied by functional changes which frequently are associated with symptomatic complaints, such as back pain. Undeniably, these structural alterations also may lead to the topic of this book, spinal stenosis.

This chapter derives heavily from a number of key publications describing the general anatomy and pathologic anatomy of age-related changes in the lumbar spine.*

The Initial Event in Disc Degeneration

There is frequent speculation as to the nature of the "initial event" in disc degeneration. While substantial research has addressed this issue, it is probably the case that a number of quite different initiating events, at a microscopic or molecular level, possibly affecting different components of the disc, can lead to gross structural changes which may have remarkably similar appearances. Therefore, we should not fall into the trap of believing, at this stage, that, in the case of the spine, similar pathologic changes equate with identical pathogenesis.

THE NUCLEUS PULPOSUS

Age-Related Changes in the "Normal" Nucleus

By the third decade of life, the nucleus normally has finally lost its earlier gelatinous consistency but

References 4, 5, 6, 8, 10, 12, 15, 26, 28, 29, 35, 36, 39.

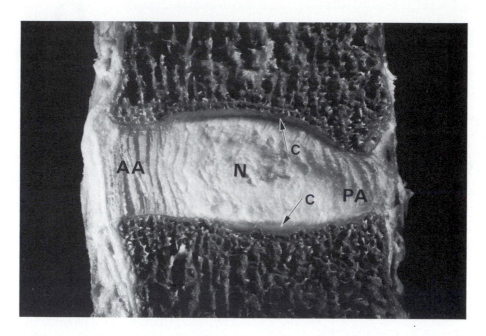

FIG 6–1.
Sagittal section of a bisected normal lumbar disc in a young adult. It shows that the nucleus *(N)*, while no longer gelatinous and turgescent as in adolescence, is clearly demarcated from the layered anterior *(AA)* and posterior *(PA)* annulus. The cartilage end plates *(C)*, separating the nucleus from the bone end plates above and below, are clearly seen. The attachment of the annular fibers directly to the bone of the vertebral rim, without an intervening layer of cartilage, can also be visualized.

still is quite well demarcated from the annulus (Fig 6–1); is semisolid through loss of some of its water content and increase in its collagen content; and shows a reduction in the number of cells present. By middle age, the nucleus feels dry and has a solid rubbery consistency; merges with the inner annulus so that its boundaries are not readily distinguished; contains more collagen and fewer cells; and may show brown discoloration.

Accompanying and Superimposed Pathologic Changes

While these "normal" age-related changes may remain unaccompanied by other changes, particularly in the presence of significant degrees of osteoporosis affecting the vertebral bodies, it is frequently the case that a spectrum of other changes becomes superimposed with increasing frequency as age advances. Given that these changes are associated with structural failure of key components of the disc, attempts at repair through the formation of granulation and scar tissue, and osteoarthritis in the posterior intervertebral joints, it is difficult to avoid classifying these additional changes as pathologic consequences or accompaniments of the aging process.

Of importance, in the presence of disc protrusions (prolapses, herniations), in the form of Schmorl's nodes (vertical protrusions) which are present in about 50% of spines overall,[5, 6, 14, 29] and posterior protrusions (prolapsed intervertebral discs) which affect about 15% of spines,[1] the "degenerative" changes occur at an earlier age and are generally more advanced in involved discs when compared with discs without protrusions.[14, 35, 36]

The Formation and Propagation of Nuclear Clefts

Macroscopically, the earliest change is the appearance of clefts which seem to originate most frequently midway between the center of the disc and the end plates, and parallel to the end plates (Figs 6–2 and 6–3). Frequently, such clefts are present in both the upper and lower parts of the disc (although single central clefts are not uncommon). Once formed, these clefts tend to propagate posteriorly and posterolaterally, and upper and lower clefts frequently merge. The clefts extend to involve the annulus, thereby causing disruption, thinning, and splitting of the annular layers. Indeed, clefts extending in the posterior direction often penetrate the annulus completely to reach the peridural space of the

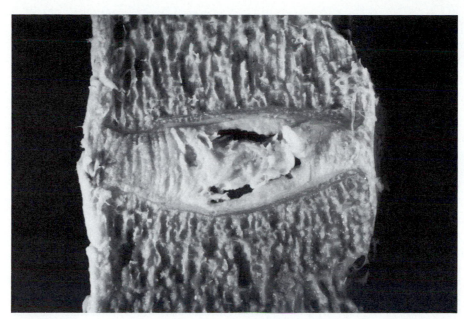

FIG 6–2.
Sagittal section of a lumbar disc showing nuclear clefts which have formed parallel to the end plates and have merged posteriorly *(right)*. At this stage, the clefts have not extended to involve the annulus.

spinal canal (Fig 6–3). Less frequently, the clefts may extend through the anterior regions of the annulus (Figs 6–4 and 6–5). Occasionally, merging of clefts leads to the complete isolation of portions of the nucleus (with or without attached portions of

cartilage end plate) which then act as free fragments within nuclear cavities (see Fig 6–5), and may be extruded posteriorly to impinge on the nerve root.

Also, propagating nuclear clefts frequently extend toward the cartilage end plates where they may

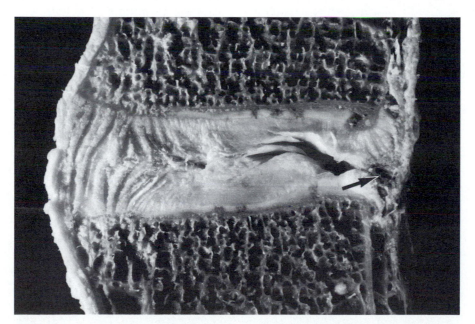

FIG 6–3.
Sagittal section of a lumbar disc showing a central nuclear cleft which has propagated posteriorly and has completely penetrated the posterior annulus. Ingrowth of new blood vessels along the margins of the cleft has commenced in

the outer annulus *(arrow)*. Blood vessels can be seen to have grown across the cartilage and bone end plates in other regions of the disc.

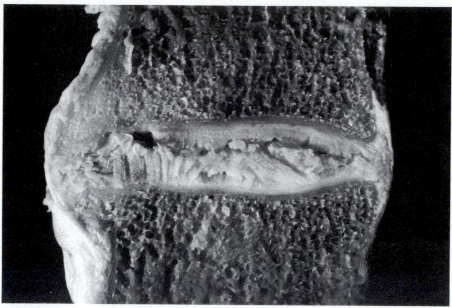

FIG 6–4.
Sagittal section of a lumbar disc showing a cleft which has extended deeply into the anterior and posterior annulus. There has been a reduction in disc height, and osteophyte formation has taken place anteriorly *(left).*

undermine the attachment of the cartilage to the bony end plate. When they pass into the annulus, they may extend to the bone of the vertebral body rim to which the annulus fibers are attached. If they extend to the bone in these situations, the clefts often are continuous with cracks which extend through the bone to reach the bone marrow where a chronic inflammatory reaction may be observed.

While not all clefts propagate to the same degree in all persons, the outcome for many is that cleft propagation results eventually in the formation of cavities, or potential cavities, varying in complexity

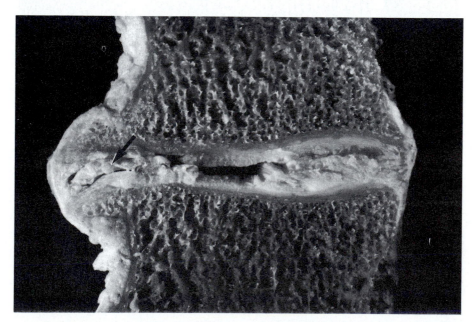

FIG 6–5.
Sagittal section of a lumbar disc showing an extensive cavitated cleft containing a free fragment of nucleus *(arrow)* which is lying within an extension of the cleft in the anterior annulus. There has been marked loss of disc height. Large osteophytes have formed anteriorly *(left)*, and smaller osteophytes are present posteriorly.

and shape within the affected discs (Figs 6–5 and 6–6). These advanced changes are associated with substantial loss of disc tissue, sclerosis of opposing vertebral body bone, and marked osteophyte formation (see Fig 6–6).

Microscopy of Cleft Formation

Microscopy[36] shows that cleft formation usually begins in the posterior region of the nucleus, near its junction with the annulus. Cleft formation is associated with other changes in the nucleus, including loss of metachromasia and a decline in the number of viable cells. Large clefts, particularly those extending into the annulus, may show "fibrillation" and "fissuring" of the cleft margins accompanied by the formation of chondrone-like clusters of chondrocyte-type cells, to show appearances closely mimicking the changes seen on the articular surfaces of joints in early osteoarthritis. Occasionally, the margins of clefts may acquire a synovial-type lining closely resembling the lining of a bursa.

Vascular Ingrowth Associated With Cleft Formation

When clefts have penetrated deeply through the annulus, it is not uncommon to observe the presence of new blood vessels extending along the mar-

gins of a cleft[36, 39] (see Fig 6–3). Sometimes, these new vessels, accompanied by nerves, extend into the central nuclear region by this route. This is one way in which the normally avascular and aneural inner annulus and nucleus zones of the disc can acquire a blood and nerve supply. Infrequently, this ingrowth may be associated with areas of calcification and ossification in the nucleus.

Epidemiology of Disc Degeneration

Epidemiologic data have demonstrated that the prevalence of radiographic signs of disc degeneration (the presence of osteophytes or loss of disc height) is greater in adult males than females. A correlation of data from 16 published reports, relating graded macroscopic changes in discs to age and sex, has corroborated this observation[22] and shown that the male lumbar disc starts to degenerate in the second decade of life, significantly earlier than the female disc. Moreover, male discs are generally more degenerate than female discs at any age beyond 10 years.[22] The cause of earlier disc degeneration in males is not known, but possible contributory factors include differences in disc size, disc nutrition, mechanical loading, ultrastructure, and nutrition or biochemical composition.[22] In both sexes, some 97% of discs show clear evidence of degeneration by the age of 50 years.

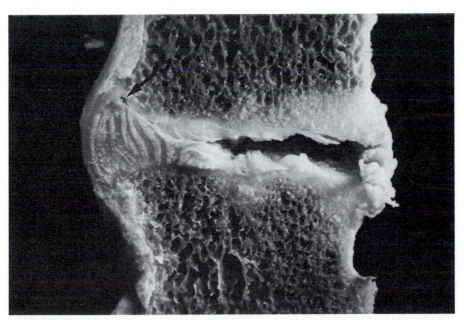

FIG 6–6.
Sagittal section of a lumbar disc showing marked loss of nuclear and annular tissue from the posterior region of the disc *(right)*; dense sclerosis of the bone on each side of a large cleft; and large posterior osteophytes. Anteriorly, the cleft communicates with a rim lesion *(arrow)*.

Cumulative pathologic data[22] show that more L3–4 discs degenerate than at the L1–2 and L2–3 levels, and mild degrees of radiographic change also occur more frequently at the L3–4 level.[3, 16] There are no significant differences in pathologic grades between the L3–4, L4–5, and L5–S1 discs. However, severe radiographic changes with osteophytes and marked disc narrowing occur most frequently at the L5–S1 level, where they are present three times more often than at the L4–5 level.[16] It is important to note that when radiography shows significant disc narrowing and osteophyte formation, the corresponding disc will always show advanced degeneration; however, marked degeneration may be present in the absence of these radiographic changes, and a normal radiograph does not exclude degeneration of a disc.[10]

THE ANNULUS FIBROSUS

Structure of the Normal Annulus

The normal annulus is constructed of concentric layers (Fig 6–7) of collagen fibers which sweep diagonally from the outer rims of adjoining vertebral bodies. The collagen fibers of each distinct layer are parallel, but the fibers of succeeding layers are arranged at tilt angles of about 70 degrees to each other. Presumably owing to the fact that the axis of rotation of the spine is close to the posterior annulus, the anterior and anterolateral annulus is much thicker than the posterior and posterolateral annulus (see Fig 6–7).

Types of Tears of the Annulus

Macroscopically, grossly identifiable lesions in the annulus tend to accompany age-related degenerative changes in the nucleus. These grossly observed clefts of the annulus generally are termed "tears," although it is rarely the case that trauma can be incriminated in their formation with any certainty, and they are just as likely to result from degeneration or fatigue failure, or a combination of both processes.

There are three principal categories of annulus tears or clefts (Fig 6–8): (1) radiating tears (sometimes called "radiating ruptures"; (2) concentric or circumferential clefts; and (3) rim lesions (sometimes misleadingly called "annular tears" as though they are the only type of tear sustained by the annulus) which often are so small as to be identifiable only by microscopy.

Radiating Tears

Radiating tears[12, 15] commonly are present by the fourth or fifth decade, and particularly affect the

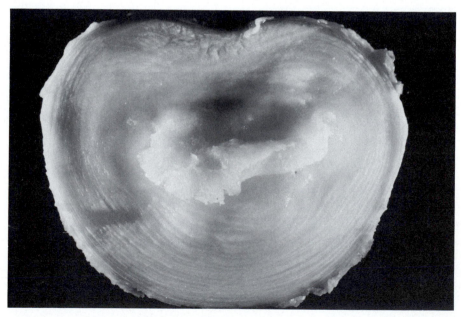

FIG 6–7.
Horizontal section through a lumbar disc at the age of 20 years. It shows the concentric layering of the normal annulus. The annulus is much thicker anteriorly *(bottom)* than posteriorly. Because it is still semigelatinous and turgescent at this age, the nucleus bulges spontaneously above the cut surface.

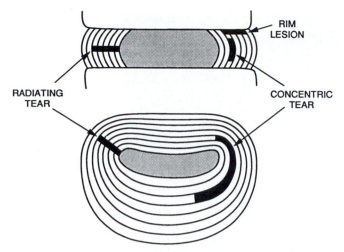

FIG 6–8.
Diagram showing the location of radiating tears, concentric tears, and rim lesions within the annulus.

posterolateral zones of the lower lumbar discs (Fig 6–9). Not infrequently, they extend into, or through, the annulus. When the annulus is involved in this process, commonly there is vascular ingrowth along the margins of the tear,[15, 36] but there is no convincing evidence that this leads to healing since scar tissue has not been convincingly demonstrated.

The question which has to be addressed is, "Are radiating tears part of nuclear cleft formation which commonly accompanies age-related changes in the nucleus, or are they the result of a separate process?" While it is not possible to be dogmatic, it is my opinion that radiating tears and nuclear clefts are part of the same process in most instances, and both are the consequence of a combination of progressive desiccation of the disc and failure of its components due to repeated loading and, perhaps, episodes which may be regarded as traumatic in nature.

Concentric (Circumferential) Tears

Concentric (circumferential) tears[35, 36] of the annulus (Figs 6–10 and 6–11) are commonly present by the fourth decade, and appear to originate within the annulus, although they may sometimes communicate with radiating clefts or rim lesions.

Possibly contributing to their formation are changes in the annulus which occur early in life, since a range of microscopic changes can be identified in the annulus from adolescence onward.[36] These changes are in the form of fragmentation of fibers, mucinous degeneration of fibers, focal nodular hyalinization of fibers, mucinous pools and cyst formation between layers of the annulus, and microscopic separation of the layers of the annulus.[36]

Once established, clefts tend to propagate, subsidiary clefts appear in adjoining layers of the annulus, and clefts may eventually merge and communicate with cavities within the annulus (see Fig 6–11).

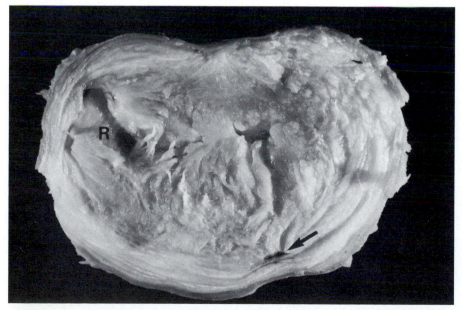

FIG 6–9.
Horizontal section of a disc showing a radiating tear *(R)* involving the nucleus and the posterolateral annulus. A small rim lesion is present within the anterior annulus *(arrow)*.

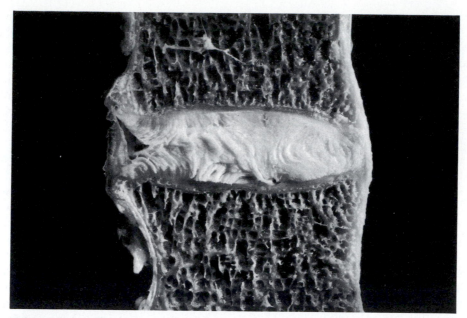

FIG 6–10.
Sagittal section of a lumbar disc showing part of a concentric tear within the outer anterior annulus *(left).*

It would appear that circumferential tears occur most frequently in the posterolateral region of the annulus,[18] and it has been postulated that repeated minor trauma may induce these tears to enlarge and coalesce to form one or more radial tears which may predispose to disc herniations.[18]

While vascular ingrowth along the margins of clefts, even with microscopic clefts,[35, 36, 39] may occur, there is no convincing evidence that this progresses to healing by scar tissue formation. Thus, once formed, these clefts appear to enlarge inexorably at varying rates of progression.

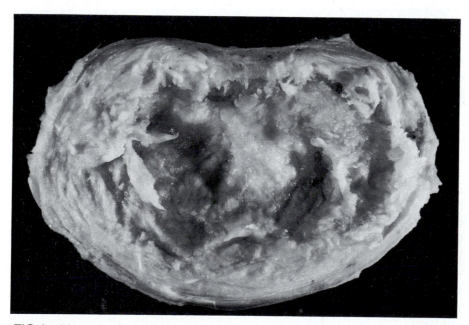

FIG 6–11.
Horizontal section through a lumbar disc showing concentric tears involving various parts of the annulus. Some tears communicate with an extensive nuclear cleft.

Rim Lesions (Annular Tears)

Rim lesions[13, 29, 39] commonly are located in the anterior or anterolateral annulus, close to the insertion of the annulus fibers into the bone of the marginal rim of the vertebral body (Figs 6–6, 6–9, and 6–12). Frequently, they are detectable only by careful naked-eye examination of cadaveric specimens, or may require microscopy to identify them, but occasional larger lesions may be recognized radiographically by the presence of the vacuum phenomenon, vertebral rim sclerosis with or without a cup-shaped defect in the rim, and osteophytes confined to one side of the defect.[13]

While they may occasionally show ingrowth of vascular granulation tissue, evidence of healing by scar tissue formation is lacking.[36] They are rare in subjects under the age of 30 years, but increase in frequency thereafter so that they are commonly present after the age of 50 years.[13]

It is considered that rim lesions occur as a result of traumatic avulsion of the annular attachment, with, in some instances, the site being already weakened by degenerative processes.

The importance of rim lesions arises from the fact that experimental studies show that they can initiate progressive disc degeneration and spondylosis in previously normal discs, and that they can initiate concentric tears of the annulus.[23] This explains why rim lesions often may be found to communicate with early concentric tears (Fig 6–13).

DISC HEIGHT

Age-Related Reduced Disc Height

There is no doubt that in the presence of advanced age-related changes it is commonly the case that there is a reduction in disc height (see Figs 6–4, 6–5, 6–6, and 6–21). While the evidence supporting this is now overwhelming,[22] some authors have maintained that disc thinning is not a feature of age-related degenerative change.[32] This latter view may have its origin in the fact that significant degrees of osteoporosis affecting the vertebral bodies, a condition encountered with particular frequency in postmenopausal women, seem to afford substantial protection against age-related disc degeneration. Indeed, in severe osteoporosis associated with characteristic codfish vertebrae, there is substantial ballooning of the discs.

Thinning of the disc (which should be distinguished from the rare condition described as "isolated disc resorption"[34]) is encountered frequently in advanced spondylosis. Probably it is the result of

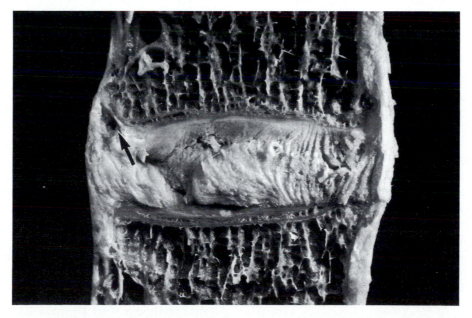

FIG 6–12.
Sagittal section of a lumbar disc showing a rim lesion *(arrow)* formed by the separation of the anterior annular fibers from their attachment to the bone of the vertebral rim. The nucleus shows a cleft extending anteriorly through the inner annulus, but not communicating (in this disc) with the rim lesion.

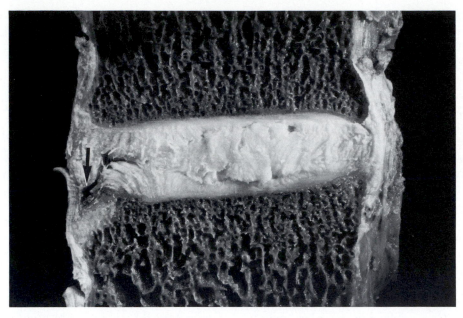

FIG 6–13.
Sagittal section of a lumbar disc showing a rim lesion *(arrow)* with localized sclerosis of the adjoining vertebral bone. The rim lesion communicates with a concentric tear of the annulus. The nucleus shows the formation of early clefts parallel and close to the upper and lower end plates.

several processes, including progressive loss of water content of the nucleus, increasing collagenization of the nucleus, cleft formation in the nucleus and annulus, protrusion of disc tissue, circumferential annular bulging, and ossification advancing from the end-plate zone.

Effects of Reduced Disc Height

Clearly, whatever causative factors are involved in the reduction in disc height, any reduction in disc thickness must have important implications for the biomechanics of the affected spinal motion segment in addition to those resulting from other age-related changes in disc structure.

Because the functional and structural integrity of the posterior intervertebral (apophyseal) joints at each level is dependent upon the functional and structural integrity of the intervertebral disc at the same level, it follows that disc thinning has a substantial influence on the initiation and progression of degenerative and arthritic changes in the posterior intervertebral joints. In addition, loss of disc height must be accompanied by subluxation of the facets of the posterior intervertebral joints at the same level (see Fig 6–22).

THE END-PLATE REGION

Age-Related Changes

The end-plate region not only acts as a major supporting and attachment structure for the disc but also plays a critically important role in maintaining disc nutrition. Consequently, structural changes in the end plate have very important implications for disc structure and function.

As aging progresses, and in association with the nuclear and annular changes previously described, a spectrum of features may be observed in the end-plate region which become more frequent and marked during the third decade. Thus, in addition to the commonly present Schmorl's nodes (see Fig 6–21), which have been reported to be present with equal frequency in subjects above and below the age of 50 years,[14] other changes may be encountered with increasing frequency during the third decade, affecting either or both of the cartilage and bone components of the end plate.[5]

The Cartilage End Plate

Early changes in the cartilage end plate are fissure formation; horizontal cleft formation, which may be accompanied by intrusions of nuclear material between the cartilage and bone end plates; death of chondrocytes; vascular penetration, which may extend into the nucleus (see Fig 6–3); and extension of calcification and ossification from the bony end plate. Later, and especially after the fifth decade, there is frequent extensive or total loss of the cartilage end plate, and many clefts and fissures are present in the residual cartilage, which may communicate with nuclear clefts.[36]

The Bone End Plate

After the age of 50 years, the bone end plate adjoining the cartilage end plate may be breached by clefts passing through the cartilage (Fig 6–14). These clefts rarely contain any nuclear material and appear to be quite separate from the process involved in the formation of Schmorl's nodes.

When the marginal bone end plate (the site of insertion of the annular fibers) is breached in a similar way, such breaches often are in continuity with nuclear clefts which have extended through the annulus and, as is commonly the case, diverge toward the upper or lower bony rim region where they come into contact with the bone of the annular attachment.

End-Plate Disorganization

In addition to breaches in the bony end plate, advanced age-related changes in the disc often are accompanied by the formation of islands of cartilage in the bony end plate, microfractures in trabeculae, irregular new bone formation, and the formation of double end plates.[39] The end result of this process is substantial structural disorganization producing end plates of varying irregularity and thickness, with probable marked impairment of disc nutrition. Radiographically, a classic pattern of bandlike sclerosis along the vertebral end plate is a characteristic consequence of advanced disc degeneration.

THE MARGINS OF THE VERTEBRAL BODIES

Marginal Osteophyte Formation

As the discs undergo age-related "degenerative" changes, osteophytic outgrowths develop as spikes and flanges from the margins of the vertebral bodies. In general, the more advanced are the changes in the disc, the larger and more extensive is the development of osteophytes (see Figs 6–4 through 6–6, 6–21, and 6–22). In particular, progressive reduction in disc thickness usually is associated with the formation of increasingly large osteophytes.

While the osteophytes occur earlier and grow to a larger size in the anterolateral regions, osteophytes

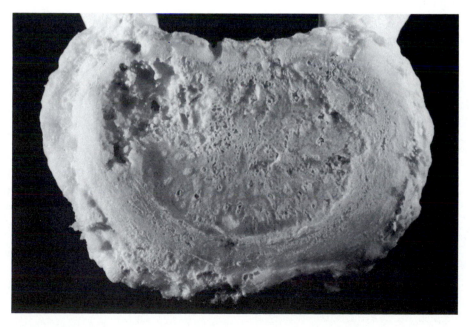

FIG 6–14.
End plate of a lumbar vertebral body following the removal of soft tissues. It shows osteophytic new bone extending outward from the circumference of the vertebral rim, including the posterolateral regions. Also visible is the irregular cavitation of the bone end plate and vertebral rim associated with the presence of a radiating tear.

of substantial size may involve the posterior regions of the vertebral bodies (see Fig 6–14). Posterior osteophytes may contribute to central stenosis when the lumbar spinal canal is already narrowed, and posterolateral osteophytes may contribute to the symptomatology of lateral stenosis when osteophytes have also formed on the margins of the posterior intervertebral joints (see Figs 6–19 through 6–22).

Possible Causes of Osteophyte Formation

The nature of osteophyte formation remains largely speculative. It has been suggested that disc degeneration leads to tilting of the vertebral bodies and anterior squeezing of the disc which then bulges forward and elevates the adjoining periosteum to stimulate new bone formation.[4] However, microscopy does not provide convincing supporting evidence for this concept, but indicates that osteophytes form, at least initially, by endochondral ossification taking place in the outer attachment region of the annulus following chondrocytic change in the fibrocytes of this zone.[39] The stimulus to this chondroid metaplasia, and that which causes progressive growth of osteophytes, presently remains speculative.

Nonfusion of Large Osteophytes

While the osteophytes of degenerative spondylosis may grow to a large size and those arising from adjoining vertebral bodies may come into contact, it is very rarely the case that true fusion of such osteophytes takes place despite this apparently being the case radiographically. The misleading radiographic appearance of fusion results from the undulating and complex nature of the junction between the contacting, but still separate, osteophytes.

THE BONE OF THE VERTEBRAL BODY

Loss of Bone With Aging

The remodeling of bone which results in changes in the end plates and in the formation of marginal osteophytes is influenced substantially by age-related degeneration of the discs. Largely separate factors are involved in the changes which take place in the cancellous bone of the vertebral bodies as age advances.

In the majority of, if not all, people, the normal aging process is accompanied by progressive reduction in the volume of cancellous bone from the skeleton commencing in middle age in both sexes.[33] In women, this loss commences with the menopause and the rate and amount of the decline is greater than in men. If the peak bone mass of an individual is low, then the process of normal bone loss with aging, or accelerated bone loss due to any cause, may result in osteoporosis.

The primary reason for the loss of bone is a reduction in the size and number of transversely orientated trabeculae during aging, with increased stresses imposed on the remaining vertically orientated trabeculae.[38]

Osteoporosis

Osteoporosis has a particular importance for the bone of the vertebral body, since substantial bone loss may lead to fracture-collapse.

The importance of osteoporosis is not only the risk of collapse of vertebral bodies but its association with the presence of increased numbers of healing trabecular microfractures[11, 38] (which may give rise to back pain). As noted earlier in this chapter, its presence often is associated with lesser degrees of disc degeneration in osteoporotic individuals when compared with those having normal amounts of bone in their vertebral bodies.

While it is conceivable that the amount of cancellous bone in osteoporosis may be reduced to a level which impairs the stiffness of the vertebral body to a degree where the loading transmitted to the discs, and consequently the wear and tear on the discs, is below some critical point, this hypothesis does not satisfactorily address several issues. For example, it would appear that age-related disc "degeneration" commences during the second or third decades in most persons, whereas osteoporosis does not become significant until the fifth decade or later in many who develop it. This could suggest that some of the factors, probably genetic but yet undetermined, which influence the peak bone mass attained by an individual are related to the factors concerned with age-related disc degeneration.

THE POSTERIOR INTERVERTEBRAL (APOPHYSEAL, FACET) JOINTS

Relationship Between Disc Degeneration and Osteoarthritis of the Posterior Intervertebral Joints

Comprehensive studies[20, 21] have established a strong link between age-related disc degeneration and osteoarthritis of the posterior intervertebral joints, and it has been convincingly shown that changes in the disc always precede changes in the posterior intervertebral joints, and not vice versa[3, 39]; that when disc degeneration becomes significant, changes always are present in the posterior intervertebral joints at the same level[9, 18, 39]; and, in the presence of advanced disc degeneration, the posterior intervertebral joints at the same level will always show the changes of advanced osteoarthritis.

Clearly, when other conditions complicate or accelerate the onset of age-related disc degeneration, such as kyphosis, scoliosis, spondylolisthesis, vertebral body collapse, or disc protrusion, severe degrees of osteoarthritis may develop in the posterior intervertebral joints. In most circumstances, the severity of osteoarthritis is inversely related to the preservation of disc structure.[39]

Differences Between the Posterior Intervertebral Joints and Other Synovial Joints

The posterior intervertebral joints differ from most other synovial joints in several important respects. Thus, unlike other joints, from an early age, substantial and increasing amounts of subchondral bone are formed such that this bone normally is densely sclerotic by the second decade[31, 39] (Figs 6–15 and 6–16). It has been reported that this thickening of the subchondral bone plate increases with age to maturity and decreases in old age, with the thinning of the subchondral plate with aging being quite dramatic in some instances and occurring earlier in the inferior facet.[31] However, the report of a decrease in subchondral bone with aging did not correlate these changes with graded degeneration of the discs, and it is my experience that sclerosis often persists in aged individuals in the presence of the advanced disc degeneration of osteoarthritis of the posterior intervertebral joints.[37] Clearly, this sclerosis often seen with degenerate discs could be part of the sclerosis characteristic of osteoarthritis, rather

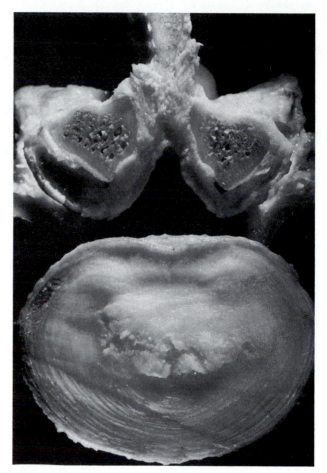

FIG 6–15.
Horizontal section through a lumbar disc and associated posterior intervertebral joints at the age of 20 years. It shows a normal intervertebral disc, and the dense bone which normally underlies the articular cartilage of the posterior intervertebral joints.

than persistence of the normal subchondral sclerosis seen in young posterior intervertebral joints.

The density of bone in the subchondral region of the posterior intervertebral joints is somewhat similar to the bone density of the patella, and, in both locations, appears to be a response to very substantial stresses being transmitted across the joint surfaces in these locations. Moreover, in the case of the posterior intervertebral joints, biomechanical studies have reported that the pressure between the facets increases significantly with narrowing of the disc space and increasing extension.[7]

There is a progressive change from a flat to a wedge shape in the subchondral bone plate of the superior facet, but wedging does not appear until late in adult life in the inferior facet and is seen only at the L4–5 level.[31]

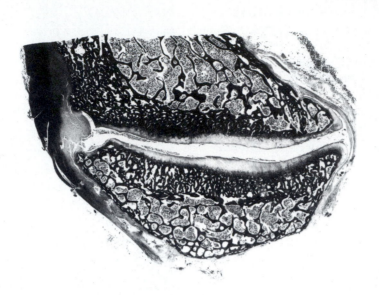

FIG 6–16.
Low-power microscopic view of a horizontal section through a posterior interverte-bral joint at the age of 20 years. It shows the dense bone which normally underlies the articular cartilage at this age.

While characteristic osteoarthritic changes, which include areas of total loss of articular cartilage (Fig 6–17), frequently are encountered in association with advanced disc degeneration, the posterior intervertebral joints also differ from other osteoar-thritic joints in that often the joint surfaces retain an extensive covering of articular cartilage despite large marginal osteophytes having formed[35, 36, 39] (Figs 6–18 through 6–20). Indeed, the retention of articular cartilage until late in the course of the condition,

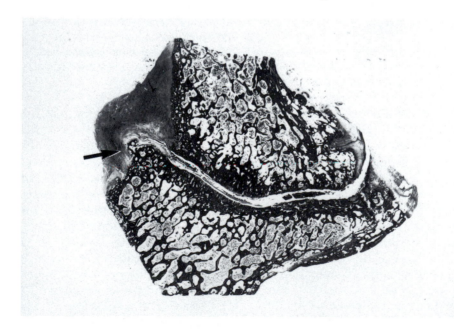

FIG 6–17.
Low-power microscopic view of a horizontal section through a posterior intervertebral joint from an elderly person with advanced degeneration of the disc at the same level. Changes of osteoarthritis are present, with almost total loss of the articular cartilage, and there is bulging of the capsular tissue medially where it overlies an osteophyte *(arrow)* aris-ing from the concave superior facet.

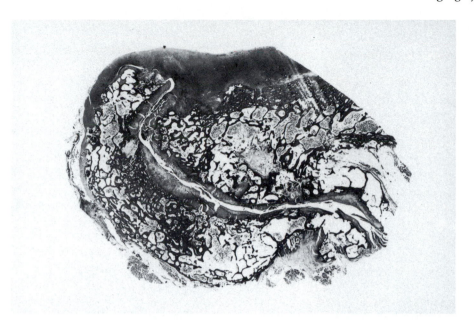

FIG 6–18.
Low-power microscopic view of a horizontal section through a posterior intervertebral joint from an elderly person with advanced disc degeneration at the same level. Articular cartilage showing varying degrees of osteoarthritic change still covers most of the articulating surfaces. Very large osteophytes project from the medial and lateral margins of the concave superior facet, and the lateral margin of the convex inferior facet. Note that the medial superior facet *(left)* wraps around the inferior facet.

combined with the formation of osteophytes and sclerotic subchondral bone early in the course of the condition, suggests that remodeling of the bone due to changing mechanical stresses may be the principal response associated with the earlier phases of age-related disc degeneration. The full spectrum of osteoarthritic changes, including cartilage loss and cyst formation, would then supervene when the degenerative changes in the disc had progressed to a certain level.

The osteophytes, which form frequently by middle age, are present at the attachment of the ligamentum flavum or capsule, and are common as beaklike extensions from the anteromedial margin of the superior facet into the ligamentum flavum.[31] The osteophytes are often accompanied by enlarged synovial fat pads which form cushions between the osteophyte and the inferior facet.[31]

Impingement of Osteophytes and Pseudarthrosis Formation

When osteoarthritic changes are advanced, osteophytes may impinge upon the dorsal surfaces of the laminae of the neural arches, and pseudarthroses may form at these impingement sites.[35] Contributing to this impingement is the subluxation of the posterior intervertebral joints which results from reduction in the height of the intervertebral disc. Despite impingement occurring, bony ankylosis is rarely encountered in spines showing age-related changes alone.

Impaction Fractures of the Subchondral Bone Plate

In addition to the development of densely sclerotic bone underlying the articular surfaces, another indicator of the substantial stresses imposed on the posterior intervertebral joints is the occasional finding of a breach in the bone plate underlying the articular cartilage with herniation of a portion of the articular cartilage into the bone through the breach.[39] This feature may be found in the absence of significant degrees of disc degeneration or osteoarthritis of the posterior intervertebral joints, and suggests that it is the result of traumatic herniation following fracture of the subchondral bone plate. This conclusion is supported by the report of small fractures of the facets identified by stereoscopic radiography.[30]

The rudimentary fibrous invaginations extending from the dorsal and ventral capsules of the posterior intervertebral joints, and the so-called menisci at the superior and inferior poles of these joints, consist of fat-filled synovial reflections, some of

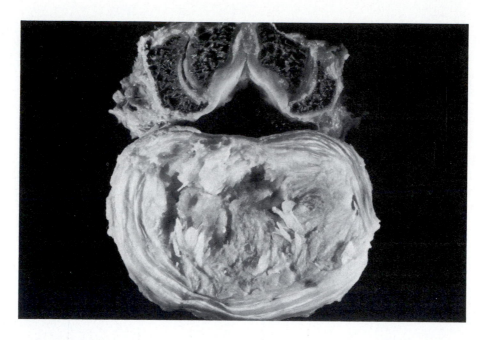

FIG 6–19.
Horizontal section through a lumbar disc and associated pair of posterior intervertebral joints from an elderly person with advanced disc degeneration. The posterior intervertebral joints show focal loss of articular cartilage, and osteophyte formation. There is narrowing and elongation of the lateral recesses resulting from the combination of osteoarthritic changes in the posterior intervertebral joints, and osteophytic outgrowths from the adjoining posterolateral margins of the vertebral body.

which contain dense fibrous tissue.[2] Irregular fibrocartilaginous inclusions may be present in the posterior aspect of the joint,[31] and occasional small bony nodules may be present within the base of meniscal reflections.[37] While there has been debate as to the possible role of these "menisci" in acute back pain,[2, 20, 21] their possible roles in age-related and arthritic changes in the posterior intervertebral joints have not been considered despite possible roles in joint lubrication, nutrition, or biomechanics.

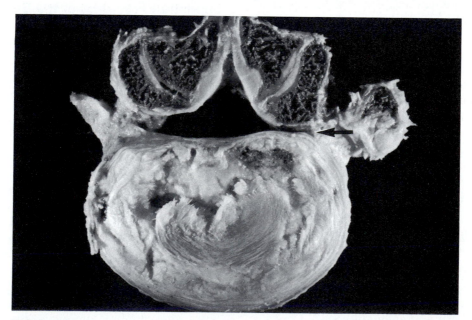

FIG 6–20.
Marked unilateral stenosis *(arrow)* resulting from advanced osteoarthritic changes in the posterior intervertebral joint and osteophytic new bone extending posterolaterally from the vertebral rim.

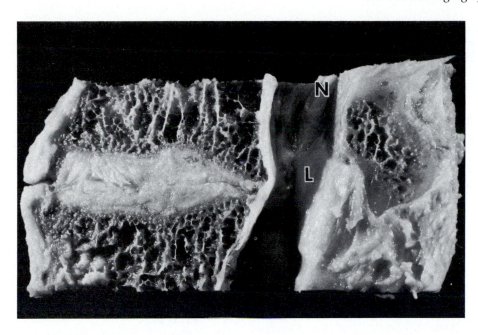

FIG 6–21.

Sagittal section of a lumbar motion segment showing moderate central narrowing of the spinal canal resulting from posterior osteophytes arising from the vertebral body associated with advanced disc degeneration, together with bulging of the capsule and ligamentum flavum *(L)* associated with osteoarthritis of the underlying posterior intervertebral joint. The exit of the nerve root *(N)* is markedly narrowed by the osteophytes and ligamentous bulging.

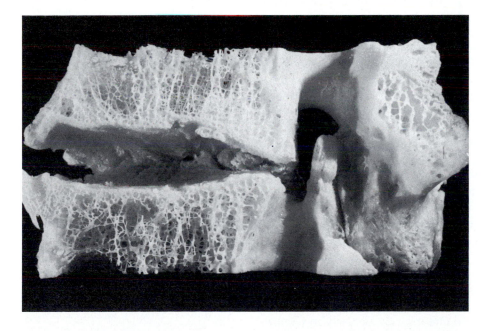

FIG 6–22.

Sagittal section of the lumbar motion segment shown in Figure 6–21 following removal of the soft tissues. It shows the marked narrowing of the intervertebral foramen by a large osteophyte arising from the inferior facet of the posterior intervertebral joint and by subluxation of the facets due to loss of disc height. Contributing to the narrowing of the foramen is osteophytic new bone arising from the posterior margin of the upper vertebral body. There are large osteophytes arising from the margins of both vertebral bodies anteriorly. The bony end plates show Schmorl's nodes and marked disorganization associated with advanced disc degeneration.

CONCLUSIONS

As outlined in the foregoing part of this chapter, the normal aging process is, in the spine, associated with a range of changes which appear to be initiated within the substance of the disc. With respect to the site of the earliest changes, it would seem that the process of degeneration can be initiated from within either the nucleus or the annulus. As the degenerative process involving the disc progresses, inevitably it will be accompanied by arthritic changes in both posterior intervertebral joints at the same level as any disc showing degenerative changes.

Advanced degenerative changes in the disc, often complicated by the presence of vertical or posterior disc protrusions, are accompanied by the formation of flangelike or spiked osteophytes arising from the margins of the vertebral bodies and osteophytes developing at the margins of the intervertebral joints as part of the osteoarthritic process.

The osteophytes arising from the posterolateral margins of the vertebral bodies and from the posterior intervertebral joints, which are a characteristic feature of advanced age-related spinal changes, are a major contributor to the development of acquired "degenerative spinal stenosis" through their impingement on the various zones of the nerve root canals[17, 25] (Figs 6–19 through 6–22). Also contributing to this lateral stenosis is the reactive proliferation of capsular and soft tissues, including the ligamentum flavum, overlying osteophytes arising from the posterior intervertebral joints[35] (see Fig 6–21); changes in the nerve root microcirculation leading to edema; fibrous scarring around the nerve roots[27]; and, perhaps, the deposition of fibrin as a result of minor trauma to small blood vessels, possibly by osteophytes, and its persistence due to impaired fibrinolytic activity leading to fibrous scar tissue formation.[19, 24]

Osteophytes arising from the posterior margins of the vertebral bodies, again formed frequently as part of the aging process, may contribute to the development of central stenosis, particularly in circumstances where the spinal canal already is developmentally narrow.

REFERENCES

1. Andrae R: Über Knorpelknötchen am hinteren Ende der Wirbelbandscheiben im Bereiche des Spinalkanals. *Beitr Pathol Anat* 1929; 82:464–474.
2. Bogduk N, Engel R: The menisci of the lumbar zyga- pophyseal joints: A review of their anatomy and clinical significance. *Spine* 1984; 9:454–460.
3. Butler D, Trfimow JH, Andersson GBJ, et al: Discs degenerate before facets. *Spine* 1990; 15:111–113.
4. Collins DH: *The Pathology of Articular and Spinal Diseases.* London, Edward Arnold, 1949.
5. Coventry MB, Ghormley RK, Kernohan JW: The intervertebral disc: Its microscopic anatomy and pathology. II. Changes in the intervertebral disc concomitant with age. *J Bone Joint Surg [Am]* 1945; 27:233–247.
6. Coventry MB, Ghormley RK, Kernohan JW: III. Pathological changes in the intervertebral disc. *J Bone Joint Surg [Am]* 1945; 27:460–474.
7. Dunlop RB, Adams MA, Hutton WC: Disc space narrowing and the lumbar facet joints. *J Bone Joint Surg [Br]* 1984; 66:706–710.
8. Eckert C, Decker A: Pathological studies of intervertebral discs. *J Bone Joint Surg [Am]* 1947; 29:447–454.
9. Farfan HF: Effects of torsion on the intervertebral joints. *Can J Surg* 1969; 12:336–341.
10. Friberg S, Hirsch C: Anatomical and clinical studies on lumbar disc degeneration. *Acta Orthop Scand* 1949; 19:222–242.
11. Hansson T, Roos B: Microcalluses of the trabeculae in lumbar vertebrae and their relation to the bone mineral content. *Spine* 1981; 6:375–380.
12. Harris RI, Macnab I: Structural changes in the lumbar intervertebral discs. Their relationship to low back pain and sciatica. *J Bone Joint Surg [Br]* 1954; 36:304–322.
13. Hilton RC, Ball J: Vertebral rim lesions in the dorsolumbar spine. *Ann Rheum Dis* 1984; 43:302–307.
14. Hilton RC, Ball J, Benn RF: Vertebral end-plate lesions (Schmorl's nodes) in the dorso-lumbar spine. *Ann Rheum Dis* 1976; 35:127–132.
15. Hirsch C, Schajowicz F: Studies on structural changes in the lumbar annulus fibrosus. *Acta Orthop Scand* 1953; 22:184–231.
16. Hult L: Cervical, dorsal and lumbar spinal syndromes. *Acta Orthop Scand [Suppl]* 1954; 17:1–102.
17. Kirkaldy-Willis WH: The relationship of structural pathology to the nerve root. *Spine* 1984; 9:49–52.
18. Kirkaldy-Willis WH, Wedge JT, Jong-Hing K, et al: Pathology and pathogenesis of lumbar spondylosis and stenosis. *Spine* 1978; 3:319–328.
19. Kliniuk PS, Pountain GD, Keegar AL, et al: Serial measurements of fibrinolytic activity in acute low back pain and sciatica. *Spine* 1987; 12:925–928.
20. Lewin T: Osteoarthritis in lumbar synovial joints: a morphologic study. *Acta Orthop Scand (Suppl)* 1964; 73:1–112.
21. Lewin T, Moffett B, Viidik A: The morphology of the lumbar synovial joints. *Acta Morphol Neerl Scand* 1962; 4:299–319.
22. Miller JAA, Schmatz C, Schultz AB: Lumbar disc degeneration: Correlation with age, sex, and spine level in 600 autopsy specimens. *Spine* 1988; 13:173–178.
23. Osti O., Vernon-Roberts B, Fraser RD: Annulus tears and intervertebral disc degeneration: An experimental study using an animal model. *Spine* 1990; 15:762–767.
24. Pountain GD, Keegan AL, Jayson MIV: Impaired fibrinolytic activity in defined chronic back pain syndromes. *Spine* 1987; 12:83–86.

25. Rauschning W: Normal and pathologic anatomy of the lumbar root canals. *Spine* 1987; 12:1008–1019.
26. Ritchie JH, Fahrni WH: Age changes in lumbar intervertebral discs. *Can J Surg* 1970; 13:65–71.
27. Rydevik B, Brown MD, Lundborg G: Pathoanatomy and pathophysiology of nerve root compression. *Spine* 1984; 9:7–15.
28. Saunders JBM, Inman VT: Pathology of the intervertebral disk. *Arch Surg* 1940; 40:389–416.
29. Schmorl G, Junghanns H: *The Human Spine in Health and Disease,* Besemann EF (trans). New York, Grune & Stratton, Inc, 1971.
30. Sims-Williams H, Jayson MIV, Baddeley H: Small spinal fractures in back pain patients. *Ann Rheum Dis* 1978; 37:262–265.
31. Taylor JR, Twomey LT: Age changes in lumbar zygapophyseal joints: Observations on structure and function. *Spine* 1986; 11:739–745.
32. Twomey L, Taylor J: Age changes in lumbar intervertebral discs. *Acta Orthop Scand* 1985; 56:496–499.
33. Twomey L, Taylor J, Furniss B: Age changes in the bone density and structure of the lumbar vertebral column. *J Anat* 1983; 136:15–25.
34. Venner RM, Crock HV: Clinical studies of isolated disc resorption in the lumbar spine. *J Bone Joint Surg [Br]* 1981; 63:491–494.
35. Vernon-Roberts B: Pathology of intervertebral discs and apophyseal joints, in Jayson MIV (ed): *The Lumbar Spine and Back Pain,* ed 3. London, Churchill Livingstone, 1987.
36. Vernon-Roberts B: Disc pathology and disease states, in Ghosh P (ed): *The Biology of the Intervertebral Disc,* vol 2. Boca Raton, Fla, CRC Press, 1988.
37. Vernon-Roberts B: Unpublished observations.
38. Vernon-Roberts B, Pirie CJ: Healing trabecular microfractures in the bodies of lumbar vertebrae. *Ann Rheum Dis* 1973; 32:406–412.
39. Vernon-Roberts B, Pirie CJ: Degenerative changes in the intervertebral discs and their sequelae. *Rheumatol Rehabil* 1977; 16:13–21.

7

Anatomy and Compression Pathophysiology of the Nerve Roots of the Lumbar Spine*

Kjell Olmarker, M.D., Ph.D.
Keisuke Takahashi, M.D., Ph.D.
Björn Rydevik, M.D., Ph.D.

There is no consistent anatomic definition of the term *nerve root* presented in the literature. We propose that the part of the nervous system located outside the spinal cord and surrounded by cerebrospinal fluid and meninges should be termed *nerve root* (Fig 7–1). Nerve root should also be equivalent to the term *spinal nerve root*. The part of the nerve system caudal to the point where the subarachnoid space terminates, i.e., where the nerve tissue is no longer surrounded by cerebrospinal fluid, should be termed *spinal nerve* (Fig 7–1 and 7–2). The spinal nerve has a microscopic organization similar to the nerves distal to the spine, i.e., in the plexus formations and in the extremities, and should be regarded as a peripheral nerve.[25, 31, 64] The dorsal root ganglion may be surrounded completely, partially, or not at all by cerebrospinal fluid. It is therefore better regarded as a unique region of the nervous system, and thus not necessarily as part of either the nerve root or the spinal nerve.

This chapter is based on research supported by the Swedish Medical Research Council (projects no. 8685 and 9758).

ANATOMY OF THE NERVOUS ELEMENTS OF THE LUMBAR SPINE

Gross Anatomy of Spinal Nerve Roots

The spinal cord, in the earliest embryologic stages of life, initially has a length that corresponds to the spinal column. The different spinal cord segments are thus located close to the respective vertebral segments at this stage, and the nerve roots are relatively short owing to the short distance between the spinal cord and the intervertebral foramen. However, when the individual grows, there will be a discrepancy between the lengths of the spinal cord and the vertebral column. This relative elevation of the end of the spinal cord, called the *conus medullaris,* as compared to the vertebrae is called the *ascencus spinalis* and is completed within the first decade of life. In the fully grown individual, the conus medullaris is located at the level of the L1 vertebra. This means that the nerve roots from the lowest spinal

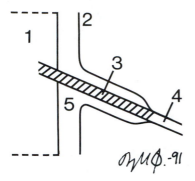

FIG 7–1.
Schematic presentation of the various spinal nerve structures. The nerve root (3) leaves the spinal cord (1) and is surrounded by cerebrospinal fluid (5) within the dura (2). When the dura joins the nerve root distally, the spinal nerve (4) is formed.

cord segments pass within the lumbar and sacral spine to their corresponding intervertebral foramina (see Fig 7–2). This bundle of nerve roots, without the presence of the spinal cord, has been said to resemble the tail of a horse and has therefore been named the *cauda equina* ("tail of horse").

Information between the spinal cord and the periphery travel in both directions. Motor or efferent impulses travel in nerve roots that leave the spinal cord from its anterior aspect, and sensory or afferent information reaches the spinal cord via nerve roots that join the spinal cord on its posterior aspect (Fig 7–3). The ventral nerve roots are therefore also referred to as *motor nerve roots* and the posterior roots as *sensory nerve roots*. This separation of in- and outgoing information to motor and sensory nerve roots is generally known as the law of Magendie. The cell bodies of the axons in the motor roots are located in the anterior horn of the gray matter of the spinal cord. The corresponding cell bodies for the axons in the sensory roots, however, are located in an enlargement of the sensory roots called the *dorsal root ganglia* (DRG), which are located near the intervertebral foramina.[14] The dorsal root ganglia are enclosed by a capsule formed by both a multilayered connective tissue sheath similar to the perineurium of the peripheral nerve, and a loose connective tissue layer called the *epineurium*.[2, 25]

The nerve roots of the cauda equina are enclosed by a sac that is formed by an extension of the cranial dura, called the *spinal dura* (see Fig 7–2). Within this sac there is cerebrospinal fluid in which the nerve roots float relatively freely.[46] However, there are extensions of the arachnoid from the dura to the nerve roots that preserve a strict anatomic relationship between the different nerve roots[66] (Fig 7–4). The loca-

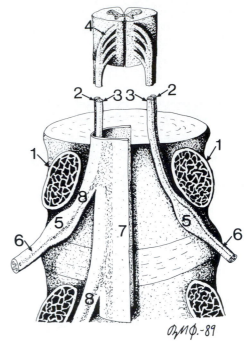

FIG 7–2.
Drawing of the intraspinal course of a human lumbar spinal nerve root segment. The vertebral arches have been removed by cutting the pedicles *(1)*, and the opened spinal canal can be viewed from behind. The ventral *(2)* and dorsal *(3)* nerve roots leave the spinal cord as small rootlets *(4)* that converge caudally into a common nerve root trunk. Just prior to leaving the spinal canal, there is a swelling of the dorsal nerve root, the dorsal root ganglion *(5)*. Caudal to the dorsal root ganglion, the ventral and the dorsal nerve roots mix and form the spinal nerve *(6)*. The spinal dura encloses the nerve roots both as a central cylindrical sac *(7)*, and as separate extensions, the root sleeves *(8)*. (From Olmarker K: *Spinal Nerve Root Compression. Experimental Studies on Effects of Acute, Graded Compression on Nerve Root Nutrition and Function, With an in Vivo Compression Model of the Porcine Cauda Equina* (thesis). Gothenburg University, 1990. Used by permission.)

tion of the nerve roots within this sac is generally referred to as *intrathecal*.[66] One to two vertebral segments above the intervertebral foramen where a nerve root pair is supposed to leave the spine, the nerve roots are instead enclosed by a lateral extension of the dura called the *root sleeve*[47] (see Fig 7–2). This location of the nerve roots is referred to as *extrathecal*.[5] The takeoff angles of the nerve roots from the thecal sac to the neural foramen in the coronal plane are shown in Figure 7–5. Note that the takeoff angle for the lumbar nerve roots is about 40 degrees, as opposed to the S1 nerve root which has been found to have an approximate 20-degree takeoff an-

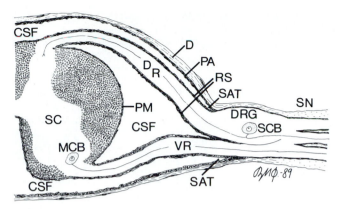

FIG 7–3.
Cross section of a segment of the spinal cord *(SC)*, a ventral *(VR)* and a dorsal *(DR)* spinal nerve root. The cell bodies *(MCB)* of the motor axons, which run in the ventral nerve root, are located in the anterior horn of the gray matter of the spinal cord. The cell bodies *(SCB)* of the sensory axons, which run in the dorsal nerve root, are located in the dorsal root ganglion *(DRG)*. The ventral and dorsal nerve roots blend just caudal to the dorsal root ganglion, and form the spinal nerve *(SN)*. The spinal cord is covered with the pia mater *(PM)*. This sheath continues out on the spinal nerve roots as the root sheath *(RS)*. The root sheath reflects to the pia-arachnoid *(PA)* at the subarachnoid triangle *(SAT)*. Together with the dura *(D)*, the pia-arachnoid forms the spinal dura. The spinal cord and nerve roots are floating freely in the cerebrospinal fluid *(CSF)* in the subarachnoid space. (From Olmarker K: *Spinal Nerve Root Compression. Experimental Studies on Effects of Acute, Graded Compression on Nerve Root Nutrition and Function, With an in Vivo Compression Model of the Porcine Cauda Equina* (thesis). Gothenburg University, 1990. Used by permission.)

gle only.[5] The root sleeve with its content of meninges, cerebrospinal fluid, and nerve tissue has been termed the *nerve root complex*.[30]

When the nerve roots approach the intervertebral foramen, the root sleeve gradually encloses the nerve tissue more tightly. The subarachnoid space and the amount of cerebrospinal fluid surrounding each nerve root pair will thus be gradually reduced in a caudad direction. Compression injury of a nerve root may induce an increase in permeability of the endoneurial capillaries, which may result in edema formation.[37, 50] This can lead to an increase in the intraneural fluid pressure,[19, 23, 53] and a subsequent impairment of the nutritional transport to the nerve roots.[20, 27, 28] Such a mechanism might be particularly important at locations where the nerve roots are tightly enclosed by connective tissue. There might thus be a more pronounced risk for such an "entrapment syndrome" within the nerve roots at

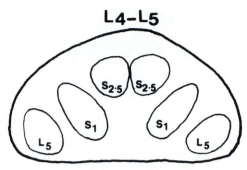

FIG 7–4.
The intrathecal nerve root organization. Schematic presentation of individual roots at the L4–5 cross-sectional disc level showing the L5 root in the anterolateral position. The S1 root is displaced medially forming a diagonal layer (V configuration). The S2–5 roots remain dorsal to the midline. (From Wall EJ, Cohen MS, Massie JM, et al: *Spine* 1990; 15:1244–1247. Used by permission.)

the intervertebral foramen than more central in the cauda equina.[48] The dorsal root ganglion, with its content of sensory nerve cell bodies, tightly enclosed by meninges, might be particularly susceptible to edema formation.[53]

Microscopic Anatomy of Spinal Nerve Roots

The endoneurium of the nerve roots, which is the compartment where the axons are located, is of

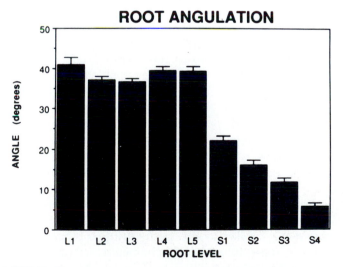

FIG 7–5.
The takeoff angle of the nerve root in the coronal plane at various levels. The nerve root angles remain approximately 40 degrees from L1 to L5, with a sudden drop to 22 degrees at S1. The lower sacral root angles decrease progressively thereafter. (From Cohen MS, Wall EJ, Brown RB, et al: *Spine* 1990; 15:1248–1251. Used by permission.)

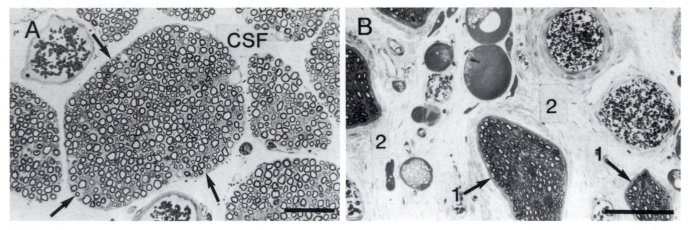

FIG 7–6.
A, the axons of the spinal nerve roots are located in the endoneurium, which is enclosed only by the thin root sheath *(arrows)* and cerebrospinal fluid *(CSF)* (cauda equina from pig; stain: Richardsson; bar = 100 μm). **B,** the endoneurium of the peripheral nerves is similar to that of the nerve roots. In the peripheral nerve, however, the axons are enclosed by the perineurium *(1)* and the epineurium *(2).* Blood vessels are located between the different nerve fascicles in the epi- neurium (tibial nerve from rabbit; stain: Richardsson; bar = 100 μm). (From Olmarker K: *Spinal Nerve Root Compression. Experimental Studies on Effects of Acute Graded Compression on Nerve Root Nutrition and Function, With an in Vivo Compression Model of the Porcine Cauda Equina* (thesis). Gothenburg University, 1990. Used by permission.)

similar structure to the endoneurium of the peripheral nerves[10] (Fig 7–6). In addition to the axons, there are blood vessels, fibroblasts, and collagen fibers in the endoneurium.[11] The amount of collagen in nerve roots is five times less than in peripheral nerves, but six times greater than in the spinal cord.[59] There is incomplete knowledge whether any lymphatic vessels exist within the endoneurium or in both nerve roots and peripheral nerves.[61]

Between the axons in the endoneurium and the cerebrospinal fluid is a thin layer of connective tissue called the *root sheath.* The root sheath has certain similarities to the pia mater that covers the spinal cord. Usually there are two to five cellular layers, which differ histologically between the outer and the inner layers.[13, 58] The cells of the outer layers resemble the pia cells of the spinal cord in the proximal part of the nerve roots and the arachnoid cells in the distal part of the nerve roots. These layers form a loose connective tissue sheath. The inner cell layers are more similar to the perineurium of peripheral nerves, with the histologic characteristics of a structure with barrier properties.[25] In addition, there is also an interrupted basement membrane which encloses the different cells. However, the root sheath is probably not an efficient diffusion barrier. In recent experiments, it has been shown that there is almost a free passage of even relatively large molecules.[17, 49, 68]

In the lumbosacral spine, the spinal dura en- closes the nerve roots and the cerebrospinal fluid. When the two layers of the cranial dura enter the spinal canal, the outer layer blends with the periosteum of that part of the laminae of the cervical vertebrae which face the spinal canal. Together with the arachnoid the inner layer forms the spinal dura. In contrast to the root sheath, the spinal dura is an effective diffusion barrier. The barrier properties are provided by a connective tissue sheath between the dura and the arachnoid called the *neurothelium.*[2] Similar to the inner layer of the root sheath, the neurothelium shows resemblances to the perineurium of the peripheral nerves. It is suggested that the neurothelium and the inner root sheath layers actually form the perineurium when the nerve root is transformed to a peripheral nerve upon leaving the spinal canal.[2, 25]

Vasculature of Spinal Nerve Roots

There has been no consistent terminology of the different vessels of the nerve roots, perhaps owing to the fact that the nerve root vessels have been described in papers dealing mainly with the vascularization of the spinal cord. However, in recent works by Crock and Yoshizawa[8] and Parke and co-workers,[41, 42] a new nomenclature of the different vessels, with respect to location and distribution, has been suggested. A summary of the existing knowledge on nerve root vasculature follows.

When the segmental arteries approach the intervertebral foramen they divide into three different branches: (1) an anterior branch, which supplies the posterior abdominal wall and lumbar plexus; (2) a posterior branch, which supplies the paraspinal muscles and facet joints; and (3) an intermediate branch, which supplies the content of the spinal canal.[8] A branch of the intermediate branch joins the nerve root at the level of the dorsal root ganglion. There are usually three branches from this vessel: one to the ventral root, one to the dorsal root, and one to the vasa corona of the spinal cord. The branch to the vasa corona of the spinal cord, called *medullary feeder artery,* is inconsistent. There are only 7 or 8 remaining of the original 128 from the embryologic period of life. Thus these vessels each supply more than one segment of the spinal cord.[18] The main medullary feeder artery in the thoracic region of the spine was discovered by Adamkiewicz in 1881 and still bears his name.[1] The medullary feeder arteries run parallel to the nerve roots but do not directly participate in the blood supply to the nerve root since there are no connections between these vessels and the vascular network of the nerve roots.[42] They have therefore been referred to as the *extrinsic vascular system* of the cauda equina.[41]

The vascular system of the nerve roots is formed by branches from the intermediate branch of the segmental artery distally, and by branches from the vasa corona of the spinal cord proximally. As opposed to the medullary feeder arteries, this vascular network has been named the *intrinsic vascular system* of the cauda equina.[42, 44] The distal branch to the dorsal root first forms the ganglionic plexus within the dorsal root ganglion. The vessels run within the outer layers of the root sheath, called *epipial tissue.*[64] The vessels from the periphery and from the spinal cord anastomose in the proximal one third of the nerve roots.[41] The anastomosing region has been suggested to have a less developed vascular network and could under such circumstances be a particularly vulnerable site of the nerve roots.[41] However, this is an issue of some controversy in the literature.[7]

The main intrinsic vessels of the nerve root, located in the root sheath, send steep branches into the nerve root which form new vessels that run parallel to the axons and in turn provide branches to the capillary networks (Fig 7–7). Unlike peripheral nerves, the venules do not course together with the arteries in the nerve roots but instead usually have a "spiraling course" in the deeper parts of the nerve tissue.[42]

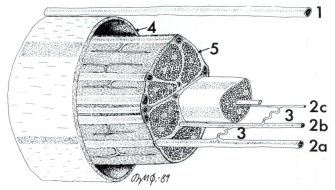

FIG 7–7.
The arterioles within the cauda equina may be referred to either the extrinsic *(1)* or the intrinsic *(2)* vascular system. From the superficial intrinsic arterioles *(2a)* branches continue almost at right angles down between the fascicles. These vessels often run in a spiraling course, thus forming vascular "coils" *(3)*. When reaching a specific fascicle they branch in a T-like manner, with one branch running cranially and one caudally, forming interfascicular arterioles *(2b)*. From these interfascicular arterioles small branches enter the fascicles where they supply the endoneurial capillary networks *(2c)*. The arterioles of the extrinsic vascular system run outside the spinal dura *(4)* and have no connections with the intrinsic system by local vascular branches. The superficial intrinsic arterioles *(2a)* are located within the root sheath *(5)*. (From Olmarker K: *Spinal Nerve Root Compression. Experimental Studies on Effects of Acute, Graded Compression on Nerve Root Nutrition and Function, With an in Vivo Compression Model of the Porcine Cauda Equina* (thesis). Gothenburg University, 1990. Used by permission.)

Between the lumen of the capillaries and the axons in the endoneurial space there is a barrier. This barrier is located in the endothelial cells of the capillaries and is thus similar to the blood-nerve barrier seen in peripheral nerves.[65] However, the barrier in the nerve root has been found to be relatively weak.[39, 40] There is experimental evidence that normal leakage of serum albumin from nerve root capillaries to the endoneurium does exist, but such leakage is less than in the dorsal root ganglion and in the epineurium of peripheral nerves.[17, 37, 39, 40] However, the capillaries in the dorsal root ganglion are fenestrated,[3, 16, 40] and the barrier present in the capillaries in the epineurium of peripheral nerves is less efficient than in the endoneurium.[22, 50] Thus, the blood-nerve barrier of nerve roots does not seem to be as well developed as in peripheral nerves, which implies that edema may be formed more easily in nerve roots.

COMPRESSION PATHOPHYSIOLOGY OF THE NERVE ROOTS OF THE LUMBAR SPINE

The spinal nerve roots are relatively well protected from external trauma by surrounding structures. However, since the nerve roots do not possess the same amount and organization of protective connective tissue sheaths as peripheral nerves, the spinal nerve roots may be particularly sensitive to mechanical deformation due to intraspinal disorders such as disc herniations or protrusions, spinal stenosis, degenerative disorders, and tumors.[26, 48]

Experimental Compression of Spinal Nerve Roots

In previous experimental studies on the effects of compression on nerve roots it was found that the nerve roots were very sensitive and that they seemed to be less resistant to compression than peripheral nerves, but no critical pressure levels in terms of impairment of basic physiologic events in the nerve roots were determined.[12, 57] However, more detailed analyses in this regard have recently been performed utilizing a newly developed model based on the pig cauda equina.[30, 31] Compression is induced by inflating a plastic balloon that is fixed to the spine (Fig 7–8). The inflation pressure may be varied between 0 and 600 mm Hg and the pressure level is continuously monitored by an attached manometer.

In this model, the cauda equina may be viewed through the translucent balloon. This makes it possible to study the flow in the intrinsic blood vessels at various pressure levels.[37] The experiment is designed so that the pressure is increased by 5 mm Hg every 20 seconds. The blood flow and diameters of the intrinsic vessels can simultaneously be observed in a vital microscope which is placed just dorsal to the compression balloon (Fig 7–9). The average occlusion pressure for the arterioles was found to be slightly below and directly related to the systolic blood pressure. The blood flow in the capillary networks was intimately dependent on the blood flow of the adjacent venules. This indicates that venular congestion induces a "retrograde stasis" of capillary networks, which has been hypothesized as a plausible pathophysiologic mechanism in peripheral nerve compression disorders such as the carpal tunnel

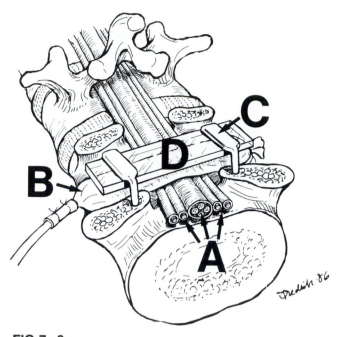

FIG 7–8.
Schematic drawing of experimental model. The cauda equina *(A)* is compressed by an inflatable balloon *(B)* that is fixed to the spine by two L-shaped pins *(C)* and a Plexiglas plate *(D)*. (From Olmarker K, Rydevik B, Holm S: *Spine* 1989; 14:579–583. Used by permission.)

syndrome.[60] The average occlusion pressures for the venules showed large variations. However, pressures as low as 5 to 10 mm Hg were sufficient to induce occlusion in some venules. When considering that venular occlusion may be present at such low levels it also seems likely to assume that capillary stasis may occur to a certain extent at these pressure levels as a result of the observed retrograde stasis mechanism.

In the same experimental setup, the effects of gradual decompression, after initial acute compression was maintained for only a short while, were studied.[34] It was seen that the average pressure for starting the blood flow was slightly lower for arterioles, capillaries, and venules. However, with this protocol it was found that there was not a full restoration of the blood flow until the compression was lowered from 5 to 0 mm Hg. This observation underlines the previous impression that vascular impairment is present even at low pressure levels.

Although there may be a compression-induced vascular impairment at low pressure levels, there is still another nutritional pathway that must be considered. Recently it was found that the nerve roots also derive a major nutritional contribution from the

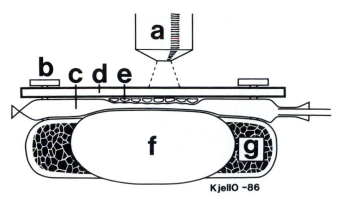

FIG 7-9.
Schematic drawing of a cross section of the spine at the compression zone. The blood vessels in the nerve roots of the cauda equina are observed with the aid of a vital microscope *(a)*. Two L-shaped pins *(b)* fix an inflatable balloon *(c)* and a Plexiglas plate *(d)* to the spine. When inflated, the balloon compresses the nerve roots *(e)* toward the Plexiglas plate. *f* is the intervertebral disc and *g*, vertebral bone. (From Olmarker K, Holm S, Rydevik B, et al: *Neuro-Orthopaedics* 1991; 10:83–87. Used by permission.)

diffusion directly from the surrounding cerebrospinal fluid.[49] To assess the compression-induced effects on the total contribution to the nerve roots, an experiment was designed where[3]H-labeled methylglucose was allowed to be transported to the nerve tissue in the compressed segment both via blood vessels and via cerebrospinal fluid diffusion after systemic injection.[36] The results showed that no compensatory mechanism from cerebrospinal fluid diffusion could be expected at the low pressure lev-

els. On the contrary, compression of 10 mm Hg was sufficient to induce a 20% to 30% reduction of the transport of methylglucose to the nerve roots, as compared with controls (Fig 7–10).

In the studies using vital microscopy presented above, it was seen that there is a rapid restoration of blood flow when a short compression period is ended. However, it is known from experimental studies on peripheral nerves that compression may also induce an increase in vascular permeability, leading to an intraneural edema formation.[50] Such edema may increase the endoneurial fluid pressure,[19, 23, 28, 53] which in turn may impair the endoneurial capillary blood flow and thus jeopardize the nutrition of the nerve roots.[20, 27, 28] Since the edema usually persists for some time after the removal of a compressive agent, edema may negatively affect the nerve root for a longer period than the compression itself. The presence of intraneural edema is also related to subsequent formation of intraneural fibrosis,[51] and may in this way contribute to the slow recovery seen in some patients with nerve compression disorders.[15]

To assess this clinically important question, the distribution of Evans blue–labeled albumin (EBA) in the nerve tissue was analyzed after compression at various pressures and at various durations.[37] Different parts of the cauda equina, both within and without the compression zone, were examined by fluorescence microscopy (Fig 7–11). This enables a mapping of the distribution of EBA in the nerve tissue. Edema, i.e., extravasation of the relatively large

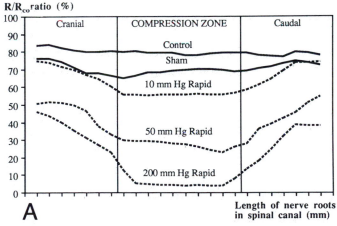

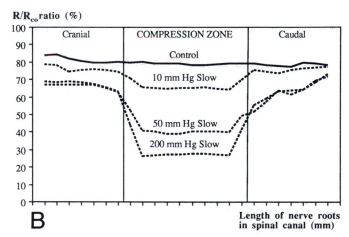

FIG 7-10.
The graphs represent average concentration in nerve roots of methylglucose as a percentage of blood concentration *(R/R_{CO}* ratio) as related to different levels of the nerve roots in the spinal canal. **A,** data from various pressure levels us- ing a rapid compression onset. **B,** same type of data using a slow compression onset. See text for further explanation. (From Olmarker K, Rydevik B, Hansson T, et al: *J Spinal Dis* 1990; 3:25–29. Used by permission.)

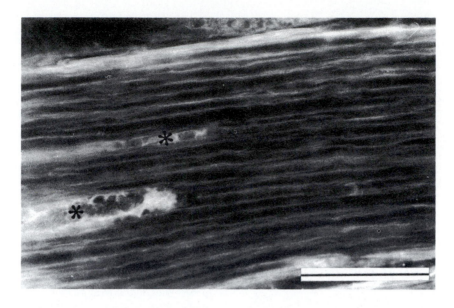

FIG 7–11.
Photograph of a longitudinal section of a single nerve root with intraneural edema. The Evans blue–labeled albumin (EBA) *(white)* is located between the axons *(black)* in all parts of the endoneurium visible in the picture. Two endo- neurial vessels to the *left* in the picture *(asterisks)* contain EBA *(white)* and blood cells *(black)* (bar = 100 μm). (From Olmarker K, Rydevik B, Holm S: *Spine* 1989; 14:579–583. Used by permission.)

albumin molecule, was seen at 50 mm Hg for 2 minutes. Higher pressure levels and longer duration increased the magnitude of the edema. The edema was most pronounced at the edges of compression in all experimental series.

By stimulating the cauda equina proximal to the compression site via screw electrodes in the sacrum and recording a muscle action potential (MAP) by two electrodes in the tail muscles, the effects of compression on impulse propagation of the motor nerve fibers was studied[32, 43, 54] (Fig 7–12). During a 2-hour compression period, a critical pressure level for inducing a reduction of MAP amplitude seems to be located between 50 and 75 mm Hg. Higher pressure levels (100–200 mm Hg) may induce a total conduction block with varying degrees of recovery after compression release. To study the effects of compression on sensory nerve fibers, the electrodes in the sacrum were instead used to record a compound nerve action potential after stimulating the sensory nerves in the tail, i.e., distal to the compression zone. The results showed that the sensory fibers are slightly more susceptible to compression than are motor fibers.[43, 54]

Onset Rate of Compression

One factor that has not previously been considered, not even in the considerable research on pe- ripheral nerves, is the onset rate of the compression. The onset rate, i.e., the time from compression start until full compression, may vary clinically from, perhaps, fractions of seconds in traumatic conditions to months or years in association with degenerative processes. Even in the clinically rapid onset rates there may probably be a wide variation in onset rates. With the presented model it was possible to

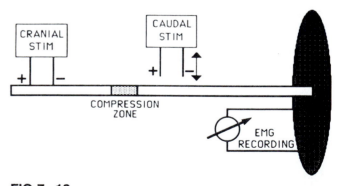

FIG 7–12.
Experimental setup. The cauda equina is stimulated either via two AO cortex screws fixed in the sacral lamina *(cranial stim)* or intermittently via a retractable electrode *(caudal stim)* (see text for details). The impulse propagation of the cauda equina is registered as an electromylogram *(EMG)* by two subdermal electrodes placed in muscles in the tail. (From Olmarker K, Holm S, Rydevik B: *Spine* 1990; 15:416–419. Used by permission.)

vary the onset time of the applied compression. Two onset rates have been investigated. Either the pressure is preset and compression is started by flipping the switch of the compressed air system used to inflate the balloon, or the compression pressure level is slowly increased during 20 seconds. The first onset rate was measured to be 0.05 to 0.1 second, which thus provides a rapid inflation of the balloon and a rapid compression onset.

Such a rapid onset rate was found to induce more pronounced effects on edema formation,[37] methylglucose transport,[36] and impulse propagation[32] than the slow onset rate. Regarding methylglucose transport, the results presented in Figure 7–10 show that the levels within the compression zone are more reduced at the rapid than at the slow onset rate at corresponding pressure levels. There was also a striking difference between the two onset rates when the segments outside the compression zones were considered. In the slow onset series the levels approached baseline values closer to the compression zone than in the rapid onset series. This may indicate the presence of a more pronounced edge zone edema in the rapid onset series, with a subsequent reduction of the nutritional transport also in the nerve tissue adjacent to the compression zone.

The effects of the two onset rates on impulse propagation are illustrated in Figure 7–13.[32] For each of the three applied pressures the impairment of nerve conduction was always most pronounced for the rapid onset rates.

For the rapid onset compression, which, of course, is more closely related to spine trauma or disc herniation than to spinal stenosis, it has been seen that a pressure of 600 mm Hg maintained for only 1 second is sufficient to induce a gradual impairment of nerve conduction during the 2 hours studied after the compression was ended.[35] Overall, the mechanisms for these pronounced differences between the different onset rates are not clear, but may be related to differences in displacement rates of the compressed nerve tissue toward the uncompressed parts owing to the viscoelastic properties of the nerve tissue.[52] Such phenomena may lead to not only structural damage to the nerve fibers but also to structural changes in the blood vessels with subsequent edema formation. The gradual formation of intraneural edema may also be closely related to the described observations of a gradually increasing difference in nerve conduction impairment between the two onset rates.[32, 35]

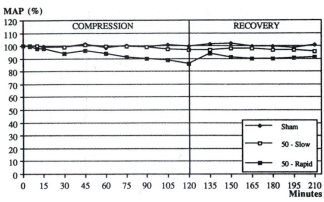

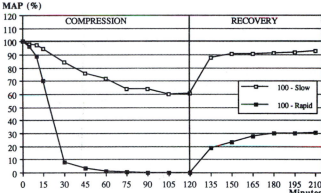

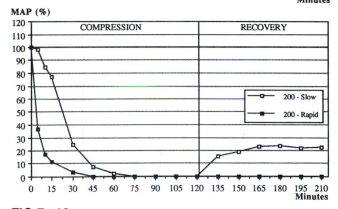

FIG 7–13.
Average amplitude of fastest conducting nerve fibers expressed as a percentage of the baseline value. The diagrams show the results of 2 hours of compression and 1.5 hours of recovery for sham compression and for rapid and slow onset of compression at 50, 100, and 200 mm Hg. *MAP* = muscle action potential. (From Olmarker K, Holm S, Rydevik B: *Spine* 1990; 15:416–419. Used by permission.)

Multiple Levels of Nerve Root Compression

There is a clinical impression that patients with spinal stenosis at more than one level may have more pronounced symptomatology than patients with only one level.[45] The presented model was

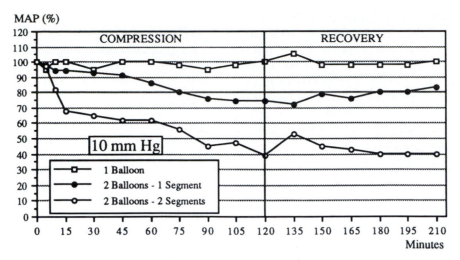

FIG 7–14.

The illustration shows the same type of recordings as in Figure 7–13. In this case, a pressure of 10 mm Hg was used. One or two balloons were applied. In experiments using two balloons, the balloons were placed either one or two vertebral segments apart. (From Olmarker K, Holm S, Rydevik B: *Clin Orthop*, in press 1991. Used by permission.)

found to be suitable to address this interesting clinical question. The use of two balloons at two adjacent disc levels, which resulted in a 10-mm uncompressed nerve segment between the balloons, induced a much more pronounced impairment of nerve impulse conduction than had been previously found at corresponding pressure levels.[33] For instance, a pressure of 10 mm Hg in two balloons induced a 60% reduction of nerve impulse amplitude during 2 hours of compression, whereas 50 mm Hg in one balloon showed no reduction (Fig 7–14).

The mechanism for the difference between single and double compression may not be based simply on the fact that the nerve impulses have to pass more than one compression zone at double-level compression. There may also be a mechanism based on the local vascular anatomy of the nerve roots. Unlike peripheral nerves, there are no regional nutritive arteries from surrounding structures to the intraneural vascular system in spinal nerve roots.[22, 31, 42, 44] Compression at two levels might therefore induce a nutritionally impaired region between the two compression sites. In this way, the segment affected by the compression would be widened from one balloon diameter (10 mm) to two balloon diameters including the interjacent nerve segment (30 mm). This hypothesis was partly confirmed in an experiment on continuous analyses of the total blood flow in the uncompressed nerve segment located between two compression balloons. The results showed that a 64% reduction of total blood flow was induced when both balloons were inflated to 10 mm Hg.[62] At a pressure close to the systemic blood pres-

sure there was complete ischemia in the nerve segment. Preliminary data from a study on the nutritional transport to the nerve tissue at double-level compression have demonstrated that there is a reduction of this transport to the uncompressed nerve segment located between the two compression balloons that is similar to the reduction within the two compression sites.[6] There is thus experimental evidence that the nutrition to the nerve segment located between two compression sites in nerve roots is severely impaired, although this nerve segment itself is uncompressed.

Regarding nerve conduction,[33] it was also evident that the effects were much enhanced if the distance between the compression balloons was increased from one vertebral segment to two vertebral segments. However, this was not the case in the nutritional transport study where the methylglucose levels in the compression zones and in the uncompressed intermediate segment were similar with double compression over one and two vertebral segments.[6] This indicates that the nutrition to the uncompressed nerve segment located between two compression sites is affected almost to the same extent as at the compression sites, regardless of the distance between the compression sites, but that functional impairment may be directly related to the distance between the two compression sites. The impairment of nutrition to the nerve segment between the two compression balloons thus seems to be a more important mechanism than the fact that the nerve impulses have to overcome two compression sites in double-level compression.

Clinical Implications

Compression may induce impairment of the conducting properties of spinal nerve roots.[32, 43, 54] In patients, such abnormalities may be associated with loss of sensory and motor function. The symptomatology of sciatica may also relate to hyperfunction of the neuromuscular system, such as hyperesthesia and muscle fasciculations. Pain may be one component of such hyperfunction of sensory axons. Pain may, however, also be considered as a general reaction to tissue injury, recorded by the central nervous system, or even as a dysfunction of normal inhibitory axons.

As presented, there is thus substantial knowledge about different critical levels of pressure for inducing changes in nerve root nutrition and function. These critical levels are of great interest for the understanding of basic pathophysiologic mechanisms of compression-induced changes in nerve roots. However, such absolute pressure levels may be of relatively less significance in chronic situations. When nerve tissue is compressed, there will be a gradual displacement of the nerve tissue from the compressed segment to the uncompressed segments.[24, 29] If the pressure is of an extremely slow onset rate, as, for instance, in spinal stenosis, there may be an adaptation of the nerve tissue to the applied pressure. In cadaveric experiments, Schönström and colleagues found that when a hose clamp is tightened around a human cadaveric cauda equina specimen, there is a critical cross-sectional area of the dura sac when the first signs of a pressure increase are recorded by a catheter placed in the compression zone.[55] This cross-sectional area was approximately 65 to 75 mm^2, which was also found to correlate to the corresponding measurement on computed tomography scans on spinal stenosis patients.[56] When the hose clamp was further tightened the pressure increased. However, owing to creep phenomena in the nerve tissue, the pressure dropped with time. When the pressure did not normalize within 10 minutes, the "sustained size" was registered and was found to be in the range of 45 to 55 mm^2. [55] This indicates that even in acute compression, there is an adaptation of the nerve tissue to the applied pressure. In a longer perspective, this probably means that the nerve may also be reorganized in its microstructural elements, which will result in a nerve with a smaller diameter. Under such circumstances, with a gradually decreasing nerve diameter, the pressure acting on the nerve will be reduced to a certain extent.

In a cadaveric study on a spinal stenosis case, Watanabe and Parke[67] found that although the cauda equina diameter had been substantially reduced, there were still nonoccluded vessels present, although reduced in number, as seen by ink perfusion. Also in an experimental study, although with initially acute compression but which was prolonged for up to 3 months, there were vessels noted in the compressed segment as seen by ink perfusion.[9] This suggests that, although initially exposed to a certain pressure, the cauda equina nerve roots may reorganize and in this way the external pressure may become reduced so that there may be at least some blood supply present. From experimental studies on the spinal cord it is known that when an extremity is used, there is an increase in the blood flow in the corresponding spinal cord segments.[4] This suggests that to function properly the nerve tissue must be able to increase the local blood supply as an answer to an increased nutritional demand. When considering the spinal stenosis situation, with the reduced nerve diameter and with only some functioning vessels, it seems that this part of the cauda equina may have difficulties in achieving such an increase in the blood supply. It has therefore been suggested that the mechanism in spinal stenosis is not so much based on compression on nerve tissue as it is an incapability of increasing the local blood supply within the nerve roots.[37] This might explain why there may be no symptoms at rest, but at exercise the symptoms will develop within seconds to minutes. The time for onset of symptoms may be related both to the degree of stenosis and to the local vascular situation within the cauda equina. From the experiments on acute in vivo compression of the cauda equina that were presented above, it was evident that nutritional impairment was seen even at extremely low pressure levels.[36, 38] This could explain why minimal changes in the demand for nutrients or increasing pressure on the nerve roots due to, for instance, changes in posture may induce neurogenic claudication.

In an experiment on continuous analyses of blood flow in the cauda equina during compression and recovery, there was a delay between compression onset and the reduction of total blood flow in the cauda equina.[62] The blood flow decreased 1 to 3 minutes after onset of compression. When the compression was ended, there was a recovery of blood flow over approximately 1 to 5 minutes until complete restoration. This onset time and the time for restoration may well be related to the time for symptomatic onset and relief in patients with neurogenic claudication upon ending exercise.

When considering nerve root compression disorders with a longer duration of nutritional deficit or at higher pressure levels, such as disc herniation or spinal trauma, there may well be other pathogenetic aspects to consider. In such cases there may be more permanent changes induced owing to the prolonged nutritional impairment, which may be related to intraneural edema formation and perhaps also to intraneural fibrosis. At higher pressure levels there is also an enhanced risk of direct structural damage to tissues within the nerve roots, such as axons and endoneurial capillaries, which may further compound the injury to the nerve roots and thereby lead to more severe symptoms for the patient.

SUMMARY

Spinal nerve roots are often involved in spinal disorders such as trauma, disc herniation, and spinal stenosis. Compression of spinal nerve roots may induce a sequence of events including impairment of nutrition, increase in microvascular permeability leading to intraneural edema formation, blockage of axonal transport, and alterations in nerve function. The mechanisms in clinical nerve root compression syndromes such as neurogenic claudication are probably even more complex. However, available experimental data indicate that compression-induced disturbances in the blood supply to the nerve roots of the cauda equina play a central role in the production of the symptoms associated with spinal stenosis, i.e., neurogenic claudication.

REFERENCES

1. Adamkiewicz A: Die Blutgefässe des menschlichen Rückenmarkes. I. Die Gefässe der Rückenmarkssubstanz. *Sitzungsb Akad Wiss Wien Math Naturwissenschaften CI* 1881; 84:469–502.
2. Andres KH: Über die Feinstruktur der Arachnoidea und Dura mater von Mammalia. *Z Zellforsch* 1967; 79:272–295.
3. Arvidson B: Distribution of intravenously injected protein tracers in peripheral ganglia of adult mice. *Exp Neurol* 1979; 63:388–410.
4. Blau JN, Rushworth G: Observations on the blood vessels of the spinal cord and their responses to motor activity. *Brain* 1958; 81:354–363.
5. Cohen MS, Wall EJ, Brown RB, et al: Cauda equina

anatomy. Part II: Extrathecal nerve roots and dorsal root ganglia. *Spine* 1990; 15:1248–1251.
6. Cornefjord M, Olmarker K, Takahashi K, et al: Impairment of nutritional transport at double level cauda equina compression, in *Transactions of the International Society for the Lumbar Spine.* Heidelberg, Germany, 1991.
7. Crock HV, Yamagishi M, Crock MC: *The Conus Medullaris and Cauda Equina in Man.* New York, Springer-Verlag, 1986
8. Crock HV, Yoshizawa H: The blood supply of the lumbar vertebral column. *Clin Orthop* 1976; 115:6–21.
9. Delamarter RB, Bohlman HH, Dodge LD, et al: Experimental lumbar spinal stenosis. Analysis of the cortical evoked potentials, microvasculature and histopathology. *J Bone Joint Surg [Am]* 1990; 72:110–120.
10. Gamble HJ: Comparative electron-microscopic observations on the connective tissues of a peripheral nerve and a spinal nerve root. *J Anat* 1964; 98:17–25.
11. Gamble HJ, Eames RA: Electron microscopy of human spinal nerve roots. *Arch Neurol* 1966; 14:50–53.
12. Gelfan S, Tarlov IM: Physiology of spinal cord, nerve root and peripheral nerve compression. *Am J Physiol* 1956; 185:217–229.
13. Haller FR, Low FN: The fine structure of the peripheral nerve root sheath in the subarachnoid space in the rat and other laboratory animals. *Am J Anat* 1971; 131:1–20.
14. Hasue M, Kunogi J, Konno S, et al: Classification by position of dorsal root ganglia in the lumbosacral region. *Spine* 1989; 14:1261–1264.
15. Hoyland JA, Freemont AJ, Jayson MIV: Intervertebral foramen venous obstruction. A cause of periradicular fibrosis? *Spine* 1989; 14:569–573.
16. Jacobs JM, MacFarlane RM, Cavanagh JB: Vascular leakage in the dorsal root ganglia of the rat, studied with horseradish peroxidase. *J Neurol Sci* 1976; 29:95–107.
17. Kobayashi S, Yoshizawa H, Hachiya Y, et al: Blood-nerve barrier in spinal nerve roots, in *Transactions of the International Society for the Study of the Lumbar Spine.* Heidelberg, Germany, May 1991.
18. Lazorthes G, Gouaze A, Zadeh JO, et al: Arterial vascularization of the spinal cord. Recent studies of the anastomotic substitution pathways. *J Neurosurg* 1971; 35:253–262.
19. Low PA, Dyck PJ: Increased endoneurial fluid pressure in experimental lead neuropathy. *Nature* 1977; 269:427–428.
20. Low PA, Dyck PJ, Schmelzer JD: Chronic elevation of endoneurial fluid pressure is associated with low-grade fiber pathology. *Muscle Nerve* 1982; 5:162–165.
21. Low PA, Nukada H, Schmelzer JD, et al: Endoneurial oxygen tension and radial topography in nerve edema. *Brain Res* 1985; 341:147–154.
22. Lundborg G: Structure and function of the intraneural microvessels as related to trauma, edema formation, and nerve function. *J Bone Joint Surg [Am]* 1975; 57:938–948.
23. Lundborg G, Myers R, Powell H: Nerve compression injury and increased endoneurial fluid pressure: A "miniature compartment syndrome." *J Neurol Neurosurg Psychiatry* 1983; 46:1119–1124.

24. MacGregor RJ, Sharpless SK, Luttges MW: A pressure vessel model for nerve compression. *J Neurol Sci* 1975; 24:299–304.

25. McCabe JS, Low FN: The subarachnoid angle: An area of transition in peripheral nerve. *Anat Rec* 1969; 164:15–34.

26. Murphy RW: Nerve roots and spinal nerves in degenerative disk disease. *Clin Orthop* 1977; 129:46–60.

27. Myers RR, Mizisin AP, Powell HC, et al: Reduced nerve blood flow in hexachlorophene neuropathy. Relationship to elevated endoneurial fluid pressure. *J Neuropathol Exp Neurol* 1982; 41:391–439.

28. Myers RR, Powell CC: Galactose neuropathy: Impact of chronic endoneurial edema on nerve blood flow. *Ann Neurol* 1984; 16:587–594.

29. Ochoa J, Fowler TJ, Gilliat RW: Anatomical changes in peripheral nerves compressed by a pneumatic tourniquet. *J Anat* 1972; 113:433.

30. Olmarker K: *Spinal Nerve Root Compression. Experimental Studies on Effects of Acute, Graded Compression on Nerve Root Nutrition and Function, With an in Vivo Compression Model of the Porcine Cauda Equina* (thesis). Gothenburg University, Sweden, 1990.

31. Olmarker K, Holm S, Rosenqvist A-L, et al: Experimental nerve root compression. Presentation of a model for acute, graded compression of the porcine cauda equina, with analyses of neural and vascular anatomy. *Spine* 1991; 16:61–69.

32. Olmarker K, Holm S, Rydevik B: Importance of compression onset rate for the degree of impairment of impulse propagation in experimental compression injury of the porcine cauda equina. *Spine* 1990; 15:416–419.

33. Olmarker K, Holm S, Rydevik B: More pronounced effects of double level compression than single level compression on impulse propagation in the porcine cauda equina. *Clin Orthop*, in press 1991.

34. Olmarker K, Holm S, Rydevik B, et al: Restoration of blood flow during gradual decompression of a compressed segment of the porcine cauda equina. A vital microscopic study. *Neuro-Orthopaedics* 1991; 10:83–87.

35. Olmarker K, Lind B, Holm S, et al: Continued compression increases impairment of impulse propagation in experimental compression of the porcine cauda equina. *Neuro-Orthopaedics* (in press) 1991.

36. Olmarker K, Rydevik B, Hansson T, et al: Compression-induced changes of the nutritional supply to the porcine cauda equina. *J Spinal Dis* 1990; 3:25–29.

37. Olmarker K, Rydevik B, Holm S: Edema formation in spinal nerve roots induced by experimental, graded compression. An experimental study on the pig cauda equina with special reference to differences in effects between rapid and slow onset of compression. *Spine* 1989; 14:569–573.

38. Olmarker K, Rydevik B, Holm S, et al: Effects of experimental graded compression on blood flow in spinal nerve roots. A vital microscopic study on the porcine cauda equina. *J Orthop Res* 1989; 7:817–823.

39. Olsson Y: Topographical differences in the vascular permeability of the peripheral nervous system. *Acta Neuropathol* 1968; 10:26–33.

40. Olsson Y: Studies on vascular permeability in peripheral nerves. IV. Distribution of intravenously injected protein tracers in the peripheral nervous system of various species. *Acta Neuropathol (Berl)* 1971; 17:114–126.

41. Parke WW, Gamell K, Rothman RH: Arterial vascularization of the cauda equina. *J Bone Joint Surg [Am]* 1981; 63:53–62.

42. Parke WW, Watanabe R: The intrinsic vasculature of the lumbosacral spinal nerve roots. *Spine* 1985; 10:508–515.

43. Pedowitz RA, Garfin SR, Hargens AR, et al: Effects of magnitude and duration of compression on spinal nerve root conduction. *Spine* (in press) 1991.

44. Petterson CÅV, Olsson Y: Blood supply of spinal nerve roots. An experimental study in the rat. *Acta Neuropathol* 1989; 78:455–461.

45. Porter RW: Personal communication, 1991.

46. Rauschning W: Computed tomography and cryomicrotomy of lumbar specimens. A new technique for multiplanar anatomic correlation. *Spine* 1983; 8:170–180.

47. Rauschning W: Normal and pathologic anatomy of the lumbar root canals. *Spine* 1987; 12:1008–1019.

48. Rydevik B, Brown MD, Lundborg G: Pathoanatomy and pathophysiology of nerve root compression. *Spine* 1984; 9:7–15.

49. Rydevik B, Holm S, Brown MD, et al: Diffusion from the cerebrospinal fluid as a nutritional pathway for spinal nerve roots. *Acta Physiol Scand* 1990; 138:247–248.

50. Rydevik B, Lundborg G: Permeability of intraneural microvessels and perineurium following acute, graded nerve compression. *Scand J Plast Reconstr Surg* 1977; 11:179–187.

51. Rydevik B, Lundborg G, Nordborg C: Intraneural tissue reactions induced by internal neurolysis. *Scand J Plast Reconstr Surg* 1976; 10:3–8.

52. Rydevik B, Lundborg G, Skalak R: Biomechanics of peripheral nerves, in Nordin M, Frankel VH (eds): *Basic Biomechanics of the Musculoskeletal System*. Philadelphia, Lea & Febiger, 1989; pp 75–87.

53. Rydevik B, Myers RR, Powell HC: Pressure increase in the dorsal root ganglion following mechanical compression. Closed compartment syndrome in nerve roots. *Spine* 1989; 14:574–576.

54. Rydevik BL, Pedowitz RA, Hargens AR, et al: Effects of acute graded compression on spinal nerve root function and structure: An experimental study on the pig cauda equina. *Spine* 1991; 16:487–493.

55. Schönström N, Bolender NF, Spengler DM et al: Pressure changes within the cauda equina following constriction of the dural sac. *Spine* 1984; 9:604–607.

56. Schönström N, Bolender N, Spengler DM: The pathomorphology of spinal stenosis as seen on CT scans of the lumbar spine. *Spine* 1985; 10:806–811.

57. Sharpless SK: Susceptibility of spinal nerve roots to compression block. The research status of spinal manipulative therapy. NIH workshop, Feb 2–4 1975, in Goldstein M (ed): *National Institute of Neurological and Communication Diseases and Blindness Monograph no. 15.* Bethesda, MD, 1975, pp 155–161.

58. Steer JM: Some observations on the fine structure of

rat dorsal spinal nerve roots. *J Anat* 1971; 109:467–485.

59. Stodieck LS, Beel JA, Luttges MW: Structural properties of spinal nerve roots: Protein composition. *Exp Neurol* 1986; 91:41–51.

60. Sunderland S: The nerve lesion in the carpal tunnel syndrome. *J Neurol Neurosurg Psychiatry* 1976; 39:615–626.

61. Sunderland S: *Nerves and Nerve Injuries,* ed 2. Edinburgh, Churchill Livingstone, 1978.

62. Takahashi K, Olmarker K, Rydevik B, et al: Double level cauda equina compression: Continuous monitoring of intraneural blood flow, in *Transactions of the International Society for the Lumbar Spine.* Heidelberg, Germany, 1991.

63. Verbiest H: A radicular syndrome from developmental narrowing of the lumbar spine vertebral canal. *J Bone Joint Surg [Br]* 1954; 36:230–237.

64. Waggener JD, Beggs J: The membraneous coverings of neural tissues: An electron microscopy study. *J Neuropathol* 1967; 26:412–426.

65. Waksman BH: Experimental studies of diphtheritic polyneuritis in the rabbit and guinea pig. III. The blood-nerve barrier in the rabbit. *J Neuropathol Exp Neurol* 1961; 20:35–77.

66. Wall EJ, Cohen MS, Massie JM, et al: Cauda equina anatomy. Part I: Intrathecal nerve root organisation. *Spine* 1990; 15:1244–1247.

67. Watanabe R, Parke WW: Vascular and neural pathology of lumbosacral spinal stenosis. *J Neurosurg* 1986; 64:64–70.

68. Yoshizawa H, Kobayashi S, Hachiya Y: Blood supply of nerve roots and dorsal root ganglia. *Orthop Clin North Am* 1991; 22:195–212.

8

The Applied Anatomy of Spinal Circulation in Spinal Stenosis

H. V. Crock, A.O., M.D., F.R.C.S.

Most surgeons who operate on the spine have two practical concerns which relate to its blood supply and venous drainage. The first of these is to control hemorrhage in the spinal canal and the second is to avoid damaging the artery of Adamkiewicz. However, those who treat patients with spinal vascular malformations must apply a more detailed knowledge of the vascular anatomy of the spinal cord.

Viewed in perspective the anatomy of spinal circulation is central to the understanding of the genesis of various syndromes seen in patients with spinal stenosis, ranging from unilateral and bilateral leg pain to cauda equina claudication. It is important also in the radiologic interpretation of radiculograms with particular reference to vascular engorgement of the cauda equina, root edema, and arachnoiditis in spinal stenosis. Knowledge of this anatomy is required not only from an academic point of view but it should be the guiding principle in the use of practical techniques which are safe and effective for the relief of spinal stenosis.

The first detailed account of the arterial supply of the human spinal cord—Thomas Willis's *Cerebri anatome*—was based on injection studies in fetal spines.[14] Willis indicated that the injection and dissection of these spines was easy because they were still largely cartilaginous, but he went on to comment, "in the adult this work would be nearly impossible." He established the fact that segmental arteries supplied the cord, both anteriorly and posteriorly, joining, respectively, the anterior spinal artery and the paired posterior longitudinal spinal arteries. *His prediction about the difficulty of demonstrating the blood supply of the spinal cord in the adult was correct, accounting, even today, for the controversy that continues to surround this subject.* The blood supply of the spinal cord and meninges is intimately related to that of the vertebral column as a whole and the relationships between them should always be borne in mind during spinal operations.

In this chapter the salient features of the arterial supply and venous drainage of the vertebral column and spinal cord in adult humans are described, and illustrated by photographs made from dissections of injected vertebral columns. All these injections were made into intact bodies post mortem as recommended by Gillilan.[7] The entire vertebral columns were removed before the pathologists conducted their investigations. The material in this chapter is presented in didactic fashion and therefore details of the techniques of injection, of the preparation of specimens, and of their ultimate dissection are not discussed. These details can be found in our previously published works.[3, 4]

THE ARTERIES OF THE VERTEBRAE

The vertebral bodies are all supplied by branches of arteries which course around the middle of the front and sides of each vertebra. In the lumbar spine these are the lumbar arteries, pairs of which arise from the dorsal wall of the abdominal aorta. Likewise in the thoracic spine, paired thoracic arteries arise from the aorta. The upper two thoracic vertebrae are usually supplied by superior intercostal branches of the subclavian arteries. The cervical vertebrae are supplied by branches analogous to the lumbar and thoracic arteries but springing for the most part from anterior and posterior vertebral body branches which arise from the vertebral arteries.

As each lumbar artery courses around the middle of the front and sides of the vertebral body, *applied to the periosteum*, it gives off innumerable small branches which penetrate the bone. These can be classified into three easily recognizable groups: The first are centrum branches which penetrate the vertebral body like the spokes of a wheel, forming an arterial grid best seen in horizontal sections through the middle of the vertebral body. From this grid, within the substance of the centrum, vertical branches pass upward and downward to contribute, respectively, to the capillary circulation of the upper and lower vertebral end plates. The second and third groups are formed by small branches which course vertically upward and downward from the upper and lower sides of the lumbar artery. Fine anastomoses occur between these ascending branches

on one vertebra and the descending branches on the adjacent higher one as they cross the outer surface of the intervertebral disc. Just below and above the levels of each vertebral end plate many of these ascending and descending branches penetrate the vertebral body passing toward the vertebral end plates where they contribute to the capillary beds.

As the main stem of each lumbar artery approaches the intervertebral foramen inferior to the vertebral pedicle, it gives off three sets of branches which enter the intervertebral foramen. *The first are the anterior intraspinal arteries* which form an arterial arcade on the posterior surface of each vertebral body, fusing at the center with the arterial arcade of the opposite side (Fig 8–1). From this arcuate system vertebral end-plate branches penetrate at each extremity of the vertebral body, while centrally, radiate branches contribute to the arterial grid of the centrum.

The second group are neural arterial branches destined to supply each nerve root ganglion and to give rise to the anterior and posterior radicular arteries

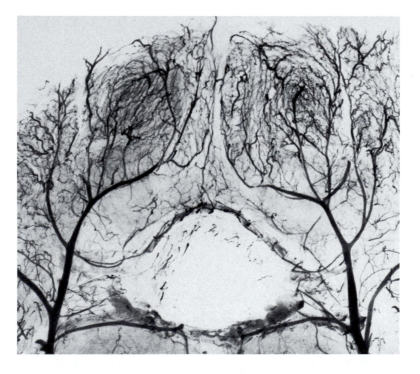

FIG 8–1.
A detailed photograph of a thin transverse section from the lumbar spine of an adult at the level of the intervertebral foramina. The arteries have been injected with a suspension of barium sulfate. Note the distribution of the anterior and posterior intraspinal branches of the lumbar artery with the neural arterial branches in between. The main stems of the lumbar arteries are then continued across the lamina on each side applied to its periosteum and up the sides of the spinous process. Throughout their courses they give branches into the bone from their deep surface and major branches into the paraspinal muscles on their outer surfaces. (From Crock HV: *Practice of Spinal Surgery.* Heidelberg, Springer-Verlag, 1983, p 111. Used by permission.)

which penetrate the dural root sleeves and course along the spinal nerve roots to reach the spinal cord. Of all the vessels supplying the human skeleton and spinal cord, these are the most difficult to study. Many of them are fine and run long courses between their origins at the level of the intervertebral foramen and their terminations on the surface of the spinal cord. They are not easily filled by injection media and readily rupture during dissection. They can only be definitively outlined after high-quality vessel filling has occurred and the spines have been fixed and processed by the Spalteholz clearing method before dissection. This renders even the most delicate and slender vessels semirigid, permitting dissection in the fluid medium without risk of their rupture. There is no other reliable method which can be used to follow the course of a long fine radicular artery. Because the method is so time-consuming and unpleasant to use, it is rarely employed. Failure to use it lies at the root of much of the academic controversy concerning the blood supply of

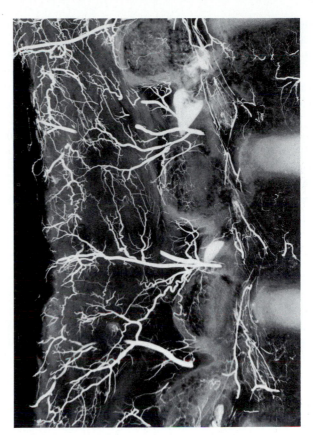

FIG 8–3.
A thin sagittal section from the lumbar spine of an adult at the level of the intervertebral foramina. The paraspinal muscles are intact. The arteries have been injected with a barium sulfate suspension. The specimen is partly decalcified. The stems of the posterior branches of three adjacent lumbar arteries can be seen related to the pars interarticularis of their respective vertebrae. Note the close proximity of the neural branches of the lumbar arteries *which can be easily damaged by the use of diathermy anterior to the pars interarticularis.* Note also the articular branches and the ramifications of the arteries within the paraspinal muscles.

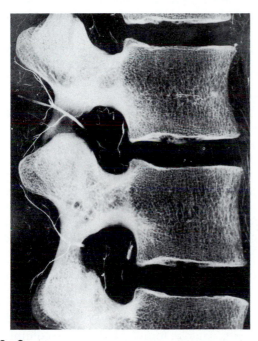

FIG 8–2.
A radiograph of a thin undecalcified sagittal section of the lumbar spine of an adult. The regional arteries have been injected with barium sulfate. The stems of the posterior branches of two lumbar arteries can be seen as they course backward behind the intervertebral foramina. These arteries are constant lateral relations of the pars interarticularis of each lamina. (From Crock HV, Yoshizawa H: *The Blood Supply of the Vertebral Column and Spinal Cord in Man.* New York, Springer-Verlag, 1977, p 20. Used by permission.)

the spinal cord. *The specimens depicted in the figures in this chapter have all been prepared according to this demanding protocol.*

The third group are the posterior lumbar intraspinal arteries which supply the laminae, spinous processes, and pedicles. These form an arcuate arcade on the anterior surface of each lamina, like a mirror image of the arterial arcade on the posterior surface of the vertebral bodies (see Fig 8–1). Having given off these three sets of intraspinal branches, the lumbar artery then crosses the pars interarticularis of each lamina and applied to the periosteum courses across the lamina to the base of each spinous process, terminating at its tip, supplying branches to the facet joints, the outer surfaces of the lamina and spinous process, and to the paraspinal muscles (Figs 8–1 through 8–3).

The scale of vessels supplying the thoracic and cervical vertebrae becomes smaller from below upward, but the general description of their distribution around and within the vertebrae is spatially identical to those in the lumbar vertebrae. The only major regional difference in the origin of vessels supplying the spinal cord is in the neck where the anterior and posterior radicular arteries arise from the vertebral arteries.

THE VERTEBRAL VEINS

The vertebral end-plate capillary beds drain via subchondral venules into a complex of veins within the vertebral bodies. The first of these is a horizontally placed *subarticular collecting vein system* which drains posteriorly into the anterior internal vertebral venous plexus in the spinal canal and peripherally into veins which accompany the principal arteries supplying the vertebral bodies.[5] These vertebral veins pass into the vena cava in the lumbar region, into the azygos system in the thorax, or into venae comitantes of the vertebral arteries in the neck. Other large vertically orientated veins formed beneath the vertebral end plates course upward or downward from their respective end plates toward the centrum to form *Batson's plexus*, which mirrors but dwarfs the arterial grid described above. Branches of Batson's plexus drain into *the internal vertebral venous plexus* in the spinal canal from the center of each vertebral body and into corresponding vertebral veins on its outer surfaces.[2]

Within the spinal canal *the internal vertebral venous plexus* is arranged in arcuate form overlying and obscuring the arterial arcades which have been described above. These spinal canal veins surround the dural sac lying on the periosteum of the vertebral bodies and laminae. Described as *the anterior and posterior internal vertebral venous plexuses*, they anastomose and surround the nerve root sleeves to drain into external vertebral veins outside the intervertebral foramina. The vertebral venous system is capacious and may hold a significant part of the blood volume of the body. It contains no valves apart from primitive ones between it and the intradural veins of the spinal cord and cauda equina which ultimately enter the internal vertebral venous plexus in the axillary region of each dural nerve root sleeve.[11]

THE ORIGIN OF ARTERIES SUPPLYING THE SPINAL CORD AND CAUDA EQUINA

Segmental blood vessels appear in the earliest stages of vertebral development.[13] Commencing in the cervical area, a centrally placed arterial channel is formed anteriorly by the confluence of branches from the right and left vertebral arteries. This is the *anterior median longitudinal arterial trunk* of the spinal cord.[6] Posteriorly, right and left *posterolateral longitudinal arterial trunks* of the spinal cord arise either from branches of the vertebral or posteroinferior cerebellar arteries over the medulla oblongata. These three principal arterial trunks on the surface of the spinal cord course along its length to the tip of the conus medullaris where they anastomose around its sides. Between each of these vessels on the surface of the cord there are transversely orientated anastomoses, the *vasa corona*.

At the level of each intervertebral foramen arising from the vertebral arteries in the neck, from the thoracic arteries in the thorax and from the lumbar arteries in the lumbar spine, *anterior and posterior radicular arteries arise*. These pass along their respective nerve roots—uninterrupted in their courses—to join the three main surface arteries of the spinal cord (Fig 8–4). The segmental distribution of these vessels as described by Willis in fetal spinal cords is maintained in the adult (Figs 8–5 and 8–6).

The dimensions of the radicular arteries vary from vertebral level to vertebral level and from right to left sides of the spinal cord. The larger radicular arteries are usually found in the thoracolumbar region arising between the T1 and L1 vertebrae on the right side of the spine. The largest of them is traditionally termed the *great radicular artery of Adamkiewicz*.[1, 12] Fine side branches pass off from these arteries at regular intervals. Springlike convolutions are found along the length of all of them (Fig 8–7). The overriding importance that is attached to this single vessel by most surgeons seems to obscure the more important observation that the blood supply of

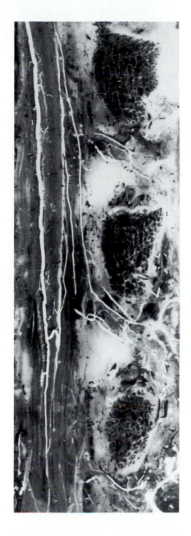

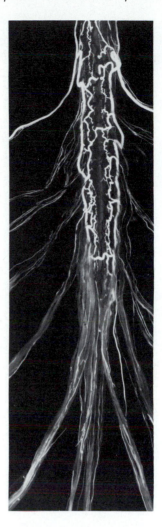

FIG 8–4.

A dissection showing the origin and distribution of a posterior radicular artery from a woman aged 29 years. The lower portion of the spinal cord and conus medullaris is viewed from in front following removal of most of the vertebral bodies. The spinal cord has been rotated slightly to the *left* of the figure to bring the posterior longitudinal arterial trunk into view. On the *right-hand side* of the figure, three pedicles are shown. At the intervertebral foraminal level between the lower two pedicles, the main stem of a lumbar artery is seen in the region of the pars interarticularis of the lamina at that level. The origin of the posterior radicular artery from that vessel just inside the intervertebral foramen is seen and its course is followed from its origin, uninterrupted, to the posterior longitudinal arterial trunk of the cord, which it joins at the upper level of the superior pedicle on this photograph (Spalteholz preparation dissected by Dr. M. Yamagishi). (From Crock HV, Yamagishi M, Crock MC: *The Conus Medullaris and Cauda Equina in Man, an Atlas of the Arteries and Veins.* New York, Springer-Verlag, 1986, p 45. Used by permission.)

FIG 8–5.

A dorsal view of the lower thoracic cord and conus medullaris from a man aged 41 years, showing the posterolateral longitudinal arterial trunks of the cord with the transversely orientated circumferential vasa corona between them. The specimen has been prepared to display only the posterior filaments of the cauda equina and their radicular arteries. Note the segmental distribution of these vessels as they join the longitudinal arterial channels on either side. Many of them are of very small caliber, but two large posterior radicular arteries can be seen at the top of the photograph. (From Crock HV, Yamagishi M, Crock MC: *The Conus Medullaris and Cauda Equina in Man, an Atlas of the Arteries and Veins.* New York, Springer-Verlag, 1986, p 32. Used by permission.)

the spinal cord remains segmental throughout life. This interpretation was widely accepted until late in the 16th century but eventually gave way to the view that in the adult it was not segmental, following the work of Adamkiewicz[1] and Kadyi.[8]

Using the techniques alluded to above there is

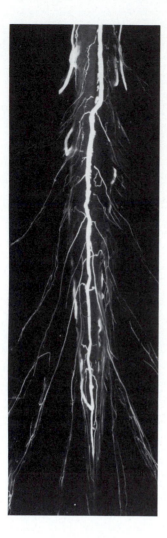

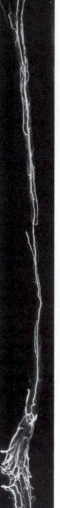

FIG 8–7.
A photograph of a single lumbar nerve root ganglion *(bottom)* and the anterior nerve filaments of the cauda equina cut just below the level of the conus medullaris *(top)* from a man aged 32 years (arterial injection with barium suspension, Spalteholz preparation). Multiple fine arteries form a plexus around and within the nerve root ganglion. By contrast, a single fine anterior radicular artery, having its own discrete origin, courses upward toward the spinal cord. This vessel is gently convoluted, giving off side branches regularly along its uninterrupted course to the conus medullaris. (From Crock HV, Yamagishi M, Crock MC: *The Conus Medullaris and Cauda Equina in Man, an Atlas of the Arteries and Veins.* The New York, Springer-Verlag, 1986, p 69. Used by permission.)

FIG 8–6.
A photograph of the anterior surface of the same specimen shown in Figure 8–5 showing the anterior median longitudinal arterial trunk and on the *left-hand side* at the tip of the conus, the junction with the posterolateral longitudinal arterial trunk on that side. The specimen has been prepared to display only the anterior filaments of the cauda equina and their radicular arteries. Each group of filaments of the cauda equina forming the anterior nerve root has running along it a vessel which in this specimen passes directly into the main anterior median longitudinal arterial trunk on the surface of the cord. (From Crock HV, Yamagishi M, Crock MC: *The Conus Medullaris and Cauda Equina in Man, an Atlas of the Arteries and Veins.* New York, Springer-Verlag, 1986, p 33. Used by permission.)

no doubt that the radicular arterial supply of the spinal cord is segmental in the human adult (see Figs 8–5 and 8–6). Furthermore, there is no strong anatomic evidence to support the view that the blood supply of the cauda equina is tenuous in its upper third[10] (Figs 8–8 and 8–9).

THE VENOUS DRAINAGE OF THE SPINAL CORD AND CAUDA EQUINA

The intrinsic veins of the spinal cord drain into principal longitudinal channels which lie in the midline on its anterior and posterior surfaces. These are the anterior median and the dorsal median longitudinal venous trunks of the spinal cord (Figs 8–10 and 8–11). They are thin-walled vessels of much larger caliber than the principal surface arteries of the cord. Their course is frequently tortuous. Vasa corona pass around the sides of the cord joining the anterior and posterior median longitudinal venous trunks.

Along each spinal nerve root, dorsal and ventral radicular veins run with their corresponding arteries (Fig 8–12). While these veins run variable courses

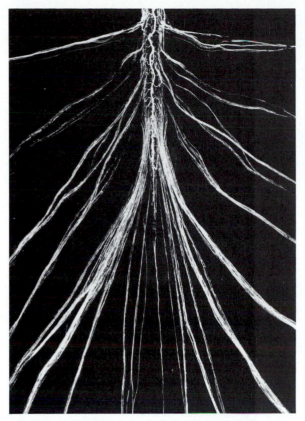

FIG 8–8.
A photograph of the anterior surface of the distal third of the spinal cord, conus medullaris, and cauda equina from a man aged 41 years. In this specimen, the filaments of the cauda equina have been widely separated. The arteries of the cauda equina run an uninterrupted course from their origins at the level of the intervertebral foramina to the surface of the cord. (From Crock HV, Yamagishi M, The Crock MC: *The Conus Medullaris and Cauda Equina in Man, an Atlas of the Arteries and Veins.* New York, Springer-Verlag, 1986, p 21. Used by permission.)

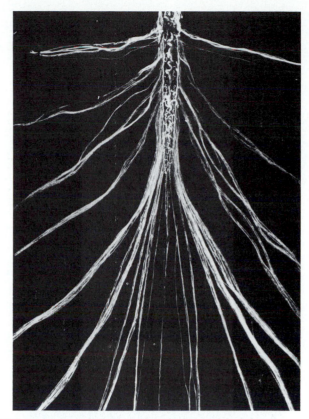

FIG 8–9.
A photograph of the dorsal aspect of the distal third of the spinal cord, conus medullaris, and cauda equina from a man aged 41 years, from the specimen illustrated in Figure 8–8. The posterolateral longitudinal arterial trunks, which in this specimen are rather fine, are clearly seen forming a loop distally at the tip of the conus, where they anastomose with the anterior median longitudinal arterial trunk of the spinal cord. (From Crock HV, Yamagishi M, The Crock MC: *The Conus Medullaris and Cauda Equina in Man, an Atlas of the Arteries and Veins.* New York, Springer-Verlag, 1986, p 23. Used by permission.)

from the surface of the cord before joining individual spinal nerves, each eventually penetrates the dural sac in the region of the axilla of the dural root sleeve and emerges in the epidural space to join the internal vertebral venous plexus (Figs 8–13 and 8–14). There is a primitive valve mechanism in radicular veins at the sites of their entry into the internal vertebral venous plexus which prevents retrograde flow of blood into them. This accounts for the fact that in vivo vascular injection studies of the spinal cord circulation fail to fill the intradural veins of the cauda equina. *The direction of venous flow in the cauda equina is centrifugal.* In cases of foraminal or nerve root canal stenosis, obstruction of sections of the internal vertebral venous plexus prevents venous outflow from the intradural veins of the cauda

equina and leads to intradural venous dilatation and root edema. In extreme cases of longstanding cauda equina claudication, this chronic venous obstruction may lead to one form of arachnoiditis of the cauda equina. Venous dilatation and root edema may be identified in radiculograms. Ooi et al.,[9] using myeloscopy during stress testing, have demonstrated a marked increase in the size of intradural radicular veins in patients with symptomatic spinal stenosis.

Large veins in the lamina and pedicles also drain into the internal vertebral venous plexus (Fig 8–15). The anastomoses between pedicle veins and those of emerging nerve roots in the intervertebral foramen assume great importance in operations combining spinal canal decompression with pedicle screw in-

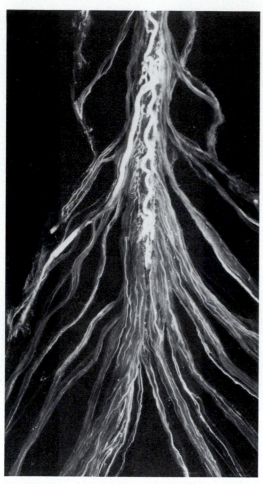

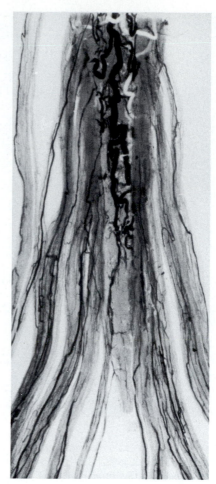

FIG 8–10.
A photograph of the posterior surface of the spinal cord from a man aged 21 years showing the posterior median longitudinal venous trunk over the conus medullaris. From this channel, directly, or from the vasa corona which encircle the cord, venous channels pass down to accompany each of the filaments of the cauda equina. (From Crock HV, Yoshizawa H: *The Blood Supply of the Vertebral Column and Spinal Cord in Man.* New York, Springer-Verlag, 1977, p 61. Used by permission.)

sertion and spinal fusion. Damage to both systems simultaneously can lead to serious neurologic deficits after operation.

PRACTICAL APPLICATIONS IN SURGERY FOR SPINAL STENOSIS

The most vulnerable vessels in operations for spinal stenosis are those which supply the paraspi-

FIG 8–11.
A photograph of the conus medullaris and cauda equina showing the venous system filled with blood. On the *right side* of the figure the posterolateral longitudinal arterial channel of the spinal cord has been filled with a barium sulfate suspension. The complexity of the veins in the upper part of the cauda equina can be clearly seen.

nal muscles. Multilevel lumbar canal decompressions may be very time-consuming taking between 2 to 4 hours. The uninterrupted use of self-retaining retractors in such cases may lead to extensive muscle necrosis and subsequent dense scar formation. This potentially serious complication may be prevented altogether by removing the retractors for short periods at intervals of 30 to 40 minutes throughout the length of the operation.

The "neural" intraspinal arterial branches to the spinal cord and cauda equina arise only millimeters anterior to the pars interarticularis, inferior to individual vertebral pedicles. Damage to these vessels may occur during the early stages of exposure of the roof of the spinal canal if excessive force is used

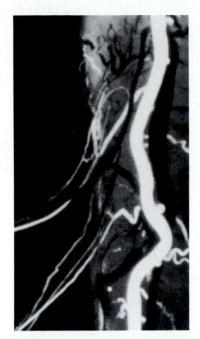

FIG 8–12.
A detailed photograph of the anterior surface of the conus medullaris from a girl aged 13 years. The dissection shows the interrelationships between two anterior radicular arteries where they join the median longitudinal channel of the spinal cord with the corresponding veins. (From Crock HV, Yamagishi M, Crock MC: *The Conus Medullaris and Cauda Equina in Man, an Atlas of the Arteries and Veins.* New York, Springer-Verlag, 1986, p 30. Used by permission.)

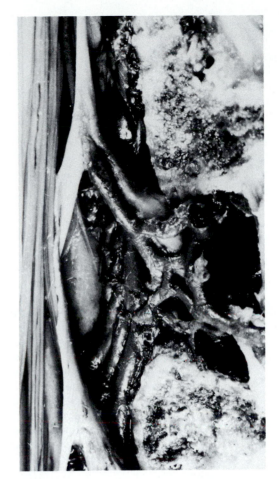

FIG 8–13.
A photograph of a dissection to show details of the anterior internal vertebral venous plexus in a man aged 71 years. In the *top left-hand side* of the figure, the dural edge is shown with a large radicular vein lying alongside. This vein emerges in the axilla between the dural sheath and the emerging nerve root to enter the internal vertebral venous plexus, segments of which are of greater diameter (dissected by H Yoshizawa). (From Crock HV, Yoshizawa H: *Clin Orthop* 1976; 115:6–21; and *The Blood Supply of the Vertebral Column and Spinal Cord in Man.* New York, Springer-Verlag, 1977, p 52. Used by permission.)

while separating the paraspinal muscles. In attempting to control the heavy bleeding which may then occur, the use of coagulating diathermy anterior to the pars interarticularis must be avoided.

In the literature dealing with operative technique in the treatment of spinal stenosis, attention is usually focused on the amount of bone which needs to be removed in order to relieve the stenosis. Spinous processes are still frequently removed and only a small central laminectomy is performed at one or more levels. This limited dissection may be followed by neurologic deficits such as footdrop and symptoms of claudication may persist, as the essential vascular decompressions in the nerve root canals and intervertebral foramina have been incomplete.

The primary aim in decompressing the spinal canal is to relieve venous obstruction in the nerve root canals and intervertebral foramina. Hemorrhage within the canal should be controlled with pledgets and some form of hemostatic agent such as Spongostan (Johnson & Johnson Products, Inc., New Brunswick, N.J.). Electrocoagulation, even with bi-

polar equipment, should be avoided. The cauda equina veins are slender where they enter the internal vertebral venous plexus and can be easily destroyed if coagulating diathermy is used in that area, leading to sequelae such as regional paresis or intractable pain (see Figs 8–13 and 8–14).

The interrelationships of the blood supply of the vertebral column, spinal cord, and cauda equina become important when posterior spinal fusion and pedicle screw fixation are added to decompressive procedures. Reports of paraplegia following lumbo-

A

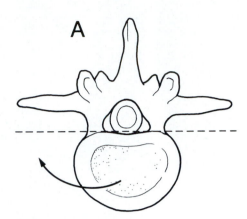

B

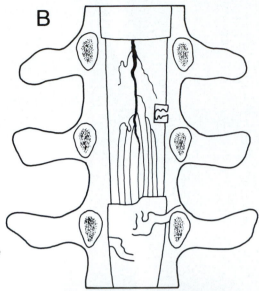

FIG 8–14.
A, a diagram to show the plane of section through the vertebral column at the base of the pedicles, the contents of the spinal canal remaining in situ. **B,** a drawing depicting the spinal canal viewed from in front following removal of the vertebral bodies by coronal section through the bases of the pedicles as depicted in **A.** The anterior wall of the dural sac has been removed except in the lower third where portions of the anterior internal vertebral venous plexus lie on its surface. On the *right,* just above the pedicle of the central lamina, a small segment of the anterior dural wall is also depicted with a fragment of the anterior internal vertebral venous plexus. The vessels on the anterior surface of the conus and cauda equina are outlined. **C,** a photograph of the anterior surface of the conus medullaris and upper third of the cauda equina viewed from in front orientated as depicted in **A** and **B.** On either side of the conus in an extradural position, the internal vertebral venous plexus has been filled with barium sulfate. The anterior median longitudinal venous channel of the spinal cord is filled with blood and two large right- and left-sided anterior radicular veins can be seen coursing from this channel distally over one and a half vertebral segments on the right and two and a half vertebral segments on the left, respectively. These veins diminish in caliber as they approach their exit points in the axillary regions of individual nerve root sheaths where they enter the internal vertebral venous plexus. (From Crock HV, Yamagishi M, Crock MC: *The Conus Medullaris and Cauda Equina in Man, an Atlas of the Arteries and Veins.* New York, Springer-Verlag, 1986, p 63. Used by permission.)

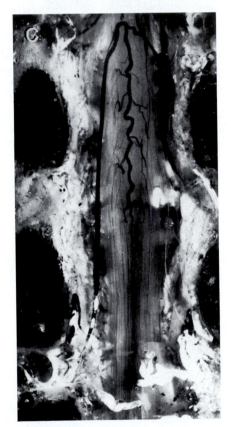

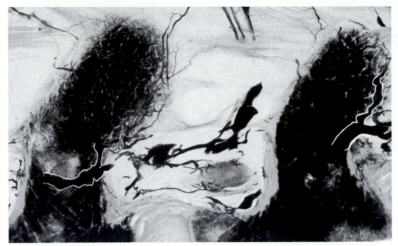

FIG 8–15.
A detailed photograph of a specimen cut in the sagittal plane through the intervertebral foramen at the level of the pedicles from a man aged 68 years. Details of the venous drainage of nerve roots in the foramen and their relationships to the anterior and posterior radicles of the internal vertebral venous plexus are shown. Note also the important relationships between veins in the pedicles and radicles of the internal vertebral venous plexus in the intervertebral foramen. The margins of the pedicular veins have been outlined in white. (From Crock HV, Yamagishi M, Crock MC: *The Conus Medullaris and Cauda Equina in Man, an Atlas of the Arteries and Veins.* New York, Springer-Verlag, 1986, p 68. Used by permission.)

sacral operations of this type appear occasionally. The theoretical basis of this disaster almost certainly lies in the combination of arterial injuries to the paraspinal muscles and to the neural intraspinal branches of the lumbar arteries, compounded by thrombosis of the pedicle veins extending to involve the internal vertebral venous plexus and lumbar radicular veins. In some of these cases the paraplegia may recover, suggesting that its basis may have been an isolated disturbance of the venous systems of the vertebral column and spinal cord.

REFERENCES

1. Adamkiewicz AA: Die Blutgefässe des menschlichen Rückenmarkes: Die Gefässe der Rückenmarkesoberfláche. *Sitzungsbericht Akad Wiss Math Naturwissenschaften* 1882; 85:101–130.
2. Batson OV: The function of the vertebral veins and their role in the spread of metastases. *Ann Surg* 1940; 112:138–149.
3. Crock HV, Yamagishi M, Crock MC: *The Conus Medullaris and Cauda Equina in Man, an Atlas of the Arteries and Veins.* New York, Springer-Verlag, 1986.
4. Crock HV, Yoshizawa H: *The Blood Supply of the Vertebral Column and Spinal Cord in Man.* New York, Springer-Verlag, 1977.
5. Crock HV, Yoshizawa H, Kame S: Observations on the venous drainage of the human vertebral body. *J Bone Joint Surg [Br]* 1973; 55:528–533.
6. Dommisse GF: *The Arteries and Veins of the Human Spinal Cord from Birth.* Edinburgh, E & S Livingstone Ltd, 1975.
7. Gillilan LA: The arterial blood supply of the human spinal cord. *J Comp Neurol* 1958; 110:75–103.
8. Kadyi H: *Ueber die Blutgefässe des menschliche Rückenmarkes; nach einer im XV. Bande der Denkschriften der mach. naturw. Classe der Akademie der Wissenschaften in Krakau erschienenen Monographie, aus dem Polnischen übersetzt vom Verfasser.* Lemberg, Poland, Gubrynowicz & Schmidt, 1889.
9. Ooi Y, Mita F, Satoh Y: Myeloscopic study on lumbar spinal canal stenosis with special reference to intermittent claudication. *Spine* 1990; 15:544–549.
10. Parke W, Gammel K, Rothman RH: Arterial vascularization of the cauda equina. *J Bone Joint Surg [Am]* 1981; 63:53–61.
11. Suh TH, Alexander L: Vascular system of the human spinal cord. *Arch Neurol Psychiatry* 1939; 41:659–677.
12. Tanon L: *Les artères de la moelle dorso-lombaire* (thesis). Paris, Vigot, 1908.
13. Uhtoff HK: *The Embryology of the Human Locomotor System.* Heidelberg, Springer-Verlag, 1990.
14. Willis T: *Cerebri anatome.* London, 1664.

9

Biomechanics of Spinal Stenosis

Malcolm H. Pope, Ph.D., Dr.Med.Sci.
Leon Grobler, M.D.

DEFINITIONS

A workable definition of *lumbar stenosis* is a narrowing of the vertebral canal or intervertebral foramina due to bony or soft tissue components. The abnormal narrowing in the former case will lead to compression of the dural sac and in the latter case will cause compression of the exiting nerve root or dorsal root ganglion. Narrowing of the canal may involve one or more levels and all or just part of the canal. At the disc interspace, compression may be due to posterior vertebral osteophytes, hypertrophic facet joints (a problem of the unstable and the aging spine) or to a disc protrusion. The far-out syndrome, described by Wiltse et al.,[64] involves compression of the L5 nerve root between the ala of the sacrum and the transverse process of L5.

INDICATIONS FOR SURGERY

Decompression

Operations for spinal stenosis are common. Decompression is generally regarded as being necessary if there is a neurologic deficit with pressure on the spinal cord and nerve roots and segmental signs of degenerative changes that coincide with the clinical findings. Thus, the goal of decompressive surgery is to eliminate the cause of neural impingement, relieve the symptoms of leg pain and lower extremity weakness, while minimizing the risk of instability. Decompression is indicated relatively more often in the presence of lateral canal stenosis since this is more likely to remain symptomatic and responds less favorably to conservative therapy. It is less indicated in the absence of unequivocal neurologic signs or if performed for back pain only.[9, 23, 27, 54] Abnormal disc bulging may be an important finding although one must note that all healthy discs bulge under axial compressive loading. Bilateral decompression of radiologically proven central stenosis is usually indicated despite unilateral symptomatology.

Instability following decompression is always a concern. However, there is a virtual guarantee against postsurgical instability if osteophytes have produced a spontaneous arthrodesis. Likewise, a loss of disc space height can indicate reduced segmental motion (Fig 9–1). Obviously, some concern for relative vertebral instability exists if there is degenerative spondylolisthesis. In general, compression is less severe at lumbar levels than higher up in the vertebral canal since the cauda equina starts below L2 and there is more space in the lumbar canal. Disc space narrowing and symptoms on hyperextension are suggestive, but by no means diagnostic findings. When the spinal canal has a constriction

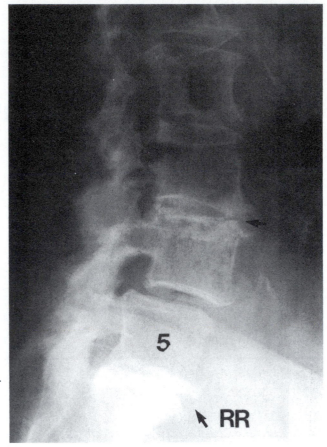

FIG 9−1.
This patient presented with symptomatic spinal stenosis secondary to L4−5 degenerative spondylolisthesis. The L4−5 level is more prone to increased slippage because of the rigid system created by disc space narrowing at the L3−4 and L5−S1 levels.

causing pressure that requires bilateral decompression, decompressive laminotomy or laminectomy may be necessary. Laminotomy maintains mechanical stability but is sometimes technically difficult owing to the narrow interlaminar space or if there is ossification of the ligamentum flavum. Laminectomy is easier to perform and has less morbidity. Laminectomy is also preferable if bilateral decompression is necessary at multiple levels, if disc surgery is performed at the same time, and for cases with previous decompression at an adjoining level. Buckling and hypertrophy of the ligamentum flavum necessitates adequate removal of this structure as part of the decompressive procedure.[15]

Anterior midline compression by a disc may be decompressed by bilateral laminectomy, or occasionally by multiple posterior laminectomies. Anterior and posterior compression may occur as the result of a combination of posterior vertebral osteophytes or protruded discs anteriorly and ligamentum flavum involvement and facet joint osteoarthritis posteriorly (Fig 9−2). Adequate decompression is usually obtained by bilateral laminectomy, but sometimes a partial vertebral body resection is necessary. If the compression is more extensive, multiple bilateral laminectomies will probably be required.

The importance of the posterior structures in providing axial, translational, and rotational stiffness has been well documented experimentally.[39, 45] Bilateral laminectomy at several levels carries a higher risk of vertebral instability than a one-level laminectomy. This risk has been incompletely studied biomechanically. However, it is self-evident that the excision of spinous processes and interspinous ligaments, which bilateral laminectomy entails, reduces vertebral stability. White and Panjabi[62] note that instability will not be a problem if the functional integrity of the three columns—the intervertebral disc (and vertebral body), and the two facet joints—are preserved. Consequently, no instability usually occurs when the lateral half to one third of the articular processes on one side is preserved and no discectomy is carried out. Functional integrity of the motion segment usually exists if there is a loss of disc space height accompanied by increased osteophyte formation (Fig 9−3). Calcified annulus fibro-

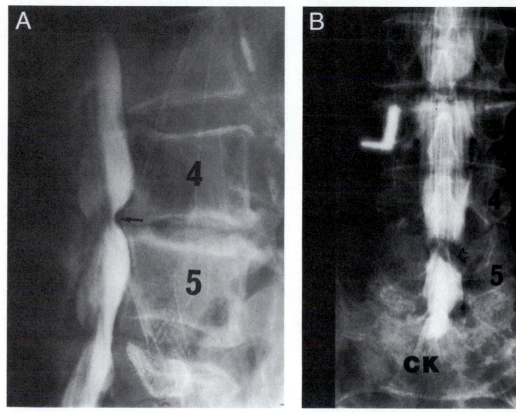

FIG 9–2.
A and **B,** this 86-year-old man presented with the symptomatology of spinal stenosis and at surgery was found to have compression due to facet joint disease as well as an extruded disc fragment (unusual at this age). The disc herniation is shown by the *open arrow* **(B).**

sus, joint capsule, ligamentum flavum, and severe disc space narrowing protects against postoperative instability.[20] White and Panjabi[62] suggest that in subtotal facetectomy, remodeling of the residual portion of the articular process may restore some stability. The probability of instability of a motion segment is greater when bilateral facetectomy and discectomy are performed. The chance is increased further if the continuity of the posterior longitudinal ligament is interrupted along the midsagittal plane. If a motion segment is preoperatively unstable, bilateral laminectomy that extends laterally may increase the instability, especially if the pars interarticularis is damaged (Fig 9–4). This is particularly true when a discectomy is performed simultaneously. Careful decision making is crucial when deciding on the extent of decompression.

Panjabi et al.[43] showed that the lumbar intervertebral foramen tends to close during extension (Fig 9–5). Procedures that tend to increase the normal lordosis may aggravate the situation. Thus, decom-

pression of the foramen may be indicated, especially in degenerative spinal stenosis where a dynamic foraminal component is suspected.[46] Care should also be taken when using internal fixation to preserve the normal lumbar lordotic pattern (Fig 9–6,A–C).

In one of the few biomechanical studies, Stokes[55] performed load-displacement studies on lumbar spine specimens to determine the effect of sequential unilateral and bilateral division of the pars intraarticularis (see also Stokes et al.[56]). Division of the pars interarticularis caused a significant increase in axial rotation and a smaller increase in lateral bending. There was no increase in anteroposterior (AP) shear, so it was to be assumed that facetectomy or laminectomy will not lead to an increased risk of spondylolisthesis. However, it is more likely that the amount of facet resected along with the orientation of the facet will have a major effect on the stability.

Goel et al.,[11, 12] using whole lumbar spine specimens, studied the effects of partial laminectomy

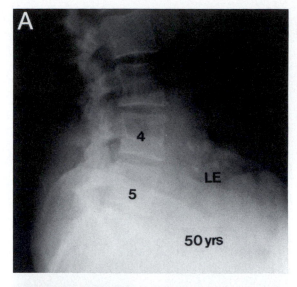

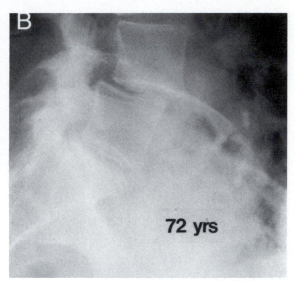

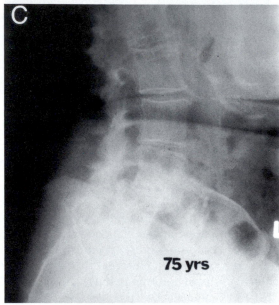

FIG 9–3.
A–C, after presenting with symptoms at the age of 50 years, this patient shows radiologic evidence of progressive disc space narrowing over 25 years. Even wide segmental decompression at the L4–5 level will not necessitate stabilization.

and facetectomy along with denucleation of the disc. The injuries were induced in the following way:

1. Partial laminectomy: Soft tissues were debrided from the posterior aspect of L4 and L5. A hemilaminectomy was performed at the L4–5 level by first excising the ligamentum flavum and then the inferior aspect of the lamina of L4 and the superior aspect of L5.

2. Partial facetectomy: The second sequential injury procedure consisted of a partial L4–5 facetectomy. The medial aspect of the lateral overhang of the right apophyseal joint at L4–5 was transected.

3. Subtotal discectomy: The annulus was identified and a subtotal discectomy was performed.

4. Total discectomy: Complete excision of the nucleus.

The three-dimensional, load-displacement behavior of the five vertebral bodies (L1–L5) of a specimen in flexion, extension, lateral bending, and axial twisting were determined for a maximum 3.0 Nm moment. It was found that there was an increased primary flexion for a given moment which was accompanied by additional AP shear. Translational instability was found to be greater with total than with subtotal discectomy (Table 9–1).

Progressive postoperative slippage has been reported clinically ranging from 28% to 100%,[22, 34] depending on the extent of decompression and preop-

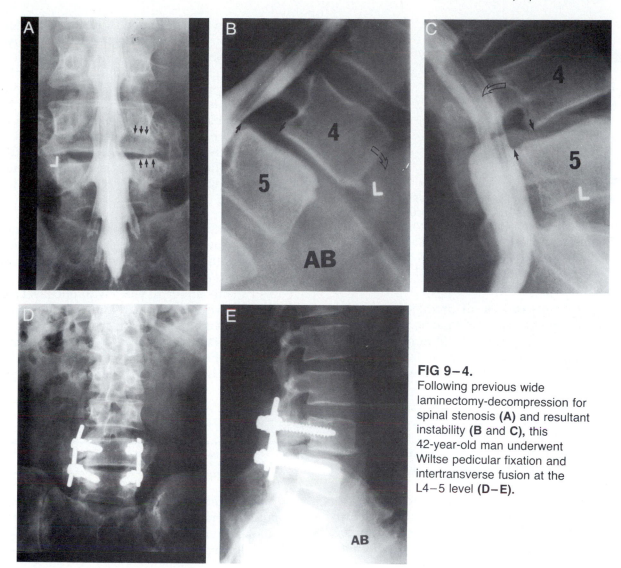

FIG 9–4.
Following previous wide laminectomy-decompression for spinal stenosis **(A)** and resultant instability **(B and C)**, this 42-year-old man underwent Wiltse pedicular fixation and intertransverse fusion at the L4–5 level **(D–E)**.

erative stability. While this obviously is not the rule but the exception, it illustrates the risk of instability following laminectomy. Three structures play an important role in the integrity of the motion segment, i.e., the pars interarticularis, intervertebral disc, and zygapophyseal joints. Excessive removal of the pars or stress fracture due to osteopenia can result in progressive slip. The facet joint is biplanar with the medial half in the coronal plane (resists forward displacement) and the lateral half in the sagittal plane (resists axial rotation). If medial facetectomy is excessive, there is a potential for increased forward displacement, and excess lateral facetectomy could result in rotational instability (Fig 9–7,A). The angle of the facet joints on computed tomography may influence decision making in deciding the extent of de-

compression and the necessity for internal stabilization (Fig 9–7,B, C). Adequate decompression is nevertheless our primary goal but one should realize the potential for instability.

Fusion

The use of a fusion after spinal decompression is very common, especially in degenerative spondylolisthesis.[4, 17, 25, 38, 42, 47] Decompression for lateral recess stenosis does not require fusion if unilateral.[42] The surgical choice is one of type of fusion (placement), type of bone (allograft or autograft), and necessity for supplementary mechanical fixation (see Chapter 28). All surgery to the motion segment should be considered potentially damaging to its ki-

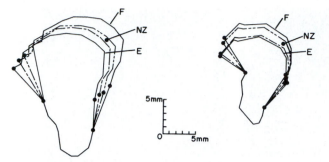

FIG 9–5.
Changes in size of the intervertebral foramen when in the neutral zone *(NZ)*. Size increases in flexion *(F)*, and decreases in extension *(E)*. (Adapted from White AA, Panjabi MM: Biomechanical considerations in the surgical measurement of the spine, in *Clinical Biomechanics of the Spine*, ed 2. Philadelphia, JB Lippincott, 1990, pp 511–634.)

nematics and thus capable of producing long-term changes. Fusion can also lead to abnormal kinematics at adjacent motion segments. In terms of the type of fusion material, iliac bone graft is usually preferred (see Chapter 30). However, the morbidity at the donor site can be quite bothersome.[5, 33, 58, 66] Some surgeons make judicious use of the bone removed during the laminectomy for the fusion. From a biomechanical standpoint, allografts are as good as autografts. Polymethyl methacrylate (PMMA), which is discussed later, should be avoided as part of a "fusion procedure."

The indications for fusion are controversial and discussed further in Chapter 31. Callahan et al.[3] recommended fusion after every laminectomy to prevent abnormal motion and progressive deformity.

Tile,[60] however, recommends fusion only for selected patients (those with segmental instability, degenerative spondylolisthesis, or significant prior low back pain). Feffer et al.[6] found that patients with degenerative spondylolisthesis who had decompressive surgery had better outcomes if they also had a fusion. Kornblatt and Jacobs[29] found that rigid internal fixation resulted in an improved fusion rate. West et al.[61] reported a 92% fusion rate and early return to activities using pedicular fixation. White and Panjabi[62] suggested fusion after decompression in the following cases:

1. Patients under 75 years of age with stenosis and having a bilateral laminectomy removing more than 50% of the total facet joints at one level (Fig 9–8).
2. Patients under 50 years with one-level stenosis having bilateral laminectomy and discectomy and loss of articular process.
3. Patients under 75 years in whom a significant portion (30%–40%) of the annulus fibrosis is removed at the time of decompression.

IATROGENIC STENOSIS

Spinal fusion and disc excision are extremely common operations but they are not without complications. Frymoyer and Selby[8] reported hypermobility following disc excision and Frymoyer et al.[7]

TABLE 9–1.

Level of Significant Changes in Motion at Various Motion Segments (With Respect to Normal Specimen Behavior)*

Load Type	Primary Motion	After Stabilization of L4–5		
		L3–4	L4–5	L5–S1
FLX	R_x	↑	↓	WI
	T_z	—	—	—
EXT	R_x	↓	↓	—
	T_z	↓	—	—
RLB	R_z	—	—	—
	T_x	—	—	—
LLB	R_z	—	—	—
	T_x	—	—	—
LAR	R_y	—	—	—
RAR	R_y	—	—	—

* ↑ = an increase in motion at $P < .05$; ↓ = a decrease in motion at $P < .05$; — = no significant change in motion; WI = a weak increase in motion at $P < .1$ or $P < .2$; FLX = flexion; EXT = extension; RLB = right lateral bending; LLB = left lateral bending; LAR = left axial rotation moment; RAR = right axial rotation moment.

A

B

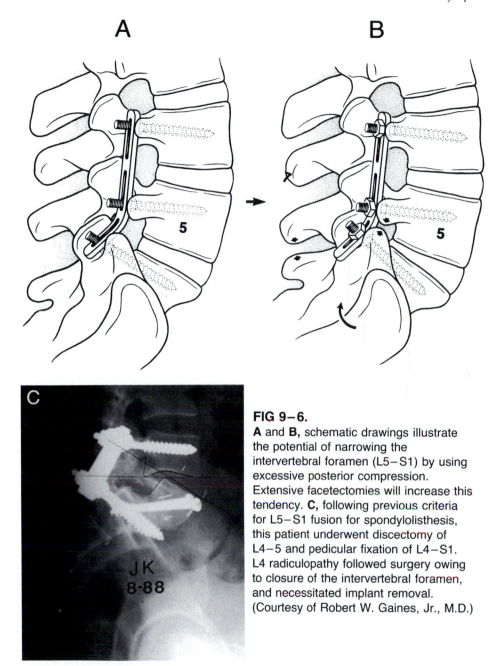

C

JK
8-88

FIG 9–6.
A and **B,** schematic drawings illustrate the potential of narrowing the intervertebral foramen (L5–S1) by using excessive posterior compression. Extensive facetectomies will increase this tendency. **C,** following previous criteria for L5–S1 fusion for spondylolisthesis, this patient underwent discectomy of L4–5 and pedicular fixation of L4–S1. L4 radiculopathy followed surgery owing to closure of the intervertebral foramen, and necessitated implant removal. (Courtesy of Robert W. Gaines, Jr., M.D.)

noted traction spurs, hypermobility, and disc narrowing above fusions. Using sophisticated stereoradiographic techniques, Stokes et al.[57] and Tibrewal et al.[59] noted increased coupled motion above the fusion, a possible precursor of remodeling. Harris and Wiley[18] reported spondylolysis above fusions and related this to stress concentration. Leong et al.[36] noted that greater than half of the discs adjacent to fusions went on to early disc degeneration, while Louis[40] found a higher incidence of herniated discs at such levels. Hutter[21] suggested that fusion

should be considered at the initial excision of degenerated or protruding disc material since most patients develop foraminal scar stenosis following decompression procedures.

Given these complications, it is perhaps no surprise that Lipson,[37] Hutter,[21] and Hirabayashi et al.[19] reported spinal stenosis above the fusion level. The last-named also reported an increased rate of spinal stenosis at levels both above and below anterior fusions which they attributed to increased stresses.[19] As further evidence of higher stresses at

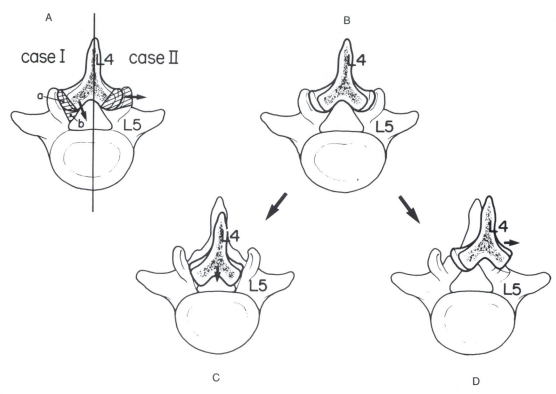

FIG 9–7.
A, by removing an excess amount of the coronal part of the superior facet and the inferior facet of L4, an increased tendency for forward displacement may occur (case I). Likewise, if an excessive portion of the sagittal component is removed (case II), rotational instability may occur: *a,* L4 medial facet; *b,* L5 lateral facet. **B,** normal relationship of L4 to L5. There is anterior and lateral stability. **C,** if the facet joint is angled in the sagittal plane, there is a greater tendency for forward displacement after even moderate decompression. Internal fixation may be indicated in these cases. Similar to case I. **D,** axial placement of the facet joints will give enough stability provided decompression is not extended more laterally than the pedicle. Similar to case II. Enough facet joint should be left intact to prevent progressive slippage.

adjacent levels, Kahanovitz et al.[24] reported frequent facet joint changes. Goel et al.[14] suggest that the 5% incidence of spinal stenosis following fusion may be due to increased stresses around the facets. These stresses were determined by means of a finite element model and are discussed in Chapter 31. It is proposed that the stresses induce osteoarthritis and thus cause bone hypertrophy. These stresses, perhaps in conjunction with other factors, may result in hypertrophy in bony elements overlying the existing nerve roots.

The primary surgical choice, of type of fusion, should be a biomechanical decision. As noted by White and Panjabi,[62] the fusion mass should be placed, if possible, at the maximum distance from the instantaneous axis of rotation in order to be more effective in preventing movement around the axis. Thus, a fusion located on the tips of the spinous processes is more effective than one that is

placed closer to the axis of rotation, as shown in Figure 9–9. This principle also applies to axial rotation and lateral bending. Thus, an anterior bone graft has relatively less leverage than a posterior one with regard to its efficacy in preventing motion.

A related consideration is that of the effect of the placement of the fusion in allowing elastic deformation of the reconstituted motion segment. It is clear that a fusion that involves the spinous processes, lamina, and transverse processes is more rigid than one that involves only the spinous processes (Fig 9–9). In some careful experimental work, Rolander[48] demonstrated that after posterior fusion motion will still take place with the physiologic forces that are applied to the motion segment.

Lee et al.[35] loaded motion segments in vitro in which they had simulated posterior, bilateral lateral, and anterior fusions. All three fusion types increased the axial and bending stiffness. The anterior

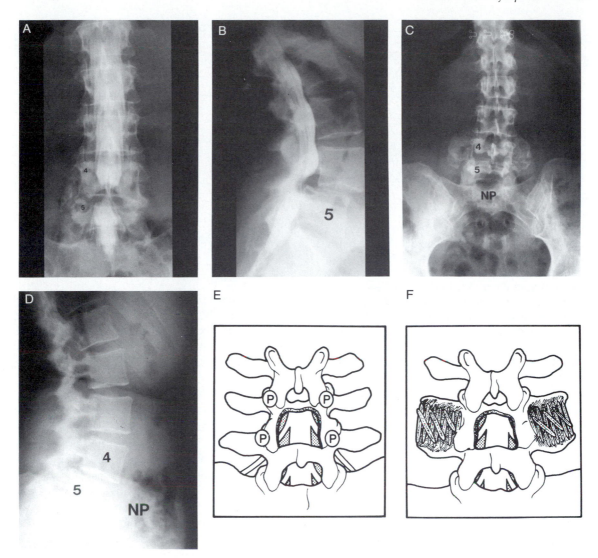

FIG 9–8.
A and **B,** a 50-year-old woman presented with symptomatic spinal stenosis due to grade I degenerative spondylolisthesis at L4–5. **C** and **D,** bilateral subtotal laminectomy and fusion at the L4–5 level resulted in an excellent clinical and radiologic outcome. **E** and **F,** schematic reproduction of the procedure performed. *P* = pedicle.

fusions were the stiffest, followed by the bilateral lateral and the posterior. All types or fusions had increased stress at the adjacent segments, especially in the facet joints, but the bilateral lateral fusion had the least effect on the adjacent unfused segments. The posterior fusion permitted anterior motion and was associated with the highest stresses on the adjacent segments. Naturally, it is the posterolateral fusion that normally has to be used in the case of decompression for spinal stenosis.

INTERNAL FIXATION

Internal fixation is used in conjunction with fusion to afford immediate stability. Internal fixation is also said to increase the fusion rate (see Chapter 28). The goals of an internal fixation device are to realign the vertebra, maintain alignment, prevent instability, and permit fusion. However, given the plethora of internal fixation devices available, judicious choice is essential and the biomechanical ra-

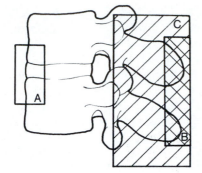

FIG 9-9.
To prevent flexion movement, fusion at **B** is more effective than fusion at **A** because it is farther from the instantaneous axis of rotation, other factors being constant. Fusion mass **C** will provide more rigidity than fusion mass **B** because the vertebrae are more supported and thus deflection is prevented. (Adapted from White AA, Panjabi MM: Biomechanical considerations in the surgical measurement of the spine, in *Clinical Biomechanics of the Spine*, ed 2. Philadelphia, JB Lippincott, 1990, pp 511-631.

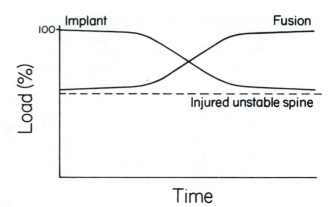

FIG 9-10.
Schematic of ideal fusion consolidation and implant fatigue.

tionale should be carefully reviewed. As Ashman et al.[1] point out, the basic objective is to provide sufficient stability to enhance fusion. However, there are obvious limitations imposed by the type of surgery. Harrington rods and Knodt rods are typically contraindicated in stenosis surgery since they apply flexion and kyphosis and require several levels for fixation. Likewise, there is only a limited role for sublaminar wiring, because often the laminae are removed.

A given internal fixation system should have undergone both experimental and clinical studies and should have had extensive component analysis, as well as functional evaluation. Systems for internal fixation are presently subject to Food and Drug Administration (FDA) regulations in the United States. Whitecloud[63] has nicely summarized the FDA regulations facing spinal implants in the United States. FDA assigns devices to class I, II, or III, with class I being of minimal risk. Spinal implants are class III, and generally the newer ones must obtain an IDE (investigational device exemption) before being used on patients. An IDE is a carefully supervised clinical trial. In an alternative, called the 510(K) process, a manufacturer submits documentation that a device is equivalent to a commercialized pre-1976 device. However, this is rarely applicable to a new spinal fixation system.

One of the most important considerations in the biomechanical test of an internal fixation device is that of fatigue. The loads are shared by the spine operated on, the internal fixation device, and the

fusion mass. As shown in Figure 9-10, the fusion mass initially has no strength and the load is taken by the fixation system. Hopefully, the implant will not fatigue before the fusion is complete. Obviously, if the implant is too stiff, too weak, or has poor fatigue characteristics, the fusion rate will be compromised. The grafted area would be exposed to too little load or motion, the graft would resorb, and no fusion healing would occur. Another consideration is that during the early stages of healing, when new vessels are forming to vascularize the fusion site and find a pathway across the site, a more rigid construct is desirable. As healing progresses a less rigid construct, which will allow more loads to the fusion mass, is desired. Nagel et al.[41] found, when performing in vivo experiments on sheep in which spine fusions had been performed, that a 36% strain in the bone graft resulted in nonunion, whereas a strain of 10% allowed the bone graft to fuse. Thus there appears to be a model strain distribution.

Sublaminar wiring techniques are obviously not indicated in the case of a laminectomy but may have limited applications if only the lateral recess is decompressed. Even so, some clinicians feel that wires under the lamina should be avoided when other options are available. When selecting wires, adequate tensile strength is the most important factor. The wires of larger diameter are stronger. When wiring is used, it is usually in conjunction with implants with segmental wiring (Hartsill, Luque double "L," C-rod). This technique involves a wire that encircles the lamina and the device. The wires form a strong attachment, and stiffen the spine. However, entry into the spinal canal has inherent risks which must be considered in relation to the advantages.

Screw Fixation

King[26] described facet screw fixation to improve arthrodesis. Kornblatt and co-workers[28, 29] found that in posterolateral lumbosacral fusions, the use of facet joint screws affixed to the pelvis decreased the pseudarthrosis rate and also the time required for fusion. Boucher[2] and Pennal et al.[44] also used screws through the facets and into the alae. Obviously, there is little applicability of this technique in the case of laminectomy.

However, screws are an important structural component in the pedicle fixation devices. These systems have recently been extensively studied. Krag et al.[30, 31] and Zindrick et al.[67] studied the pullout strength of pedicular screws. Intrapedicular and transpedicular fixation of the spine was developed by Roy-Camille and co-workers.[49–51] The advantage of the pedicle fixation device is that fixation can be achieved without the involvement of more than one vertebra above and below the level of the defect. The significant problems of hook and rod dislocation are also eliminated. The other advantages are that the devices have relatively high stiffness, allow distraction and compression, and have a great deal of adjustability. The most comprehensive design rationale is given by Krag et al.[30–32]

One method to increase the pullout strength is to optimize the design of the screw itself. For a given major diameter (limited by the pedicle size), pitch, minor diameter, and tooth shape can be varied. Krag et al.[30, 31] evaluated the effect of these variables. A smaller minor diameter and a smaller pitch appeared to increase pullout strength in most cases. It was concluded that the thread type was not important. Wittenbert et al.[65] has similar findings. Krag et al.[30, 31] concluded that the pullout strengths of the designs tested (700–2,000 newtons) were adequate for pedicle fixation.

Skinner et al.[53] found that an increase in the major screw diameter was related to greater pullout strength. It was also noted that the placement of the transpedicular screw into the vertebral end plate significantly increased the pullout strength. Screws that penetrated the anterior cortex of the vertebral body had no greater pullout strength than those placed into the vertebral body, and this technique should be avoided because of the risk to adjacent structures. Krag et al.[30, 31] established that the pullout strength at 50% depth was 75% to 77% (depending upon load type) of that at 80% depth; strength for screws at 100% ("to the far cortex") depth was 124% to 154% of that at 80%. They showed that an increase in depth of penetration from 50% to 80% is accompanied by a 30% gain in screw placement strength. They recommended that the increased strength of deeper screw placement must be balanced against possible increased operative risk. Zindrick et al.[67] noted that for the sacral fixation, screws directed straight anteriorly into the ala were not as rigidly fixed as those aimed laterally into the ala at 45° or medially into the first sacral pedicle. Wittenbert et al.[65] and George et al.[10] found that there was no significant difference in pullout strength based on whether or not a probe or drill was used to provide the entryway for the pedicle screw.

Zindrick et al.[67] and Wittenbert et al.[65] found that in pullout strength studies osteoporosis was a significant factor. This is an important consideration in older patients. Zindrick et al.[67] also found that large-diameter screws engaging the cortex of the anterior vertebral body provided the greatest strength. They also found that PMMA was helpful in restoring fixation to loose screws and that pressurized cement doubled the required pullout force. However, the possibility of unintentional neural element encroachment and the major difficulty in removing the PMMA later, if necessary, are significant drawbacks to this strengthening method. It should be noted that PMMA has no adhesive qualities and forms a poor attachment to bone because of a fibrous membrane that develops between it and the bone. Biomechanical study of surgical constructs suggest that the weak link is the attachment of the cement to the bone. Nonetheless, this is an alternative in the osteoporotic spine.

Krag et al.[30, 31] made extensive studies of the morphology of the vertebrae. It was found that the pedicle-axis angle is 0 to 10 degrees in the lower thoracic spine, and gradually increases caudally throughout the lumbar region (Fig 9–11). The data of Saillant[52] are shown for comparison: good agreement exists except for L1–4. Figure 9–12 shows that the pedicle diameter increases below L2. Pedicles smaller than 5 mm were seldom encountered below T10 and pedicles 8 mm or larger were encountered in significant numbers at all levels, from 35% at T9 up to 100% at L5.

Krag et al.[30, 31] also measured (see Fig 9–13) screw path length (chord length) for both 0- and the 15-degree approach angles. It was found that a slightly longer path length always results from the 15-degree approach. It was also found that the path length is almost constant over the vertebral levels studied.

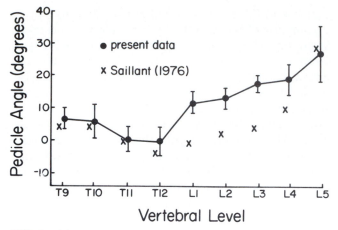

FIG 9–11.
Pedicle axis angle relative to the sagittal plane for each vertebral level. Means ±1 SD are shown, compared with means *(x)* from Saillant.[52] (Adapted from Krag MH, Beynnon BD, Pope MH, et al: *Clin Orthop* 1986; 203:75–98.)

Flexible Fixation

Flexible systems have had limited use in the spine. One early device was the Gruca-Weiss spring, which has no place in the treatment of spinal stenosis.

Recently, Graf[16] has introduced an alternative flexible fixation system. The Graf system involves a pedicle implant which is connected to the adjacent one by Dacron-type bands allowing for some degree of flexibility (Fig 9–14). The Graf system includes limited surgery, is easy to apply, and does not involve a fusion. It has been used with excellent results in patients with rotational instability and decompression. Despite extensive usage in Europe this method still needs to be evaluated in long-term follow-up studies. A controlled prospective clinical study and additional biomechanical studies are in the planning to assess the clinical use of this concept.

COMPARATIVE TESTING

Many authors have compared the relative stability of different fixation systems. However, there is no great consensus on the optimal test method or the best injury model and few are relevant to decompression.

Wittenbert and associates[65] recently completed a comparative study in the calf lumbar spine using a burst fracture model. The implant systems tested were as follows: (1) AO Fixateur Interne (with 5-mm Schanz screws); (2) Steffee plates (with 7-mm screws); (3) Harrington distraction rods; and (4) Luque plates (with 6.5-mm cannulated screws).

The AO system was significantly less stiff than the Luque system. There were no other significant differences in the stiffness of the implants. The Harrington and Luque systems both allowed significantly less posterior distraction than did the AO fixateur interne and the Steffee systems.

In some very relevant studies, Goel et al.[13] destabilized specimens at the L4–5 level to stimulate bilateral decompression. These are discussed in Chapter 31.

FIG 9–12.
Pedicle diameter means ±1 SD for each vertebral level, measured three different ways and compared with means *(x)* from Saillant.[52] (Adapted from Krag MH, Beynnon BD, Pope MH, et al: *Clin Orthop* 1986; 203:75–98.)

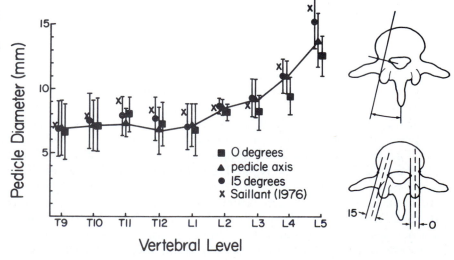

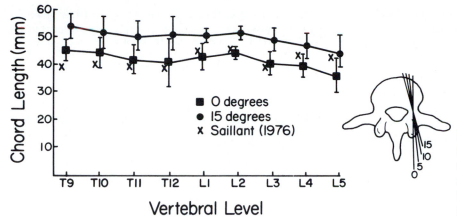

FIG 9–13.
Screw path length (chord length) measured along a line at 0 and 15 degrees relative to the sagittal plane. (Adapted from Krag MH, Beynnon BD, Pope MH, et al: *Clin Orthop* 1986; 203:75–98.)

SUMMARY

Lumbar spinal stenosis has become more prominent as a disease entity owing to improved methods of diagnosis, heightened diagnostic suspicion among physicians, the increase in the geriatric population, and the higher expectations of that population to maintain a high level of pain-free activity, even after "retirement age." Surgical procedures are also done more readily on the older age group as a result of improved surgical techniques and postoperative care. This inevitably results in a new set of rules in decision making, in a higher rate of potential complications, and requires more careful consideration and planning of the treatment options.

The goal of surgery in spinal stenosis is to decompress the neural elements while minimizing the risk of instability. This goal necessitates a thorough knowledge of the factors responsible for stability as well as a more-than-working knowledge of the potential effects of "wide decompression." We should think of stability when decompressive surgery is done for spinal stenosis.

Indications for spinal stabilization in this group

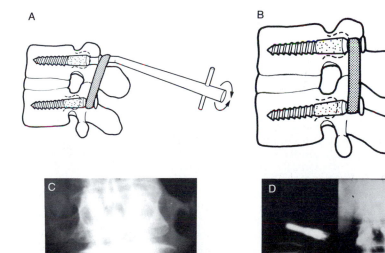

FIG 9–14.
A and **B**, schematic drawing of the pedicular screw and the method of tension band attachment. **C** and **D**, preoperative and postoperative radiographs of the flexible fixation system. (From Graf H, 1990. Used by permission.)

of patients is still very much empiric and needs to be assessed in prospective studies conducted in liaison with both clinicians and basic scientists. Correlates need to be developed in assessing the potential for instability after removal of different anatomic structures, (i.e., facet joints, interspinous ligaments, and intervertebral discs). The assessment and treatment of dynamic spinal stenosis is one of the most challenging clinical enigmas and sets the stage for close cooperation between clinician and engineer.

The era of internal fixation has brought a new dimension of factors for the spinal surgeon to consider. The effect of rigid fixation on the adjoining levels, the placement and type of bone graft to be used, and the influence of the bone density (osteopenia) on the fixation are but a few important considerations to address in this patient population.

A knowledge of the principles of both experimental and clinical studies is essential to make valid decisions on the pros and cons of the vast number of internal fixation devices made available to the surgeon by a continuously expanding industry. A thorough knowledge of the FDA guidelines in evaluating these systems will simplify the decision-making process for the surgeon.

Despite the refinement of biomechanical stabilization devices and extensive metallurgic knowledge, biological fusion is required for ultimate stability! Extensive research is being carried out to find the perfect implantable bone graft substitute and this creates a new dimension of biomechanical problems and questions.

The treatment of spinal stenosis calls for a thorough realization and knowledge of the biomechanical factors important in spinal stabilization—emphasizing once more the symbiotic coexistence of the clinician and biomechanical engineer in treating spinal problems.

REFERENCES

1. Ashman RB, Bechtold JE, Edward T, et al: In vitro spine implant mechanical testing protocol. *J Spinal Dis* 1989; 2:274–280.
2. Boucher HH: A method of spinal fusion. *J Bone Joint Surg [Br]* 1959; 41:248.
3. Callahan RA, Johnson RM, Margolis RN, et al: Cervical facet fusion for control of instability following laminectomy. *J Bone Joint Surg [Am]* 1977; 59:991.
4. Cauchoix MD, Benoist M, Chassaing V: Degenerative spondylolisthesis. *Clin Orthop* 1976; 115:122–129.
5. Dodd CAF, Ferguson CM, Freedman L, et al: Allograft versus autograft bone in scoliosis surgery. *J Bone Joint Surg [Br]* 1988; 70:431–434.
6. Feffer HL, Wiesel SW, Auckler JM, et al: Degenera-tive spondylolisthesis: To fuse or not to fuse. *Spine* 1985; 10:287.
7. Frymoyer JW, Hanley EN Jr, Howe J, et al: A comparison of radiographic findings in fusion and nonfusion patients two or more years following disc surgery. *Spine* 1979; 4:435.
8. Frymoyer JW, Selby DK: Segmental instability: Rationale for treatment. *Spine* 1985; 10:280.
9. Garfin S, Glover M, Booth R, et al: Laminectomy: A review of the Pennsylvania Hospital experience. *J Spinal Dis* 1988; 1:116–133.
10. George DC, Krag MK, Johnson CC, et al: Hole preparation techniques for transpedicle screws. *Spine* 1991; 16:181–184.
11. Goel VK: Three-dimensional motion behavior of the human spine—A question of terminology. *J Biomech Eng* 1987; 109:353.
12. Goel VK, Goyal S, Clark C, et al: Kinematics of the whole lumbar spine—effect of discectomy. *Spine* 1985; 10:543.
13. Goel VK, Weinstein JN, Found EM Jr: Biomechanics of lumbar and thoracolumbar spine surgery, in Goel VK, Weinstein JN (eds): *Biomechanics of the Spine: Clinical and Surgical Perspective.* Boca Raton, Fla, CRC Press, 1990, pp 181–232.
14. Goel VK, Weinstein JN, King Liu Y, et al: Biomechanics of spine stabilization, in Weinstein JN, Wiesel SW (eds): *The Lumbar Spine.* Philadelphia, WB Saunders Co, 1990, pp 195–211.
15. Grabias S: Current concepts review. The treatment of spinal stenosis. *J Bone Joint Surg [Am]* 1980; 62:308–313.
16. Graf H: Personal communication, 1990.
17. Hanley EN Jr: Decompression and distraction-derotation arthrodesis for degenerative spondylolisthesis. *Spine* 1986; 11:269–276.
18. Harris RI, Wiley JJ: Acquired spondylolysis as a sequel to spine fusion. *J Bone Joint Surg [Am]* 1963; 45:1159.
19. Hirabayashi K, Maruyama T, Wakano K, et al: Postoperative lumbar canal stenosis due to anterior spinal fusion. *Keio J Med* 1981; 30:133.
20. Hopp E, Tsou PM: Postdecompression lumbar instability. *Clin Orthop* 1988; 227:143–151.
21. Hutter CG: Spinal stenosis and posterior lumbar interbody fusion. *Clin Orthop* 1985; 193:103.
22. Johnsson KE, Willner S, Johnsson K: Post-operative instability after decompression for lumbar spinal stenosis. *Spine* 1986; 11:107–110.
23. Johnsson KE, Willner S, Patterson H: Analysis of operated cases with lumbar spinal stenosis. *Acta Orthop Scand* 1981; 52:427–433.
24. Kahanovitz N, Bullough P, Jacobs RR: The effect of internal fixation without arthrodesis on human facet joint cartilage. *Clin Orthop* 1984; 189:204.
25. Kaneda K, Kazama H, Satoh S, et al: Followup study of medial facetectomies and posterior-lateral fusion with instrumentation in unstable degenerative spondylolisthesis. *Clin Orthop* 1986; 203:159–167.
26. King D: Internal fixation for lumbosacral fusion. *J Bone Joint Surg [Am]* 1948; 30:560.
27. Kirkaldy-Willis WH, Paine KW: Lumbar spinal stenosis. *Clin Orthop* 1974; 99:30.
28. Kornblatt MD, Casey MP, Jacobs RR: Internal fixation

in lumbosacral spine fusion. A biomechanical and clinical study. *Clin Orthop* 1986; 203:141.

29. Kornblatt MD, Jacobs RR: The effect of bracing and internal fixation on lumbar spine fusion in 100 consecutive cases: A preliminary report. Presented at the 12th International Society for the Study of the Lumbar Spine, Sydney, Australia, April 14–19, 1985.

30. Krag MH, Beynnon BD, Pope MH, et al: An internal fixator for posterior application to short segments of thoracic, lumbar, or lumbosacral spine. *Clin Orthop* 1986; 203:75.

31. Krag MH, Beynnon BD, Pope MH, et al: An internal fixator for posterior application to short segments of the thoracic, lumbar, or lumbosacral spine: Design and testing. *Clin Orthop* 1986; 203:75–98.

32. Krag MH, Pope MH, Wilder DG: Mechanisms of spine trauma features of spinal fixation methods. Part I: Mechanisms of injury, in Ghista D (ed): *Spinal Cord Injury Medical Engineering*. Springfield, Ill, Charles C Thomas, Publisher, 1986, pp 133–157.

33. Kurz LT: Complications of harvesting iliac bone underrecognized. *Orthopaedics Today* 1987; 7:1.

34. Lee CK: Lumbar spinal instability (olisthesis) after extensive posterior spinal decompression. *Spine* 1983; 8:429.

35. Lee CK, Langrana NA, Yang SW: Lumbosacral spinal fusion: A biomechanical study. *Spine* 1984; 6:574.

36. Leong JC, Chun SY, Grange WJ, et al: Long term results of lumbar interveretebral disc prolapse. *Spine* 1983; 8:793.

37. Lipson SJ: Degenerative spinal stenosis following old lumbosacral fusions. *Orthop Trans* 1983; 7:143.

38. Lombardi JS, Wiltse LL, Reynolds J, et al: Treatment of degenerative spondylolisthesis. *Spine* 1985; 9:821–827.

39. Lorenz M, Patwardhan A, Vanderly R Jr: Load bearing characteristics of lumbar facets in normal and surgically altered spinal segments. *Spine* 1983; 8:122.

40. Louis R: Single-staged posterior lumbo-sacral fusion by internal fixation with screw plates. Presented at 12th International Society for the Study of the Lumbar Spine. Sydney, Australia, April 14–19, 1985.

41. Nagel FJ, Seals DR, Hanson P: Time to fatigue during isometric exercise using different muscle masses. *Int J Sports Med* 1988; 9:313–315.

42. Nasca RJ: Rationale for spinal fusion in lumbar spinal stenosis. *Spine* 1989; 14:451–454.

43. Panjabi MM, Takuta K, Goel VK: Kinematics of lumbar intervertebral foramen. *Spine* 1983; 8:348–357.

44. Pennal GF, McDonald GA, Dale GG: A method of spinal fusion using internal fixation. *Clin Orthop* 1964; 35:86.

45. Posner I, White AA, Edwards T, et al: A biomechanical analysis of the clinical instability of the lumbar and lumbosacral spine. *Spine* 1982; 7:374.

46. Rauschning W, Lee CK, Glenn W: Lateral lumbar spinal canal stenosis: Classification, pathologic anatomy and surgical decompression. *Spine* 1988; 13:313–320.

47. Reynolds JB, Wiltse LL: Surgical treatment of degenerative spondylolisthesis. *Spine* 1979; 4:148–149.

48. Rolander SD: Motion of the lumbar spine with special reference to stabilizing effect of posterior fusion. *Acta Orthop Scand [Suppl]* 1966; 90:1.

49. Roy-Camille R, Saillant G, Berteaux D, et al: Osteosynthesis of thoracolumbar spine fractures with metal plates screwed through the vertebral pedicles. *Reconstr Surg Traumatol* 1976; 15:2.

50. Roy-Camille R, Saillant G, Berteaux D, et al: Early management of spinal injuries, in McKibbin B (ed): *Recent Advances in Orthopaedics*. New York, Churchill Livingston, 1979, pp 21–30.

51. Roy-Camille R, Saillant G, Berteaux D, et al: Vertebral osteosynthesis using metal plates. Its different uses (in French). *Chirurgie* 1979; 105:597.

52. Saillant G: Anatomical study of vertebral pedicles. Surgical application (in French). *Rev Chir Orthop* 1976; 62:157.

53. Skinner R, Transfeldt EE, Maybee J, et al: Experimental testing and comparison of screw design variables in transpedicular screw fixation: A biomechanical study. Presented at the American Academy of Orthopaedic Surgeons 55th Annual Meeting, Atlanta, 1988.

54. Spengler D: Degenerative stenosis of the lumbar spine: Current concepts review. *J Bone Joint Surg [Am]* 1987; 69:305–308.

55. Stokes IAF: Mechanical function of the facet joints in the lumbar spine. *Clin Biomech* 1988; 3:101.

56. Stokes IAF, Counts DC, Frymoyer JW: Experimental instability in the rabbit lumbar spine. *Spine* 1989; 14:68–72.

57. Stokes IAF, Wilder DG, Frymoyer JW, et al: Assessment of patients with low back pain by biplanar radiographic measurement of intervertebral motion. *Spine* 1981; 6:233.

58. Summers BN, Eisenstein SM: Donor site pain from the ilium a complication of lumbar spine fusion. *J Bone Joint Surg [Br]* 1989; 71:677–680.

59. Tibrewal SB, Pearcy MJ, Portek I, et al: A prospective study of lumbar spinal movements before and after discectomy using biplanar radiography: Correlation of clinical and radiographic findings. *Spine* 1985; 12:455.

60. Tile M: The role of surgery in nerve root compression. *Spine* 1984; 9:57.

61. West J, Bradford D, Ogilvie J: Steffee instrumentation: Two year results. Presented at Scoliosis Research Society, 23rd Annual Meeting, Baltimore, September 1988.

62. White AA, Panjabi MM: Biomechanical considerations in the surgical measurement of the spine, In *Clinical Biomechanics of the Spine*, ed 2. Philadelphia, JB Lippincott Co, 1990, pp 511–631.

63. Whitecloud TS: Clinical trials for spinal implants. *J Spinal Dis* 1989; 2:285–287.

64. Wiltse LL, Guyer RD, Spencer CW, et al: Alar transverse process impingement of the L5 spinal nerve: The far-out syndrome. *Spine* 1984; 9:31–41.

65. Wittenbert RH, Lee KS, Coffee MS, et al: The effect of screw design and bone mineral density on transpedicular fixation in human and calf vertebral bodies. Presented at Seventh Meeting of European Society of Biomechanics, Aarhus, Denmark, 1990.

66. Younger EM, Chapman MW: Morbidity at bone graft donor sites. *J Orthop Trauma* 1989; 3:192–195.

67. Zindrick MR, Wiltse LL, Widell EH, et al: A biomechanical study of intrapeduncular screw fixation in the lumbosacral spine. *Clin Orthop* 1986; 203:99.

PART II

Pathogenesis

10

The Three-Joint Complex

Tommy H. Hansson, M.D., Ph.D.
Nils R. Schönström, M.D., Ph.D.

In a series of studies we wanted to clarify certain aspects of, particularly, central spinal stenosis that we believe still are controversial or not fully understood. These aspects are: (1) Where in the spinal canal is the likelihood for encroachment upon the nerve structures greatest? (2) Which structures or tissue components cause the encroachment? (3) Is there a critical size below which further constriction will cause pathophysiologic disturbances explaining the symptoms and signs of spinal stenosis? (4) How do motion and loading of the spine influence the available space in the spinal canal?

PATHOPHYSIOLOGY AND PATHOMECHANICS

The taxonomy of spinal stenosis includes several completely different entities. Regardless of whether the genesis of spinal stenosis is congenital or developmental, and the location central or lateral, the classic symptoms of this condition are the same, i.e., claudication, pain, weakness, and numbness. Characteristically the symptoms appear in conjunction with physical activities or postural changes. Wilson[32] found that sensory symptoms in most cases preceded the motor symptoms and also that the pain usually is paresthetic in quality. Physical activities beyond the initial discomfort, however, could result in pronounced motor weakness.

Several authors have described the apparent discrepancy between symptoms and signs in patients with spinal stenosis. This discrepancy is most obvi-ous if the spinal stenosis patient is examined without any relation to physical activities or posture changes.

Another peculiarity with spinal stenosis symptoms is that some subjects are able to continue their activities if they perform these in certain postures, typically in forward flexion. This posture dependency in eliciting symptoms has by some clinicians been included in the battery of examination tests for spinal stenosis, e.g., the so-called stoop and bicycle tests.[5] The history, in combination with a thorough physical examination is in most cases indicative of the diagnosis of spinal stenosis (see Chapter 17). To allow a definite morphologic diagnosis, however, information from other diagnostic tools has to be incorporated.

Insufficient blood supply through damaged (syphilitic) vessels causing ischemia of the medulla was one early explanation for the symptoms and signs of spinal stenosis.[1, 4, 9, 20] Presently most investigators who are trying to approach the pathophysiology of spinal stenosis tend to favor mechanical factors. Most probably these mechanical factors are directly interfering with the nerves, either in the spinal canal proper or in the root canals. Even if the detailed pathophysiology in causing the symptoms and signs of spinal stenosis is unknown, it is reasonable to believe that the mechanical pressure causes disturbances in the blood circulation or nutrition, or both, of the nerves or nerve roots. These effects are discussed further in Chapter 7. As Wilson and collaborators pointed out,[33] the mechanical interference can be brought about either by a change in posture, e.g., extension of the lumbar spine (postural stenosis), or by physical activities (ischemic stenosis).

Degenerative changes in the three-joint complex (the disc and the facet joints) can cause a direct mechanical encroachment upon the nerves centrally in the spinal canal proper or laterally in the root canals. That both soft and bony tissues can contribute to this encroachment has been well established. Encroachment by soft tissue in degenerative stenosis has been reported repeatedly.[2, 7, 14-16, 34]

In degenerative cases of spinal stenosis, bony osteophytes, located especially at the edges of the facet joints or around the end plates at the rim of the intervertebral disc, might also exert direct mechanical pressure on the adjacent nerve structures.

WHERE IS THE ENCROACHMENT?

In the congenital type of stenosis described primarily by Sarpyener,[21] as well as in the developmental type first described by Verbiest,[30] the bony ring of the spinal canal is the space-limiting structure conflicting with the abundant nerves and nerve roots.

Schönström and co-authors convincingly demonstrated through examination of consecutive computed tomographic (CT) sections of stenotic spines that the risks for encroachment are greatest at the disc level, or more precisely at the level of the disc-joint complex (Fig 10–1). They estimated that at least from a dynamic standpoint, more than 90% of

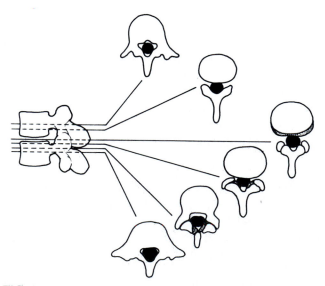

FIG 10–1.
Transverse sections of a lumbar spine segment showing the structures of the spinal canal at different levels.

all the changes which possibly could affect the structures within the spinal canal were present at or around the disc-joint complex. In the same study the authors also found that, at the level of the disc-joint complex, the walls of the spinal canal were made up of both the upper and the lower neigboring vertebrae.[22] The latter observation clearly emphasized that the bony ring or the bony canal of each vertebra, which consists of the posterior wall of the vertebral body, the pedicles, and the laminae, contributes only to a minor degree to the wall of the spinal canal at the joint complex level. In most clinical studies it has been observed that the bony ring of the spinal canal, as in congenital or developmental stenosis, is the cause of the constriction only in a minority of all stenotic cases (<10%). Degenerative changes at the joint level, on the other hand, are responsible for the constriction in more than 90% of all stenotic spines.[8, 22] In other words, the bony canal in itself is rarely the encroaching structure (except in congenital and developmental stenosis).

The bony measurements of the spinal canal are therefore relevant only in developmental spinal stenosis, whether of congenital or achondroplastic origin.

WHAT IS CAUSING THE ENCROACHMENT?

As shown in Figure 10–2 the predominating structures outlining the spinal canal at the joint level are the disc, the facets from the lower vertebra, the joint capsules from both facet joints, the ligamentum flavum, and the most caudal part of the lamina from the cranial vertebra. It is quite evident that the disc, through a disc herniation or just by bulging into the spinal canal, is the structure which has the greatest potential for occupying available space in the spinal canal.

A thick ligamentum flavum was earlier believed to be an important space-occupying factor not only in spinal stenosis but also in other back disorders, such as disc herniations. The thickness was believed to be caused by hypertrophy. No one has been able to demonstrate a true hypertrophy of the ligament, however.[34, 35] The normal ligamentum flavum has been found to be prestressed (in tension).[17, 25] In the absence of hypertrophy it is likely that the thickening of the ligamentum flavum is a straightforward mechanical phenomenon in which the highly elastic

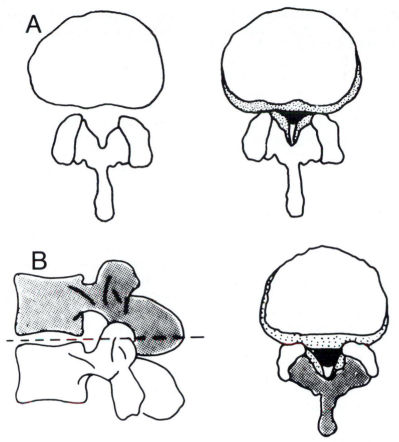

FIG 10–2.
A and **B,** the structures surrounding the cauda equina at the three-joint level, and the difference between the "bony spinal canal" and the "soft tissue spinal canal" at this level.

ligament when allowed to relax retracts and bulges into the spinal canal. In contrast to the rigid bony ring of the spinal canal, the abundance of soft tissues at the joint complex level no doubt make this region more prone to variations in both shape and size. The prerequisites for the occurrence of dynamic as well as postural changes of the shape and size of the canal are therefore better met at the joint level than at any other spinal level.

IS THERE A CRITICAL SIZE OF THE CAUDA EQUINA?

Numerous studies have been performed to address this question. When does a protruding disc, osteophytes at the rim of the disc, a "hypertrophied" yellow ligament, or all in combination encroach upon the nerve tissues? Verbiest measured the size of the canal with a stenosimeter during surgery.[31] Although hardly meant to be definitions of spinal stenosis, his suggestion that an anteroposterior (AP) diameter of less than 10 mm marked "absolute" stenosis and an AP diameter between 10 and 12 mm marked "relative" stenosis frequently was used as such. These measures were readily transferred to, and used to interpret, among others, the myleographic pictures of the spinal canal in patients with stenotic problems.

To assess objectively the size of the spinal canal and the presence of stenosis, the most frequently used diagnostic techniques are ultrasonography, plain radiography, positive contrast myelography, CT, and magnetic resonance imaging (MRI).

Ultrasonography

Ultrasonography has been used to determine both the diameter of the spinal canal and its cross-sectional area.[10, 19] Porter and collaborators reported that the measures obtained through ultrasonographic examinations could predict not only spinal stenosis but also other types of back pain. Although ultrasonography reflects the size of the dural sac, the accuracy and precision of this technique have been found to be so low that its use in the individual case is questionable.[10] Other techniques have evolved replacing sonography, at least for the time being.

Plain Radiography

Plain radiography still has an unsurpassed value in spinal stenosis. It can reveal metabolic diseases of the bone which might be of importance for the diagnosis of spinal stenosis. In addition, it can reveal post-traumatic and postoperative changes, and the degree of degenerative changes as well as infections and neoplasms (see Chapter 18). The presence of stenosis might be strongly suggested from the radiographs but for the exact diagnosis they are usually insufficient.

The AP diameter of the bony spinal canal can be determined with standard radiographic technique.[6] Since the bony canal with few exceptions, however, is not the reason for the encroachment, the value of the bony measurements is restricted.

Positive Contrast Myelography

Positive contrast myelography has long been a useful method to diagnose spinal stenosis. One advantage compared to more recent techniques is that myelography can be performed with the subject standing. The standing position will load the spine and can therefore "provoke" changes otherwise invisible.

In comparison to CT and MRI one of the advantages of this technique is that the appearance and, to some extent, function of the entire spine can be captured in one picture. Through relatively simple modifications of technique, the capacity of myelography in diagnosing spinal stenosis can be profoundly improved. This has been demonstrated by, among others, Sortland and co-workers[28] who included flexion-extension films in their examination. This permits examinations of the spine in a quasidynamic situation which can reveal, e.g., posturally induced changes.

It has also been suggested that loading of the spine in combination with myelography will add important information, especially about the behavior of the discs in the stenotic spine.[27]

Others have let the patient undergoing myelography flex the spine while sitting to allow the contrast to pass beyond a block when present.[12] In this way it is possible to depict the canal distal to the block, which increases the value of the examination.

Computed Tomography

The use of CT has added new possibilities in obtaining information about the morphology of the spinal canal.[22] Measures not possible to obtain through positive contrast myelography became available. Since it was believed that a close correlation existed between the bony canal and its content, a lot of interest was initially focused on the bony surroundings of the spinal canal. Normal values were presented for the AP and interpedicular diameters of the bony canal as well as the transverse areas.[29] Schönström and collaborators[22] found no correlations between the size of the bony spinal canal and the size of the dural sac in a CT study that was performed in order to reveal the pathomorphology of the spinal canal in stenotic spines. On the contrary, they found that many patients with nondisputable clinical claudication symptoms had bony canals which were close to normal in size. Their results seemed to indicate that the size of the dural sac (cross-sectional area) is the measure that best reflects the symptoms and signs of spinal stenosis.

Magnetic Resonance Imaging

MRI can reveal multilevel stenosis in one sequence. There are indications that sagittal T1-weighted images tend to underestimate the degree of stenosis, whereas T2-weighted images overestimate a stenotic condition. It is possible that MRI can indicate the duration and extent of compression and thus add information beyond the capacities of other techniques. We believe that MRI as well as CT can be used for determination of the critical size of the cauda equina.

Measurements

As discussed above, a direct mechanical pressure is the probable cause of the clinical symptoms in spinal stenosis. In central spinal stenosis the cauda equina, with few exceptions, is compressed asymmetrically (Fig 10–3). A diameter measure of the cauda is therefore unlikely to accurately represent the shape of the compressed nerve structures. Since both CT and MRI techniques can easily depict the spinal canal and the cauda equina in transverse sections, the cross-sectional area seemed to be a measure which in a more appropriate way reflected the size of the spinal canal and the cauda equina or

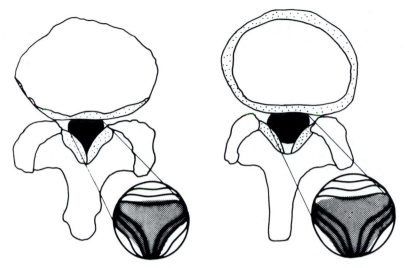

FIG 10–3.
This drawing indicates the asymmetric shape of the cauda equina in a stenotic patient.

the spinal cord. In a couple of experiments we evaluated the minimal cross-sectional area of the cauda below which a further constriction would cause increased intrathecal pressure. To that purpose we excised intact dural sacs from fresh cadavers. Each specimen was mounted in its proximal end while the distal end was hanging freely. Through a small incision in the dura a pressure-sensitive catheter was inserted in among the nerve roots. A circular clamp was then applied around the cauda at levels corresponding to each disc space (about 5 mm below the exit of the L2, L3, and L4 nerve roots, respectively). The tip of the pressure-sensitive catheter was placed at the same level.

While the pressure was continuously recorded, the clamp was gradually constricted. At the first sign of a pressure increase, defined as *the critical size,* the size of the clamp was determined.[23] In this experiment the cerebrospinal fluid (CSF) could not be contained in the dural sac. Since the CSF might have some pressure-modulating effects in an intact system, we chose to repeat the experiment in a somewhat modified fashion. This time we exposed the intact cauda equina (CSF included) in situ in the bodies of recently deceased subjects. The critical size was once again determined with a similar technique but now in a system which contained CSF.[24] The results from the two experiments were very similar. At the L3–4 level in the first experiment the mean critical size was 71.5 ±13.3 mm^2, while in the second study it was 77.4 ±13.3 mm^2. The studies were performed both in Sweden and in the United States and included both men and women as well as black and white subjects. The apparent similarities and the relatively minor variations found made us suggest that the cauda equina of the human spine is approaching its critical size when it has a cross-sectional area less than 80 mm^2.

In order to evaluate the clinical relevance of our critical size measure, the preoperative cross-sectional area of the dural sac was analyzed retrospectively in a group of subjects operated on for central spinal stenosis.[23] The average area in this group of patients was 90 ±24 mm^2, which seemed to confirm the validity of a critical size of around 80 mm^2. More recently, Rydevik and Ohlmarker have found experimentally that previously existing very low pressures among the nerve roots will disturb the venous return of blood from the cauda (personnel communication, 1991).

Our experiments also indicated that there was a strong tendency for a time-related reduction of externally applied pressures among the nerve roots of the externally compressed cauda.[24] The significance of this tissue creep is not yet well understood.

HOW DO MOTION AND LOADING OF THE SPINE INFLUENCE THE SIZE OF THE SPINAL CANAL?

Loading of the human spine will compress the discs and typically result in a bulging or protrusion of the disc into the spinal canal. The magnitude of disc compression during everyday loading exposures was recently determined *in vivo.*[11] The disc levels measured were L3–4 and L4–5. The measurements took place in healthy volunteers. A special linkage transducer system, the intervertebral motion device, (IMD), was developed. The IMD was attached to Kirschner-wires which were drilled into adjacent spinous processes in the lumbar spine in order to guarantee rigid fixation. Although the motions were determined in nondegenerated spines, the shrinkage (creep) of a single disc could exceed 1 mm after 5 minutes of upright sitting.

The resulting bulge of the disc has not been determined *in vivo.* *In vitro*, however, several studies have demonstrated that axial loading of vertebral motion segments increases the bulge or protrusion of the tested disc.[3, 13] The considerable loss of disc height *in vivo* indicates that even normal exertions and motions might increase bulging or disc protrusion.

As mentioned before it is well known empirically that different postures of the spine, e.g., extension, and also loading of the spine, e.g., carrying an object, can provoke the typical symptoms of spinal stenosis in certain subjects. That the shape of the spinal canal varies in different positions was demonstrated by Sortland and co-workers[28] when they performed positive contrast myelography examinations

in both flexion and extension. Dimension changes in the spinal canal have been found also in anatomic studies of the spine.[16] A bulging disc, a buckling ligamentum flavum, and an alteration (relative) in the position of two adjacent vertebrae (as in olisthesis) all have been thought to be able to change the shape of the spinal canal more or less momentarily.

In order to estimate these possible changes we performed a CT study on cadaveric lumbar spines.[26] The spines were mounted in a special loading device which allowed predetermined static loading in compression or distraction. In addition to the axial loading the spine could simultaneously be kept in all positions from full flexion to full extension (Fig 10–4). After the amount of loading and sagittal rotation had been selected, the device, including the spine, was placed in the gantry of a CT scanner. All spines were tested in: (1) 250-newton axial compression, (2) 250-newton axial distraction, (3) 200-newton axial compression in flexion, and (4) 200-newton axial compression in extension, all while the CT examination took place.

The cross-sectional area was the most important parameter in this study. Note, however, that this experiment was performed in order to evaluate the invasion from outside of the different structures lining the spinal canal. The cross-sectional area in this study therefore describes the spinal canal proper. The loading during testing was chosen to corre-

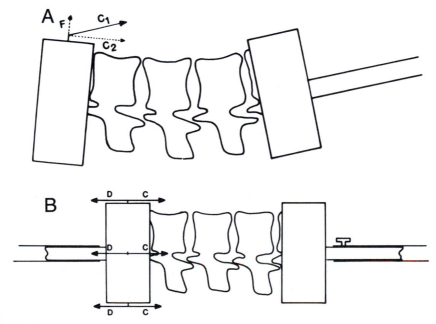

FIG 10–4.
A, B, the loading device allowing flexion-extension during simultaneous compression or distraction.

spond to the differences in physiologic loading of the spine between upright standing and a supine position (500 newtons).

The cross-sectional area of the spinal canal changed on average by 50 ±30 mm² when comparisons were made between distraction and compression, representative of lying on the back vs. standing upright. When the spines were moved from full flexion to full extension while loaded as in a standing position the cross-sectional area of the spinal canal was reduced on average by 40 ±20 mm². In this study it was evident that the disc was responsible by far for most of the reduction of the available space in the spinal canal. The findings confirmed the earlier assumptions of possible significant dynamic changes within the spinal canal.

The results in this study made us conclude that in a subject with an already relatively stenotic spine, i.e., an available cross-sectional area in the spinal canal of, e.g., 100 mm², extension of the spine can reduce this space below the critical size (80 mm²) and thus cause the classic symptoms of spinal stenosis. The posture and load variations in the size of the spinal canal ought to be considered also in CT and MRI evaluations. During these examinations the subjects are positioned supine on the examination table. This will consequently "de-load" the spine in comparison to standing upright and probably relieve some bulging and thus pressure from the cauda.

CONCLUSION

Encroachment upon the nerve structures in the spinal canal most likely occurs at the level of the three-joint complex. The encroachment is usually caused by a bulging or protruding disc, a bulging ligamentum flavum, and degenerative changes at the facets. When the cross-sectional area of the cauda equina is less than 80 mm²—the critical size—there are both experimental and clinical indications of disturbances among the nerve roots which might explain the symptoms and signs of spinal stenosis. The size of the spinal canal changes significantly when the spine is extended or loaded. These size variations might explain the postural dependency of the stenotic symptoms in some subjects.

REFERENCES

1. Bergmark G: Intermittent spinal claudication. *Acta Med Scand Suppl* 1950; 245:30–36.
2. Blau JN, Logue V: Intermittent claudication of the cauda equina. An unusual syndrome resulting from central protrusion of a lumbar intervertebral disc. *Lancet* 1961; 1:1080–1086.
3. Brinckmann P, Horst M: The influence of vertebral body fracture, intradiscal injection, and partial discectomy on the radial bulge and height of human lumbar discs. *Spine* 1985; 10:138–145.
4. Déjérine I: La claudication intermittente de la moelle épinière. *Presse Med* 1911; 19:981–984.
5. Dyck P, Pheasant HC, Doyle JB, et al: Intermittent cauda equina compression syndrome. Its recognition and treatment. *Spine* 1977; 2:75–81.
6. Eisenstein S: The morphometry and pathological anatomy of the lumbar spine in South African Negros and Caucasoids with specific reference to spinal stenosis. *J Bone Joint Surg [Br]* 1977; 59:173–180.
7. Epstein JA, Epstein BS, Lavine L: Nerve root compression associated with narrowing of the lumbar spinal canal. *J Neurol Neurosurg Psychiatry* 1962; 25:165–176.
8. Getty CJM: Lumbar spinal stenosis. The clinical spectrum and the results of operation. *J Bone Joint Surg [Br]* 1980; 62:481–485.
9. Hunt JR: The lumbar type of intermittent claudication. *J Med Sci* 1912; 143:173–177.
10. Kadziolka R, Asztély M, Hanai K, et al: Ultrasonic measurement of the lumbar spinal canal. *J Bone Joint Surg [Br]* 1981; 63:504–507.
11. Kaigle AM, Magnusson M, Pope MH, et al: In vivo measurement of intervertebral creep: A preliminary report. *Clin Biomech* in press.
12. Kapila A, Chakeres DW: Flexed sitting maneuver for complete lumbar myelography in patients with severe spinal stenosis and apparent block. *Radiology* 1986; 160:265–267.
13. Keller TS, Hansson TH, Holm ST, et al: In vivo creep behavior of the normal and degenerated porcine intervertebral disk: A preliminary report. *J Spinal Dis* 1988; 1:267–278.
14. Kirkaldy-Willis WH: The relationship of structural pathology to the nerve root. *Spine* 1984; 9:49–52.
15. Kirkaldy-Willis WH, Paine KWE, Cauchoix J, et al: Lumbar spinal stenosis. *Clin Orthop* 1974; 99:30–50.
16. Kirkaldy-Willis WH, Wedge JH, Yong-Hing K, et al: Pathology and pathogenesis of lumbar spondylosis and stenosis. *Spine* 1978; 3:319–328.
17. Nachemson AL, Evans JH: Some mechanical properties of the third human lumbar interlaminar ligament. *J Biomech* 1968; 1:211–220.
18. Porter RW, Hibbert C, Wellman P: Backache and the lumbar spinal canal. *Spine* 1980; 5:99–105.
19. Porter RW, Wicks M, Ottewell D: Measurement of the spinal canal by diagnostic ultrasound. *J Bone Joint Surg [Br]* 1978; 60:481–484.
20. Ratinov G, Jiminez-Pabon E: Intermittent spinal ischemia. *Neurology* 1961; 11:546–549.
21. Sarpyener MA: Congenital structure of the spinal canal. *J Bone Joint Surg [Br]* 1945; 27:70–79.
22. Schönström NR, Bolender NF, Spengler DM: The pathomorphology of spinal stenosis as seen on CT scans of the lumbar spine. *Spine* 1985; 10:806–811.
23. Schönström N, Bolender NF, Spengler DM, et al: Pressure changes within the cauda equina following

constriction of the dural sac. An *in vitro* experimental study. *Spine* 1984; 9:604–607.

24. Schönström N, Hansson T: Pressure changes following constriction of the cauda equina. An experimental study *in situ*. *Spine* 1988; 4:385–388.

25. Schönström NR, Hansson TH: Thickness of the human ligamentum flavum as a function of load: an *in vitro* experimental study. *Clin Biomech* 1991; 6:19–24.

26. Schönström N, Lidahl S, Willén J, et al: Dynamic changes in the dimensions of the lumbar spinal canal. An experimental study *in vitro*. *J Orthop Res* 1989; 7:115–121.

27. Schumacher, M. Die Belastungsmyelographie. *Fortsch Geb Rontgenstr Nuklearmed Erganzungsband* 1986; 145:642–648.

28. Sortland O, Magnaes B, Hauge T: Functional myelography with metrizamide in the diagnosis of lumbar spinal stenosis. *Acta Radiol Suppl* 1977; 355:42–54.

29. Ullrich CG, Binet EF, Sanecki MG, et al: Quantitative assessment of the lumbar spinal canal by computed tomography. *Radiology* 1980; 134:137–143.

30. Verbiest H: A radicular syndrome from developmental narrowing of the lumbar vertebral canal. *J Bone Joint Surg [Br]* 1954; 36:230–237.

31. Verbiest H: Further experiences on the pathological influence of a developmental narrowness of the bony lumbar vertebral canal. *J Bone Joint Surg* 1955; 37:576–583.

32. Wilson CB: Significance of the small lumbar spinal canal: Cauda equina compression syndromes due to spondylosis. Part 3: Intermittent claudication. *J Neurosurg* 1969; 31:499–506.

33. Wilson CB, Ehni G, Grollmus J: Neurogenic intermittent claudication. *Clin Neurosurg* 1971; 18:62–85.

34. Yamada H, Ohya M, Okada T, et al: Intermittent cauda equina compression due to narrow spinal canal. *J Neurosurg* 1972; 37:83–88.

35. Yong-Hing K, Reilly J, Kirkaldy-Willis WH: The ligamentum flavum. *Spine* 1976; 1:226–234.

11

Degenerative Spondylolisthesis

J. W. Frymoyer, M.D.

A German obstetrician, Hermann Friedrich, Kilian,[38] first described spondylolisthesis in 1854. Soon thereafter, Lambl[44] identified a neural arch defect, and Robert[66] concluded that it was this defect which caused one vertebra to slip forward onto its neighbor. Although Naugebauer[58] showed that displacement could occur without a neural arch defect, it was generally assumed that isthmic defects were the major causation. Almost 50 years later, Junghanns[36] showed unequivocal evidence of spondylolisthesis with an intact neural arch, as he reanalyzed Schmorl's collection of vertebral specimens. He coined the term "pseudospondylolisthesis," but his observations were largely ignored by clinicians. Macnab[51] can be credited with the first complete, clinically useful description wherein symptoms and signs are correlated with radiographic findings and surgical outcomes. He renamed the condition "spondylolisthesis with an intact neural arch." Newman and Stone[61] coined the description "degenerative spondylolisthesis," which remains the preferred terminology (Fig 11–1).

In recent years it has become recognized that degenerative spondylolisthesis is a very common occurrence, particularly in older populations. Furthermore, the importance of this condition as a cause of clinical symptoms has become increasingly obvious. Patients may complain of axial skeletal pain or spinal stenosis manifested by sciatica or neurogenic claudication. Therefore, this condition is included in classifications of both spondylolisthesis (Table 11–1), and spinal stenosis[3] (Table 11–2). However, the lesion most commonly occurs as an asymptomatic radiographic finding. In addition to the isolated, primary condition, degenerative spondylolisthesis can occur in association with degenerative scoliosis, or secondarily above spinal fusions. A similar radiographic picture is also produced by extensive lumbar decompressions.

It is the purpose of this chapter to focus on these multiple presentations from the perspectives of epidemiology, pathophysiology, clinical symptoms and signs, radiographic imaging, and treatment.

EPIDEMIOLOGY

The most complete analysis of the epidemiology of degenerative spondylolisthesis has been provided by Valkenburg and Haanen,[79] who analyzed spinal radiographs from the Dutch community of Zoetermeer. They identified an age-related increasing prevalence of the condition, as shown in Table 11–3. A surprisingly high prevalence of 10% was found in females over the age of 60 years, but many of the subjects were totally asymptomatic. Farfan[12] analyzed autopsy specimens, which may or may not be representative of a Canadian population, and found the prevalence to be 4.1%.

Based on analysis of anatomic specimens and patients, Rosenberg[68] identified certain factors associated with an increased risk of degenerative spondylolisthesis (see Fig 11–1). The lesion is most common at L4–5; the prevalence is four times greater when L5 is hemisacralized; females are affected four times more often than males; and diabetics have a

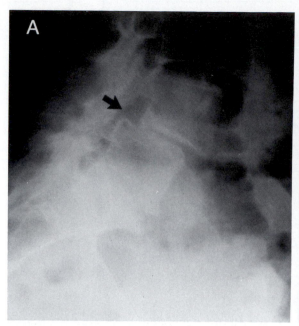

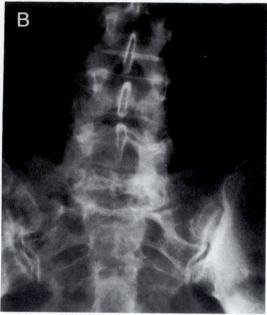

FIG 11–1.
This 72-year-old woman presented with low back pain and mild neurologic claudication. **A,** the lateral radiograph shows a typical forward translation of L4 on L5, which is 25% of the vertebral body width. Note the disc space narrowing and the absence of an apparent defect in the pars interarticularis. At L5–S1 the disc is narrowed and there are large osteophytes present suggesting this is a "stable seg-ment." **B,** the AP radiograph shows the very elongated transverse processes of L5, which is producing sacralization. Sclerosis of the facet joints is also suggested. The combination of the patient's age, sex, location of lesion, and L5–S1 stabilization makes it highly probable that this is a degenerative lesion.

fourfold increased prevalence. These observations confirmed Newman and Stone's,[61] and Newman's[60] earlier studies. The magnitude of forward slippage correlated with the degree of intervertebral disc degeneration at the affected level, but displacement rarely exceeded 25% to 30% of vertebral body width.[69]

It has also become recognized that degenerative spondylolisthesis can occur at levels other than L4–5 and L5–S1. Forward slips are identified at L3–4, most commonly when the patient has had a prior fu-sion which extends form L4 vertebra to the sacrum[4] (Fig 11–2). Instability accompanied by forward displacement of L3 on L4 was identified in 20% of males[22] whose spinal fusion had been performed at least 10 years previously. A similar finding was present in 30% of subjects where 30 years had elapsed since their spinal fusions.[46] However, this radiographic finding often occurred without clinical symptoms or signs. The condition also can arise following extensive surgical decompressions, but there is not yet enough reliable information to determine the frequency of that occurrence (Fig 11–3). It can be argued that this last presentation more appropriately is a variant of isthmic spondylolisthesis, because it is most common when the pars interarticularis has been sacrificed as part of the decompression.

The natural history of the primary lesion remains largely unknown, nor is it clear precisely what factors are associated with the development of symptoms. Feffer et al.[14] thought the rate of progression was 2 mm every 4 years, but final displacements rarely exceeded 33% of vertebral body width. Moreover, the severity of patient symptoms corre-

TABLE 11–1.

Classification of Spondylolisthesis*

Type I	Dysplastic spondylolisthesis
Type II	Isthmic spondylolisthesis
Type III	Degenerative spondylolisthesis
Type IV	Traumatic spondylolisthesis
Type V	Pathologic spondylolisthesis

*From Grobler LJ, Wiltse LL: Congenital and acquired osseous deformities of the lumbar spine presenting in the adult, including the classification, non-operative, and operative treatment of spondylolisthesis, in Frymoyer JW (ed): *The Adult Spine: Principles and Treatment.* New York, Raven Press, 1991. Used by permission.

TABLE 11–2.

Classification of Spinal Stenosis*

1. Congenital-developmental stenosis
 a. Idiopathic
 b. Achondroplastic
2. Acquired stenosis
 a. Degenerative
   i Central portion of spinal canal
   ii Peripheral portion of canal, lateral
     recesses and nerve root canals (tunnels)
   iii Degenerative spondylolisthesis
 b. Combined
  Any possible combinations of
  congenital-developmental stenosis,
  degenerative stenosis and herniations of
  the nucleus pulposus
	c. Spondylolisthetic, spondylolytic
	d. Iatrogenic
	   i Post laminectomy
	   ii Post fusion (anterior and posterior)
	   iii Post chemonucleolysis
	e. Post traumatic, late changes
	f. Miscellaneous
	   i Paget's disease
	   ii Fluorosis

*From Arnoldi CC, et al.: *Clin Orthop* 1976; 115:130–139. Used by permission.

lated poorly with the rate of progression or degree of displacement (Fig 11–4). These clinical observations are similar to the epidemiologic findings reported by Valkenburg and Haanan.[79]

PATHOPHYSIOLOGY

Since the original comprehensive description by Macnab,[52] a body of knowledge has been gathered about the pathophysiology of degenerative spondylolisthesis. A useful starting point is Kirkaldy-Willis's[39] description of what has become known as the "degenerative cascade" (Figs 11–5 and 11–6). Based on the analysis of autopsy specimens, he proposed that there is a point in the degenerative process where the mechanical properties of the discs, ligaments, and facets are characterized by decreased stiffness, or "segmental instability." During that phase intermittent or continuous back pain may become prominent.[40] The physiologic condition and altered mechanical properties may also promote a stabilizing mechanism through the production of vertebral body and facet osteophytes, leading to decreased back symptoms. However, restabilization may be associated with symptoms of spinal stenosis, as the spinal canal's cross-sectional area is reduced by facet

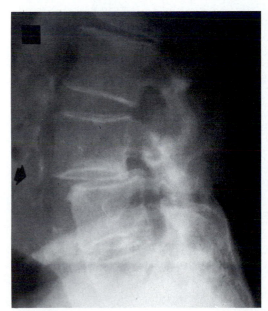

FIG 11–2.
This 70-year-old woman had spinal fusion performed from L4 to the sacrum 18 years previously for low back pain. She presented with neurologic claudication and anterior thigh pain. Lateral radiographs demonstrate displacement of L3 on L4 above the prior fusion *(arrows)*. Note the presence of a solid posterior arthrodesis and the calcification of the L4–5 disc space.

TABLE 11–3.

The Age-Related Prevalence of Degenerative Spondylolisthesis in the Dutch Community of Zoetermeer*

	Percentages According to Age Group					
	35	45	55	65	75	Total (%)
Men						
(Pseudo) spondylolisthesis						
Grade 2	1.3	2.7	7.0	5.5	7.0	4.1
Grade 3/4	0.9	1.5	1.8	3.0	2.3	1.7
Total grade 2+	2.2	4.2	8.8	8.5	9.3	5.8
Women						
(Pseudo) spondylolisthesis						
Grade 2	1.2	2.2	10.6	11.5	17.5	7.1
Grade 3/4	0.8	0.9	1.2	2.9	7.8	2.0
Total grade 2+	2.0	3.1	11.8	14.4	25.3	9.1

*From Valkenburg HA, Haanen HCM: The epidemiology of low back pain, in White AA, Gordon SL (eds): *American Academy of Orthopaedic Surgeons Symposium on Idiopathic Low Back Pain.* St Louis, Mosby-Year Book, Inc, 1982, pp 9–22. Used by permission.

overgrowth, combined with hypertrophy or collapse of the ligamentum flavum.

These observations of gross anatomic specimens correlate with the known biomechanical events that occur with aging and degeneration.[21] The loss of nuclear matrix proteoglycans and water, combined with an increase in the collagen content, tends to stiffen the vertebral motion segments. These morphologic, chemical, and biomechanical events are often termed "physiologic stabilization." However, these analyses do not answer the fundamental question, Why do some vertebrae undergo forward slippage, while others with equivalent degeneration do not?

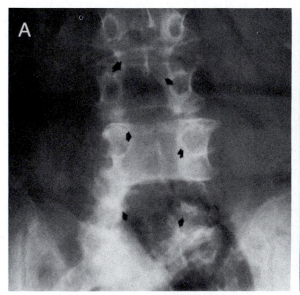 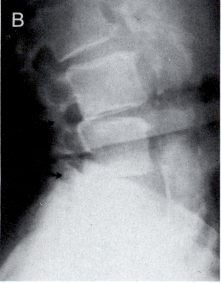

FIG 11–3.
This 74-year-old woman presented with severe low back pain and recurrent neurogenic claudication. She had undergone decompression of an L4–5 degenerative spondylolisthesis elsewhere. Recurrent claudication led to decompression at the L3–4 level, followed within 6 months by severe back pain. **A,** the AP radiograph demonstrates the extent of the prior decompression. **B,** the lateral radiograph shows the original degenerative spondylolisthesis, as well as a new lesion at L3–4 which has occurred since her second decompression.

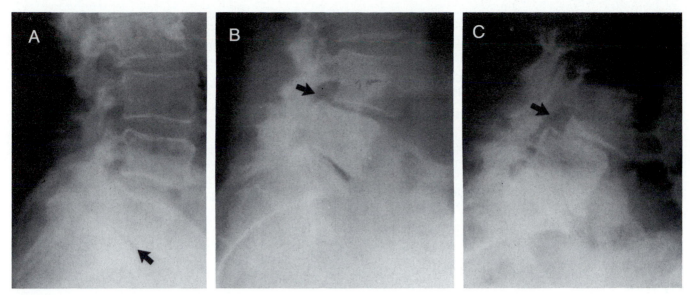

FIG 11–4.
A–C, this 72-year-old woman has been followed by me over the past 10 years. She originally presented with mild low back pain and a minimal slip as shown in **A.** Note that the magnitude of displacement is no more than 3 mm, the disc space is wide, and a small traction spur is seen projecting off the inferior body of L4. The L5–S1 disc space appears narrowed and there is a suggestion of a vacuum sign, a sure indicator of advanced degeneration and possibly stabilization. **B,** is 6 years later, the displacement has increased and is now readily visible. The disc space has further narrowed at both L4–5 and L5–S1, where a vacuum sign is now apparent. Her symptoms in this interval have only mildly increased, but she noted some increased "muscle fatigue" in both legs with walking. **C,** 4 years later and 10 years after **A,** she now has modest low back pain and claudication after walking 1 mile. No neurologic deficits are evident. Her radiographs show further disc space narrowing at L4–5 and L5–S1, where the presence of a large anterior osteophyte is now visible.

Despite the intuitive appeal of Kirkaldy-Willis's model, it has proved far more difficult to establish the clinical criteria for instability. The use of flexion-extension or lateral bending radiography,[41, 55] applications of compression or traction loads,[17] biplanar radiography either using bony landmarks or implanted tantalum markers,[77] and bracing trials have all been utilized and criticized.[78] Clinical classifications have been devised,[18, 19, 24] which include degenerative spondylolisthesis (Table 11–4).

Despite the clinical problems encountered in assessing stability, all studies to date indicate that a requisite for degenerative spondylolisthesis is the presence of an abnormal mechanical environment which selectively shifts stresses to the affected spinal motion segment. By definition, abnormal displacement must have occurred to permit the development of this deformity and, hence, instability has been present at some time. Most commonly, this condition occurs when adjacent motion segments are abnormally stable. The evidence supporting this view is the commonality of a stabilized motion segment below the level of a motion segment with degenerative spondylolisthesis. Abnormal stabilization may be due to sacralization or hemisacralization,[60, 61, 68] or to a prior spinal fusion. A subtler cause of increased stability results from the anatomic location of L4–5 relative to the ilium. Albrook[1] first described a relationship between L4–5 disc hernias and the intercristal line, as shown in Figure 11–7. Fitzgerald and Newman[16] noted that the L4 transverse processes were often smaller in patients with degenerative spondylolisthesis, and concluded there might be fewer ligamentous attachments to provide stabilization to the L4–5 motion segment. MacGibbon and Farfan[50] carefully analyzed spinal radiographs and correlated the intercristal line and the L4 transverse process length with interdiscal degeneration. They concluded that a high-lying intercristal line, combined with small L4 transverse processes, exposed the L4–5 disc to increased shear and torsional stresses. Later, anatomic dissections[47] confirmed the anatomic importance of stabilizing ligaments. This perspective, that L4–5 is inherently less stable than L5–S1, is also suggested by the propensity for progression of L4–5 isthmic spondylolisthesis in the

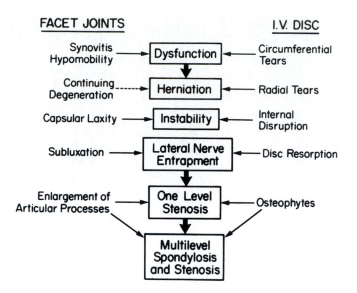

FACET JOINTS   I.V. DISC

FIG 11–5.
Kirkaldy-Willis's conceptualization of the stages of degeneration. (From Kirkaldy-Willis WH: *Managing Low Back Pain.* New York, Churchill Livingstone Inc, 1983, p 47. Used by permission.)

adult, in comparison to L5–S1 isthmic defects which rarely progress after skeletal maturity[27] (Fig 11–8).

Grobler and Wiltse[28] have suggested yet another mechanism which might produce a stabilizing effect on L5–S1, and thus shift stresses to L4–5. They propose that L5–S1 disc degeneration occurs earlier than L4–5 degeneration. As the L5–S1 level physiologically stabilizes, forces are then shifted to L4–5. Although their view is strengthened by clinical and imaging studies,[2, 76] Miller et al.[53] have shown that the rate of degeneration starts at about the same time at L5–S1 and L4–5, and that L3–4 proceeds at the same rate with aging. This is probably more the result of their selection than a reflection of the true prevalence and development.

Finally, altered mechanical stresses can be produced by an operation which artificially stabilizes motion segments. Conversely, an extensive laminectomy can destabilize a previously stable motion segment. Stabilization is produced typically by a prior

NATURAL HISTORY OF SPINAL DEGENERATION

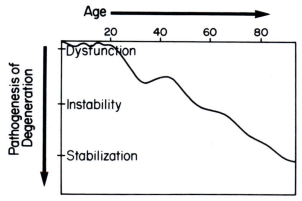

FIG 11–6.
The appearance of symptoms as a function of the stages of degeneration. (From Kirkaldy-Willis WH: *Managing Low Back Pain.* New York, Churchill Livingstone Inc, 1983, p 47. Used by permission.)

TABLE 11–4.

Classification of Lumbar Degenerative Instabilities Based on the Nature of the Deformity and the Preexistent Treatment*

A. Primary instabilities
  1. Axial rotational instability
  2. Translational instability
  3. Retrolisthetic instability
  4. Progressing degenerative scoliosis
  5. (?)Disc disruption syndrome
B. Secondary instabilities
  1. Post–disc excision (subclassified according to the pattern of instability as described under primary instabilities)
  2. Post–decompressive laminectomy
    a. Accentuation of preexistent deformity
    b. New deformity, i.e., no deformity existed at the time of original decompression; further subclassified as for primary instabilities
  3. Post–spinal fusion
    a. Above or below a spinal fusion, subclassified as for primary instabilities
    b. Pseudarthrosis

*From Frymoyer JW: Segmental instability, in Weinstein JN, Wiesel SW (eds): *The Lumbar Spine.* Philadelphia, WB Saunders Co, 1990. Used by permission.

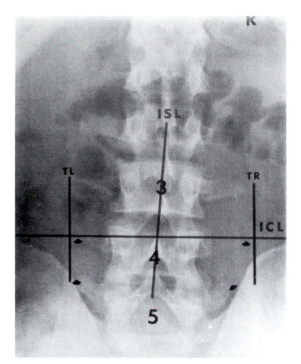

FIG 11–7.
This AP radiograph describes the relationship of the L4–5 disc to the intercristal line drawn between the posterior superior iliac crests, as constructed according to MacGibbon and Farfan.[50] The line connecting the transverse processes and the line connecting the spinous processes are also thought by them to have significance for the etiology of osteoarthritis. (For a detailed explanation, the reader is referred to Frymoyer JW, Newberg A, Pope MH, et al: Spine radiographs in patients with low-back pain. An epidemiological study in men. *J Bone Joint Surg [Am]* 1984; 66: 1048–1055, from which this figure is reproduced with permission of the publisher.)

spine fusion from L4 to the sacrum. As noted, altered mechanics with increased shear follows fusion, both as measured clinically,[77] and after laboratory simulations.[63, 67]

Acquired instability occurs most commonly when facets are sacrificed as part of a wide decompression. Current evidence suggests that this occurs when more than 50% of both facets, an entire facet, or the pars interarticularis is sacrificed. However, there is some evidence this can occur with far less invasive procedures. Twenty percent of females who have undergone disc excisions at L4–5 show later evidence of "instability" as measured by flexion-extension spinal radiographs.[22] Goldner[25] concluded that this condition was sufficiently common that serious consideration should be given to spinal fusion when females undergo L4–5 disc excision. However, it should be emphasized that most of the post-

operative female patients we studied with radiographic evidence of "instability" did not have unusual symptoms of low back pain or spinal stenosis.

Although altered mechanical stresses appear to be crucial to the development of degenerative spondylolisthesis, it is far less certain which biomechanical and physiologic factors cause forward displacement. In the traditional perspective, sagittally directed shear stresses have been thought to be causative.[65, 69] For example, Epstein et al.[10] thought that disc, ligamentous, and facet degeneration shifted the axis of rotation within the nucleus pulposus dorsally toward the facet joints. Congenital or acquired variations in facet orientation have also been thought to be an underlying anatomic causation.

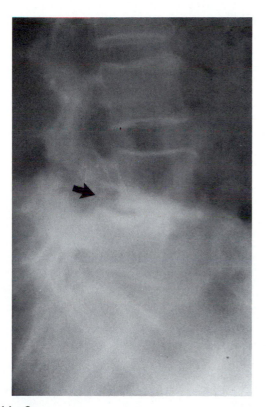

FIG 11–8.
This 56-year-old man with longstanding low back pain now has symptoms of significant spinal stenosis with neurologic claudication and L4 and L5 radiculopathy. This lateral radiograph shows a slip at L4–L5 which approximates 30% of the vertebral body width, severe disc space narrowing with end-plate sclerosis, and large anterior traction osteophytes. Note the wide L5–S1 disc space. Although this lesion could easily be mistaken for degenerative spondylolisthesis, closer scrutiny reveals a defect in the pars interarticularis of L4. This lesion represents, therefore, an isthmic lesion.

An alternative theory has been proposed by Farfan and co-workers.[12, 13] Their careful analyses of the spinal mechanics demonstrated the effects of torsional overloads on the various elements of the motion segment. They concluded that repetitive torsional overloads, usually concentrated at L4–5, could lead to "crumpling" of the neural arch and to asymmetric facet degeneration. Farfan's anatomic studies[12] provide convincing evidence that rotational deformity rather than sagittally directed displacement is present in degenerative spondylolisthesis (Fig 11–9). From this perspective, spinal stenosis is increased by the axial deformity of the spinal canal. Such a deformity could arise without any anatomic abnormality or could be promoted by facet tropism.

Finally, how do we explain the propensity of diabetics to develop this deformity? The most intriguing theory is the observation that disc degeneration is accelerated, at least in experimentally induced diabetes mellitus.[33] However, in other animal models in which diabetes occurs naturally, evidence of accelerated disc degeneration has not been identified.[56]

A summary of the available information strongly suggests that abnormal mechanical forces are important to the etiology of degenerative spondylolisthesis and occur when the adjacent caudal vertebra(e) are mechanically stabilized by congenital or acquired variants in anatomy. It seems most likely, but not yet completely proved, that torsional forces are accentuated at the next mobile level, leading to asymmetric stresses on the facets. If the other stabilizers, i.e., discs and ligaments, are in a phase of aging or degeneration which leads to decreased stiffness, slowly progressing axial deformity may occur. By comparison, the relatively rare isthmic defect at L4–5 appears to be a forward translational deformity, which has the propensity to increase in the adult, unlike its L5–S1 counterpart.[27]

CLINICAL SYMPTOMS AND SIGNS

The studies of Valkenburg and Haanan[79] suggest the most common presentation is an asymptomatic radiographic finding. This fact is of enormous importance because there is a natural tendency for clinicians to ascribe pain to radiographic abnormalities, when in fact the finding has no clinical significance. In clinical practice, the most common presentation is low back pain, reported in 80% of patients who seek medical attention.[70] Often the back pain has been episodic and recurrent over many years. Some patients may have been diagnosed as having

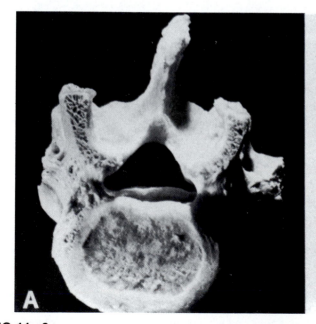
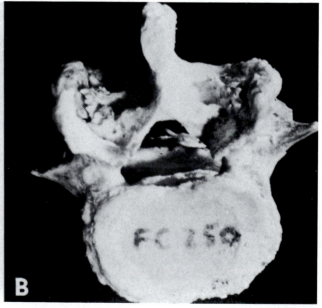

FIG 11–9.
A and **B**, this anatomic specimen is taken from a patient whose autopsy revealed a degenerative slip. On this axial view the rotational deformity of L4 on L5 is visible. Based on this type of evidence, Farfan has developed a convincing theory: the etiology of degenerative slips most likely involves a component of repetitive torsional overload in a patient who has an inherently stable L5–S1 level. (From Farfan HF: *Spine* 1980; 5:412–418. Used by permission.)

"segmental instability" based on subtle displacements identified on prior flexion-extension spinal radiographs.[23, 41, 55] Indeed, Kirkaldy-Willis and Farfan[40] reported that instability was defined by recurrent and increasingly severe back pain, precipitated by mechanical stresses of less and less magnitude. Only a few patients can identify any single precipitating cause. For example, 14% of Brown and Lockwood's[7] patients reported a traumatic antecedent event.

The pain has the usual and typical attributes of any mechanically induced lower back problem, i.e., pain is increased as a function of mechanical loads and worsens as the day progresses. Stiffness and pain often occur in getting out of bed in the morning, which has been thought to be the result of facet degeneration. However, careful analyses of pain patterns in facet degeneration make this theory less plausible.[34] Radiation into the posterolateral thighs is also a common complaint and has been interpreted as the scleratome distribution of the L4–5 motion segment.[70]

Leg symptoms, when present, tend to occur later in the disease process, usually following a prior history of back pain, and may be of two types. Frank sciatica usually arises from lateral recess stenosis affecting the L5 root, but can arise from a frank lumbar disc herniation which accompanies the spondylolisthesis (Fig 11–10). When lateral recess stenosis occurs, it is caused usually by the hypertrophied superior facet of L5 pressing the root against the L4 body, or occasionally by pedicular kinking (Fig 11–11). As already noted, Farfan[12] thinks the root is placed under increased tension by the rotational deformity. The L4 root may also be compressed by these same pathoanatomic features, leading to anterior thigh pain (femoral neuritis), rather than the classic sciatica.

The second peripheral manifestation is more typical of spinal stenosis and has the features of neurogenic claudication. This presentation is reported to occur in 42%[7] to as many as 80%[11] of patients. The underlying mechanism in this instance is thought to be vascular, and is discussed elsewhere in this book, and occurs when stenosis is more prominent in the central spinal canal (Fig 11–12). The central stenosis is thought to be the result of facet hypertrophy, disc bulging, and buckling of the ligamentum flavum, although the role of ligaments in the etiology of spinal stenosis has been ques-

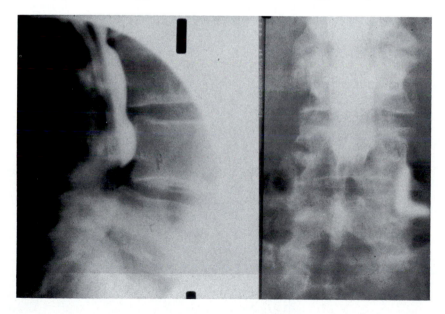

FIG 11–10.
This 65-year-old man had been evaluated over a 5-year period during which his mild low back pain and atypical leg pain was thought to be suggestive of neurogenic claudication. His claudication increased dramatically as did his back pain. Myelogram was obtained and interpreted as a virtually complete block secondary to spinal stenosis. At the time of operation the obvious tension of the L5 nerve roots' caudal sac were unrelieved by bony decompression. Exploration of the disc space revealed a huge sequestered disc fragment, which on removal resulted in complete decompression. He has remained virtually asymptomatic over the ensuing 5 years and currently walks 5 miles every day. In retrospect, the serrated border of the dye column, particularly noted at the upper border of L4, should have made me more suspicious of a disc sequestrum. In reviewing the enhanced CT, however, the disc lesion is not immediately apparent. In this instance, an MRI might have been more revealing of the disc fragment.

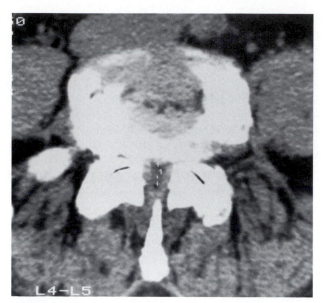

FIG 11–11.
This lumbar CT scan shows the rather typical appearance of a primary degenerative spondylolisthesis. Note the massive hypertrophy of the facets with the accompanying vacuum signs. Facet hypertrophy has rendered the lateral recesses barely visible. The neural canal is constricted by the osteophytes, as well as by ligamentous hypertrophy. Despite this profound radiographic appearance, the patient has only intermittent symptoms, usually walks 1 to 2 miles daily and does not wish to consider operative therapy.

tioned.[71] A third peripheral manifestation is the "restless legs syndrome" or "vespers curse." In this condition, patients are awakened by aching pain in the calves, restlessness of the legs, an irresistible urge to move the legs, and fasiculations. This condi-

tion is most common with degenerative spondylolisthesis, is exacerbated by congestive heart failure, and is relieved by walking and by medical management of the congestive failure.[43]

Typical of all central canal stenosis, the patients may report an increasing forward flexed posture, decreasing ability to walk, and the need to sit down when leg pain occurs. At the extreme, patients may report the need to sleep in the fetal position to relieve their symptoms. Complaints of numbness, tingling, cold feet, giving out, and altered gait with loss of balance are also reported. This instability may not only cause functional impairments, but increasingly is implicated in the etiology of hip fractures. Sometimes a limp occurs which may be due to a dropped foot, quadriceps weakness, or abductor weakness, in which case a positive Trendelenburg's sign may be elicited. The hips should be examined carefully because coexistent osteoarthritis of the hip is found in 11% to 17% of patients.[69]

Although it is convenient to isolate sciatica from claudication, there are often overlaps in the patient's symptoms suggestive of both central stenosis and lateral recess symptoms. Other variations also may occur. For example, a degenerative spondylolisthesis may be associated with degenerative scoliosis, and the patient may present with the complaint of an increasing spinal deformity. In fact, Epstein et al.[11] thought degenerative spondylolisthesis was the underlying etiology of many cases of degenerative scoliosis (Fig 11–13). When this deformity is present, multiple nerve roots may be involved, dependent on the extent and magnitude of the deformity.

Patients may also present with a cauda equina

FIG 11–12.
A myelographically enhanced CT scan demonstrates more clearly than the unenhanced CT scan the relationships of the dural sac to the bony and ligamentous components of the stenosis. Note that at the level of the degenerative spondylolisthesis, the thecal sac is severely constricted.

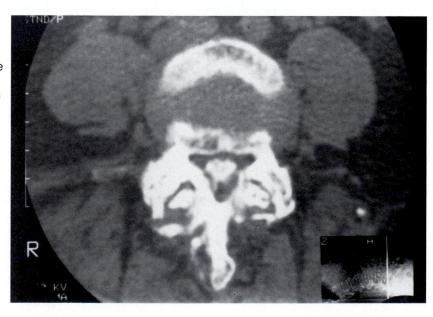

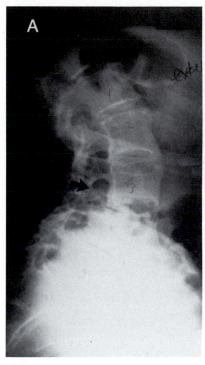
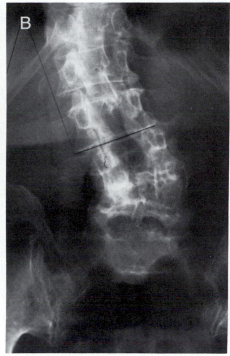
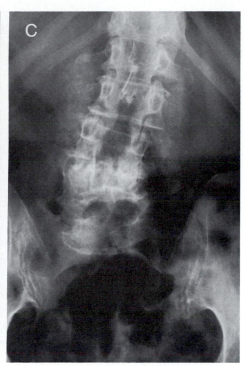

FIG 11–13.

A–C, this 76-year-old woman presented with the major challenge of a degenerative spondylolisthesis, degenerative scoliosis, and prior unsuccessful decompression. Note on the AP radiographs the completely narrowed disc space and forward slip with vacuum sign at L4–5, the acquired slip at L3–4 secondary to wide decompression **(A),** and the significant abnormality in take-off of the L4 vertebra *(arrow)* accompanying scoliosis and prior decompression **(B).** Significant osteoporosis is also present. Because of her very small frame and the virtual absence of paraspinal muscle and body fat, we did not consider the patient a candidate for pedicle fixation. Therefore, a combined procedure was carried out with anterior interbody fusions at L3–4 and L4–5, and transverse process fusion through a far-lateral Wiltse approach extended from L1 to L5. Complete relief of back and leg pain for 3 months was followed by recurrent symptoms **(C).** She is currently considering further surgical alternatives. In retrospect, we might have considered anterior instrumentation as the method of choice for surgical stabilization.

syndrome. Unlike the acute and often devastating bladder and bowel symptoms of cauda equina syndrome due to acute lumbar disc herniation, stenotic patients may have an insidious and subtle presentation[42] which may go undetected by the physician unless changes in bladder function are addressed specifically. Often the patient's complaints are misinterpreted as being due to myogenic bladder or a cystocele, particularly in the multiparous woman.

Finally, an unusual primary presentation is degenerative spondylolisthesis in association with diffuse idiopathic skeletal hyperostosis. If surgery is required, these patients present unusual challenges because of the adjacent multiple fused levels.

The second group of patients are those who have undergone prior surgical interventions, either fusion or extensive decompression. When fusion has been the prior operation, it is common for the patient to have had a rather long symptom-free interval, consistent with having obtained a solid arthrodesis. However, there is some evidence that the interval may be shortened when rigid internal fixation devices are used to facilitate the original operation.[82] Like primary degenerative spondylolisthesis, the onset of symptoms is subtle and back pain is the usual complaint. Later, neurologic symptoms may occur, most commonly affecting the L4 or L3 roots or with neurogenic claudication (see Fig 11–2).

In contrast, the onset of symptoms after extensive decompression is more rapid. Patients often report early postoperative accentuation of their back pain accompanying relief of the peripheral neurologic complaints that led to the decompression. Back pain may remain as the only symptom, or progressive displacement may be associated with new or recurrent neurologic complaints.

PHYSICAL EXAMINATION

As with all patients with spinal stenosis, the physical examination often yields little diagnostic information. Furthermore, there are relatively few signs which are specific to degenerative spondylolisthesis. Inspection may reveal a loss of lumbar lordosis, and sometimes a forward flexed posture when stenotic symptoms are severe. If rotation is significant or there is accompanying degenerative scoliosis, rotational prominence of paraspinal muscles may be present, accentuated by forward flexion. Truncal shift can also be present, manifested in pelvic obliquity and clinically identified by a plumb bob placed at C7, deviating laterally at the gluteal crease. The step deformity is a rarely observed event except in the very thin patient, and is often difficult to appreciate from palpation. Similarly, spinal tenderness, when present, is often difficult to localize precisely.

Unlike many patients with spinal degeneration, patients with degenerative spondylolisthesis often have surprisingly normal spinal mobility, other than the loss of extension. Some observers report that they can palpate the abnormal mobility at the involved level which accompanies degenerative spondylolisthesis before the deformity becomes fixed,[62] but controlled clinical observations make that finding questionable.[59]

The neurologic examination may be quite useful when a patient has isolated and unilateral radicular symptoms. Because the L5 root is commonly involved, reflex asymmetry is uncommon. Unilateral dorsiflexion weakness or sensory losses may confirm nerve involvement, but nerve root tension signs such as a positive straight leg raising test are uncommon. More commonly, the neurologic findings are unspecific and may include absent reflexes, spotty sensory losses, and peripheral atrophy without frank weakness. If bladder symptoms are present, sensory loss may be present in the perineal area, accompanied by decreased sphincter tone. However, the findings are often subtle.

The remaining examination is directed toward eliminating other possible causes, including other central nervous system diseases which cause gait disturbance, hip osteoarthritis, peripheral vascular disease, and primary or metastatic vertebral tumors. The examiner should also be alert to coexisting cervical spondylosis, which may produce a subtle myopathy.

IMAGING STUDIES

The typical features of degenerative spondylolisthesis are found in the plain anteroposterior (AP) and lateral radiographs. The lateral radiographic findings include displacement of L4 on L5 in the usual case, although after a spinal fusion the deformity occurs at the next adjacent level, and after a wide decompression at the decompressed level; varying degrees of disc space narrowing sometimes accompanied by a vacuum sign; end-plate sclerosis; and facet hypertrophy and sclerosis, although these changes may be poorly visualized. Peridiscal osteophytes may be configured as a claw or traction spur; the latter is thought to be one sign of potential instability.[52] A subtle sign indicative of a axial rotational deformity is asymmetry of the pedicle image of L4.

The AP radiograph may confirm the presence of a segmentation error including complete or hemisacralization. Facet sclerosis and asymmetry may also be present. Again, a subtle sign of axial rotational deformity may be malalignment of the spinous process of L4, but the sensitivity or specificity of this observation remains to be established.

Oblique radiographs are of minimal value, other than that facet degeneration may be more evident, and this view serves to eliminate the less common etiology of L4–5 isthmic spondylolysis as a cause of forward displacement.

In addition to static radiographs, dynamic flexion-extension views may be obtained to assess the stability of the lesion. Instability is considered to be present when displacement exceeds 4 mm.[81] An alternative approach has been described by Friberg[17] who first applies an axial compressive load, followed by an axial traction load. The difference in displacements between these two views are correlated with low back pain and instability and are thought by him to have prognostic significance.

The choice for further imaging studies is based on the patient's symptoms and the plan for treatment. Lumbar computed tomography (CT) scan, magnetic resonance imaging (MRI), and myelography may be indicated, particularly when there are peripheral neurologic symptoms unresponsive to conservative care and surgery is contemplated, or when the symptoms and clinical findings suggest the possibility of another pathologic condition.

The choice of imaging studies which will best delineate the stenosis is debated. MRI is considered by some[54] to be the method of choice, because of its noninvasive character (Fig 11–14). I favor a myelographically enhanced CT (Fig 11–15) because (a) the cross-sectional diameter of the caudal sac is still the best indicator of spinal stenosis;[72] (b) the bony architecture is best delineated by CT scan; (c) the relationship of the exiting nerve roots to facet overgrowth is most easily visualized and all possible points of compression can be established; and (d) when there is a questionable dynamic component to the stenosis, flexion-extension views can be taken with the dye in place.

The usual findings (Fig 11–16) are a wasting deformity of the dye column, diminished cross-sectional diameter of the caudal sac, facet degeneration and hypertrophy with subarticular entrapment of the L5 nerve root(s), apparent thickening of the ligamentum flavum, and bulging of the intervertebral disc. It is common to misinterpret the CT image projected from the posterior aspect of the upper body of L5 as a large disc bulge when, in fact, this is rarely present.

Electrodiagnostic studies are rarely necessary,

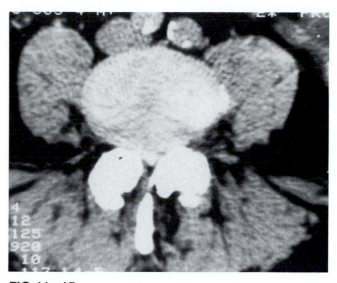

FIG 11–15.
The CT scan obtained in the patient described in Figure 11–10.

unless there is a question regarding involvement of more than one nerve root, based on the clinical symptoms and signs, or one is attempting to differentiate nerve root compressive signs from a neuropathy, often related to diabetes mellitus. Usually an electomyelogram (EMG) is sufficient, although there has been some enthusiasm for evoked somatosensory potentials, particularly in determining if a complete surgical decompression of the nerve roots has been accomplished. With isolated degenerative spondylolisthesis this is less an issue than is the case with the more diffuse, multilevel stenotic syndromes. The use of cystometrography may also be considered in a patient with suspected bladder or bowel impairment. However, the cystometrogram appears to be as useful in separating a myogenic from a neurogenic causation.

Additional studies which may be useful include a technetium bone scan if metastatic osseous tumors are a possible causation of symptoms. Occasionally, a facet block at L4–5 may be helpful in delineating a spinal causation from primary hip disease. In these instances, anesthetic block of the hip joint is more likely to give a definitive answer. Discography is of little use in these patients.

The imaging findings are similar to those identified when the deformity occurs above an old spinal fusion. When there has been prior decompression, partial or complete absence of the facets is common, and varying degrees of both dorsal and perineural scarring may be seen. If there is any question

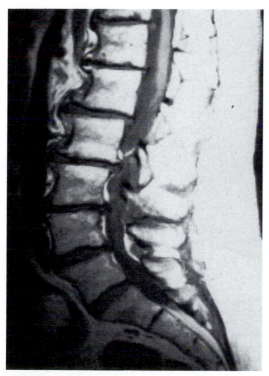

FIG 11–14.
An unenhanced MRI demonstrating a degenerative retrolisthesis.

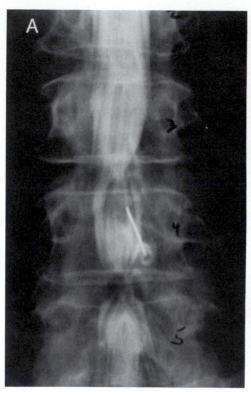
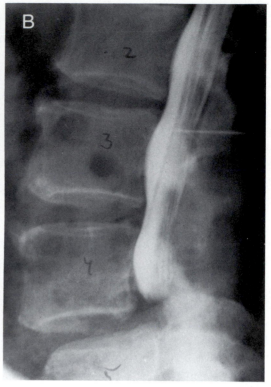

FIG 11–16.
A and **B**, A typical myelogram in a 69-year-old with claudication. Note the waisting deformity of the dye column at the L4–5 level **(A)** and the apparent complete block on the lateral view **(B)**. Decompression has resulted in relief of symptoms.

whether the perineural changes are scar or disc, a gadolinium-enhanced MRI scan is the most sensitive and specific method to differentiate these two possibilities.[54]

TREATMENT

Conservative Treatment

There are no prospective, randomized clinical trials which establish a preferred method of nonoperative treatment. Treatment, therefore, is nonspecific and consistent with conservative care of most degenerative lumbar spinal disorders. These methods include (1) nonsteroidal anti-inflammatory drugs with a caveat that the elderly patient be carefully monitored for the gastropathy associated with these drugs;[23] (2) encouragement of aerobic conditioning, on the premise that this may improve arterial circulation to the cauda;[21] since walking is often aggravating, stationary bicycles are a good alternative and usually are well tolerated, particularly if the handle-

bars and seat are set up to allow a forward flexed posture; (3) weight reduction, which is helpful, but often futile; and (4) careful management of osteoporosis, since that condition may be associated with progression of scoliosis; braces may be attempted in (5) a therapeutic trial. Despite the enthusiasm for flexion braces, such as those advocated by Rainey, many elderly patients do not tolerate immobilization well. There is no evidence for extended bed rest as a treatment method, although acute exacerbations of low back pain may respond to short-term rest. If radiculopathy is a prominent symptom, relief sometimes follows epidural block, but again, there are no well-controlled clinical trials to establish the efficacy of this treatment.

Operative Treatment

Because the natural history of a patient with degenerative spondylolisthesis is unknown, it is difficult to establish what percentage of patients will respond poorly to conservative management and require surgical intervention. If Valkenburg and Haanen's data[79] are generalizable to other populations, a very small percentage of those with radiographic evidence of degenerative spondylolisthesis require operative management. Newman[60] and Rosenberg[68] estimated that no more than 10% to 15% of patients presenting to orthopaedists for treatment later need surgical decompression. The indications for operation, listed in the order of their relative importance, are:

1. Clinical symptoms and signs of cauda equina dysfunction accompanied by a complete block at the affected level. This is an absolute indication.
2. Progressing muscular weakness that may be manifested by a dropped foot, or less commonly, quadriceps weakness. A subtler manifestation may be gait disturbance, sometimes associated with drop episodes. How this condition serves as an indication is less certain.
3. Progressive and incapacitating radicular pain or claudication. When this interferes with sleep or requires a fetal position for relief, the indication is strong. Progressive reduction of walking distance before claudication occurs is a rough but useful indicator of the magnitude of stenosis.
4. Back pain serves as the least certain indication, particularly in the early and so-called unstable phase before the deformity is clearly visible on plain spinal radiographs. Whether facet blocks or discography are useful diagnostic tests at that stage of disease is conjectural.

Surgical Alternatives

For the vast majority of patients that fulfill an indication for operative care, the basic surgical procedure is decompression. The debate centers on whether this should be accompanied by fusion or by fusion with stabilizing instrumentation (See Chapter 28).

Decompression

The extent of the decompression advocated by spinal surgeons has varied. Rosomoff[70] took a very aggressive approach in which total laminectomy and facetectomy were performed. His perspective was strengthened by Dall and Rowe,[9] who reported that 83% of their patients had symptomatic relief when this method was employed. In comparison, only 36% had relief when partial decompression was used. Instability and back pain were not reported as a later complication. However, their experience has not been duplicated by others. For example, Lombardi and Wiltse,[48] and Rosenberg[68] thought the results were poorer and back pain a greater problem when radical decompressions were performed. The approach they and others[11, 60, 64] have advocated is preservation of the articular facets with decompression accomplished by undercutting of the medial aspect of the superior articular facets.

Surgical Technique.—The patient is positioned in the prone position on any frame which allows the abdominal contents to hang freely, and which minimizes vena cava compression. A midline incision is made from the spinous processes of L4 to S1; the median raphe is incised with a cautery and subperiosteal dissection extended out to the facet joints, while preserving the capsule. Troublesome bleeding can be encountered in the vessels which cross the pars interarticularis, which is controlled by identifying a small fat pad and cauterizing the bleeder. The interspinous ligament between L4 and L5 can be preserved, although many surgeons prefer to remove it with portions of the adjacent spinous processes. I usually undercut the ligamentum flavum from the inferior aspect of L4, entering lateral to the spinous process. In some patients the dura may be adherent to the ligamentum in the midline, and a more midline approach appears to have an increased risk of dural laceration. The ligament is then removed, usually with rongeurs, progressing from medial to lateral, while protecting the dura with pledgets. The lateral expansion of the ligament beneath the facet joints is then removed with rongeurs to expose the nerve root. With the roots protected, the facets then are undercut back to the pedicles (Fig 11–17). The decompression then extends distally until the nerve root is demonstrated to be free. Some (Kirkaldy-Willis) establish nerve root canal patency with small probes of varying diameters (spondylometers); others use Woodson or Penfield probes. The upper margin of L5 is then removed until the patency of the distal canal is established. Sometimes a constriction band will be identified corresponding to the leading edge of the L5 lamina. Similarly, the inferior margin of L4 is removed until the patency is established proximally. If the interspinous ligaments and spinous processes of L4–5 have been left intact, the midline can be undercut using either a power burr or rongeurs, while protecting the dura. Frequently, there is no obvious defect on the dorsal dural sac, where the inferior aspect of L4 has compressed the caudal contents. Certainty of adequate proximal central canal decompression is present when dural pulsations are reestablished.

Although the disc may appear to bulge prominently, most surgeons do not advocate its removal

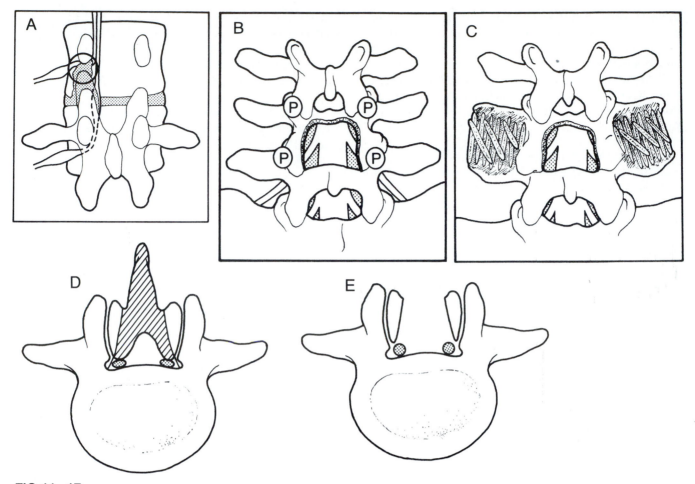

FIG 11–17.
A, the anatomic relationships of the nerve root are shown. **B,** the extent of the decompression that may be required is shown in this anatomic view (*P* = pedicles, and thus a pedicle-to-pedicle decompression has been performed). **C,** the anatomy of the intertransverse process fusion performed only at the decompressed level ("floating fusion") is demonstrated. **D,** the extent of the decompression of the lateral spinal canal with preservation of the facets through undercutting is shown. **E,** the final decompression and the relationship of the L5 nerve roots is illustrated. (**A–E** From Grobler LJ, Wiltse LL: Congenital and acquired osseous deformities of the lumbar spine presenting in the adult, including the classification, non-operative, and operative treatment of spondylolisthesis, in Frymoyer JW (ed): *The Adult Spine: Principles and Treatment.* New York, Raven Press, 1991, pp 1655–1704. Used by permission.)

on the premise that this will increase the postoperative instability.

At the completion of the decompression all bleeding should be controlled. Often, bone bleeding can be troublesome but is controlled by bone wax, if necessary. The patency of the dura can be determined by having the anesthesiologist perform a Valsalva maneuver. A free fat graft is placed over the exposed dura. A HemoVac may or may not be necessary, depending on the degree of intraoperative bleeding encountered. Closure is routine.

Postoperative Care.—The patient is mobilized within 24 hours, unless dural laceration has occurred, which fortunately, in our experience, has been rare (see Chapter 32). A light corset may be used if the patient feels this provides increased comfort. We encourage our patients to begin walking soon after the operation and set a goal of a minimum of 1 mile per day within 2 weeks, and 2 miles within 1 month. Avoidance of lifting and straining is advocated for at least 6 weeks. If the patient has significant abdominal muscular weakness, abdominal strengthening exercises are begun 1 month to 6 weeks postoperatively.

If the patient has significant residual urine after voiding or has had bladder symptoms preoperatively, intermittent catheterization is warranted until normal residual urines are established.

Fusion

Who should be fused is a far more debated question, nor is there any certain answer from the clinical experience reported in the literature. The extreme variation in surgical philosophy ranges from that of Rosomoff[70] and Dall and Rowe,[9] who advocate wide decompression and total laminectomy without fusion, to Hanley and Levy[30] who believe that routine fusion is preferable. Feffer et al.[14] compared fusion with nonfusion, and concluded the results were somewhat better with arthrodesis, but only marginally. Others[48] advocated selective fusion based on the following criteria: (1) physiologic age of less than 65 years;[64] (2) absence of peridiscal osteophytes and disc space narrowing;[11] (3) removal of more than 50% of both facets or one entire facet; or (4) accompanying L4–5 disc excision.

The rationale for fusion is based on the premise that solid arthrodesis will prevent further slip, or recurrent or increased back pain. Increased slip is observed in many patients. Most studies indicate this occurs during the first postoperative year, rarely exceeds 10% to 15% additional vertebral displacement, and rarely extends beyond 30% of vertebral body width.[7, 9, 48, 69] However, the correlation between postoperative displacement and clinical symptoms is minimal.[31, 35, 64, 74] In this respect, the clinical studies of Herron and Trippi[32] are most useful. They found that slip did not increase by more than 4 mm and the average postoperative total displacement was 8 mm. Flexion-extension radiographs showed there was less than 2 mm of translatory motion, a finding within the measurement error of radiographic techniques.

My current approach is similar to that of Reynolds and Wiltse.[64] Patients are informed that fusion will be performed if decompression requires facet sacrifice, pars violation, or disc excision. Fusion is suggested as the preferred treatment for patients younger than 65 years who wish to maintain a very active life style, or when back pain is a prominent symptom, accompanied by more than 4 mm of translation on flexion-extension or distraction-compression radiographs.

Alternatives in Fusion Techniques.—If fusion is selected, there is a wide menu of possible alternatives, the single best determinant of which is the surgeon's experience. Feffer et al.[14] have reported

that transverse process fusion is the method of choice and is accompanied by a high rate of successful arthrodesis and symptomatic relief. The technique used is well established in the literature[80] and is performed through the midline incision or sometimes through a lateral muscular incision (Wiltse) (Fig 11–18). Because the underlying biomechanics of degenerative spondylolisthesis indicates L5–S1 is usually stable, a floating fusion from L4 to L5 is sufficient. Brodsky[5] has an extensive experience with that technique for a variety of pathologic conditions, and his long-term data suggest L5–S1 uncommonly becomes the source of symptoms.

Alternative fusion techniques include interbody fusions. Cloward[8] and others have advocated the posterior interbody technique, often combining this with interspinous wiring of L4 to L5. In these expert hands, complication rates are low, but those who are less experienced should be concerned about dural scarring, graft extrusion, and long operative times, a point made by Lee.[45] Anterior interbody fu-

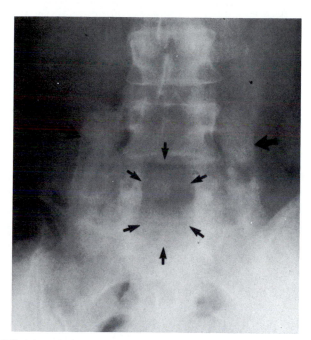

FIG 11–18.
The typical appearance of a transverse process fusion done in a 59-year-old man who is an avid golfer. Preoperatively, he had evidence of significant lateral recess stenosis, clinically and by myelographically enhanced CT scan, at L5–S1 in addition to symptoms and findings indicative of L5 root involvement (dorsiflexor weakness of both feet and sensory changes involving both L5 and S1 roots). Thus, his decompression included both levels and the fusion extended in this instance to the sacrum. He is virtually asymptomatic 6 years later.

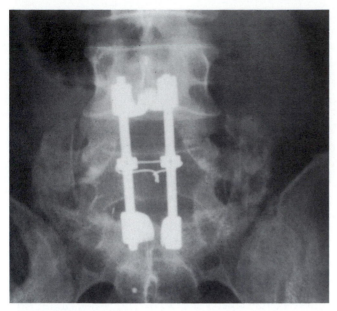

FIG 11-19.
An AP radiograph showing Knodt rods wired together spanning L4 to the sacrum, a transverse process fusion, and a wide decompression at both levels. (Courtesy of Dr. David Selby, Dallas, Texas.)

sions have also been advocated by Goldner et al.,[26] particularly in women beyond menopause. However, their case material was made up of patients who did not have any associated neurologic symptoms or who required decompression.

Internal Fixation.—There is growing experimental evidence that the rate and predictability of spinal fusion can be enhanced by internal fixation,[49] but there are yet no convincing clinical trials to prove this occurs in humans. A variety of techniques have been advocated. Hanley[29] used Harrington rods wired together; Kaneda et al.[37] adapted their anterior fixation device to this procedure, and Selby[73] has promoted the use of Knodt rods (Fig 11-19). Today, pedicle fixation devices are most promising because their point of fixation is to the strongest vertebral structure, and they are compatible with wide decompression. The number of available devices are formidable and they differ mainly in the design of the linkage system. Some of the choices include the Steffee (VSF) (Fig 11-20), Roy-Camille, Wiltse, Edwards, Zielke,[75] and Vermont systems (Fig 11-21). These systems and the technique of insertion have been reported in detail in numerous publications and are discussed further in Chapter 28. All have the potential risk for misplacement of the pedicle screw with nerve root injury, although this is some-

what less of an issue following wide decompression. When osteoporosis is present, methyl methacrylate can be used to enhance screw purchase. In this instance, it is critical to be certain that the pedicle has not been perforated because cement can leak around the nerve root.

Postoperative Care.—The basic program is similar to decompression. It is debatable whether or not a brace is necessary or improves fusion. What is known is that bracing minimally immobilizes any lumbar motion segment, and accentuated motion may actually result.[15, 57] A brace reminds the patient to avoid movements, however, and provides protection from the most excessive ones. However, patients should be encouraged to stop smoking because of a decreased rate of fusion.[6]

Surgical Results

Like all surgical procedures performed on the lumbar spine, it is virtually impossible to compare results because of the different criteria used to measure success; variations in the duration of follow-up; and when fusion is performed, varying measures of the solidarity of the arthrodesis. A review of the results reported by the numerous authors cited in this chapter leads to the following general conclusions: (1) Relief of radiculopathy or claudication occurs in 70% to 85% of patients; and (2) relief of low back pain is less predictable and is less apt to occur when a solid arthrodesis is present.

Complications

The complications which occur are similar to those seen in patients who undergo decompressive operations for spinal stenosis. Because patients are often in an older age group with other significant diseases such as arteriosclerotic cardiovascular disease, the risks are higher than for simple disc excisions. Death, ileus, urinary tract infections, and pulmonary emboli are complications of which the patient should be aware.

Local complications are those of dural laceration and cerebrospinal fluid (CSF) leak which can lead to later meningocele if unrecognized and not repaired; nerve root and caudal damage (the risk of which is increased with pedicle screw fixation), and posterior lumbar interbody fusion; failure of relief of neurologic symptoms because of inadequate decompression or recurrent symptoms resulting from inadequate decompression, new abnormalities, or epidural scarring; and new or accentuated low back pain, usually caused by instability.

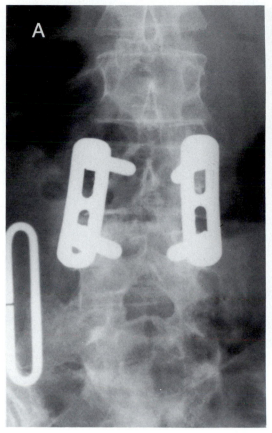 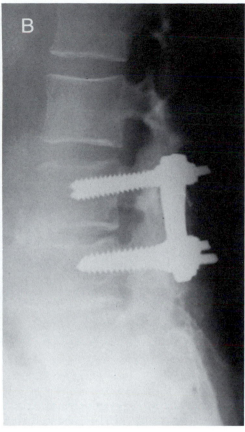

FIG 11–20.
AP **(A)** and lateral **(B)** radiographs showing pedicle fixation with the Steffee device at L4–L5 for a patient with minimal slip, but severe back pain. No decompression has been per- formed because her preoperative evaluation did not suggest any neural compression.

Surgical Management of Degenerative Spondylolisthesis Following Prior Spinal Fusion

The principles and issues of surgical management of acquired degenerative spondylolisthesis after prior spinal fusion are similar to those of the primary condition. However, it can be argued that the majority of these patients should be fused because of the adjacent long lever arm of the prior fusion.[4]

Management of Degenerative Spondylolisthesis Accompanying Scoliosis

The management of degenerative spondylolisthesis accompanying degenerative scoliosis creates other significant problems (see Fig 11–13). These issues are discussed in Chapter 14. The important points which differentiate its treatment from primary degenerative spondylolisthesis are as follows:

1. The patient may have multilevel disease affecting both the neurologic and the axial skeletal complaints. Determining the extent of decompression may be far more difficult, as in all patients with multilevel disease.

2. The decompression, at the level of the spondylolisthesis and at adjacent levels, may be followed by curve decompression, and thus spinal fusion is more likely to be required. In these multilevel fusions, establishing the extent of the fusion may be difficult and a solid arthrodesis more difficult to obtain. For these reasons, many authorities now recommend aggressive decompression and pedicle fixation as an adjunct to bone graft.[75]

Surgical Management of Degenerative Spondylolisthesis Following Prior Decompression

This condition arises under two circumstances: The first situation is when a patient has had prior decompression for degenerative spondylolisthesis and now presents with increasing back pain or recurrent neurologic claudication, or both, or, less

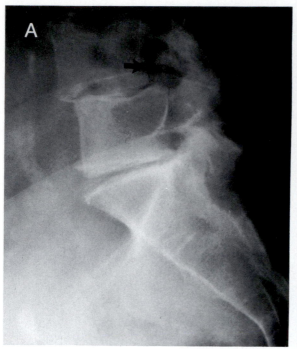
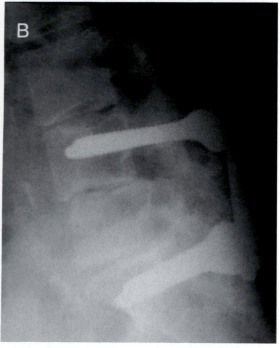

FIG 11–21.

A, preoperative radiograph of a 68-year-old woman shows typical degenerative spondylolisthesis. **B,** because of the angulated collapse of the disc space and the severe back pain accompanying neurogenic claudication, the surgeon elected fixation with the Vermont Fixator. The decompression included both L4–5 and L5–S1, accompanied by ex-

tension of the fusion because preoperative history and electrodiagnostic studies suggested L5 and S1 nerve involvement shown by myelogram-CT to be secondary to severe lateral recess stenosis at the L5–S1 level. (Courtesy of Martin Krag, M.D.)

commonly, with a true radiculopathy. The second is when a patient had decompression for a condition other than degenerative spondylolisthesis (most commonly wide decompression for spinal stenosis) and now presents with new or recurrent symptoms of back pain or recurrent neurologic claudication and radiographic evidence of a new anterior slip. As noted earlier, it can be argued that the later presentation could be classified as an isthmic rather than as a degenerative lesion.

Differential Diagnosis.—The management of both conditions is the same and the presence of either an increased slip, or a new slip, cannot be assumed immediately to be the cause of low back or neurologic symptoms. The initial differential diagnosis should include all of the conditions previously described for the differential diagnosis of primary degenerative spondylolisthesis. Once it is established that the slipped level is the likely source of symptoms, the local causation of pain can be determined. When neurologic symptoms (claudication or sciatica) predominate, the differential diagnosis in-

cludes (1) inadequate initial decompression, usually presenting as a recurrent lateral recess stenosis; (2) postoperative root or dorsal scarring, which may produce symptoms indistinguishable from central bony spinal stenosis;[4] (3) recurrent central or lateral recess stenosis from progressive slipping; (4) spinal stenosis at the adjacent level(s); (5) a postoperative meningocele from an unrecognized or incompletely treated dural tear which occurred at the time of the first decompression; or (6) the rare occurrence of a true lumbar disc herniation at the site of prior surgery.

The considerations for the initial imaging study are identical to those for the primary condition, although the preliminary examination is best accomplished with an enhanced MRI. This imaging study is most sensitive and specific in differentiating scar from other soft tissue lesions. However, I still believe a myelographically enhanced CT scan remains the procedure of choice if an operation is to be considered. If a meningocele is suspected, then it is important to have the patient stand for at least 15 to 30 minutes because the sac may not initially fill.

When back pain is the predominant symptom, or a significant accompanying symptom, the focus tends to be on progressive slip as the most likely cause. However, determining the causation of axial pain, particularly in an elderly patient with other levels of spinal arthritis, may be difficult. Tests which may be useful, but which have no well-established sensitivity or specificity, include facet blocks and flexion-extension radiographs which are particularly useful if the displacement exceeds 4 to 5 mm or, alternatively, compression-distraction radiographs.[17] A role for discography has not been established and there is evidence the test has poor sensitivity and specificity in the older patient. Because the diagnostic tests have less predictive value, it may be difficult to establish with certainty the causation of the back pain.

Treatment.—All of the conservative measures previously outlined should again be tried, unless the patient has obvious progressing neurologic deficits. If these fail, the following general principles should be adopted in the operative approach:

1. New or recurrent pathologic changes deemed to be the cause of neurologic symptoms should be surgically decompressed. However, the operative approach is much more difficult because of the inevitable presence of scarring to some degree. No attempts are made to remove scar, but the plane between the dura and scar laterally and the remaining bone is developed and, if possible, the plane of the nerve root and bone continued. Sometimes it is necessary to identify the nerve root far distally in an area where there has been no prior decompression and then work proximally. If a meningocele is present, this must be repaired, which may require fascial grafts. If scarring is the primary cause of symptoms, the chance of an operative success is diminished significantly. Brodsky[4] reported improvements of the central canal stenotic symptoms. As part of the decompression, the use of a large free fat graft is recommended.

2. The need for either wider decompression or a presentation with predominant back pain should increase the indication for an accompanying spinal fusion. Although the clinical hypothesis that internal fixation improves fusion is not proven, I believe use of a pedicle device is currently the procedure of choice (Figs 11–3 and 11–22). This has replaced the use of other fixation devices, such as the Luque quadrilateral frame (Fig 11–23).

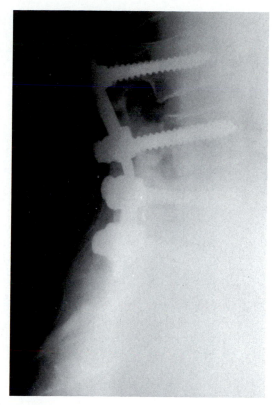

FIG 11–22.
The postoperative AP and lateral radiographs of the patient described in the legend to Figure 11–3 are shown. A four-level fusion has been performed using the Wiltse pedicle fixation device with transverse process fusion. The L5–S1 level deliberately has been left out of the fusion based on the preoperative evaluation. The patient has been relieved initially of her severe back pain. Note reduction of the deformities. In this osteoporotic patient we were able to obtain solid fixation by extending the screws anteriorly to the full depth of the vertebral body. Had we deemed fixation suboptimal, methyl methacrylate would have been used for supplemental screw fixation enhancement. I believe this approach should be reserved for patients in whom there is no alternative to adequate fixation.

SUMMARY

Degenerative spondylolisthesis is a prevalent radiographic finding, which is often asymptomatic. Symptoms, when they occur, usually become clinically evident after the sixth decade and usually include low back pain of varying intensity, neurologic claudication, or a radiculopathy. The underlying causation of the neurologic symptoms is similar to all stenotic lesions affecting the lumbar spine, but the presence of a spondylolisthetic defect compli-

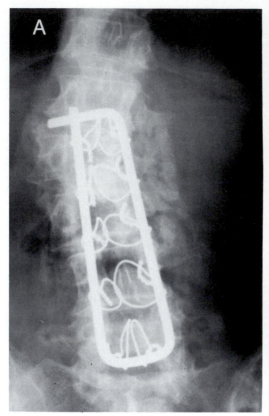

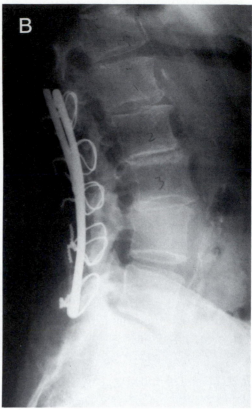

FIG 11–23.
A and **B,** this woman had a minimal degenerative spondylolisthesis accompanying a significant degenerative scoliosis. She was treated 7 years ago with the Luque quadrilateral frame and transverse process fusion with combined autograft and allograft. These AP **(A)** and lateral **(B)** radiographs were obtained 1 year postoperatively. She has been reevaluated for follow-up of her later performed total knee replacements and at most recent evaluation her spine was asymptomatic. (From Frymoyer JW: Segmental instability, in Weinstein JN, Wiesel SW (eds): *The Lumbar Spine.* Philadelphia, WB Saunders Co, 1990, p 612. Used by permission.)

cates treatment because of the potential underlying instability.

There are no currently available prospective clinical trials which establish the superiority of one or another conservative management program, but the condition seems to be responsive, in many patients, to anti-inflammatory agents, exercise, and avoidance of spinal overloads.

Surgical management for patients whose primary symptoms are neurologic appears to be effective in 70% to 85% of patients, as measured by reduction in peripheral symptoms. However, the relief of low back pain is less predictable, particularly when a patient has multilevel osteoarthritis. At present, there is no valid outcome study which establishes the superiority of decompression vs. decompression with spinal fusion. However, clinical experience suggests fusion is a reasonable option for younger patients. Particularly, those with wide disc spaces or whose preoperative motion or compression or tension radiographs demonstrate more than 4 to 5 mm of displacement. Those patients in whom adequate decompression requires the sacrifice of greater than 50% of both facets or the pars interarticularis should also be considered for fusion. Current thinking indicates that for most patients a single-level fusion ("floating fusion") is adequate. Current bias suggests pedicle fixation may be the method of choice.

Despite the growth in clinical experience with degenerative spondylolisthesis, the detailed biomechanics, physiology, and neural anatomy which cause the lesion to develop or a patient to become symptomatic remain elusive. The common occurrence of the primary lesion in females and those with segmentation abnormalities, as well as the later occurrence above old spinal fusions, suggests a primary mechanical etiology.

REFERENCES

1. Albrook D: Movements of the lumbar spinal column. *J Bone Joint Surg [Br]* 1957; 39:339–345.
2. Andersson GBJ, Schultz AB, Nathan A,: Roentgenographic measurement of lumbar intervertebral disc height. *Spine* 1981; 6:154–158.
3. Arnoldi CC, Brodsky AE, Cauchoix J,: Lumbar spinal stenosis and nerve root entrapment syndromes: Definition and classification. *Clin Orthop* 1976; 115:4–5.
4. Brodsky AE: Post-laminectomy and post-fusion stenosis of the lumbar spine. *Clin Orthop* 1976; 115:130–139.
5. Brodsky AE, Hendricks RL, Khalil MA, et al: Segmental ("floating") lumbar spine fusions. *Spine* 1989; 14:447–450.
6. Brown CW, Orme TJ, Richardson HD: The rate of pseudoarthrosis (surgical nonunion) in patients who are smokers and patients who are nonsmokers: A comparison study. *Spine* 1986; 11:942–943.
7. Brown MD, Lockwood JM: Degenerative spondylolisthesis. *Instr Course Lect* 1983; 32:162–169.
8. Cloward RB: The treatment of ruptured lumbar intervertebral discs by vertebral body fusion: Indications, techniques, after care. *J Neurosurg* 1953; 10:154–168.
9. Dall BE, Rowe DE: Degenerative spondylolisthesis. Its surgical management. *Spine* 1985; 10:668–672.
10. Epstein JA, Epstein BS, Lavine L: Nerve root compression associated with narrowing of the lumbar spinal canal. *J Neurol Neurosurg Psychiatry* 1962; 25:165–176.
11. Epstein NE, Epstein JA, Carras R, et al: Degenerative spondylolisthesis with an intact neural arch: A review of 60 cases with an analysis of clinical findings and development of surgical management. *Neurosurgery* 1983; 13:555–561.
12. Farfan HF: The pathological anatomy of degenerative spondylolisthesis: A cadaver study. *Spine* 1980; 5:412–418.
13. Farfan HF, Osteria V, Lamy C: The mechanical etiology of spondylolysis and spondylolisthesis. *Clin Orthop* 1976; 117:40–55.
14. Feffer HL, Wiesel SW, Chuckler JH, et al: Degenerative spondylolisthesis: To fuse or not to fuse. *Spine* 1985; 10:287–289.
15. Fidler MW, Plasmans CMT: The effect of four types of support on the segmental mobility of the lumbosacral spine. *J Bone Joint Surg [Am]* 1983; 65:943.
16. Fitzgerald J, Newman P: Degenerative spondylolisthesis. *J Bone Joint Surg [Br]* 1976; 58:184–192.
17. Friberg O: Lumbar instability: A dynamic approach by traction-compression radiography. *Spine* 1987; 12:119–129.
18. Frymoyer JW, Pope HH, Wilder DG: Segmental instability, in Weinstein JN, Wiesel SW (eds): *The Lumbar Spine.* Philadelphia, WB Saunders Co, 1990, pp 612–636.
19. Frymoyer JW: Segmental instability, in Frymoyer JW (ed): *The Adult Spine: Principles and Practice,* Raven Press, New York, 1991, pp 1873–1891.
20. Frymoyer JW, Gordon SL: *New Perspectives on Low Back Pain.* Park Ridge, Ill, American Academy of Orthopaedic Surgeons, 1989.
21. Frymoyer JW, Hanley EN, Hone J, et al: A comparison of radiographic findings in fusion and nonfusion patients ten or more years following lumbar disc surgery. *Spine* 1979; 4:435–440.
22. Frymoyer JW, Pope MH: Segmental instability, in Wiesel SW (ed): *Seminars in Spine Surgery.* Philadelphia, WB Saunders Co, in press.
23. Frymoyer JW, Moskowitz RW: Spinal degeneration, in Frymoyer JW (ed): *The Adult Spine: Principles and Practice,* New York, Raven Press, 1991, pp 611–634.
24. Frymoyer JW, Selby DK: Segmental instability: Rationale for treatment. *Spine* 1985; 10:280–286.
25. Goldner JL: The role of spine fusion: Question 6. *Spine* 1981; 6:293–303.
26. Goldner JL Urbaniak JR, McCollum DE: Anterior disc excision and interbody spinal fusion for chronic low back pain. *Orthop Clin North Am* 1971; 2:543–568.
27. Grobler LJ, et al: L4–5 isthmic spondylolisthesis: Clinical and radiological review of 52 cases. Presented at the Meeting of the International Society for the Study of the Lumbar Spine, Kyoto, Japan, 1989.
28. Grobler LJ, Wiltse LL: Congenital and acquired osseous deformities of the lumbar spine presenting in the adult, including the classification, non-operative, and operative treatment of spondylolisthesis, in Frymoyer JW (ed): *The Adult Spine: Principles and Treatment.* New York, Raven Press, 1991, pp 1655–1704.
29. Hanley EN: Decompression and distraction-derotation arthrodesis for degenerative spondylolisthesis. *Spine* 1986; 11:269–276.
30. Hanley EH, Levy JA: Surgical treatment of isthmic lumbosacral spondylolisthesis: Analysis of variables influencing results. *Spine* 1989; 14:48–50.
31. Herron LD, Pheasant HC: Bilateral laminotomy and discectomy for segmental lumbar disc disease. Decompression with stability. *Spine* 1983; 8:86–97.
32. Herron LD, Trippi AC: L4-5 degenerative spondylolisthesis. The results of treatment by decompressive laminectomy without fusion. *Spine* 1989; 14:534–538.
33. Holm S: Does diabetes induce degenerative processes in the lumbar intervertebral disc? Presented at the meeting of the International Society for the Study of the Lumbar Spine, Kyoto, Japan, 1989.
34. Jackson RP, Jacobs RR, Montesano PX: 1988 Volvo Award in Clinical Sciences. Facet joint injection in low-back pain. A prospective statistical study. *Spine* 1988; 13:966–971.
35. Johnsson K-E, Willner S, Johnsson K: Post operative instability after decompression for lumbar spinal stenosis. *Spine* 1986; 11:107–110.
36. Junghanns H: Spondylolisthesen ohne Spalt in Zwischengelenkstück. *Arch Orthop Unfallchirurgie* 1930; 29:118–127.
37. Kaneda K, Kurakami C, Minami A: Free vascularized fibular strut graft in the treatment of kyphosis. *Spine* 1988; 13:1273–1277.
38. Kilian HF: *Schilderungen neuer Backenformen und ihrer Verhalten im Leben.* Mannheim, Bassermann & Mathy, 1854.
39. Kirkaldy-Willis WH: *Managing Low Back Pain.* New York, Churchill Livingstone, Inc, 1983.
40. Kirkaldy-Willis WH, Farfan HF: Instability of the lumbar spine. *Clin Orthop* 1982; 165:110–123.
41. Knutsson F: The instability associated with disc de-

generation in the lumbar spine. *Acta Radiol* 1944; 25:593–609.

42. Kostuik JP, Harrington I, Alexander D, et al: Cauda equina syndrome and lumbar disc herniation. *J Bone Joint Surg [Am]* 1986; 68:386–391.

43. LaBan MM: Restless legs syndrome associated with diminished cardiopulmonary compliance and lumbar spinal stenosis—A motor concomitant of "vespers curse." *Arch Phys Med Rehabil* 1990; 71:384–388.

44. Lambl DL: Zehn Thesen über Spondylolisthesis. *Zentralbl Gynakol Urol* 1855; 9:250.

45. Lee C: Lumbar spinal instability (olisthesis) after extensive posterior spinal decompression. *Spine* 1983; 8:429–433.

46. Lehmann TR, Spratt KF, Tozzi JE, et al: Long-term follow-up of lower lumbar fusion patients. *Spine* 1987; 12:97–104.

47. Leong JCY, et al: The biomechanical functions of the iliolumbar ligament in maintaining stability of the lumbosacral junction. *Spine* 1987; 12:669–674.

48. Lombardi JS, Wiltse LL: Treatment of degenerative spondylolisthesis. *Spine* 1985; 10:821–827.

49. McAfee PC, Farey ID, Sutherlin CE, et al: Device-related osteoporosis with spinal instrumentation. *Spine* 1989; 14:919–926.

50. MacGibbon B, Farfan HF: A radiographic survey of various configurations of the lumbar spine. *Spine* 1979; 4:258–266.

51. Macnab I: Spondylolisthesis with an intact neural arch: The so-called pseudo-spondylolisthesis. *J Bone Joint Surg [Br]* 1950; 32:325–333.

52. Macnab I: The traction spur—an indicator of segmental instability. *J Bone Joint Surg [Am]* 1971; 53:663–670.

53. Miller JA, Schmatz C, Schultz AB: Lumbar disc degeneration: Correlation with age, sex, and spine level in 600 autopsy specimens. *Spine* 1988; 13:173–178.

54. Modic MT, Steinberg PH, Ross JS, et al: Degenerative disk disease: Assessment of changes in vertebral body marrow with MR imaging. *Radiology* 1988; 166:193–199.

55. Moran FP, King T: Primary instability of lumbar vertebrae as a common cause of low back pain. *J Bone Joint Surg [Br]* 1957; 39:6–22.

56. Moskowitz RW, Ziv I, Denko CW, et al: Spondylosis in sand rats: A model of intervertebral disc degeneration and hyperostosis. *J Orthop Res* 1990; 8:401–411.

57. Nachemson AL, Schultz A, Andersson G: Mechanical effectiveness studies of lumbar spine orthoses. *Scand J Rehabil Med* 1983; 9:139–149.

58. Naugebauer F: Die Entstehung der Spondylolisthesis. *Centralbl Gynakol* 1881; 5:260–261.

59. Nelson MA, Allen P, Clamp SE, et al: Reliability and reproducibility of clinical findings in low back pain. *Spine* 1979; 4:97–101.

60. Newman PH: Surgical treatment for spondylolisthesis in the adult. *Clin Orthop* 1976; 117:106–111.

61. Newman PH, Stone K: The etiology of spondylolisthesis. *J Bone Joint Surg [Br]* 1963; 45:39–59.

62. Paris SV: Physical signs of instability. *Spine* 1985; 10:277–279.

63. Quinnell RC, Stockdale HR: Some experimental observations of the influence of a single lumbar floating fusion on the remaining lumbar spine. *Spine* 1981; 6:263–267.

64. Reynolds JB, Wiltse LL: Surgical treatment of degenerative spondylolisthesis. *Spine* 1979; 4:148–149.

65. Rissanen PM: Comparison of pathological changes in intervertebral disc and interspinous ligaments of the lower part of the lumbar spine in the light of autopsy findings. *Acta Orthop Scand* 1964; 34:54–65.

66. Robert K: Eine eigentümliche angeborene Lordose, wahrscheinlich bedingt durch eine Verschiebung des Körpers des letzten Lendenwirbels auf die vordere Fläche des ersten Kreuzbeinwirbels. *Monatsschrift Geburtsheilkd Frauenkrankheit* 1855; 5:891–894.

67. Rolander SD: Motion of the lumbar spine with special reference to the stabilizing effect of posterior fusion. *Acta Scand Orthop Suppl* 1966; 90:1–144.

68. Rosenberg NJ: Degenerative spondylolisthesis: Predisposing factors. *J Bone Joint Surg [Am]* 1975; 57:467–474.

69. Rosenberg NJ: Degenerative spondylolisthesis: Surgical treatment. *Clin Orthop* 1976; 117:112–120.

70. Rosomoff HL: Lumbar spondylolisthesis: Etiology of radiculopathy and role of the neurosurgeon. *Clin Neurosurg* 1980; 27:577–590.

71. Schönström N: *The Narrow Lumbar Spinal Canal and the Size of the Cauda Equina in Man. A Clinical and Experimental Study.* Goteborg, Sweden, Department of Orthopaedics, Goteborg University, Sahlgren Hospital, 1988.

72. Schönström NSR, Bolender NF, Spengler DM: The pathomorphology of spinal stenosis as seen on CT scans of the lumbar spine. *Spine* 1985; 10:806–811.

73. Selby D: Internal fixation with Knodt's rods. *Clin Orthop* 1986; 203:179–184.

74. Shenkin HA, Nash CJ: Spondolylisthesis after multiple bilateral laminectomies and facetectomies for lumbar spondylosis. *J Neurosurg* 1979; 50:45–47.

75. Simmons EH, Capicotto WN: Posterior transpedicular Zielke instrumentation of the lumbar spine. *Clin Orthop* 1988; 236:180–191.

76. Spangfort EV: The lumbar disk herniation: A computer-aided analysis of 2,504 operations. *Acta Orthop Scand Suppl* 1972; 142:1–95.

77. Stokes IAF, Frymoyer JW: Assessment of patients with low back pain by biplanar radiographic measurement of intervertebral motion. *Spine* 1981; 6:233–240.

78. Stokes IAF, Frymoyer JW: Segmental motion and instability. *Spine* 1987; 12:688–691.

79. Valkenburg HA, Haanen HCM: The epidemiology of low back pain, in White AA, Gordon SL (eds): *American Academy of Orthopaedic Surgeons Symposium on Idiopathic Low Back Pain.* St Louis, Mosby-Year Book, Inc, 1982, pp 9–22.

80. Wiltse LL, Bateman JG, Duey, R: Experiences with transverse process fusions in the lumbar spine. *J Bone Joint Surg [Am]* 1962; 44:1013–1014.

81. Woody J, Lehmann T, Weinstein J, et al: Excessive translation on flexion-extension radiographs in asymptomatic populations. Presented at the meeting of the International Society for the Study of the Lumbar Spine, Miami, 1988.

82. Zucherman J, Hsu K, White A, et al: Early results of spinal fusion using variable spine plating system. *Spine* 1988; 13:570–579.

12

Spinal Stenosis in Children, Achondroplasia, and Spinal Deformity

Kim W. Hammerberg, M.D.

Disabling back pain is an infrequent complaint in children and adolescents, though episodic pain may be fairly common. Balague et al. report that up to one third of healthy children experience back pain associated with an increase in physical activity or starting a rigorous sport.[2] In most situations, a one-time, self-limited episode of back pain can be approached with expectant observation. Conversely, recurrent or persistent back pain should not be dismissed. In a series of 100 children, Hensinger reported an identifiable cause in 85% of patients.[25] However, lumbar spinal stenosis was not included in his series. In fact, there is a distinct paucity of literature concerning symptomatic lumbar stenosis in children and adolescents. Obviously spinal stenosis exists in children as evidenced by the presence of congenital stenosis in adults (Fig 12–1).

At birth, the spinal canal is already approximately 65% of the adult size in both transverse and midsagittal diameters. By 4 to 5 years of age, the spinal canal has essentially reached its mature caliber.[26, 44, 49] Thus, by age 5, the canal is narrow and the predisposition toward symptoms has been established. One must remember that developmental stenosis is an anatomic anomaly and not a clinical diagnosis. As Verbiest has stated, stenosis of the lumbar canal is a conditional but not an absolute determinant of symptoms.[59] Idiopathic developmental stenosis appears well tolerated until secondary changes further reduce the volume of the spinal canal. In the older person, symptoms are often produced by degenerative changes superimposed on a narrow canal (Chapters 10 and 11). In children and young adults the onset of symptoms is usually due to a disc her-

niation. In the presence of developmental spinal stenosis, even a minor disc protrusion can result in severe and intractable neural compression.

The type of spinal stenosis found in children is congenital, except for spondylolisthesis. The stenosis can be classified as either idiopathic developmental, as described by Verbiest in 1954,[57] or associated with various skeletal dysplasias as typified by achondroplasia.[1] The cause of idiopathic developmental stenosis is uncertain. The perplexing question is how a small canal can be associated with a normal-sized vertebral body. Verbiest postulates that stenosis develops as a result of a growth disturbance of the posterior elements.[60] Perinatal nutrition has been implicated by some investigators as having a role in developmental stenosis.[10] Genetics appears to influence the development of stenosis because familial occurrences have been reported.[45, 56] Others suggest that environmental factors such as repetitive microtrauma are responsible for the development of stenosis.[5]

IDIOPATHIC DEVELOPMENTAL STENOSIS

Incidence

Although Verbiest first used the term *idiopathic developmental stenosis*, his series did not include children.[57, 58] In 1945 and 1947, Sarpyener described 13 children with symptomatic congenital stricture of the spinal canal.[47, 48] These children presented with

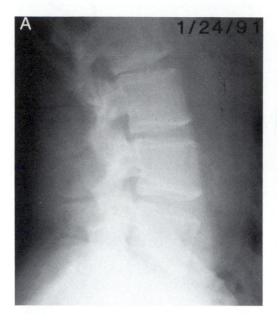

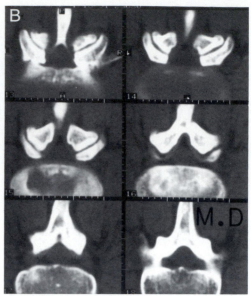

FIG 12–1.
A, lateral radiograph of an 18-year-old man with complaints of low back and posterior thigh pain. Although able to play recreational basketball, this patient has a standing tolerance of only 15 minutes. The radiograph demonstrates extremely short pedicles in the lower lumbar spine. **B,** CT scan demonstrates congenital spinal stenosis with enlarged facets, and thickened laminae and flavum resulting in a trefoil-shaped canal.

urinary incontinence, lower limb deformity, or flaccid paralysis, individually or severally. Although 7 of these patients had an associated spinal bifida occulta, 6 had no bony abnormality of the spine. The congenital stricture was described as a ringlike narrowing of the canal at one or more levels, with a myelographic block usually at the level of L2 or L3. These children experienced remarkable neurologic recovery following wide multilevel decompressive laminectomies. The congenital stricture described by Sarpyener is consistent with our current concept of idiopathic developmental stenosis. He also conjectured that congenital strictures of the intervertebral foramina may cause pressure against the nerve roots, thus describing lateral recess stenosis as well.[48] In a similar series, Dharker et al. reported 60 cases of developmental lumbar stenosis of which 6 patients were children.[12] These two series are the largest in the English literature concerning idiopathic lumbar stenosis in children.

The overall incidence of stenosis was determined by Eisenstein to be 6% in a study of 433 skeletons.[14] He did not make a distinction between acquired and developmental narrowing, however. The true incidence of idiopathic developmental stenosis remains uncertain, as there are few reports concerning stenosis in children.[11] However, there are numerous reports of disc herniations in the young even though they account for only 1% of the patients undergoing disc surgery. These reports frequently mention associated bony anomalies, including spinal stenosis.

In 1950, Key described 4 young patients with typical disc syndromes and mentioned that the roentgenograms demonstrated "occasional congenital anomalies" but did not elaborate.[30] Bradford and Garcia, in 1969 in a paper on disc herniations in children and adolescents, noted that 9 of their 30 patients had radiographic abnormalities, including hypoplastic lamina and congenital narrowing of the canal.[7] Gurdjian et al., in 1961, analyzed 1,176 cases of disc herniation and recognized the presence of lateral recess entrapment in some of their younger patients.[21] These early series were prior to the availability of computed tomographic (CT) imaging. It is probable that the incidence of spinal stenosis was much higher in these series than was then recognized.[23]

In 1980, Kurihara and Kataoka reviewed 70 operative cases of lumbar disc herniations in children and found congenital structural abnormalities in 20.[37] They commented on the relatively high incidence of symptomatic disc herniation in Japanese children as compared to whites. They theorized that the tendency to develop sciatica might be higher because in the Japanese the spinal canal is smaller than that of the white.

In a more recent (1984) series, Epstein et al. reviewed 25 children with symptomatic lumbar disc herniation.[19] They found evidence of central lumbar stenosis in 5 patients and lateral recess stenosis in 11 patients. Thus, over 50% of this group had spinal stenosis. This report stresses the importance of recognizing associated anomalies of the spine such as stenosis in teenage children with herniated lumbar discs.

Treatment

The initial management of symptomatic stenosis in children should be conservative (see Chapter 26). As with adults, these measures include bed rest, nonsteroidal anti-inflammatory medications, and corset immobilization. If satisfactory improvement is achieved, an active exercise program is initiated. Attendance at a low back school may be beneficial, but these programs are directed more toward the rehabilitation of chronic low back pain patients than children. Epidural steroids may be helpful if the pain has a large radicular component. The child and family should be counseled on the chronic nature of this problem. The child should be discouraged from activities which place high demands on the lumbar spine, such as vigorous sports and physically demanding occupations, in hopes of limiting future degenerative changes. The prognosis for avoiding surgery in a child with symptomatic stenosis is probably poor.

The treatment of symptomatic, high-grade, multilevel stenosis, as described by Sarpyener,[47, 48] is by wide multilevel decompressive laminectomies. As in an adult, the facets should be preserved, if possible, to provide some stability. The lateral recess can be decompressed by undercutting the medial one third of the superior facet.[5] The child must be followed periodically throughout growth for the possible development of spinal deformity, especially kyphosis, or instability.

An alternative to multilevel laminectomy is multilevel laminoplasty which may avoid the complications of late deformity and instability. Laminoplasty was first described by Raimondi and colleagues in 1976.[46] In their discussion, they described the use of this technique for the decompression of a 12-year-old with congenital lumbar stenosis. This technique involved bilateral osteotomies medial to the facet joints, unroofing the spinal canal. After completion of surgery, the posterior arch was trimmed down and replaced. The use of laminoplasty to enlarge the spinal canal has been reported frequently for the treatment of spinal cord tumors and ossification of the posterior longitudinal ligament, usually in the cervical or thoracic regions. The laminoplasty was usually accompanied by posterolateral fusion. However, the technique of multilevel laminoplasty can be adapted and applied to the decompression of symptomatic lumbar stenosis in children.

The surgical treatment of a young patient who presents with symptoms of nerve root compression due to a bulging disc and developmental stenosis is controversial (Fig 12–2). Some authors advocate a two-level laminectomy and excision of the intervening disc, on the basis that nerve root entrapment can be avoided should subsequent degenerative changes develop.[4, 43] Epstein et al. recommend disc excision and lateral recess decompression through wide bilateral interlaminar laminotomies.[16] Others recommend only addressing the secondary abnormality responsible for the production of symptoms. Kornberg et al. suggested that the development of degenerative changes from simple disc excision is unpredictable, and that the destabilizing effect of multilevel laminectomies in a young active person may accelerate the degenerative process.[32] They conclude that simple disc excision is the treatment of choice for the young patient with developmental lumbar stenosis and a disc protrusion.

I agree with a more limited approach that addresses the secondary abnormality which produces the symptomatology. These situations may be an excellent indication for microsurgical techniques or percutaneous methods of disc excision.

STENOSIS IN ACHONDROPLASIA

Natural History

Spinal stenosis is a well-recognized problem in achondroplasia. Normally, the interpedicular distance increases from L1 to L5. In an achondroplastic child, the interpedicular distance remains the same or decreases in the lower lumbar spine[39] (Fig 12–3). Thus, in the achondroplastic child the spinal canal is narrowed in both the midsagittal and transverse diameters, unlike idiopathic developmental stenosis in which the canal is usually narrowed only in its midsagittal diameter. Additionally, the facet joints in the lumbar spine are relatively large resulting in an ex-

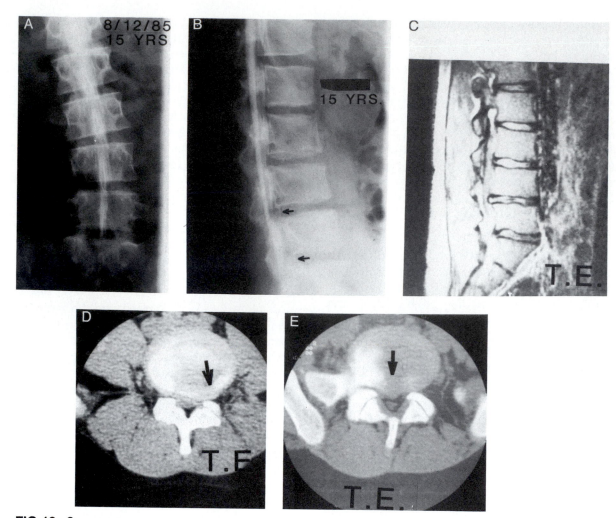

FIG 12–2.
A and **B,** anteroposterior (AP) and lateral myelogram of a 15-year-old boy presenting with acute left leg pain. The AP radiograph demonstrates a sciatic scoliosis and a narrow column of dye in the lower lumbar canal. The lateral radiograph demonstrates disc protrusions at two levels. Note the reversal of normal lumbar lordosis perhaps in an attempt to "open up" the canal. **C,** sagittal magnetic resonance imaging (MRI) confirms disc protrusions at the two lower levels. **D** and **E,** CT scans at the L4–5 and L5–S1 levels, respectively, demonstrate congenital stenosis with acute disc herniations.

tremely stenotic neural canal with little tolerance for secondary narrowing, as from bulging discs or degenerative changes (Fig 12–4).

Anchondroplastic patients are able to tolerate the stenosis until a secondary process further compromises the canal space. As with idiopathic stenosis, this is usually a disc protrusion in younger patients or a degenerative process in older ones.[15, 20] Unique to the achondroplastic child, spinal stenosis may be exacerbated by spinal deformity, specifically thoracolumbar kyphosis and lumbar hyperlordosis.[40, 50, 63]

The achondroplastic newborn commonly dem-

onstrates an increased lumbosacral angulation and a gentle thoracolumbar kyphosis. As the child grows, the lumbosacral angulation increases until the sacrum may be horizontally orientated and the thoracolumbar kyphosis spontaneously improves (Fig 12–5). Often this lumbar hyperlordosis is exacerbated by hip flexion contractures, further reducing the volume of the spinal canal. In a few achondroplastic children, the gentle thoracolumbar kyphosis typical of the newborn may be associated with apical vertebral hypoplasia. This combination results in a progressive kyphosis after the start of ambulation, and may lead the older child and adolescent to se-

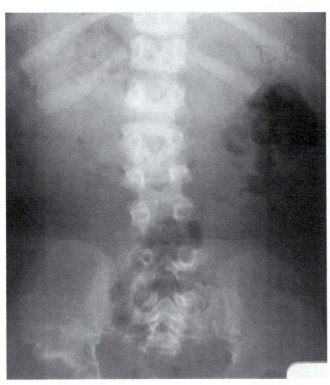

FIG 12–3.
Anteroposterior radiograph of a 4-year-old achondroplastic child. The interpedicular distance narrows from L1 to L5.

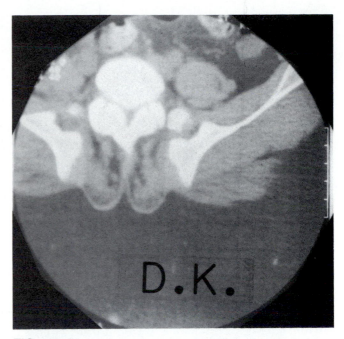

FIG 12–4.
CT scan through the L5 level of a 7-year-old asymptomatic achondroplastic child, the same patient as in Figure 12–3. The lamina and facets are extremely thickened resulting in a markedly narrow trefoil canal.

vere deformity and neurologic compromise (Fig 12–6).

The developmental stenosis of achondroplasia, narrowed interpedicular distance, shortened pedicles, thickened lamina, and foraminal stenosis does not allow any further compromise of the neural elements. Hyperlordosis will compromise the narrowed lower lumbar canal. Progressive thoracolumbar kyphosis will decrease the already narrow upper lumbar spine.

Lutter and Langer have identified four patterns of neurologic symptoms observed in achondroplastic patients.[41] Type I is described as a slow onset progressive paraplegia. This type is frequently seen in association with an acute thoracolumbar kyphosis. Type II is characterized by intermittent claudication with the chief symptoms being pain and paresthesias. Lumbar hyperlordosis is usually observed with this neurologic pattern, but not necessarily thoracolumbar kyphosis. Type III is acute onset of nerve root compression consistent with a disc herniation. Type IV is acute onset paraplegia associated with trauma or a kyphosis. Types I, II, and IV have been observed in children. Early intervention is urged be-

cause of the progressive nature of the neurologic compromise regardless of the type.

The most efficacious treatment of symptomatic spinal stenosis in achondroplastic children is prevention of deformity. The initial management should be an orthosis, with the goal of preventing the progression of, or correcting, the hyperlordosis and hyperkyphosis.

Lumbar Hyperlordosis

Many achondroplastic children and adolescents complain of low back pain when standing for any length of time. It is speculated that the hyperlordotic lumbar spine places increased pressure on the lumbar facets.[42] The developmental stenosis is compromised by the hyperlordosis and may cause neurogenic claudication in some children. Orthotic management is aimed at reducing the hyperlordosis. As with degenerative stenosis, relative lumbar flexion can open up the spinal canal and foramina sufficiently to relieve symptoms.

The brace is worn full-time until correction of the hyperlordosis is achieved. The brace can then be worn at night as a maintenance device. The flexion contractures of the hips must be addressed by

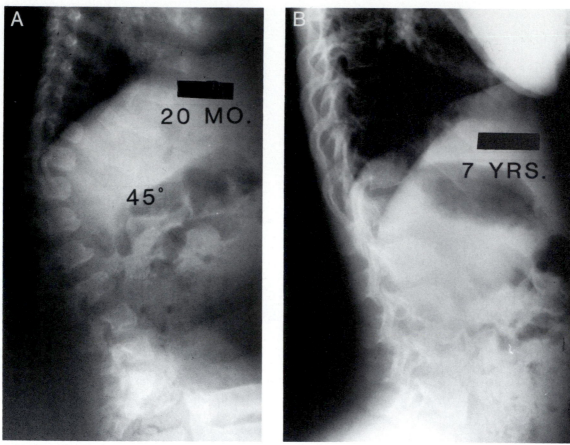

FIG 12–5.
Lateral radiographs of an achondroplastic child. **A,** at 20 months of age, a 45-degree kyphosis is noted at the thoracolumbar junction. **B,** by 7 years of age, the kyphosis has resolved with fairly normal development of the vertebral bodies.

stretching to avoid recurrence of the hyperlordosis when the orthosis is discontinued.

Patients with more significant neurologic deficits are managed by wide decompressive laminectomies. These patients generally exhibit type II neurologic symptoms. The laminectomies should not extend above L2 since this can exacerbate any potential thoracolumbar kyphosis (Fig 12–7). The laminectomies should be wide, while preserving the facets if at all possible. The facets can be undercut to enlarge the lateral recesses and release the foramina.[40] On occasion, complete facet resection is necessary, thereby increasing the potential for postoperative kyphosis or spondylolisthesis. In these instances, if progression of the deformity is noted, an anterior fusion is recommended, as suggested by Lutter et al.[42]

Thoracolumbar Hyperkyphosis

Neurologic compromise has been recognized as a frequent complication in adults with achondropla-
sia. Recently, neurologic compromise has been appreciated as common in children, especially when associated with a thoracolumbar hyperkyphosis.[24] Approximately 10% of achondroplastic children develop a major progressive thoracolumbar kyphosis.[31] Untreated, the kyphosis can result in back pain, sciatica, urinary incontinence, and paraplegia.

Achondroplastic children identified as having a nonresolving or progressive kyphosis should be braced. A thoracolumbar sacral orthosis (TLSO) should provide hyperextension to the thoracolumbar kyphosis. If a concomitant lumbar hyperlordosis is present, the TLSO can also address this problem. The TLSO is worn full-time until correction of the kyphosis is achieved. The orthosis can then be worn at night as a maintenance device.

Progression of a kyphosis beyond 30 degrees is an indication for surgical intervention. In a very young child, i.e., less than 3 or 4 years old, a posterior fusion alone may be indicated for a kyphosis of approximately 30 degrees. The intention is that

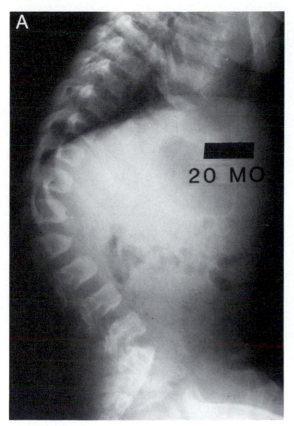 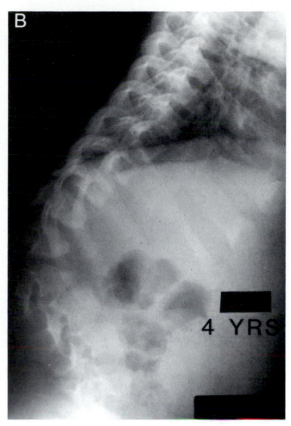

FIG 12–6.
A, another 20-month old child with a moderate thoracolumbar kyphosis. **B,** the kyphosis has increased dramatically by age 4 years secondary to hypoplasia of the apical vertebrae.

some spontaneous correction of the kyphosis may be obtained with a solid posterior fusion and continued anterior vertebral body growth.

In a larger kyphosis, in an older child or an adult, both anterior and posterior fusion should be performed (Fig 12–8). The anterior surgery includes disc excision, interbody fusion, and strut grafting. The strut graft must be placed in the weight-bearing line as determined by the sagittal vertical axis. The posterior fusion should include one level above and one below the measured kyphosis. Instrumentation which penetrates the spinal canal, such as Luque wires or Harrington hooks, should be avoided.

Achondroplastic children or adults demonstrating spinal cord compromise need anterior decompression in addition to the anterior fusion. These patients usually demonstrate type I and, on occasion, type IV neurologic symptoms. The techniques of anterior spinal cord decompression have been delineated in detail elsewhere.[8] Laminectomy in the region of the kyphosis is contraindicated because it will potentiate the kyphotic deformity, and does not provide adequate decompression.

STENOSIS IN SPINAL DEFORMITY

Natural History

Spinal deformity rarely produces significant symptoms in children unless associated with a secondary process such as tumor or infection. Spinal deformity associated with a developmental stenosis, as in achondroplasia, may become symptomatic in late childhood or adolescence, as previously discussed.

In adults, pain has a well-established correlation with deformity, especially scoliosis.[2, 13, 17] The origin of the pain, however, is often not well defined.[62]

Lumbar and thoracolumbar curvatures are much more likely to produce symptoms of low back pain than single thoracic curvatures. Curvatures greater than 45 degrees are clearly related to an increase in back pain.[35] Additionally, the back symptoms in these patients appear to be more refractory to conservative treatment than the "usual" backache.[28]

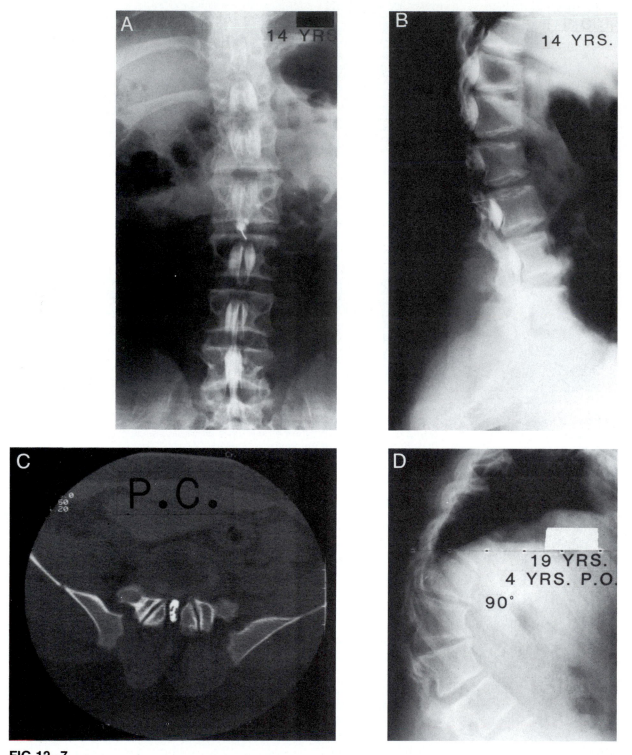

FIG 12–7.
A and **B,** AP and lateral myelograms demonstrate extreme stenosis in this 14-year-old achondroplastic child with marked neurogenic claudication. **C,** CT scan at the L5–S1 disc level demonstrates marked residual narrowing despite midline laminectomies. **D,** the laminectomies were extended superiorly across the thoracolumbar junction which resulted in the exacerbation of the kyphosis. Anterior strut fusion has been recommended.

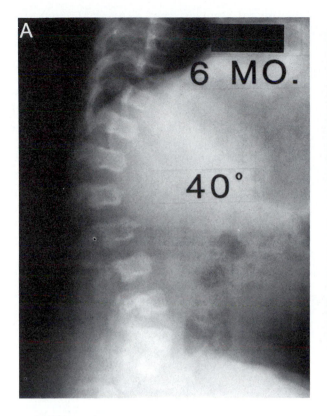

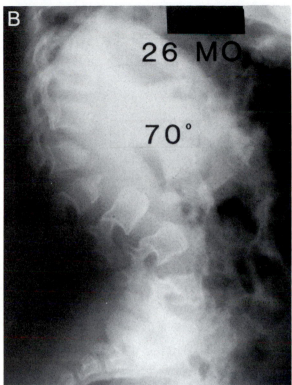

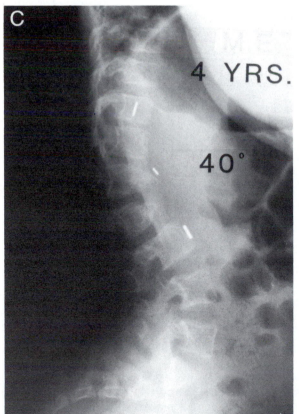

FIG 12–8.
A, a 6-month-old child with a 40-degree thoracolumbar kyphosis. **B,** the kyphosis had increased to 70 degrees by 26 months of age. Hypoplasia of the apical vertebrae is noted. **C,** the kyphosis has been partially corrected and stabilized by an anterior fibular strut graft and posterior fusion.

Scoliosis can lead to symptomatic acquired stenosis of the lumbar spine. The stenosis may be either central or lateral recess and foraminal. The mechanism by which the stenosis develops is the same as the typical degenerative stenosis abetted by progression of the spinal deformity. The volume of the spinal canal normally decreases with aging secondary to the degenerative changes.[53] Also with aging, there may be slow but continuous progression of scoliosis. The progression can be exacerbated by osteoporotic compression fractures later in life.[9] The malalignment of the lumbar spine results in asymmetric loading of the trijoint complex and accelerates the degenerative process.

Central stenosis develops as a result of disc degeneration, annular prolapse, ligament buckling, and laminar shingling. Lateral recess and foraminal stenosis may result from facet hypertrophy compounded by facet subluxation due to the curvature.

Foraminal stenosis may also result from disc collapse, pedicle approximation, and facet subluxation. Nerve entrapments may be caused by pedicular kinking of one or more roots. This is especially true in curvatures with a rotatory lateral olisthesis of one vertebral body on another. The root is kinked by the downward pedicle migration in the concavity of the curve as the disc degenerates, the curve progresses, and rotation increases (Fig 12–9).

Stenosis and root entrapment may occur from progression of an adolescent curve in adulthood or from a senescent scoliosis arising de novo from asymmetric disc collapse in later life.

Lateral recess and foraminal stenosis generally occur in the concavity of the curves. Symptomatic stenosis arising from the convexity of the curve is distinctly rare. The most common nerve root symptoms are in the sciatic nerve distribution arising from the side opposite the major deforming curve. This

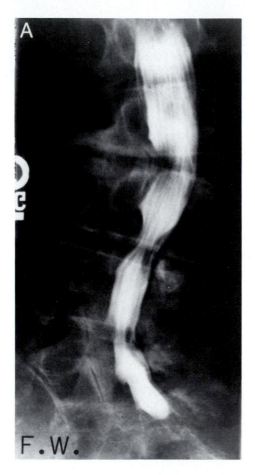
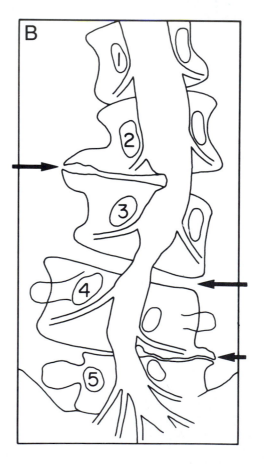

FIG 12–9.
A and **B,** AP myelogram and line drawing demonstrating a degenerative scoliosis in a 75-year-old woman. At the L2–3 level, lateral recess stenosis on the left is noted from asymmetric disc collapse, facet hypertrophy, and reactive osteophyte formation. At the L3–4 level central stenosis results from the rotatory listhesis and annular prolapse. At the L4–5 level, the downward migration of the right L4 pedicle kinks the L4 nerve root in the foramen.

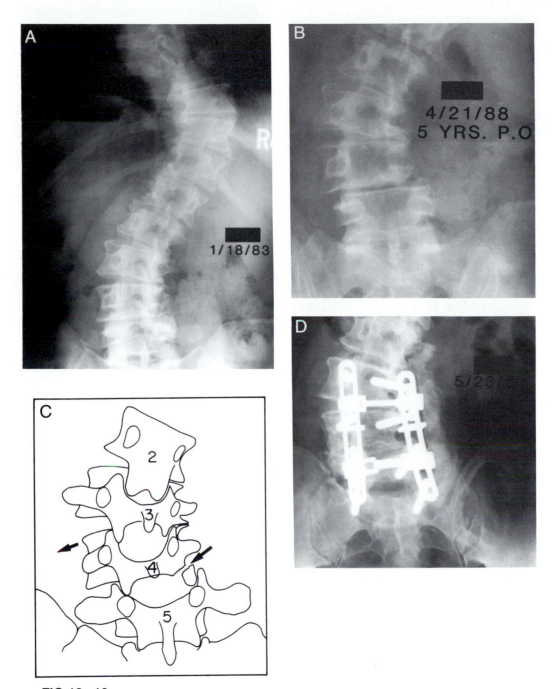

FIG 12–10.
A, standing posteroanterior (PA) radiograph of an adult with idiopathic scoliosis. This patient had complained of right radicular pain arising from the concavity of the compensatory lumbosacral curve. **B** and **C,** At 5 years post-operation, there has been increased rotary and lateral listhesis at L4–5 secondary to a fracture of the right L4 pars interarticularis. **D,** the deformity has been stabilized by pedicular instrumentation and posterior fusion. The fate of the interspaces above the fusion mass is worrisome.

entrapment occurs in the concavity of the fractional, compensatory lumbosacral curve.[22] Nerve root symptoms in the femoral nerve distribution are less common, and usually arise from the concavity of the major lumbar curve.

Treatment

The management of progressive incapacitating low back pain secondary to stenosis associated with scoliosis presents a dilemma for low back surgeons. The initial management, as with all types of stenosis, is conservative. Nonsteroidal anti-inflammatory medication, epidural steroid injections, and a supervised physical therapy program will often alleviate the initial complaints. Exercises are designed to improve muscle tone, increase range of motion, and increase muscle strength. Facet injections under fluoroscopic control may be both diagnostic and therapeutic. A well-molded orthosis may be extremely beneficial.[6, 54] The intent of the orthosis is primarily to reduce the lumbar kyphosis that accompanies thoracolumbar and lumbar curves, and not to reduce the scoliosis.

The surgical treatment of spinal stenosis associated with scoliosis must be approached with trepidation. Scoliosis and lateral olisthesis are recognized as preoperative indicators of potential instability following decompression procedures.[27] In a few select patients with end-stage degenerative changes, as proposed by Kirkaldy-Willis, central or lateral decompression may suffice without acceleration of further collapse.[5, 18] Such an end stage is characterized by bony spurs, spondylophytes, and calcified annulus, facet capsules, and ligamentum flavum.

In general, the removal of posterior restraints by decompressive laminectomy in the presence of a scoliosis will only increase the mechanical instability.[3] Symptoms may be relieved temporarily, but will recur with progression of the deformity. Preservation of the facets does not provide adequate stability by itself. Fracture through the pars interarticularis has been observed as a result of the increased loads in the concavity of a curvature (Fig 12–10).

Central stenosis is not as common as lateral stenosis or root entrapment syndromes. As stated, the stenosis results from annular prolapse, ligament buckling, laminar shingling, and facet hypertrophy. This type of stenosis is usually located in the junctional region between the major curvature and the fractional compensatory curvature (Fig 12–11). Frequently, a relative kyphosis exists in this region as

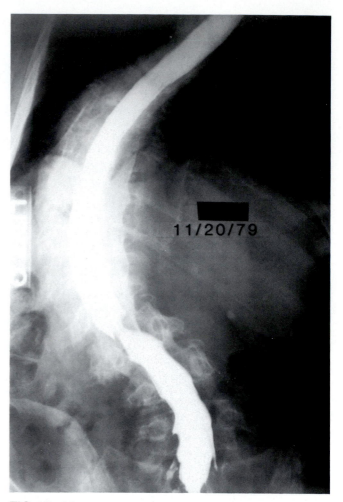

FIG 12–11.
Marked central stenosis is noted at the junction of the thoracic curve, previously fused in situ, and the compensatory lumbar curve.

well. The objectives of the surgical treatment of central stenosis associated with scoliosis are the decompression of the neural elements, and realignment and stabilization of the spinal column. The means by which these objectives can be accomplished are dependent on multiple factors including the patient's age, health, magnitude of curvature, bone quality, and degree and extent of stenosis.

Decompression should be generous and thorough. An attempt should be made to preserve the facets but only if it does not compromise the decompression. Preservation of the facets lends some degree of stability to the spine, but is not adequate by itself. Instrumentation and fusion must accompany the decompression to avoid instability, progressive deformity, and worsened symptoms (Fig 12–12). A discussion of instrumentation and fusion techniques involves a review of the treatment of adult scoliosis

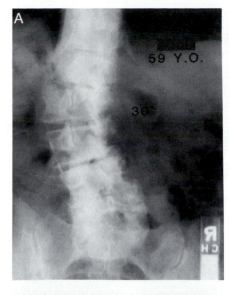

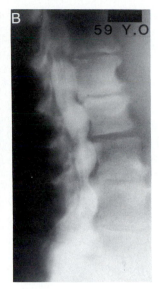

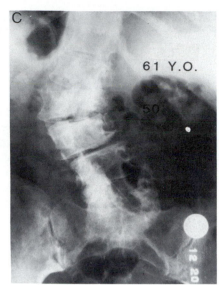

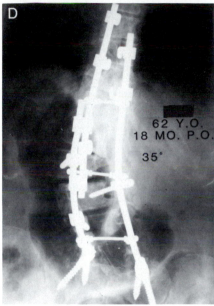

FIG 12–12.
A, a 59-year-old woman with a mild degenerative scoliosis and neurogenic claudication. **B,** lateral myelogram confirms multilevel spinal stenosis as a result of asymmetric disc collapse, annular prolapse, and facet hypertrophy. **C,** 2 years following decompressive laminectomies the degenerative scoliosis has progressed and symptoms of low back and lower extremity pain have markedly increased. **D,** relief of symptoms was achieved following further decompression, and partial correction and stabilization of the deformity.

and can be found elsewhere.[29, 33, 36, 55] The basic principles of the reconstruction are to realign the spine, both in the frontal and sagittal planes, and to provide sufficient stability to encourage a solid fusion.

Lateral recess and foraminal stenosis in association with scoliosis produce nerve root entrapment syndromes as previously discussed. In these situations, correction of the major curvature will often provide relief of the symptoms. A formal decompression of the lateral recess or foramina is usually not necessary. Sciatic nerve symptoms are relieved by the spontaneous correction of the fractional lumbosacral curve with opening of the concave foramina. Symptoms arising from the concavity of the ma-

jor curve are similarly benefited by opening the foramina, reducing the rotation and lateral olisthesis, and relieving the pedicular kinking.[34, 50, 52] The techniques of instrumentation are determined by the magnitude and nature of the curvature, and require great experience in the treatment of adult scoliosis.

Simmons and Jackson in 1979 reported good success in correction of the curvature and in relief of root entrapment symptoms by anterior Dwyer instrumentation.[52] Winter and others have suggested that more reliable and predictable results can be achieved by combined anterior and posterior instrumentation.[29, 61] More recently, posterior decompression and posterior transpedicular instrumentation has resulted in good relief of symptoms and stabilization of the deformity.[51] The long-term results of transpedicular fixation are not yet available (see Fig 12–10). In general, distraction instrumentation should be avoided as it has a tendency to create kyphosis which only exacerbates symptoms arising from lumbar stenosis.[38]

In conclusion, there is little role for decompression alone in lumbar stenosis associated with spinal deformity. Central stenosis requires not only decompression but also realignment and stabilization of the curvature. Most nerve root entrapment syndromes, whether arising from the major or fractional curve, can be relieved by correction of the scoliosis without simultaneous decompression.

REFERENCES

1. Arnoldi CC, Brodsky AE, Cauchoix J, et al: Lumbar spinal stenosis and nerve root entrapment. *Clin Orthop* 1976; 115:4–5.
2. Balague F, Dutoit G, Waldburger M: Low back pain in school children. An epidemiologic study. *Scand J Rehabil Med* 1988; 20:175–179.
3. Benner B, Ehni G: Degenerative lumbar scoliosis. *Spine* 1979; 4:548–552.
4. Birkenfeld R, Kasdon DL: Congenital lumbar ridge causing spinal claudication in adolescents: Report of 2 cases. *J Neurosurg* 1978; 49:441–444.
5. Bowen V, Shannon R, Kirkaldy-Willis WH: Lumbar spinal stenosis. *Childs Brain* 1978; 4:257–277.
6. Bradford DS: Adult scoliosis; current concepts of treatment. *Clin Orthop* 1988; 229:70–87.
7. Bradford DS, Garcia A: Herniations of the lumbar intervertebral disc in children and adolescents. *JAMA* 1969; 210:2045–2051.
8. Bradford DS, Winter RB, Lonstein JE, et al: Techniques of anterior spinal surgery for the management of kyphosis. *Clin Orthop* 1977; 128:129–139.
9. Briard JL, Jegon D, Cauchoix J: Adult lumbar scoliosis. *Spine* 1979; 4:548–552.
10. Clark GA, Panjabi MM, Wetzel FT: Can infant malnutrition cause adult vertebral stenosis? *Spine* 1985; 10:165–170.
11. Danser RC, Chandler WF: Symptomatic congenital stenosis in a child. *Neurosurgery* 1982; 11:61–63.
12. Dharker SR, Roman PT, Mathai KU, et al: Congenital stenosis of the lumbar canal. A study of 60 cases. *Neurol India* 1978; 26:1–6.
13. Edgar MA, Mehta MH: Long-term followup of fused and unfused idiopathic scoliosis. *J Bone Joint Surg [Br]* 1988; 70:712–716.
14. Eisenstein S: Lumbar vertebral canal morphometry for computerized tomography in spinal stenosis. *Spine* 1983; 8:187–191.
15. Epstein NE, Epstein JA: Individual and coexistent lumbar and cervical spinal stenosis. Diagnosis and management, in Hopp E (ed): *Spine: State of the Art Reviews,* vol 1. Philadelphia, Hanley & Belfus, Inc, 1987, p 402.
16. Epstein NE, Epstein JA, Carras R: Spinal stenosis and disc herniation in a 14-year old male. *Spine* 1988; 13:938–941.
17. Epstein JA, Epstein BS, Jones MD: Symptomatic lumbar scoliosis with degenerative changes in the elderly. *Spine* 1979; 4:542–547.
18. Epstein JA, Epstein BS, Lavine LS: Surgical treatment of nerve root compression caused by scoliosis of the lumbar spine. *J Neurosurg* 1974; 41:449–454.
19. Epstein JA, Epstein NE, Marc J, et al: Lumbar intervertebral disc herniation in teenage children: Recognition and management of associated anomalies. *Spine* 1984; 9:427–432.
20. Fortunato A: Narrowing of the thoracolumbar spinal canal in achondroplasia. *J Neurosurg Sci* 1989; 33:185–196.
21. Gurdjian ES, Webster JE, Ostrowski AZ, et al: Herniated lumbar intervertebral discs. An analysis of 1176 cases. *J Trauma* 1961; 1:158–176.
22. Hammerberg KW: Scoliosis, in Goldsmith HS (ed): *Practice of Surgery.* Philadelphia, JB Lippincott Co, 1986, pp 1–59.
23. Hasso AN, McKinney JM, Killeen J, et al: Computed tomography of children and adolescents with suspected spinal stenosis. *J Comput Assist Tomogr* 1987; 11:609–611.
24. Hecht JT, Butler IJ: Neurologic morbidity associated with achondroplasia. *J Child Neurol* 1990; 5:84–97.
25. Hensinger RN: Back pain in children, in Bradford DS, Hensinger RN (eds): *The Pediatric Spine.* New York, Thieme-Stratton, 1985, pp 41–60.
26. Hinck VC, Hopkins CE, Clark WM: Sagittal diameter of the lumbar spinal canal in children and adults. *Radiology* 1965; 85:929–937.
27. Hopp E, Tsou PM: Post decompression lumbar instability. *Clin Orthop* 1988; 227:143–151.
28. Jackson RP, Simmons EH, Stripinis D: Incidence and severity of back pain in adult idiopathic scoliosis. *Spine* 1983; 8:749.
29. Johnson JR, Holt RT: Combined use of anterior and posterior surgery for adult scoliosis. *Orthop Clin North Am* 1988; 19:361–370.
30. Key JA: Intervertebral disc lesions in children and adolescents. *J Bone Joint Surg [Am]* 1950; 32:97–102.
31. Kopits SE: Orthopedic complications of dwarfism. *Clin Orthop* 1976; 114:154.
32. Kornberg J, Rechtine GR, Dupuy TE: The treatment of a herniated lumbar disc in a young adult with developmental spinal stenosis. *Spine* 1984; 9:541–545.
33. Kostuik JP: Decision making in adult scoliosis. *Spine* 1979; 4:521–525.
34. Kostuik JP: Treatment of scoliosis in the adult thoracolumbar spine with special reference to fusion to the sacrum. *Orthop Clin North Am* 1988; 19:371–381.
35. Kostuik JP, Bentivoglio J: The incidence of low back pain in adult scoliosis. *Spine* 1981; 6:268.
36. Kostuik JP, Carl A, Gerron S: Anterior Zielke instrumentation for spinal deformity in adults. *J Bone Joint Surg [Am]* 1989; 71:898–912.
37. Kurihara A, Kataoka O: Lumbar disc herniation in children and adolescents. A review of 70 operated cases and their minimum 5-year follow-up studies. *Spine* 1980; 5:443–450.

38. LaGrone MO: Loss of lumbar lordosis. A complication of spinal fusion for scoliosis. *Orthop Clin North Am* 1988; 19:383–393.
39. Langer L, Banmann P, Gorlin RS: Achondroplasia. *AJR* 1967; 100:12–26.
40. Lonstein JE: Treatment of kyphosis and lumbar stenosis in achondroplasia. *Basic Life Sci* 1988; 48:283–292.
41. Lutter LD, Langer LO: Neurological symptoms in achondroplastic dwarfs—surgical treatment. *J Bone Joint Surg [Am]* 1977; 59:87–92.
42. Lutter LD, Langer LO, Winter RB: Spinal problems in immature individuals with achondroplasia, in Hou JD (ed): *Spine: State of the Art Reviews*, vol 4. Philadelphia, Hanley & Belfors, 1990, pp 131–145.
43. Paine K, Haung P: Lumbar disc syndrome. *J Neurosurg* 1972; 137:75–82.
44. Porter RW, Hibbert C, Wellman P: Backache and the lumbar spinal canal. *Spine* 1980; 5:99–105.
45. Postacchini F, Massobrio M, Ferro L: Familial lumbar stenosis. *J Bone Joint Surg [Am]* 1985; 67:321–323.
46. Raimondi AJ, Gutierrez FA, DiRocco C: Laminectomy and total reconstruction of the posterior spinal arch in childhood. *J Neurosurg* 1976; 45:555.
47. Sarpyener MA: Congenital stricture of the spinal canal. *J Bone Joint Surg [Am]* 1945; 27:70–79.
48. Sarpyener MA: Spina bifida aperta and congenital stricture of the spinal canal. *J Bone Joint Surg [Am]* 1947; 29:817–821.
49. Schwarz GS: The width of the spinal canal in the growing vertebra with special reference to the sacrum: Maximum interpedicular distances in children and adults. *AJR* 1956; 76:476–481.
50. Siebens AA, Hungerford DS, Kirby NA: Curves of the achondroplastic spines: A new hypothesis. *Johns Hopkins Med J* 1978; 142:205–210.
51. Simmons EH, Capicotto WN: Posterior transpedicular Zielke instrumentation of the lumbar spine. *Clin Orthop* 1988; 236:180–191.
52. Simmons EH, Jackson RP: The management of nerve root entrapment syndromes associated with the collapsing scoliosis of idiopathic lumbar and thoracolumbar curves. *Spine* 1979; 6:533–541.
53. Spengler DM: Degenerative stenosis of the lumbar spine. *J Bone Joint Surg [Am]* 1987; 69:305–308.
54. VanDam BE: Nonoperative treatment of adult scoliosis. *Orthop Clin North Am* 1988; 19:347–351.
55. VanDam BE: Operative treatment of adult scoliosis with posterior fusion and instrumentation. *Orthop Clin North Am* 1988; 19:353–359.
56. Varughese G, Quartey GRC: Familial lumbar stenosis with acute disc herniations: Case reports of four brothers. *J Neurosurg* 1979; 51:234–236.
57. Verbiest H: A radicular syndrome from developmental narrowing of the lumbar vertebral canal. *J Bone Joint Surg [Br]* 1954; 36:230–237.
58. Verbiest H: Further experiences on the pathologic influence of a developmental narrowness of the bony lumbar vertebral canal. *J Bone Joint Surg [Br]* 1955; 37:576–583.
59. Verbiest H: Pathomorphological aspects of developmental lumbar stenosis. *Orthop Clin North Am* 1975; 6:177–196.
60. Verbiest H: The significance and principles of computerized axial tomography in idiopathic developmental stenosis of the bony lumbar vertebral canal. *Spine* 1979; 4:369–378.
61. Winter RB: Combined Dwyer and Harrington instrumentation and fusion in the treatment of selected patients with painful adult idiopathic scoliosis. *Spine* 1978; 3:135–141.
62. Winter RB, Lonstein JE, Denis F: Pain patterns in adult scoliosis. *Orthop Clin North Am* 1988; 19:339–345.
63. Wynne-Davies R, Walsh WK: Achondroplasia and hypochondroplasia. Clinical variations and spinal stenosis. *J Bone Joint Surg [Br]* 1981; 63:508–515.

13

Iatrogenic and Metabolic Spinal Stenosis

Thomas W. McNeill, M.D.
Gunnar B.J. Andersson, M.D., Ph.D.

Unfortunately, a significant number of the patients requiring treatment for spinal stenosis today have arrived at this state as a direct result of previous surgical or medical treatment. This is not to say that the prior treatment was poorly done or ill-advised in any way. Fusions (for any reason), laminectomies, chemonucleolysis, postinvasive discitis, fluorosis, oxalosis, and steroid-induced osteoporosis can each result in one or several of the morphologic varieties of spinal stenosis even when originally perfectly appropriate. The main purpose of this chapter is to review these causes and illustrate peculiarities associated with some of them. Metabolic stenosis of noniatrogenic origin will also be discussed.

POSTFUSION STENOSIS

Spinal fusion has been described using a variety of approaches, techniques, and for a myriad of indications.[1, 4, 11, 17, 18, 20, 21, 27] In the past, a great many spinal fusions were done. It is not the place of this chapter to debate the merits of spinal fusion per se or specific techniques of spinal fusion. (As related to stenosis, fusion is discussed in Chapters 28 through 31, 33, and 34.) Fortunately, most patients previously submitted to spinal fusion are doing well, and have not become "postfusion stenosis" patients. There are no data to indicate what percentage of patients treated in the past with spinal fusion will develop stenosis nor is there an accurate indication as to how long after the fusion stenosis can be expected

to appear. Each patient seems to be almost an individual case in this respect.

Postfusion stenosis may occur because of the fusion mass (Figs 13–1 and 13–2). It can occur centrally under the fusion mass, in the neuroforamina under the fusion, in the region of a fusion pseudarthrosis, anteriorly under the fusion, and at the level adjacent to the fusion, either proximally or distally (Figs 13–3 through 13–6). Stenosis may also occur after a burst fracture case in which fusion was performed, but decompression of the spinal canal or neuroforamina was not achieved (see Chapter 15). Lastly, prior to the common recognition of spinal stenosis, fusions were often done over a significantly stenotic segment which remained symptomatic or became symptomatic.

From a biomechanical point of view fusions have a number of long-term disadvantages[15–17, 19] (see Chapters 9 and 31). These disadvantages include accelerated degeneration of adjacent motion segments, which appears to be due to stress concentration on these segments, because when some segments have been fused, the remaining segments have to provide motion. Stenosis leading to paraplegia following fusion for scoliosis has actually been reported.[6] Changes adjacent to a fused segment should eventually be expected in every case since stresses are concentrated at the junction between a rigid and a flexible segment. Newer fixation constructs using rigid plates and screws to produce spinal fusions have, in our experience, occasionally produced examples of rapid and severe failure of an adjacent unfused segment. This complication must be balanced against the demonstrated improvement

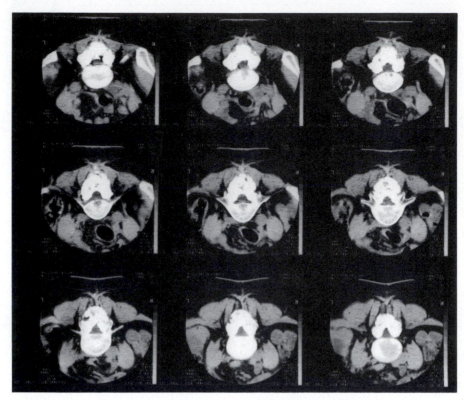

FIG 13–1.
CT indicating hypertrophy of a posterior fusion with neuroforaminal stenosis.

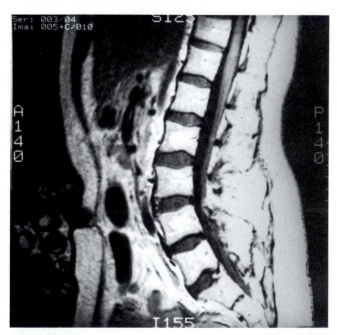

FIG 13–2.
Postfusion stenosis. MRI indicates a posterior indentation of the vertebral canal.

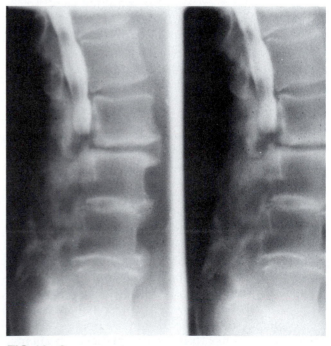

FIG 13–3.
Myelogram after a posterior fusion with stenosis above the fusion and obliteration of the neuroforamina at all levels. The myelographic findings were confirmed at surgery.

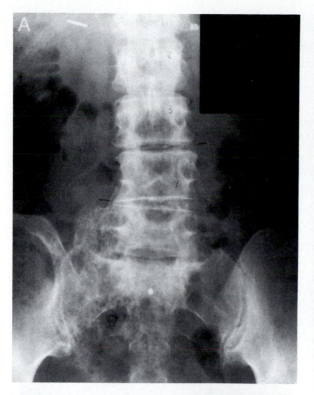

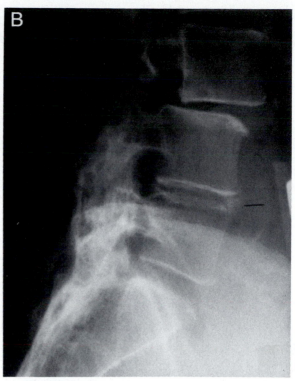

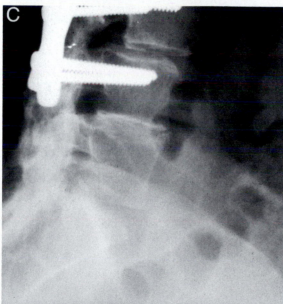

FIG 13–4.
Degenerative spondylolisthesis at the L3–4 level after a previous L4–S1 fusion. The stenosis was treated with decompression alone **(A)**. This resulted in acquired spondylolysis and further instability **(B)**. The fusion was extended to L3 using pedicle screw instrumentation **(C)**.

in the fusion rate with the use of some spinal fixation systems[14] (see Chapter 28). However, some of these systems may be too stiff.[28] Stress concentrations may also cause bony failure with a resulting acquired spondylolysis (spondylolysis aquisita) of the pars interarticularis of the vertebra adjacent to the fusion.[10]

In 1976, Brodsky[2] described the findings in 106 patients with postfusion stenosis; 57 had a solid fusion and 49 had a pseudarthrosis. Brodsky described his patients' symptoms as being "protean and nonspecific" with some dramatic examples of significant motor weakness. In our patients, difficulty with walking (pseudoclaudication) and radicular symptoms were about equally represented.[23] In another study, by Nasca,[24] postfusion and postlaminectomy

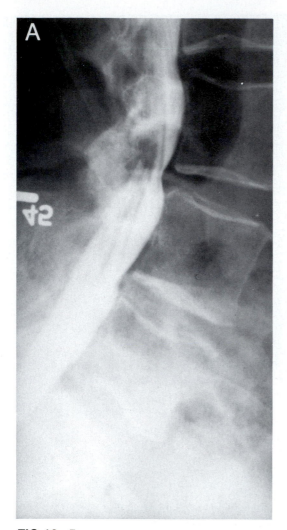
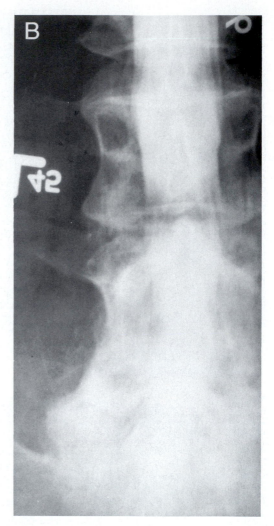

FIG 13–5.
Myelogram demonstrating stenosis above the fusion caused largely by soft tissue thickening. **A,** lateral view.
B, anteroposterior view.

patients were unfortunately grouped together; thus, no specific statement about postfusion patients can be inferred. The pathologic findings in Brodsky's patients were described as a concentric narrowing caused by extension of the fusion mass, thickening and infolding of the ligamentum flavum, hypertrophy and medial extension of the articular processes, and disc herniation, all of which occurred at the segment above the fusion mass (but which could, of course, also occur below the fusion) (see Fig 13–5). Narrowing under the fusion mass was also seen in Brodsky's series but to a lesser extent. Brodsky does not mention degenerative spondylolisthesis above a solid fusion as a cause of symptomatic spinal stenosis. However, in our experience, this is the commonest pathologic finding in patients with postfusion stenosis (see Figs 13–3, 13–4, and 13–6).

Treatment of patients with postfusion stenosis includes a surgical decompression of all of the involved neural elements. Preoperative studies should include a myelogram with water-soluble dye and a postmyelogram computed tomography (CT) study with frontal and sagittal reconstructions when available (see Chapters 19 and 22). There is presently little or no place for magnetic resonance imaging (MRI) studies in postfusion stenosis as MRI tends to "hide" dense cortical bone, and thus may give a false sense of adequate neural canal dimensions.

The surgical treatment may involve extensive removal of bone and refusion with posterolateral grafting and segmental fixation (see Fig 13–4). When the stenosis is directly under the old fusion mass, this can be difficult and tedious since the fusion mass, when placed on the laminae, may become as thick as 5 cm or more and the neuroforamina can be narrowed to 2 mm or less. This is one area of spinal sur-

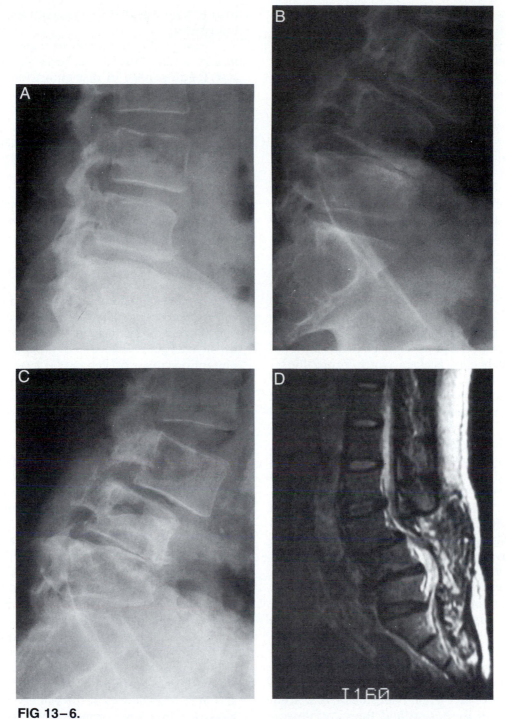

FIG 13—6.
A and **B,** lateral radiograph indicating collapse of the L4—5 segment after laminectomy.
The patient was treated with a posterolateral fusion which did not prevent further slip of L3
on L4 **(C). D,** MRI confirms the local stenosis at the level of L3. Successful treatment was
obtained with refusion and pedicle screw fixation.

gery in which the high-speed turbine burr is invaluable.

The key to the surgical exploration is to start in an area not previously included. In a typical case, in which the previous surgery was a posterior fusion from the sacrum proximally through L4, the surgery is begun at the L3–4 interspace. This space may be hidden by the proximal extension of the fusion mass, but usually some remnant of the L3 spinous process can be identified. Using a periosteal elevator, the plane between the spinous process above and the overgrown fusion mass below can be developed without too much difficulty. This portion of the fusion mass overlying the flavum of the intact segment above can easily be removed with an osteotome, rongeur, or burr. Next, the plane between the ligamentum flavum and the lamina above is developed and all or a portion of this lamina is removed. Working distally from this point, the flavum is then carefully dissected from the dura. The flavum may have lost its original character and become replaced with dense fibrous tissue which is adherent to the dura and nerve roots. Even with the greatest care, unwanted durotomy may occur when attempting to remove this tissue (see Chapter 32). The articular processes may be greatly hypertrophic, almost meeting in the midline. The medial one fourth to one half of the inferior facet may need to be removed. An osteotome is useful for this purpose. The cut is angled from proximal to distal and slightly lateral. In this way the neural elements are protected by the superior facet below. This will expose the remains of the articular cartilage which is usually severely degenerative. The superior articular facet of the proximal fused segment is often so enlarged that it envelops the nerve root. A sella punch or small Kerrison rongeur may not even fit under this portion of the joint. It may be necessary to crack the medial portion of the superior articular facet with an osteotome, and then use a blunt instrument such as a Penfield dissector to pry the facet loose (see Chapter 27). If the stenosis extends below the fusion mass, start carefully by teasing the adherent dura from the overlying thickened bone and then remove the fusion mass with a rongeur, osteotome, or burr while protecting the dura and neural elements. Open each neuroforamen from medial to lateral, along the course of the nerve root.

Additional fusion is necessary if (a) there is a pseudarthrosis present; (b) in the course of the decompression the fusion has been broken; (c) the segment above or below has been rendered unstable by the decompression (this means extending the fusion); (d) degenerative spondylolisthesis is present at the junction of the fusion and the movable segment above; and (e) the segment is demonstrably hypermobile (as in cases of segmental instability above fusions with very rigid instrumentation). Demonstration of such instability will require flexion-extension radiographs. We currently believe that the segment above a fusion should be instrumented if an extension of a previous fusion is required, because of the unfavorable biomechanical situation at that level. Extending the fusion further proximally than to the immediately adjacent segment is usually unnecessary.

Occasionally, the involved segment is below the fusion (as in previous scoliosis surgery) in which case the principles of decompression are the same, but the need for additional fusion is less frequent.

POSTLAMINECTOMY STENOSIS

Laminectomy, as such, is not likely to produce stenosis; indeed it is typically a treatment method (see Chapter 27). Brodsky[2] suggests, however, that the normal subperiosteal stripping may result in thickening of the lamina, thus causing stenosis, and he notes several examples of this presumed etiology. This is more of theoretical interest than common in clinical practice. We have not experienced this potential cause of stenosis in spite of having searched for an example. Nonetheless, laminectomy is an important precursor of stenosis because of other procedures done via the laminectomy approach. The commonest such procedure is discectomy. In the past, an aggressive discectomy with curettage of the end plates of the vertebrae was the standard of care. This often resulted in rapid narrowing of the disc space which had the secondary effect of producing facet subluxation, facet degeneration,[3] and "laminar shingling." Likewise, chemonucleolysis without laminectomy may produce the same structural changes. In the case of laminar shingling the inferior lamina slides under the lamina above, carrying with it the flavum, which in turn becomes folded under the lamina above and also shortened. This shortening of the flavum results in thickening. Laminar shingling and infolding of the flavum can produce significant central canal stenosis.

Facet subluxation leads to a secondary narrowing of the neuroforamina (see Chapter 11). This neuroforaminal narrowing would be of no consequence if enough room remained for the nerve root, and in most instances of discectomy this is the case. However, in a few instances, the loss of disc height is of sufficient magnitude to produce neuroforaminal stenosis. Plain radiographs will often give a false impression of adequate space for the nerve root. The root compression, however, typically is the result of the joint capsule (flavum) having been driven into the neuroforamen by the advancing facet. The actual nerve root compression, therefore, is caused by radiographically invisible soft tissues (see Chapter 3).

Subsequent to the inevitable disc degeneration after discal hernia (even without surgical treatment), the increased loads on the apophyseal joints frequently result in hypertrophy and degeneration of these joints. This can result in central canal stenosis and so-called lateral recess stenosis which might be better termed "subarticular" stenosis (see Chapter 2). Laminar shingling and facet hypertrophy can be seen on plain radiographs. Thus, central canal stenosis and lateral recess stenosis can be inferred from these films. CT scans will eliminate any doubt in most instances.

Postoperative deformities may also result in stenosis. The commonest deformities seen in the lumbar spine following laminectomy or discectomy are (1) shortening (as described above) with or without retrolisthesis; (2) degenerative spondylolisthesis; (3) spondylolysis aquisita; (4) rotatory subluxation; and (5) lateral tilt. Each of these deformities can produce neuroforaminal stenosis with secondary radicular symptoms (see Chapter 11).

Spondylolisthesis is a common complication of stenosis surgery. Hopp and Tsou[12] reported on 344 stenosis patients in which the reoperation rate was 17%. Sixteen patients had olisthesis and 14 had fresh disc herniations. Sienkiewicz and Flatley[25] reported on 8 patients with postoperative slip. All of these patients were female, their average age was 62, and seven of the eight slips occurred at L4–5. The procedure leading to the slip was either a bilateral facetectomy or a complete transection of the pars interarticularis. Five of these patients had had no preoperative slip while 3 patients had progression of a preexisting slip.

Farfan[7] and Troup[26] describe three mechanisms that may result in failure of the neural arch. These are flexion overload, unbalanced shear forces, and forced rotation. Spondylolysis aquisita in postoperative stenosis patients[10] is a result of these forces acting on a weakened motion segment, where the surgeon was required to remove some portion of the pars interarticularis in order to achieve adequate decompression of the involved nerve root.

Postoperative rotatory subluxation is a complication of unilateral facet excision in a mobile segment. Lateral tilt is more often seen with asymmetric disc degeneration from disc herniation or unilateral disc excisions. In both cases, stenosis occurs mainly in the lateral recess for geometric reasons.

A fusion can prevent postlaminectomy spondylolisthesis. Hopp and Tsou[12] suggest that the indications for fusion should include preoperative deformity consisting of olisthesis of 2 mm; scoliosis of 10 degrees; or a wedged disc of 20 degrees. In addition, fusion should be considered in cases with complete facetectomy, excision of the pars (or severe weakening of the pars), decompression at a level above the iliotransverse ligament, disc narrowing of 25% or more, and diabetes mellitus. In our opinion, the archetypal patient requiring fusion following decompression for spinal stenosis is an obese woman who requires a wide decompression at L4–5 and who has a small olisthesis preoperatively. However, one should consider fusion in any patient with preoperative deformity who requires wide decompression.

POSTCHEMONUCLEOLYSIS STENOSIS

Stenosis following chemonucleolysis is uncommon. A decrease in disc height is common after chemonucleolysis, however, and can result in foraminal and other types of lateral stenosis (Fig 13–7). Because of this potential complication, chemonucleolysis should not be used in patients where some degree of lateral stenosis already exists.

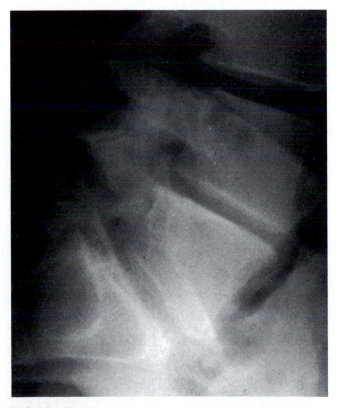

FIG 13–7.
Reduction in disc height following chemonucleolysis.

The diagnosis is usually simple. Continued or recurrent radicular pain, perhaps now involving both legs, should lead to suspicion. A CT scan (or MRI) will typically confirm the diagnosis. Treatment is similar to that of other types of lateral stenosis. Fusion may be necessary should decompression require removal of significant portions of the facet and lamina (see Chapter 9).

SPINAL INFECTION

The general categories of spinal infection include (1) pyogenic vertebral osteomyelitis; (2) discitis; and (3) granulomatous infections. Each of these types of infection can produce stenosis, but usually only the postinvasive discitis is iatrogenic in nature.

Adult pyogenic vertebral osteomyelitis is a relatively rare disease with an estimated annual incidence of about 1 in 250,000 of the population.[5] Risk factors include advanced age, male sex, diabetes, and recent genitourinary manipulation.[22] The offending organism is most often *Staphylococcus aureus* followed by *Escherichia coli*. In the past, pyogenic vertebral osteomyelitis presented as an acute illness. Today, a subacute presentation is becoming more common. Initially, the patients present with back pain unrelieved by rest. Deformity, stenosis, and radicular symptoms are late findings.

In adults, discitis is usually the result of direct inoculation.[8, 9] The onset following surgery or infection is often delayed a month or longer, and the symptoms are nonspecific except for severe back pain. Discitis results in nearly complete disc resorption (Fig 13–8). Diagnostic delay is the rule rather than the exception.

Worldwide tuberculosis remains the most common granulomatous infection of the spine. Fungal diseases are far less common. Spinal tuberculosis is slow in onset and may be difficult to diagnose in countries where it is uncommon. Risk factors include origin from an endemic region and acquired immunodeficiency syndrome (AIDS)–related complex.

Infection causes stenosis by producing deformity. Pyogenic vertebral osteomyelitis may produce destruction of bone and disc resulting in a severe variety of spondylolisthesis with significant secondary neural injury. Epidural abscess, scar, and massive disc displacement may also occur and result in spinal stenosis.

The surgical complication of discitis[22] may result in very severe shortening with severe and early neuroforaminal stenosis even after healing of the infection with autofusion (see Fig 13–8). Tuberculosis often results in a kyphotic deformity and late neural injury secondary to anterior bony impingement on the cord or cauda equina.

The treatment of each of these deformities must be individualized. In each case, the neural elements

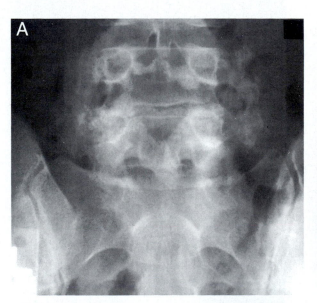
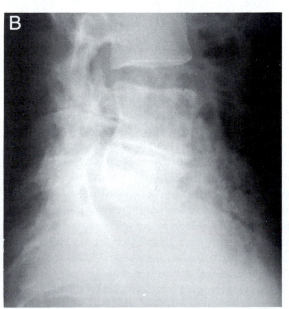

FIG 13–8.
Postdiscitis stenosis. Anteroposterior **(A)** and lateral **(B)** views post decompression and fusion for neuroforaminal stenoses caused by disc resorption (discitis).

must be decompressed and, where possible, the deformity corrected. This will often require a fusion, and a combination of anterior and posterior procedures.

IATROGENIC METABOLIC STENOSIS

Brief mention should be made of the iatrogenic metabolic diseases which may produce stenosis. Fluoride stimulates bone formation and as such may contribute to the development of spinal stenosis. Radiographs will show hypertrophic bone, sometimes with osteosclerosis. Ossification of the ligaments and intervertebral discs can be present as well. As a curiosity, oxalosis has been reported as a cause of spinal stenosis.[13] This is usually the result of a heritable metabolic defect. We have seen one case of oxalosis secondary to an iliojejunal bypass for obesity resulting in severe multilevel degenerative changes and increased severity of a preexisting stenosis. Steroid-induced osteoporosis may result in multiple compression fractures. Rarely, one of these fractures may involve the middle column resulting in an anterior compression of the neural canal and thus be a cause of symptomatic stenosis of a posttraumatic type.

NONIATROGENIC METABOLIC STENOSIS

The primary causes of metabolic stenosis are osteoporosis and Paget's disease. More rarely, stenosis can also be caused by hyperparathyroidism which can cause severe vertebral body collapse, compression, and wedging resulting in kyphosis or local gibbus and secondary stenosis. These patients typically also complain of loss of appetite, nausea, vomiting, and polydipsia, and renal stones are common as well. Treatment of the underlying disease should precede any treatment of the stenosis, except when severe neurologic deficit exists.

Osteoporosis is defined as a loss of absolute bone mass with a normal ratio of the bone's mineral and osteoid content. Spinal stenosis is a late occurrence resulting from the sometimes progressive deformity or from compression fractures. As discussed in Chapter 31, osteoporosis complicates the treatment of spinal stenosis because of the weakened bone. Instrumentation is therefore sometimes ill-advised or even contraindicated.

Paget's disease is a bone disease of unknown etiology presenting early with excessive bone resorption, and then with excessive bone formation. It is in the osteoblastic phase that stenosis can occur. The vertebral bodies may increase in size, showing a characteristic marginal sclerosis and thickened end plates (picture frame appearance). Hypertrophic narrowing of the vertebral canal and foramina can result. In addition, the weak pagetic bone can deform from loading (or sometimes fracture), causing kyphosis, canal stenosis, and neurologic compromise. Treatment is frequently conservative but sometimes wide laminectomies (with or without fusion) are required. Surgery should be done only after drug treatment has been started. These patients frequently have multiple medical problems, and are at risk for surgical complications. A specialist in metabolic bone disorders should manage the treatment of the underlying disease.

REFERENCES

1. Albee FH: Transplantation of a portion of the tibia into the spine for Pott's disease. *JAMA* 1911; 47:855.
2. Brodsky AE: Post-laminectomy and post-fusion stenosis of the lumbar spine. *Clin Orthop* 1976; 115:130.
3. Butler D, Trafimow JH, Andersson GBJ, et al: Discs degenerate before facets. *Spine* 1990; 15:111.
4. Campbell WC: An operation for extra articular arthrodesis of the sacroiliac joint. *Surg Gynecol Obstet* 1927; 45:218.
5. Digby JM, Kersley JB: Pyogenic non-tuberculous spinal infection: An analysis of thirty cases. *J Bone Joint Surg [Br]* 1979; 61:47.
6. Eismont FJ, Simone FA: Bone overgrowth (hypertrophy) as a cause of late paraparesis after scoliosis fusion. *J Bone Joint Surg [Am]* 1981; 63:1016.
7. Farfan HF: The pathological anatomy of degenerative spondylolisthesis—A cadaveric study. *Spine* 1980; 5:412–418.
8. Fernand R, Lee CK: Postlaminectomy disc space infection: A review of the literature and a report of three cases. *Clin Orthop* 1986; 209:215.
9. Fraser RD, Osti OI, Vernon-Roberts BJ: Discitis following chemonucleolysis: An experimental study. *Spine* 1986; 11:679.
10. Harris RI, Wiley JJ: Acquired spondylolysis as a sequel to spine fusion. *J Bone Joint Surg [Am]* 1963; 45:1159.
11. Hibbs RH: An operation for progressive spinal deformities. *N Y J Med* 1911; 93:1013.
12. Hopp E, Tsou PM: Post-decompression lumbar instability. *Clin Orthop* 1988; 227:143.
13. Knight RQ, Taddonio RF, Smith FB, et al: Oxalosis: Cause of degenerative spinal stenosis—a case report

and review of the literature. *Orthopedics* 1988; 11:955.

14. Kornblatt MD, Jacobs RR: The effect of bracing and internal fixation on lumbar spine fusion in 100 consecutive cases: A preliminary report. Presented at the 12th Annual Meeting of the International Society for the Study of the Lumbar Spine. Sydney, Australia, April 14–19, 1985.

15. Lee CK: Accelerated degeneration of the segment adjacent to a lumbar fusion. *Spine* 1988; 13:375.

16. Lee CK, Langrana NA: Lumbosacral spine fusion. A biomechanical study. *Spine* 1984; 9:554.

17. Lehman TR, Spratt KF, Tozzi JE, et al: Long term follow-up of lower lumbar fusion patients. *Spine* 1987; 12:97.

18. Lin PM: Posterior lumbar interbody fusion technique: Complications and pitfalls. *Clin Orthop* 1985; 193:90.

19. Lipson SJ: Degenerative spinal stenosis following old lumbosacral fusion. *Orthop Trans* 1983; 7:143.

20. McElroy KD: Lumbosacral fusion by bilateral lateral technique. Proceedings of the American Academy of Orthopaedic Surgery. *J Bone Joint Surg [Am]* 1961; 43:918.

21. Macnab I, Dall D: The blood supply of the lumbar spine and its application to the technique of intertransverse lumbar fusion. *J Bone Joint Surg [Br]* 1971; 53:628.

22. McNeill TW: Spinal infection. *Instr Course Lect* 1990; 39:515.

23. McNeill TW, Andersson GBJ, Sinkora G: Spinal stenosis: Not a single entity. Presented at the Clinical Orthopaedic Society Meeting. Chicago, 1986.

24. Nasca RJ: Surgical management of lumbar spinal stenosis. *Spine* 1987; 12:809.

25. Sienkiewicz PJ, Flatley TJ: Post-operative spondylolisthesis. *Clin Orthop* 1987; 221:172.

26. Troup JDG: The etiology of spondylolisthesis. *Orthop Clin North Am* 1977; 8:59–64.

27. Watkins MB: Posterolateral fusion of the lumbar and lumbo-sacral spine. *J Bone Joint Surg [Am]* 1953; 35:1014.

28. White AA, Panjabi MM: *Clinical Biomechanics of the Spine*, ed 2. Philadelphia. JB Lippincott Co, 1990, pp 564, 615.

14

Stenosis in Spondylolisthesis of the Lumbar Spine

Leon L. Wiltse, M.D.

Stephen L.G. Rothman, M.D.

Neil I. Chafetz, M.D.

Lumbar spondylolisthesis is a complex series of disorders which may cause a variety of neurocompressive syndromes as well as back pain. Newer imaging methods allow very exact localization of the site of neurocompression allowing the surgeon to plan a precise operation to relieve the clinical signs and symptoms.

In this chapter we demonstrate the points of likely stenosis in each type of spondylolisthesis. A classification previously published by Wiltse et al. is used.[16] We then discuss the necessary surgical treatment for each of the various types.

CLASSIFICATION OF SPONDYLOLISTHESIS

I. Congenital. In this type, the spondylolisthesis is due to congenital anomalies at the lumbosacral junction. There are three subtypes, as follows:
   Subtype A. This subtype has dysplastic articular processes at the level of olisthesis which are axially oriented and frequently combined with spina bifida (Fig 14–1).
   Subtype B. In this subtype, there is sagittal orientation of the articular processes, causing instability at the affected level (Fig 14–2).[17]
   Subtype C. There are other congenital anomalies of the lumbar spine which permit spondylolisthesis to occur. Congenital kyphosis is the principal one (Fig 14–3).[1]

II. Isthmic. The lesion is in the pars interarticularis. Here also, three subtypes can be recognized.
   Subtype A. (Lytic) Stress fracture of the pars (Fig 14–4).
   Subtype B. An elongated but intact pars secondary to healed stress fractures; this subtype has an identical etiology with subtype A above (Fig 14–5).

III. Degenerative. This type usually occurs in people past 40 years and is due to longstanding intersegmental instability (Fig 14–6).

IV. Postsurgical. This is due to partial or complete loss of posterior bony or discogenic support secondary to surgery. This can also be due to stress fractures of the inferior articular processes which are also secondary to surgery (Fig 14–7).

V. Posttraumatic (Fig 14–8). This is due to fractures at areas other than the pars and is always the result of major trauma.

VI. Pathologic. This type is due to generalized or localized bone disease. It is of little clinical importance and is mentioned only for completeness.

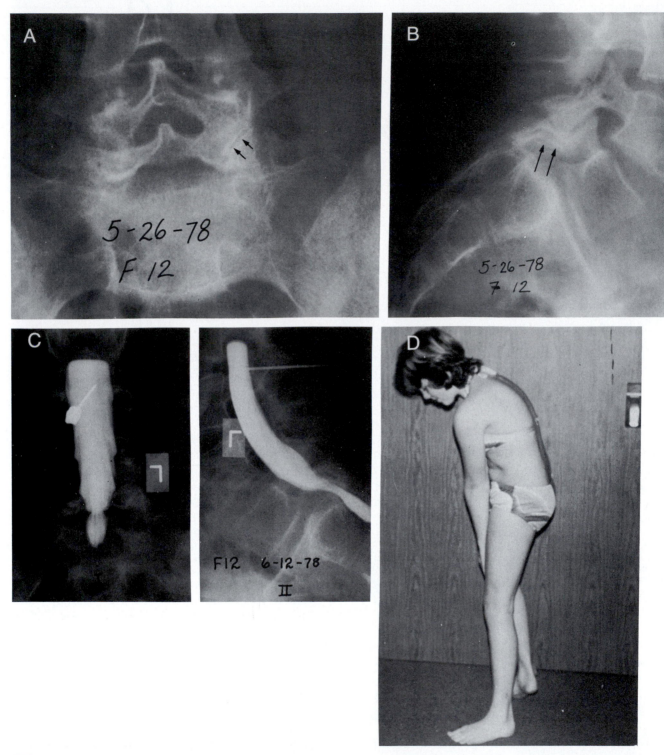

FIG 14–1.
A, anteroposterior (AP) view of congenital spondylolisthesis. Note the axial orientation of the facets *(arrows)*. **B,** lateral view of a congenital spondylolisthesis showing no more than a 25% slip *(arrows)*. **C,** myelogram of the same patient as **B,** showing the rather severe constriction of the cauda equina at the L5–S1 level. This is because both pars are intact and the laminae are dragged forward with a slip caus-ing a good deal of pinching of the cauda equina, even with this low grade of slip. **D,** a 12-year-old patient with very se-vere hamstring spasm. She cannot place her right heel on the floor and is unable to bend over more than what is shown. (**B–D** from Wiltse LL: Spondylolysis and spon-dylolisthesis, in Finneson B (ed): *Low Back Pain.* Philadel-phia, JB Lippincott Co, 1981, p 454. Used by permission.)

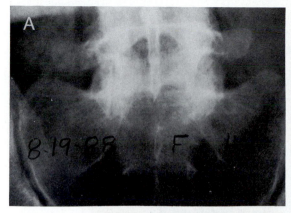

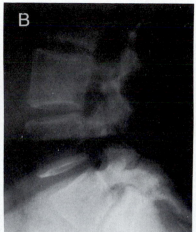

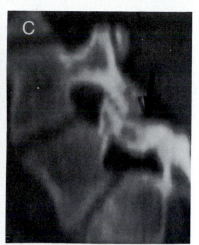

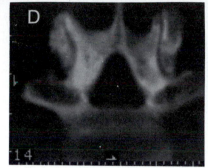

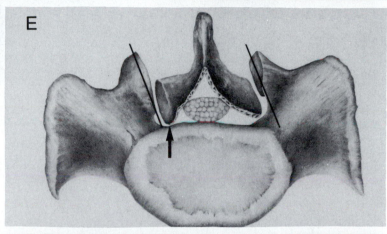

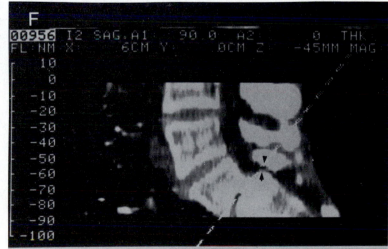

FIG 14–2.

A, AP view of congenital spondylolisthesis subtype B. Note the sagittal orientation of the facets. This orientation does not resist forward thrust well. **B,** lateral view. Note the intact pars and low degree of olisthesis. **C,** on sagittal CT, note the small amount of space between the lamina and the posterior rim of the sacrum. This is the most striking area of stenosis, but stenosis can also occur far laterally, which is characteristic of this type of spondylolisthesis. **D,** axial CT showing the sagittal orientation of the facets. Note hypoplasia of the articular processes. **E,** this drawing shows how stenosis can occur in the midline and also far laterally where inferior articular processes of L5 *(arrow)* come down on the posterior rim of S1. **F,** lateral CT re-formation demonstrating spondylolisthesis of L5 on the sacrum with an intact neural arch. Note the forward position of the lamina of L5 with respect to the posterior portion of the sacral end plate. The spinal canal is profoundly narrowed. (**B** and **E** from Wiltse LL, Rothman S: Lumbar and lumbosacral spondylolisthesis, in Weinstein JW, Wiesel SW (eds): *The Lumbar Spine.* Philadelphia, WB Saunders Co, 1990, p 478. Used by permission.)

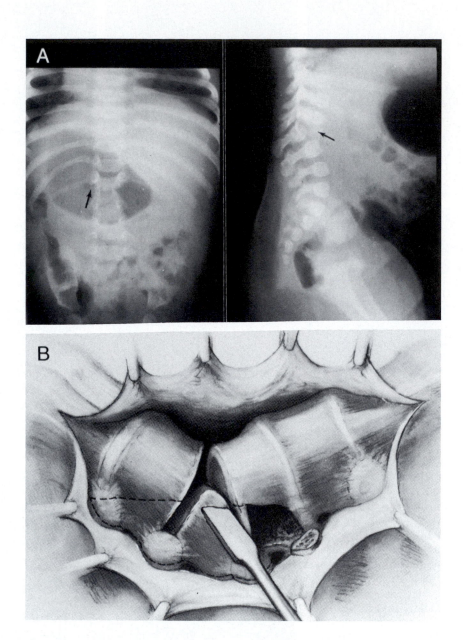

FIG 14–3.
A, AP view of congenital kyphosis between L1 and L2 in an infant. Note the total dislocation of L1 on L2. **B,** method of decompression recommended by Bunnell and MacEwen. The area of severe stenosis is obvious. The resection pictured above removes the pressure from the front of the spinal cord. Anterior and posterior fusion is added. (**B** from Bunnell W, MacEwen D: Congenital deformities of the spine, in Evarts M (ed): *Surgery of the Musculoskeletal System,* ed 2, vol 2. New York, Churchill Livingstone Inc, 1990, p 2043. Used by permission.)

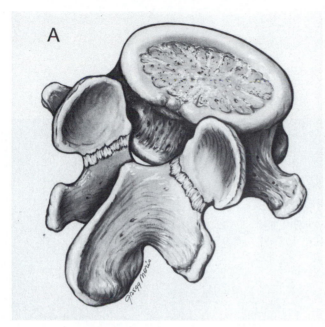

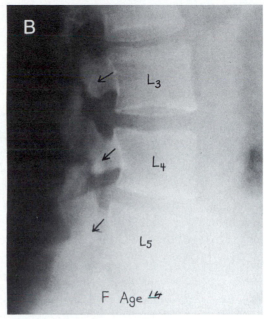

FIG 14–4.
A, a typical lesion in the pars due to a stress fracture. (From Ruge D, Wiltse L: *Spinal Disorders.* Philadelphia, Lea & Febiger, 1977, p 195. Used by permission.) **B,** lateral film showing stress fractures at three levels in a 14-year-old female gymnast. (From Wiltse LL, Rothman S: Lumbar and lumbosacral spondylolisthesis, in Weinstein JW, Wiesel SW: *The Lumbar Spine.* Philadelphia, WB Saunders Co, 1990, p 473. Used by permission.)

GENERAL DESCRIPTION OF ANATOMY

It is most useful to describe the types of neurocompressive stenotic lesions of the spine by the precise anatomic zone involved and the specific tissue or anatomic part causing the neurocompression. In describing anatomic areas, we use the term *zone* when indicating a point in the axial plane and *levels* for the cephalocaudad direction, that is, the sagittal or coronal planes.

Terms Used to Describe Areas of Neurocompression

The central canal is basically the space occupied by the dura. The neurovascular canal extends from the point where the spinal nerve leaves the dura until it exits at the lateral border of the pedicle and a centimeter or two beyond the axial plane. This includes the following zones (Fig 14–9):

1. Entrance or subarticular zone. This is the area between the medial swing of the articular processes and the posterior border of the vertebral body and the posterior margin of the annulus. This includes the lateral recess.
2. Pedicle zone. The portion of the neurovascular canal formed by the pedicles.
3. Exit zone. The extreme lateral border of the pedicles where the nerve leaves the bony canal. This zone is often called the lateral foramen.
4. Far lateral zone. This area, beyond the pedicles and thus beyond the lateral foramen, is often called the extraforaminal zone.

In the caudocephalad direction, we like the description used by Macnab and McCullock.[8] They speak of the "anatomical house." The first story is the disc level; the second, the foramen level; and the third, the pedicle level. Thus, for example, one could describe a fragment of disc as lying at the foraminal level in the entrance zone.

CANAL STENOSIS

Central canal stenosis occurs most commonly when the posterior arch of the olisthetic vertebra

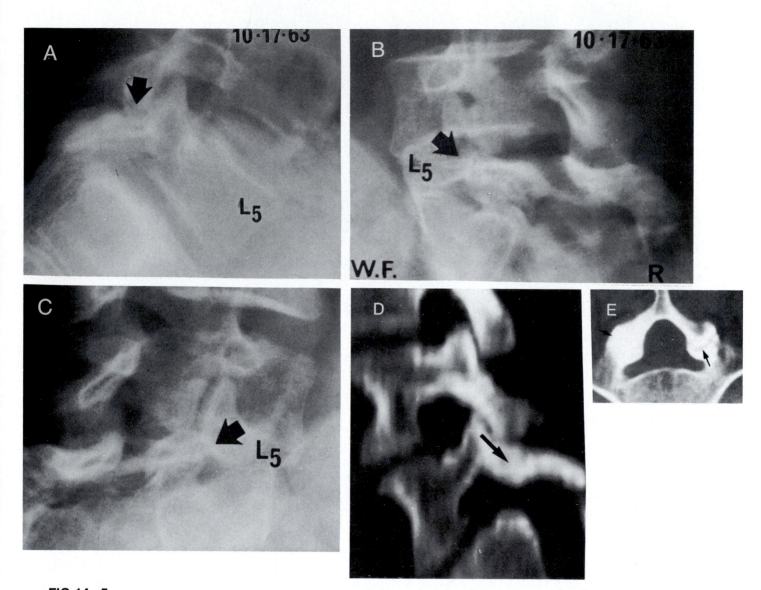

FIG 14–5.
A, bilateral healed pars interarticularis defect. **B,** lateral radiograph demonstrating hockey-stick deformity of the pars. **C,** oblique radiograph demonstrating same as **B**. **D,** lateral CT re-formation. Note the bony sclerosis and the deformity of the pars, and the distortion of the shape of the neural foramen. **E,** axial CT of a 14-year-old boy. Note that the left pars is well healed and the right is nearly healed.

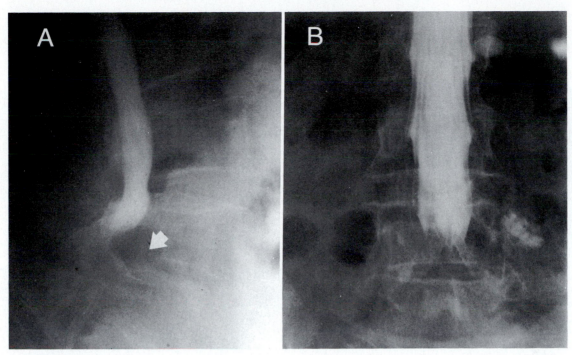

FIG 14–6.
A, lateral view showing degenerative spondylolisthesis at L4–5 in a 77-year-old woman. Note total block, yet only a relatively small amount of slip. **B,** AP view again showing total block.

moves forward along with the vertebral body (see Fig 14–2). Compression of the cauda equina occurs between the neural arch of the slipping vertebra and the posterior portion of the vertebral body of the next lowest vertebral segment. Central canal stenosis is common in all forms of spondylolisthesis when the posterior arch is intact, but not when there is wide spina bifida. It is also common in degenerative spondylolisthesis, but is very uncommon in isthmic spondylolisthesis except in extraordinary circumstances. In a few cases the loose element appears to be dragged forward by the tough scar tissue between the ends of the fractured pars. Thus it is pulled against the posterior superior rim of S1.

SUBARTICULAR OR ENTRANCE ZONE STENOSIS

We use the term *subarticular or entrance zone stenosis* to describe neurocompressive lesions within the space between the posterior body and the medial swing of the anterior processes. This type of stenosis causes neural compression of the root entrapped in the affected recess and it may be unilateral or bilateral (Fig 14–10).

PEDICLE ZONE

Figure 14–11 shows an example of end-plate osteophytes extending into the neurovascular canal in the pedicle zone at the disc level, narrowing the canal. These compress the L5 nerve.

Figure 14–12 is a drawing of the proximal stump of the pars of L5 settling down on the L5 nerve and pinching it between the rim of the body of S1. Figure 14–9,B is a parasagittal computed tomographic (CT) re-formation of that phenomenon.

EXIT ZONE STENOSIS

Lateral foraminal or exit zone stenosis is a fairly common anatomic cause of neural compression in isthmic spondylolisthesis and there is a characteristic deformity. The canals become horizontally oriented and flattened rather than remaining bean-shaped and vertically oriented (Fig 14–13). Annular fibers of the degenerative disc often bulge laterally into the foramen, further compromising the exiting nerve roots. Bony callus frequently projects down into the foramen from the fractured pars above and there is a

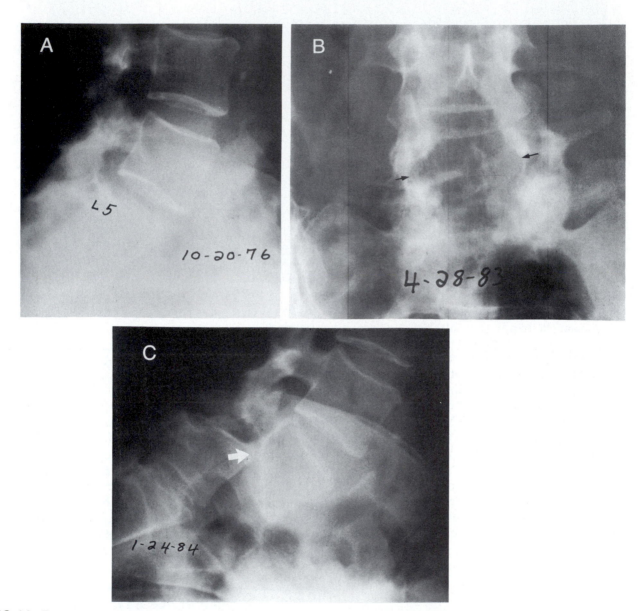

FIG 14–7.
A, radiograph taken 6½ years preoperation. **B,** post decompression. Very little lateral support was left. The articular processes were largely removed *(arrows)*. **C,** severe post-decompression slip occurred. In older people, women especially, at L4–5 one must leave at least two thirds of the articulating faces of the facets or severe postsurgical olisthesis may occur. (From Bunnell W, MacEwan D: Congenital deformities of the spine, in Evarts M (ed): *Surgery of the Musculoskeletal System,* ed 2, vol 2. New York, Churchill Livingstone Inc, 1990, p 2104. Used by permission.)

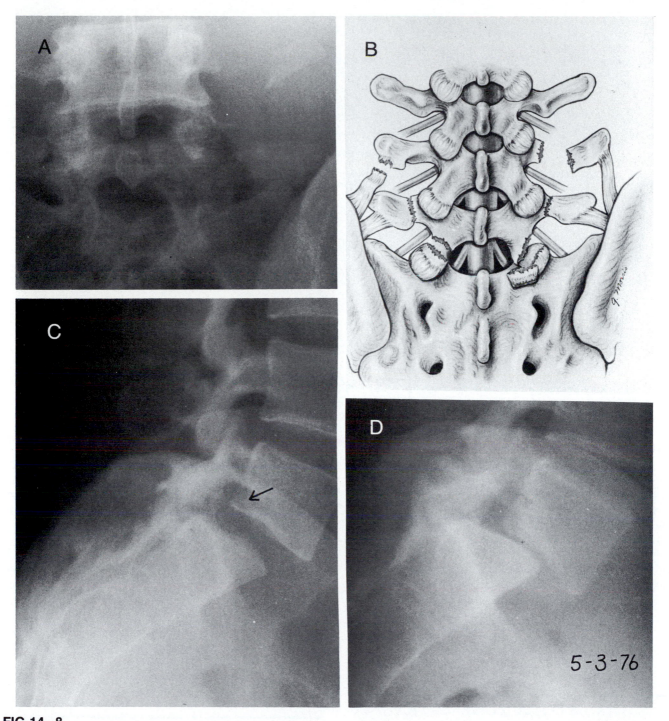

FIG 14–8.

A, traumatic spondylolisthesis. AP radiograph of a 25-year-old man who was involved in a severe car accident. Note multiple fractures but lack of pars fracture. **B,** the injuries. **C,** lateral view taken 14 days after the injury. **D,** lateral view taken 1 year after the injury and after solid fusion. Note that the slip had progressed. This case demonstrates the slow progression of olisthesis after severe injury typical of traumatic spondylolisthesis. (From Wiltse LL: *J Cont Orthop EdL,* July/1979, p 82.

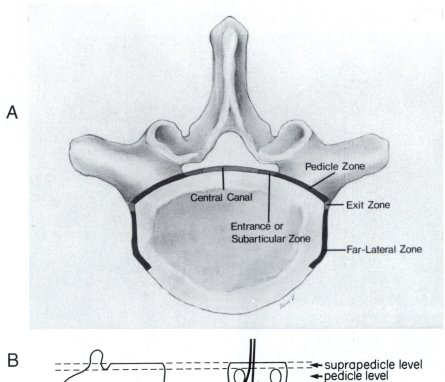

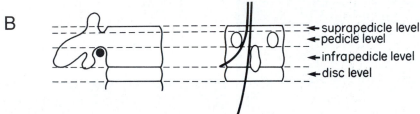

FIG 14–9.
A, axial drawing of the various zones. The central canal is largely occupied by the dura. The entrance zone is the point where the two nerve roots are encased by the dural sheath coming out of the dura and entering the neurovascular canal. The pedicle zone is that area bordered by a pedicle above and one below. The midportion of the nerve has a ganglion and beyond the ganglion is a true mixed nerve. **B,** for localizing a lesion considered from the caudocephalad direction we use "levels." Thus, an MRI report might read, "8-mm extruded disc fragment lying in the entrance zone at the infrapedicle level."

prominent bony ridge arising from the inferior end plate of the L5 vertebra associated with diffuse bulging of the disc. This bony crest tends to point upward, compressing the exiting L5 spinal nerve (Fig 14–14).

occasionally but is not truly stenosis. We recognize that neurophysiologically it may not be totally correct to speak of an "entrance zone" or "exit zone," since different impulses travel outward and inward, but in these situations we are referring to the relationship to the central and peripheral nervous system.

FAR LATERAL ZONE–EXTRA FORAMINAL COMPRESSION

The exiting nerve roots may be entrapped between the alae of the sacrum and the transverse process of the L5 vertebra. This has been previously termed the *far-out syndrome* (Fig 14–15).[15] True extraforaminal or far-lateral disc herniation also occurs

STENOSIS AS IT RELATES TO THE VARIOUS FORMS OF SPONDYLOLISTHESIS

Congenital

In all three congenital forms of spondylolisthesis the pars and thus the neural ring remain intact, at

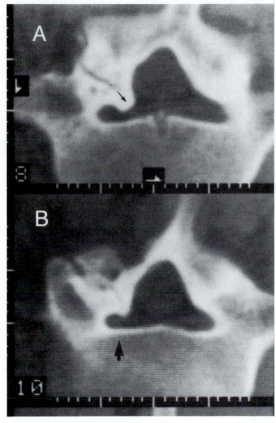

FIG 14–10.
A, axial bone window CT scan showing prominent callus in the entrance zone. **B,** the pars defect is healing on this left side but is well healed on the right. The right side does not show this build-up of new bone.

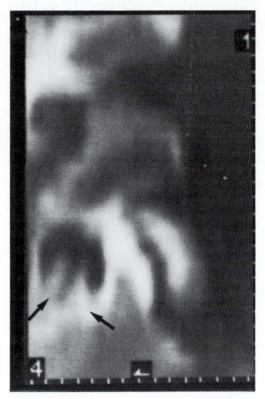

FIG 14–11.
Lateral CT reconstruction showing "railroad track osteophytes" *(arrows)*. Large bony ridges project up from the inferior end plate of L5 and the superior end plate of the sacrum. The ridges point directly up into the L5 nerve root, which sits in the anterosuperior portion of the neural canal, corresponding to the pedicle zone. (From Rothman S, Glenn WV: *Multiplanar CT of the Spine.* Baltimore, University Park Press, 1985, p 138. Used by permission.)

least at first. Sometimes the pars cracks and pulls apart after olisthesis has progressed. Typically there is central stenosis with cauda equina compression due to slippage of the entire vertebra and its neural arch.

Subtype A

In this type, the facets are orientated in a more or less horizontal plane. This position is not well adapted to stability and there is a tendency for the vertebra above to slide forward on the one below. L5–S1 is by far the most frequently affected level. The pars interarticularis is always intact (at least early) and because of this, the entire vertebral ring is pulled forward, thus compressing the cauda. The area of stenosis is principally between the posterior arch of L5 and the posterior superior border of the body of S1. This often causes cauda equina compression at an early age. Note on Fig 14–1, B that the slip is only 25%, yet neural compression in this 11-year-old child was manifested by very severe tight-

ness of the hamstrings. This was because the posterior arch of the neural ring was intact. This child had had an L4–S1 fusion a year before, which had become solid, yet her tight hamstrings remained. Simple posterior decompression of the posterior ring resulted in a complete cure within 2 weeks. Her hamstring spasm had been so severe that she had not attended school for 10 weeks before operation, but she was back in school 3 weeks post decompression.

Stenosis of the lateral canals between the lateral masses of L5 and the sacrum may also occur, but this is not the usual site of neural compression in these patients.

In patients with a wide spina bifida, severe hamstring spasm does not occur and often these vertebrae go on to a very high degree of slip and sagittal rotation without much clinical symptomatology. The lateral canals do narrow and flatten owing

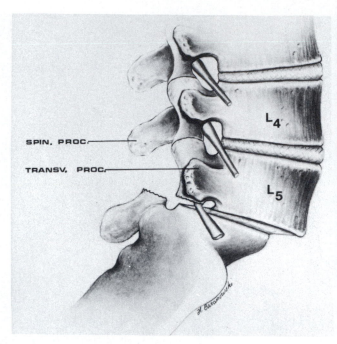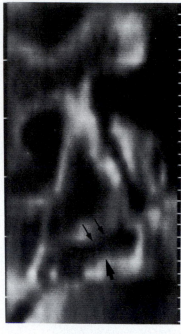

FIG 14–12.
A, the proximal stump of the pars settling down on the L5 nerve. (From Wiltse LL: *J Cont Orthop Ed,* July/1979, p 81. **B,** parasagittal CT re-formation. The *two small arrows* are on the proximal stump of the pars of L5. The *large arrow* is on the posterior rim of S1.

to the slippage, but tend not to cause radiculopathy. Because these children have few symptoms, the olisthesis and sagittal rotation of L5 often become extremely severe before the parents notice any abnormality in the child's body contour (Fig 14–16).

FIG 14–13.
Exit zone stenosis. Diagnostic representation showing exit zone stenosis in isthmic spondylolisthesis. (From Rothman S, Glenn WV: *Multiplanar CT of the Spine.* Baltimore, University Park Press, 1985, p 226. Used by permission.)

Subtype B

This type is seen most commonly in women between 30 and 50 years of age but it can occur earlier. The facets in this type are sagittally oriented and seldom subluxate more than 25%. The area of compression is between the posterior arch of L5 and the

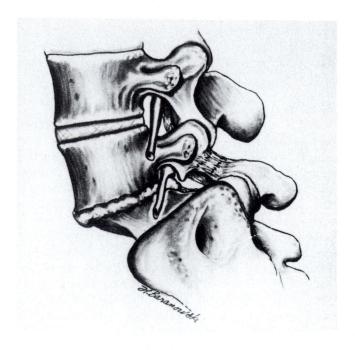

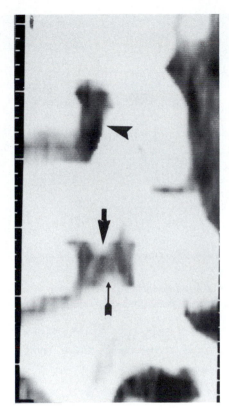

FIG 14–14.
Lateral CT re-formation showing the typical neural foraminal deformity of spondylolisthesis. Note the horizontal orientation of the foramen. An upward projecting bony ridge arises from the superior end plate of the sacrum *(small arrow)* and a second bony protuberance projects downward from the callus at the pars defect *(large arrow)*. Note that there is no fat within the neural foramen owing to diffuse annular bulge.

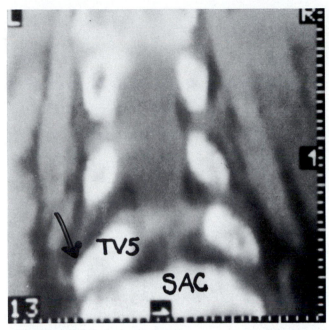

FIG 14–15.
Alar transverse process impingement. Coronal CT re-formation showing how the lateral mass and transverse process of L5 on the left *(TV5)* is jammed down onto the alae of the sacrum *(SAC)*. This patient had severe left leg pain treated by decompression on the left side only and fusion of L5 to S1. (From Wiltse LL, Guyer R, Spencer C: *Spine* 1984; 9:38. Used by permission.

posterior rim of the body of S1. Clinical signs are usually those of cauda equina compression. The lateral recesses and entire canal may also be compressed. The sagittally oriented inferior articular processes of L5 slip forward and compress the S1 nerve roots within the lateral recess and subarticular gutter. Any surgical decompression of these patients must take this anatomic fact into account.

Isthmic

Subtype A

In the great majority of patients with this type, the posterior elements remain in or near their normal location because the zygapophyseal joints at the lumbosacral segment are intact, although often hypoplastic. There is almost always adequate room for the neural elements between the arch of L5 and the posterior rim of the sacrum. However, in rare cases[2] the soft tissues attaching the fractured pars to the

neural arch are very tough and strong. The neural arch can then be pulled forward with the anterior elements causing symptoms of central stenosis. This is not common and the stenosis, when it becomes symptomatic, is in the central canal.

It can be said that isthmic spondylolisthesis is ordinarily a self-decompressing fracture as far as the central canal is concerned. The vertebra slips forward leaving the posterior elements behind. Therefore, neural compression rarely occurs within the central canal. Posterior disc herniation at the level of the spondylolisthesis of sufficient degree to cause symptoms is a rarity, occurring in approximately 4% of patients. A hard, bulging, rolled-up annulus in the area of the exit zone and just beyond is a common finding, and when combined with other factors associated with forward slip, often causes symptoms. Rarely, an extrusion occurs far laterally. Disc herniation at the L4–5 level in association with an L5 spondylolisthesis is much more common that herniations at L5–S1 and probably accounts for L5 radiculopathy in many patients.

L5 root compression occurs in the entrance zone when prominent callus forms at the pars fracture.

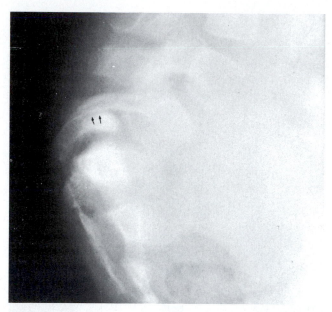

FIG 14–16.
High-grade slip in a 5-year-old girl with congenital spondylolisthesis, subtype 1A. Because she also had a wide spina bifida posteriorly, she was able to function well with little hamstring spasm. (From Wiltse LL: Spondylolysis and spondylolisthesis, in Finneson B: *Low Back Pain.* Philadelphia, JB Lippincott Co, 1981, p 452. Used by permission.)

The most common neural compressive lesion is due to horizontal flattening of the lateral canals. At least one third of symptomatic patients have objective CT or magnetic resonance imaging (MRI) evidence of moderate to severe narrowing and deformity of the canal at its exit zone (see Fig 14–12). The deformity is absolutely characteristic. The orientation of the foramina and canals, which is normally vertical, becomes horizontal as the pedicle of L5 slides forward and downward with respect to the sacrum. The higher the degree of slippage, the lower the pedicle descends. Lateral canal stenosis is further aggravated by downward projection of cartilaginous or calcified callus at the pars fracture. Because the disc degenerates prematurely, there are often lateral circumferential osteophytes arising from the inferior end plate of L5, which point upward into the L5 nerve. These bony ridges are always associated with diffuse annular bulging into the narrowed degenerated disc space. Central canal stenosis and lateral subarticular space stenosis can be caused by prominent callus from the pars interarticularis fracture. This may be primarily soft fibrous tissue or it may be calcified fibrous tissue or dense ossified bone. The bony protuberance may become so large that the

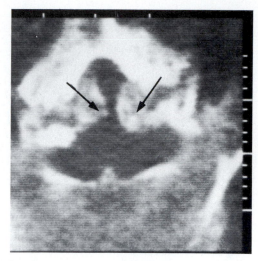

FIG 14–17.
Axial CT image demonstrating very profound extraossification at the pars fracture *(arrows)*. This produces severe canal stenosis.

spinal canal is reduced by more than 50% (Fig 14–17).

Subtype B

There is elongation of the pars with or without separation. Often the pars attenuates like taffy when being pulled until it finally separates. This represents cracking and healing of the pars with elongation. The pars is, however, in continuity. This is the same disease as isthmic subtype A. In most patients with this type, only slight to moderate slippage and neural compression are found. The lateral canals are frequently deformed and the possibility of L5 root compression does exist.

Degenerative

Degenerative spondylolisthesis is due to long-standing intersegmental instability and is most commonly found at the L4–5 segment, less commonly at L3–4 and L5–S1. It is associated with a transitional lumbosacral articulation in one of four cases.[9] Farfan[5] believes that rotary stresses initiate the lesion causing disc degeneration, which is followed by multiple small fractures of the inferior articular processes. The articular processes become irregular and eroded and the diseased facets subluxate. As the slip progresses, the articular processes become remodeled and their orientation is more horizontal. The articular processes tend to be sagittally oriented and facet tropism is quite common. It is not clear whether the tropism precedes the subluxation or is in some way caused by the remodeling. Rotary instability is an integral part of this syndrome. Subluxation is nearly always more severe on the side of the more sagittally oriented facet. Central canal stenosis is caused by two factors: (1) narrowing between the posterior arch of L4 and the posterosuperior rim of the body of L5, and (2) bunching of the ligaments, particularly the ligamentum flavum. This ligament may also become swollen. The second area of compression is in the entrance zone between the inferior articular process of L4 and the posterior body of L5. As the L4 vertebra slips forward, it compresses the L5 nerve between these two bony areas (Fig 14–18). This bunching up of the liga-

ments further narrows the lateral recesses (Fig 14–19). Occasionally, a synovial cyst communicating with the facet joint at the olisthetic level further narrows the available space for the cauda (Fig 14–20).

It is stated that often there is severe stenosis between the superior articular processes of L5 and the back of the L5 vertebral body. This is especially true in patients with congenitally small spinal canals (see Fig 14–17).[9] While there is no question that there are vertebrae with very small lateral recesses due to an exuberant superior articular process, degenerative disease, and hypertrophy, the symptom producing radiculopathy is somewhat hard to explain because the stenotic area is enclosed within the same vertebra. How can this cause pain? The most logical explanation is that traction must be exerted on the exiting nerve roots during the normal motion of the neural structures through the bony canals (Fig 14–21). This tethering of the nerves allows abnormal tugging on them. Since they are fixed in these bony canals, pain results. Tilting and translation motions, as in walking and stooping and bending forward, further compromise the roots by abnormally pulling them and compressing them against the fixed bony protuberances. Wagoner[13] and Farfan[5] have performed surgical reduction without decompression on a number of these patients with relief of the lateral gutter compressive syndrome. It is most likely that in these cases the neural compression was due to the mobile inferior articular process and the hypertrophic thickened articular capsules. By pulling these inferior articular processes posteriorly and fixing them, the compression was taken off the L5 nerve and the stability of the fusion stopped the traction.

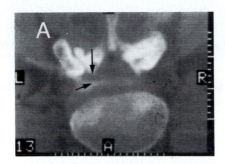

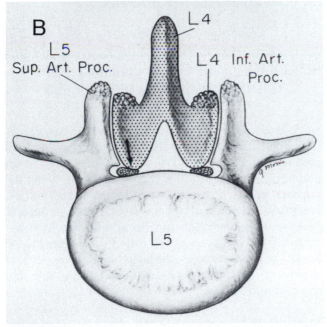

FIG 14–18.
A, axial CT of a patient with severe degenerative spondylolisthesis. Note that the inferior articular processes project forward into the subarticular gutter and compress the exiting nerves. This is much more severe on the left in this patient. **B,** diagram of the phenomenon shown in **A.**

Postsurgical

There are two main types of postsurgical spondylolisthesis. The most common is due to aggressive posterior decompression with removal of the articular processes. In a fair percentage of these patients the lack of stability allows spondylolisthesis of the vertebrae. Neural compression of the central portion of the canal is rare here because of the wide decompression which allowed the vertebra to slip in the first place. There is, however, quite often compression of the exiting nerve roots in the lateral canals. When this occurs, it is generally between the pars of the upper vertebra and the posterior rim of the lower vertebra (Fig 14–22).

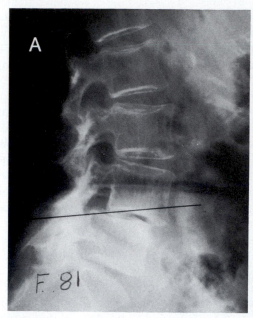
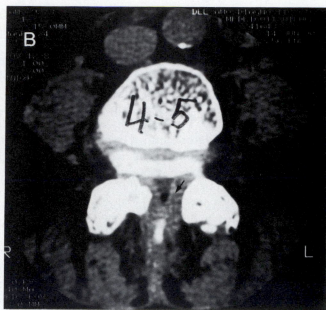

FIG 14–19.
A, lateral radiograph of an 81-year-old woman with severe degenerative spondylolisthesis. The *black line* shows the level of the axial view. **B,** axial view. *Arrow* indicates bunch-ing up of ligaments and perhaps actual hypertrophy of ligaments. Note the small canal at this level.

Posttraumatic

Because of the marked variety of injuries, the areas of compression are different with each case.

Pathologic

As in cases of traumatic spondylolisthesis, the area of stenosis is extremely variable. The area of compression depends on the type of deformity and the underlying pathologic process.

SURGERY IN SPONDYLOLISTHESIS GENERAL CONSIDERATIONS

There are two main indications for surgery in the patient with spondylolisthesis, the relief of back pain and the elimination of neurocompressive radiculopathy. Diffuse nonradicular back pain generally requires fusion of the unstable segment but not decompression. Radicular pain often requires decompression and nearly always an added fusion. If decompressive surgery is indicated, it is critical to know, preoperatively, precisely where the area of stenosis is in order to avoid destabilizing the segment unnecessarily.

Method of Fusion When No Decompression Is Necessary

Paraspinal Approach

When a fusion is done without decompression, the senior author (L.L.W.) has used the paraspinal approach exclusively since 1962.[14] Even with a unilateral decompression, a paraspinal approach is usu-

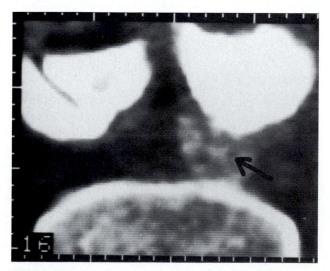

FIG 14–20.
Arrow points to a partially calcified synovial cyst from the right facet joint between L4 and L5.

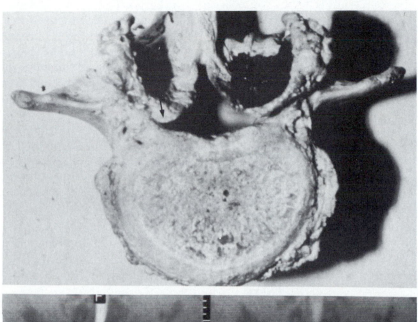

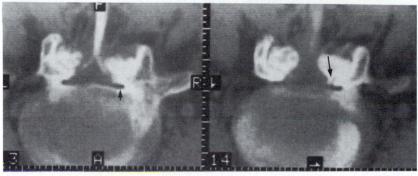

FIG 14-21.

A, anatomic specimen of L5 in a case of severe degenerative spondylolisthesis. Note how the superior articular processes have eroded posteriorly and built up anteriorly to compromise the space for the L5 nerve. The *arrow* points to the area where the L5 nerve must pass. **B,** two axial CT scans, each demonstrating stenosis of the entrance zone as shown in the anatomic specimen in **A.**

ally used. If both sides need to be totally decompressed, a midline approach is used.

Technique.—The patient is placed on any type of frame that allows the abdomen to swing free. A midline skin incision (Fig 14–23,A) is made. This incision is carried down to the level of the deep fascia and the skin is retracted about 2.5 cm laterally on either side. This is done so that the fascial incisions can be made in their proper place, which is 2 cm lateral to the midline, as shown in the figure. Once the heavy fascial layer has been cut through, two ordinary Gelpi retractors are placed so as to separate the fascia a few centimeters. There is a natural cleavage plane between the multifidus and the longissimus muscles. The finger can be plunged between these muscles at any point at or above the L4 level (Fig 14–23,B). For best deep exposure, two ordinary

Gelpi retractors, which are bent at right angles 5 cm from their tips, have proved to be very satisfactory. The laminae of the vertebrae to be fused are exposed well up onto the sloping bases of the adjacent spinous processes. The transverse processes should also be denuded of soft tissue clear out to their tips and slightly around their superior and inferior borders (Fig 14–23,C).

A note of caution should be sounded here. When working on the loose posterior element, never use a hammer or gauge. Never press hard, even with a Leksell rongeur. In high-grade spondylolisthesis, the posterosuperior rim of S1 is just in front of the cauda equina. Schoenecker et al.[12] have reported several cases of cauda equina syndrome that may be from trauma.

Only the lateral surface of the superior articular process of the most cephalad vertebra need be in-

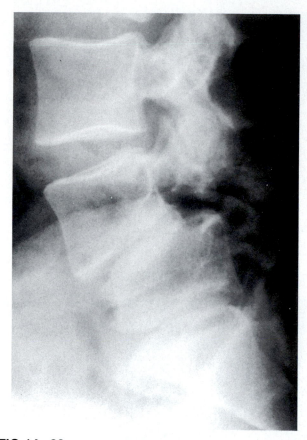

FIG 14–22.
Lateral radiograph of isthmic spondylolisthesis with increased postoperative slip amounting to 0.6 mm. Note small canal for exiting nerves. To decompress, the surgeon would need to channel the canal on both sides.

cluded in the fusion and the area should be denuded. Care should be taken not to remove the capsule or damage the adjacent joint at the top of the fusion, nor should the surgeon expose any part of the lamina of the vertebra immediately above the area to be fused. By observing these precautions any tendency for the fusion to extend upward will be avoided. Incidentally, we also believe that damage to these facets may account for some of the cases of postfusion spondylolisthesis and other problems often seen at the upper ends of the fusions.

In the case of spondylolisthesis involving a loose element, the joint cartilage between the loose element and the S1 facet should not be removed because this further destabilizes an already unstable area. In spondylolisthesis we always fuse the loose element to the S1 lamina since otherwise it may rock about with the muscle contractions and cause pain. This loose element often lies against the posterior rim of the sacrum. Thus, it should be prepared with

a rongeur that has teeth at the tip so no pressure is exerted when getting a bite on the bone. A hammer and gouge should never be used, as this has been known to damage the underlying nerves. Also, in using a Cobb elevator when taking off the soft tissue, be extremely careful not to exert pressure downward.

When should the fusion be limited to L5–S1, and when should L4 be included? Based on the degree of slip and roll, ignoring for the moment such factors as a ruptured disc at the L4 level or internal disc disruption at that level, we use the following rule of thumb: If the angle of the superior border of L5 with the horizontal, i.e., the new sacrohorizontal angle (Fig 14–23,D) is less than 55 degrees, we fuse only L5 to S1. If this angle is greater than 55 degrees, we include L4 in the fusion.[19]

Wound Closure.—Before closure, any small tags of muscle are snipped off.[18] The muscle itself is closed extremely loosely with small sutures. Both layers of the fascia are closed securely. The thoracolumbar fascia is essential to the stability of the lumbar spine. Thus nonabsorbable sutures should probably be used.

It is important to suture the skin edges to the underlying deep fascia, or blood and serum will collect under the portion of the skin that has been undermined and the area will balloon out. If this occurs, it may need to be aspirated (Fig 14–23,E).

Postoperative Management

After paraspinal fusion patients are encouraged to get out of bed when able, usually in a few days, and walk as much as they like. Patients should sit in straight-backed chairs and avoid twisting and should be trained to squat rather than bend their backs. No corsets or braces are used in children. In adults we may use a brace or a cast with a thigh extension on one side.

It is our practice in children with high-grade slip always to take a standing spot lateral radiograph of the lumbosacral joint just before operation to use as a baseline. Then, a week after the patient has been out of bed, another standing spot lateral film is taken of L5–S1. If there is any sign of slip, the child is put to bed until the fusion becomes solid. In 20 years of experience with this technique, our patients have never needed to be put back to bed because of increased slip. A few children who have had extremely tight hamstrings and sciatic scoliosis have

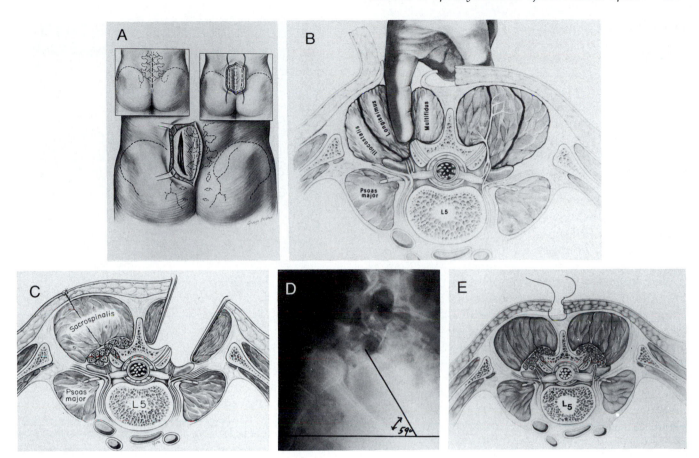

FIG 14–23.
A, midline skin incision with fascial incision 2 cm lateral to the midline. (From Wiltse LL, et al: *Clin Orthop* 1973; 91:52. Used by permission.) **B,** there is a natural cleavage plain between the multifidus and longissimus muscles, except at the L5–S1 level. (From Wiltse LL, et al: *Spine* 1988; 13: 698. Used by permission.). **C,** type of fusion done. (From Wiltse LL, et al: *J Bone Joint Surg [Am]* 1968; 15:921. Used by permission.) **D,** after a fusion from L5 to S1. Functionally the superior border of L5 becomes the new sacrohorizontal angle. **E,** wound closure. We include the fascia in the suture to prevent ballooning of the skin due to collection of fluid in the wound. (From Wiltse LL, et al: *Spine* 1988; 13:701. Used by permission.)

been kept horizontal for 2 weeks to 2 months to allow the spasms and tightness to go away. This bed rest was given not for fear of further slip but simply to let the severe pain subside.

If the loose posterior element has been removed in a patient with spondylolisthesis, further slip may occur. If the annulus has been incised for removal of a ruptured disc at the olisthetic level and the loose element has been removed, progression of slip is a virtual certainty if the patient is allowed out of bed before the fusion has solidified.

The Midline Approach for Arthrodesis in Spondylolisthesis

We have not used the midline approach to fuse isthmic or congenial spondylolisthesis since the later 1950s. However, when we perform a midline decompression for the degenerative type, we use a midline approach.

If surgery is done to decompress a nerve or nerves in spondylolisthesis, a fusion is nearly always done also.

Decompression in the Congenital and Isthmic Types

Congenital Type.—*Subtype A.*—In this type, as slip progresses, the lateral canals for the L5 nerves do not close down severely, but because the lamina is in place, instead the space between the laminae and the posterosuperior rim of the sacrum decreases and the entire remaining cauda equina at that level becomes compressed (see Fig 14–1,C). These patients often walk with a very poor gait and may occasionally even develop bowel and bladder trouble. If surgery in this type is elected in patients with a lot of leg pain and gait abnormalities, the entire lamina should be removed to decompress the cauda. However, if pain and sciatica are limited to one side only, only that side is decompressed. If fused in situ without decompression, hamstring tightness eventually disappears but this can take 1 to 3 years and patients with severe stenosis often continue to have some hamstring tightness indefinitely.

If surgery is done in a child with removal of the lamina of L5, and a lateral fusion is performed, the child is placed in a knees-to-nipples cast for 8 weeks. Otherwise, further slip is likely to occur. In an adult, pedicle screws should be used. Then the patient can be ambulatory with no cast or brace, unless there is a contraindication, such as severe L4 disc disease. Fuse only L5 to S1 if the top border of L5 is less than 55 degrees with the horizontal in the standing position. If greater than 55 degrees, include L4.

If there is a wide spina bifida of L5, one likely need not decompress.

Subtype B.—The area of stenosis is between the posterior arch of L5 (see Fig 14–2) and the posterior rim of the body of S1. Also in these cases, since the inferior articular process of L5 slips forward, it compresses the S1 spinal nerve and any decompression must take this into account (Fig 14–24). These patients seldom have spina bifida. If it is necessary to decompress the lateral canals, use pedicle screws.

Subtype C.—In this type we shall discuss only the case of congenital kyphosis according to Bunnell and MacEwen.[1] These patients should be watched very carefully and at the slightest indication of impending neurologic trouble, they should be placed in bed. If resolution of symptoms occurs, a fusion anteriorly and posteriorly will often suffice. If not, an anterior decompression is probably necessary. Figure 14–3 shows one type of decompression recommended by Bunnell and MacEwen.[1]

It should be noted that there is considerable difference of opinion as to when the surgeon should resort to decompression. Many believe that an anterior and posterior fusion should be done in all of these children very early and certainly before they have symptoms.

Isthmic.—*Subtype A.*—If, as the anterior elements slip forward, the posterior element stays in somewhere near its normal position because there is

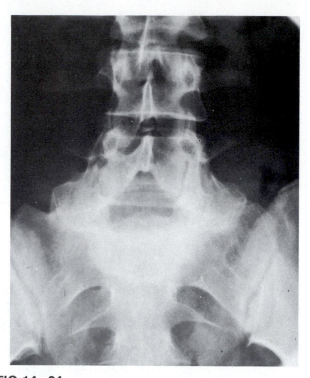

FIG 14–24.
Midline decompression (Gill operation) and fusion. This works in the rare case where it is needed in children, but in an adult, internal fixation with pedicle screws would be added.

a defect in the pars of L5, no stenosis occurs between the arch and the posterior rim of the body of S1. However, when the body and lateral masses of L5 slip forward, especially if they rotate, the proximal stump of the pars and lateral masses of L5 settle down onto the L5 spinal nerve and cause pain and hamstring spasm.

If the lateral canals must be widely decompressed in the adult, pedicle screws should be used.

Subtype B.—In these cases, the pars is elongated but intact and the posterior element remains in its normal position. The area of stenosis, if it occurs, is similar to that in isthmic subtype A, described above, and the methods of decompression are the same.

In the patient with a low-grade olisthesis in isthmic spondylolisthesis of up to 33%, unilateral sciatica with neurologic change is a common finding. If the leg pain is less than 20% of the patient's total pain and neurologic changes are mild, fusion in situ without decompression will suffice. If the sciatica is severe, and there is accompanying neurologic change, decompression of the L5 nerve is in order.

This can be done by starting medially and tracing the nerve laterally (Fig 14–25). The causes of nerve compression may be due to one or several of the following.

1. Bony callus build-up in the defect (see Fig 14–17).
2. Bony ossicles in the defect (see Fig 14–10).
3. Proximal stump of the pars settling down and pinching the L5 nerve against the body of S1 (see Fig 14–12).
4. Hard rolled-up disc bulging laterally[10] (see Fig 14–13).
5. Constriction by the sickle ligament (lumbosacral ligament) (Fig 14–26).

The nerve should be traced out laterally until it is totally decompressed all the way out. Very often the compression is due to overgrowth of osteophytes anterior to the traversing nerve (see Fig 14–11). The nerve may be compressed between this osteophyte and the posteriorly lying bone of the articular processes or pars. Usually removing the bone posteriorly decompresses the nerve adequately. However, occasionally owing to slip, the nerve is stretched over a protuberance or spur and is not be-ing compressed from posteriorly. In these cases, it is necessary to decompress anteriorly in order to remove tension from the nerve. This requires considerable care on the part of the surgeon not to damage the nerve and to save at least some of the circulation to the nerve. There is some evidence that too vigorous removal of tissue from around a nerve may cause painful claudication[3] caused by removing too much of the circulation.

There are a few cases of high-grade olisthesis in which there is such rapid progression of slip owing to decompression that the cauda equina is stretched over the top of S1 so severely that the slip must be either reduced or a wedge of bone must be removed posteriorly from the body of S1 to give the nerves more laxity (Fig 14–27).

Removal of the Loose Element Only

In 1950, Gill, at the annual meeting of the Western Orthopaedic Association in Portland, Oregon, described an operation in which the loose element is removed along with any fibrocartilaginous mass or bony fragments that might be impinging on the L5 spinal nerve[6] (Fig 14–28). Spinal stenosis was not widely recognized at that time and although Gill

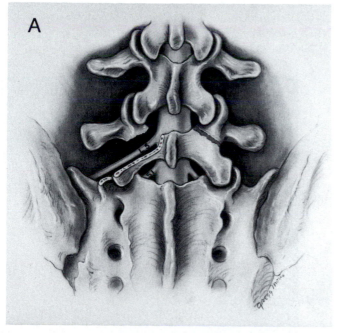

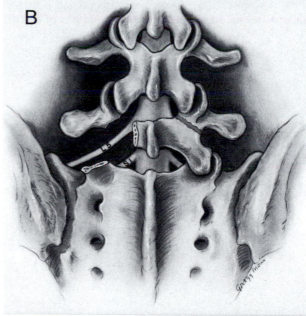

FIG 14–25.
A, decompression of the L5 nerve canal can be done and still save enough bone to fuse to. This is the most common decompression for low-grade spondylolisthesis (25% or less). **B,** unilateral Gill operation, to be used when there is a need to decompress very liberally. (From Wiltse LL, et al: *J Bone Joint Surg [Am]* 1968; 15:923. Used by permission.)

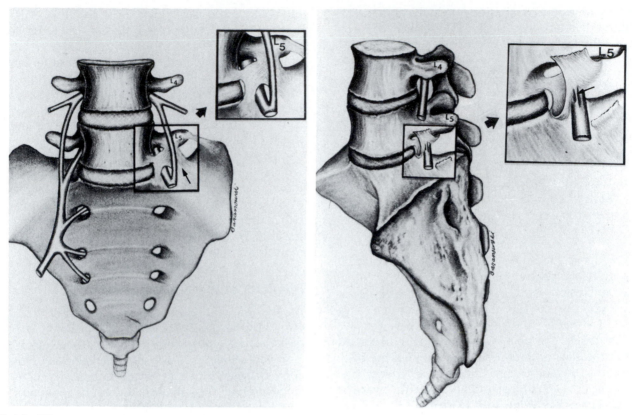

FIG 14–26.
A, *arrow* points to the lumbosacral ligament. This can constrict the nerve, causing a type of stenosis, although a soft tissue stenosis. **B,** small ligaments, shown at the tip of the *arrow*. Both the front and back hold the nerve solidly to the larger lumbosacral ligament. (From Wiltse L: The intervertebral foramina, in Watkins RG (ed): *Lumbar Discectomy and Laminectomy.* Rockville, Md, Aspen, 1987, p 213. Used by permission.)

FIG 14–27.
By taking off part of the top of the body of S1, the cauda equina can be decompressed in cases where reduction is not feasible. *Arrow* indicates line of osteotomy.

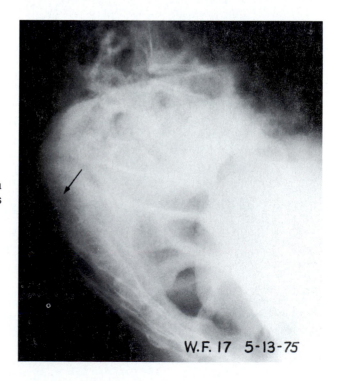

W.F. 17 5-13-75

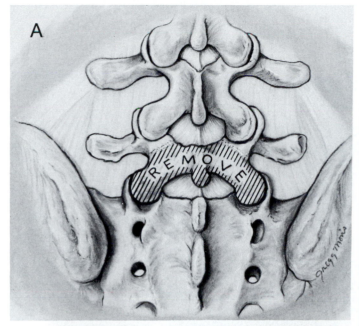

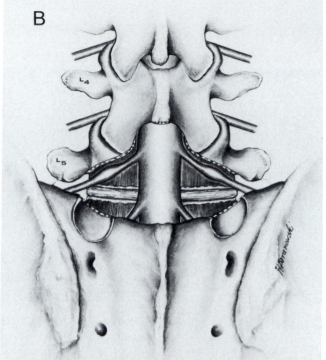

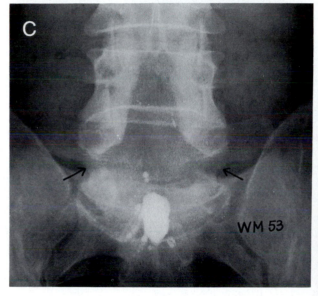

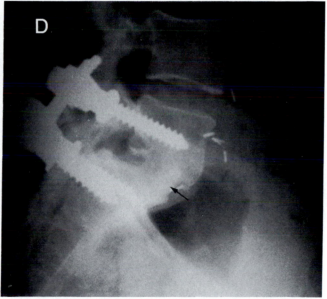

FIG 14–28.

A, the Gill operation as originally described. (From Wiltse LL: *J Cont Orthop Ed* July/1979, p 30.) **B,** bone removed by us when doing a Gill operation. The operation must decompress the lateral canals to be successful. **C,** radiograph of a Gill operation *(arrows)*. The L4 lamina had been removed in a previous operation (not part of the Gill operation). **D,** pedicle screws would virtually always be used by us at this time and probably an interbody fusion also *(arrow)*.

probably did not realize it, he was treating spinal stenosis by the operation. Over the years since his original description, the only significant change in the technique is that the nerve is channelled more widely and often the stump of the pars is removed and even the lower half of the base of the transverse process of L5. Normally we would always fuse after a Gill operation and virtually always use internal fixation. The operation is usually used in association with any reduction operation. In an adult, a Gill op-

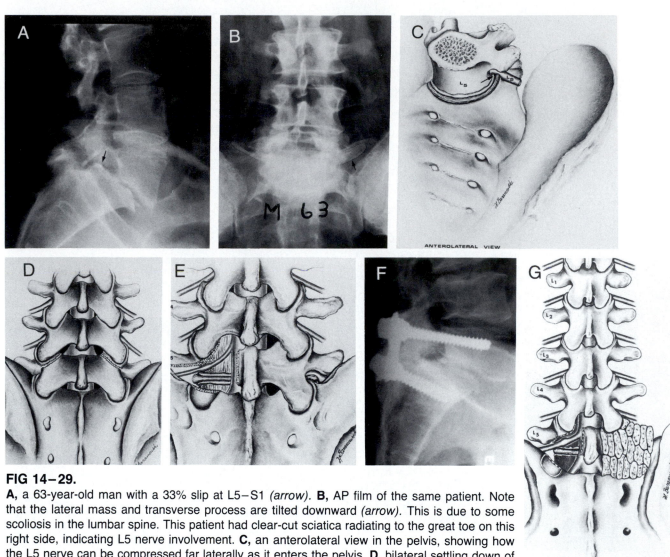

FIG 14–29.
A, a 63-year-old man with a 33% slip at L5–S1 *(arrow).* **B,** AP film of the same patient. Note that the lateral mass and transverse process are tilted downward *(arrow).* This is due to some scoliosis in the lumbar spine. This patient had clear-cut sciatica radiating to the great toe on this right side, indicating L5 nerve involvement. **C,** an anterolateral view in the pelvis, showing how the L5 nerve can be compressed far laterally as it enters the pelvis. **D,** bilateral settling down of the lateral masses and transverse processes along with pars defects. A few patients have a bilateral far-out syndrome. **E,** If a decompression is done in a case of alar transverse process impingement, it must be adequate to remove all pressure from the nerve. Often part of the pedicle either of L5 or of S1 must be removed. **F,** internal fixation with pedicle screws is usually done after decompression. **G,** in elderly people with marked narrowing of the disc space at L5–S1, especially if there is ostophytosis at that level after a unilateral decompression, we are loathe to put bone over the exposed nerves on the side of the decompression. A unilateral fusion can be done on the undecompressed side with about an 80% to 85% chance of obtaining solid fusion. (**C–E** and **G** from Wiltse LL, Guyer R, Spencer C, et al: *Spine* 1984; 9:32, 34, 35, 39. Used by permission.)

eration might be done if the patient has very severe bilateral leg pain with neurologic change. In such a case, one could do a Gill operation, fixing just the one level with pedicle screws. We would go in anteriorly, either immediately or a week or so later, and put in an anterior graft. Bank bone works well in such a case.[11] We never do a complete Gill operation for unilateral leg pain; instead, we decompress only the L5 nerve on the painful side and follow with a fusion. If the nerve must be traced all the way out, totally destabilizing that side, we would use pedicle screws at that one level and add an interbody graft.

Unless rods have been inserted, which would hold the graft bone out laterally so that it does not creep medially over on the nerve, we would not recommend laying bone over a wide gap with an exposed nerve as is always present with a Gill operation.

The Alar Transverse Process Impingement Syndrome (Far-Out Syndrome)

This syndrome, when it is secondary to spondylolisthesis, is a perfect example of stenosis between the lateral masses or even the transverse processes of L5 and the alae of S1 (Fig 14–29).

Impingement of the L5 spinal nerve is common in spondylolisthesis when there is more than a 20% slip. The leg symptoms may be either unilateral or bilateral. As the body of L5 slips forward, owing to a combination of the olisthesis, the disc bulging out laterally, and disc space narrowing, it settles down onto the nerve, pressing it against the base of the alae. The annulus is drawn taut posteriorly but bulges posterolaterally. Because the nerve is tethered out laterally, there may be some traction on it, which may also explain the severe dermatomal pain. Also, the corpora–transverse process ligament may compress the nerve.

Surgery can relieve far-lateral impingement in two ways: (1) the nerve can be decompressed by channeling out beyond the sickle ligament, or (2) the slip can be at least partially reduced in combination with lifting of the L5 vertebra cranially by an interbody graft along with fixation with pedicle screws.

Degenerative Spondylolisthesis

The principal area of stenosis in L4–5 degenerative spondylolisthesis is between the inferior articular processes of L4 (Fig 14–30) and the posterosuperior portion of the body of L5. The disc between L4 and L5 often appears quite large on MRI (Fig 14–31).

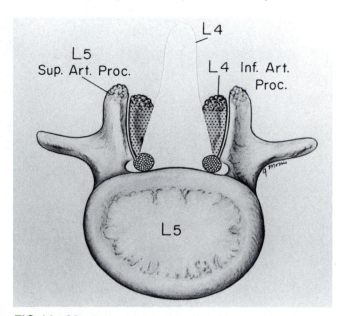

FIG 14–30.
Type of decompression done for degenerative spondylolisthesis. This is cut through near the cephalic border of the L5 vertebral body.

This nerve tissue should be decompressed by removing bone from posteriorly and not by removing the disc. If for any reason the disc is removed, pedicle internal fixation should be added or severe further olisthesis may occur. Even though the disc appears large far laterally, it still does not compress the L4 nerve in the lateral canals.

As mentioned, the other area that is often incriminated as an area of nerve compression is that between the superior articular processes of L5 (in L4–5 spondylolisthesis) and the body of L5 (see Fig 14–21). There is no question that this space gets very small. As the superior facet of L5 erodes posteriorly, bone builds up anteriorly and thus the canal gets smaller. Those of us who have decompressed cases of degenerative spondylolisthesis know that this part of the operation must be done with great care because there is so little space. The tethering of the nerve at this point along with traction could cause pain. Against this is the fact that when the L4 vertebra is pulled back into place and fixed without decompression, as Farfan[4] or Wagoner[13] has done using pedicle screw fixation, pain is reported to disappear. It may be that the fusion between L4 and L5 has stopped motion and thereby has stopped the tugging on the nerve (Fig 14–32).

Figure 14–32 documents the type of operation done in degenerative spondylolisthesis.[7] Pedicle screws were used in this case, but we usually do not

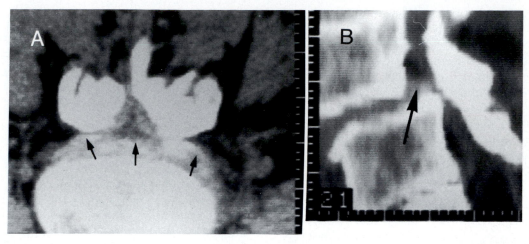

FIG 14–31.
A, lateral MRI view shows a typical bulge of a disc at L4–5 *(arrows)*. Note that the disc bulges up behind the L4 vertebral body but not beyond the posterior border of L5. This is very characteristic. The spinal canal is markedly narrowed between the lamina of L4 and the back of the disc at L5. **B,** axial CT, soft tissue window A, demonstrates profound spinal stenosis due to a combination of congenitally short pedicles, subluxation of L4 on L5, diffuse bulging of the disc, and severe paraarticular soft tissue and bony disease.

add pedicle screws to a typical degenerative spondylolisthesis operation. We may change that rule in the future.

Only one level need be fused when the olisthesis is limited to one level. We have no objection to a floating fusion. No cast, brace, or corset is used in most cases. The L4 spinal nerve lying between L4 and L5 is seldom compressed. It goes forward with the body of L4 and except post surgery if a very high-grade slip occurs, i.e., 50% or more, combined with marked disc narrowing, it escapes compression (Fig 14–33).

Postoperative Fracture of the Pars of L5 in Degenerative Spondylolisthesis

If too much bone is removed during decompression in degenerative spondylolisthesis and a fusion has not been done, postoperative fracture of the pars is common. If the pars fractures, severe slip may occur and pain is usually severe. In these cases, reduction back to the preoperative position is easily accomplished—often just putting the patient in the kneeling position at surgery allows the olisthetic vertebra to slip back. One must excise enough of both the proximal and distal pars so that the nerve is clearly visible. A posterior lumbar interbody fusion (PLIF) could be added to very good advantage. If one had elected to do an anterior lumbar interbody fusion (ALIF), we would do this before going posteriorly, but not much time should elapse between the anterior and the posterior fusion, as severe olisthesis

may result in the interim because of the instability. An anterior interbody graft does not prevent slip as it increases instability. When pedicle screw fixation is used, we use an allograft rather than an autograft for the interbody fusion with either PLIF or ALIF (Fig 14–34).

Even with a good reduction and with increased lordosis, which is desirable, compression may occur. It is a good idea to visualize the nerve to be sure there is no compression.

Surgery in Postsurgical, Traumatic, and Pathologic Spondylolisthesis

In postsurgical, traumatic, and pathologic spondylolisthesis, the area of stenosis is variable depending upon the underlying abnormality. Reformatted CT and MRI will nearly always define the area of compression precisely and the appropriate surgical decompression can be planned. The same rules apply as to the other types of spondylolisthesis described in this chapter. Simple laminectomy is rarely sufficient and spinal fusion must be added. It is important to save as much of the lamina as possible since this adds to the area for bone graft. Now that we have pedicle screws and connecting rods, the surgeon can be as radical in his decompression as necessary.

If a large amount of posterior bone is removed, adding an anterior interbody graft is essential. The interbody fusion can be done through the same ap-

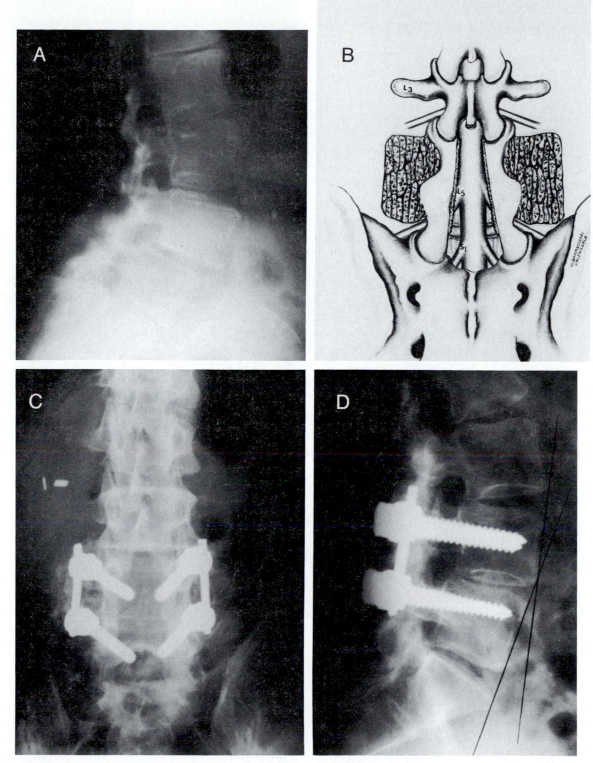

FIG 14–32.
A, lateral view of typical degenerative spondylolisthesis. **B,** type of surgery done. (From Lombardi J, Wiltse L, Reynolds J, et al: *Spine* 1985; 10:822. Used by permission.) **C,** postoperative AP film shows pedicle screws and rods in place. Note that a decompression and floating fusion has been done. **D,** lateral films showing pedicle screws in place. The use of pedicle screws is not routine with us in treating degenerative spondylolisthesis.

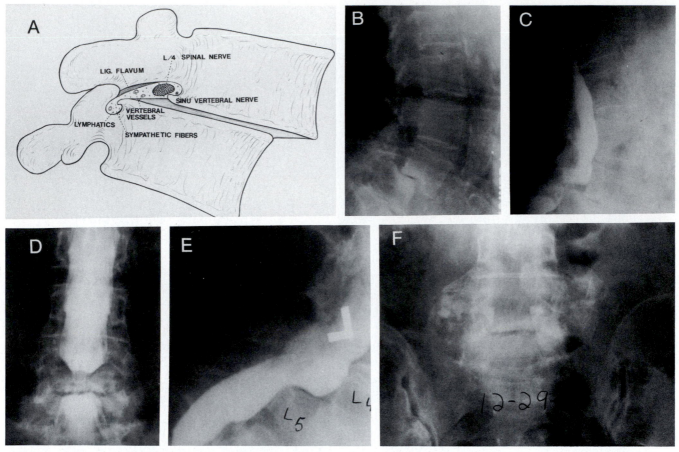

FIG 14–33.
A, this drawing demonstrates how the L4 nerve is pulled forward and does not usually become compressed. **B,** with a very high-grade slip and a very narrow disc space, it is rare that it becomes compressed and needs surgical release, as in this patient. **C,** a high-grade slip at L4–5. Note that the pedicle of L4 is jammed down on the superior posterior corner of the body of L5. **D,** preoperative myelogram. Note near-total cutoff of contrast. **E,** postoperative lateral myelogram. Note cutoff of contrast has been relieved. **F,** decompression and fusion at one level with decompression of the L4 nerve has been done.

proach as a PLIF if the surgeon is skilled in the operation, or through an abdominal approach (ALIF).

SUMMARY

Neurocompressive spinal stenosis associated with spondylolisthesis is a major surgical problem. It is, however, not the only cause of pain in these patients. Back pain without neural compression is commonly seen and must be treated appropriately. If there is no leg pain, decompression is not necessary. If severe radicular pain is present, diagnostic studies to find the area of compression are indicated. These include CT, MRI, contrast myelogra-

phy, and electromyography. It is critical to remember that in many patients, symmetric, bilateral anatomic abnormalities are seen on the CT scan or on MRI, yet the patient complains of unilateral symptoms. The surgeon must decide whether to decompress both sides or only the symptomatic side. We would normally decompress only the painful side. The surgeon must also decide whether interbody fusion should be added to the usual lateral fusion. Should internal fixation be used? These are all questions the answers to which must be tailored to the individual patient. The current diagnostic studies, when integrated with careful physical examination, will nearly always allow the appropriate surgical decision to be made. Pedicle screw fixation allows excellent judgment of the necessity for wide decompression and the maintenance of adequate

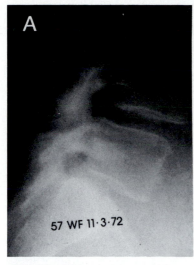
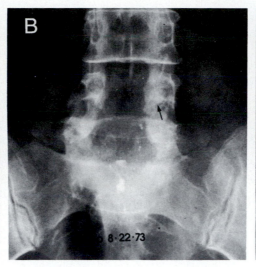
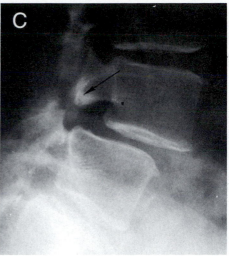

FIG 14–34.
A, preoperative lateral radiograph. Note the low degree of olisthesis. Despite this, the patient had near total block at L4–5 due to bunching and possible hypertrophy of ligaments. **B,** large midline decompression. The date of the operation was 8/22/73. Note that on the right side *(arrow)* one can see a crack in the pars. Postoperative fractures of the pars after midline decompression in osteoporosis is a frequent occurrence. **C,** note that on 3/28/74, slightly more than 8 months postoperatively, a wide defect in the pars has developed *(arrow)* and there is considerable olisthesis. These patients characteristically have severe back pain. They also frequently have sciatica due to loss of disc height. When sciatica develops, it is because the proximal stump of the pars may jam down on the L4 spinal nerve as it exits posterolaterally.

segmental stability. Present fusion techniques provide successful arthrodeses in a high percentage of cases.

It is our opinion that diagnostic modalities have now reached a degree of sophistication such that it is no longer acceptable for a surgeon to go exploring in the back. He should be able to plan ahead what he will do and only rarely digress from his plan.

REFERENCES

1. Bunnell W, MacEwen D: Congenital deformities of the spine, in Evarts M (ed): *Surgery of the Musculoskeletal System,* ed 2, vol 2. New York, Churchill Livingstone Inc. 1990, pp 2042–2443.
2. Burski G, McCall IW, O'Brien JP: Myelography in severe lumbosacral spondylolisthesis. *J Bone Joint Surg [Br]* 1970; 57:432–437.
3. Crock HV: Personal communication, 1989.
4. Farfan HF: *Mechanical Disorders of the Low Back.* Philadelphia, Lea & Febiger, 1973.
5. Farfan HF: Personal communication, 1980.
6. Gill GG, Manning JG, White HL: Surgical treatment of spondylolisthesis without spinal fusion. *J Bone Joint Surg [Am]* 1978; 33:471–476.
7. Lombardi J, Wiltse L, Reynolds J, et al: Treatment of degenerative spondylolisthesis. *Spine* 1985; 10:821.
8. Macnab I, McCulloch JA: *Backache,* ed 2. Baltimore, Williams & Wilkins Co, 1990, p 18.
9. Rosenberg NJ: Degenerative spondylolisthesis, surgical treatment. *Clin Orthop* 1976; 117:112.
10. Rothman SL, Glenn WV: CT multiplanar reconstruction in 253 cases of lumbar spondylolysis. *AJNR* 1984; 5:81–90.
11. Selby D: Personal communication, 1990.
12. Shoenecker PL, Cole HO, Herring JA, et al: Cauda equina syndrome following in situ fusion of spondylolisthesis of the lumbosacral joint. *Orthop Trans* 1987; 11:513.
13. Wagoner T: Personal communication, 1990.
14. Wiltse LL, Bateman JG, Hutchinson RH: The paraspinal sacrospinalis-splitting approach to the lumbar spine. *J Bone Joint Surg [Am]* 1968; 50:919.
15. Wiltse L, Guyer R, Spencer C, et al: Alar transverse process impingement of the L5 spinal nerve: the far out syndrome. *Spine* 1984; 9:30–41.
16. Wiltse LL, Neuman PH, Macnab I: Classification of spondylolisthesis. *Clin Orthop* 1976; 117:23–29.
17. Wiltse L, Rothman S: Lumbar and lumbosacral spondylolisthesis. in Weinstein JW, Wiesel SW (eds): *The Lumbar Spine.* Philadelphia, WB Saunders Co, 1990, pp 471–499.
18. Wiltse L, Spencer C: New uses and refinements of the paraspinal approach. *Spine* 1988; 13:696–706.
19. Wiltse L, Winter RB: Terminology and measurements in spondylolisthesis. *J Bone Joint Surg [Am]* 1983; 65:768–772.

15

Posttraumatic Stenosis of the Lumbar Spine

Dieter Grob, M.D.

Traumatic stenosis is diagnosed by computed tomography (CT) scans on admission to the trauma unit. It represents a momentary and mostly unstable equilibrium of the forces involved in this situation. These forces include the pressure of the fracture hematoma, tension of stretched ligaments (posterior longitudinal ligament), and present axial loading of the spine, etc.

Posttraumatic stenosis is the final result of the primary and secondary changes of the injury which compromise the width of the spinal canal.

In this chapter, an attempt is made to describe the anatomy of traumatic and posttraumatic stenosis and their clinical symptoms. Guidelines for treatment and prevention are also provided.

ANATOMY OF POSTTRAUMATIC STENOSIS

The localization of the stenosis is dependent on the injured and displaced structures bordering the vertebral canal. The extent of encroachment, and therefore the clinical relevance of the stenosis, is determined by the anatomic specification of the injured spine.

A primary normal width of the vertebral canal is essential for undisturbed performance of the neural structures. The available "reserve space" is reduced in congenital spinal stenosis or in degenerative stenosis present at the time of injury. Therefore, the capacity to tolerate traumatic encroachment of the spinal canal without neurologic deficits decreases with the degree of preexisting narrowing.

There are considerable variations of "normal" in measurements of stenosis. Relative measurements of the width of the spinal canal in the assessment of stenosis, therefore, give more accurate information than absolute values[2] of decreased space. This reasoning allows Hashimoto et al.[16] to postulate that neurologic involvement is likely with an obstruction of 35% or more of the spinal canal at T11–12, of 45% or more at L1, and of 55% or more at L2 or below this level. Precise information of the degree of narrowing is given by measuring the cross-sectional area of the vertebral canal, which is defined relative to the area of the vertebral canal of the level above plus the area of the vertebral canal of the level below divided by two.[17] Spinal stenosis is also dependent on the type of injury to the lumbar spine. Fracture dislocations involve neurologic deficits in 79% of patients, in contrast to burst fractures which have a 31% neurologic involvement.[6, 17] However, until now, no general fracture classification has been universally accepted. Fracture classification seems not to be an ideal predictor of posttraumatic spinal stenosis. Strict anatomic description of the injured part of a vertebra allows more precise information about possible narrowing of the spinal canal.

Fractures of the middle column with retropulsation of a fragment of the posterior wall[7, 8, 22] is re-

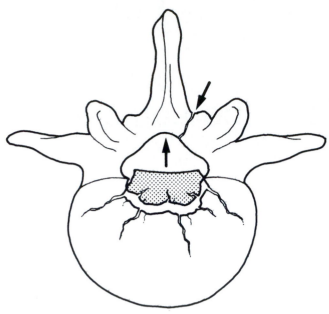

FIG 15–1.
Schematic drawing of a retropulsed fragment of the posterior wall of a vertebral body causing anterior spinal stenosis.

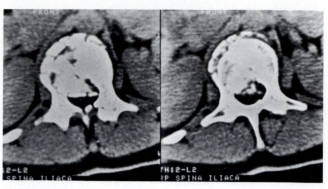

FIG 15–2.
Posttraumatic spinal stenosis by a retropulsed bony fragment.

sponsible for central spinal stenosis in the majority of the cases. Fractures that include the pedicles, the facets, or the laminae may produce lateral recess narrowing or posterior stenosis.

Bony Lesions

Central Stenosis

A fractured posterior wall may cause stenosis by a retropulsed bony fragment (Figs 15–1 and 15–2), by fracture and malalignment (Fig 15–3, A, B), or by

callus or osteophyte formation. A fractured vertebral body may cause stenosis by increasing the kyphotic deformity (Fig 15–4,A–C). Fracture of the lamina (Fig 15–5) may cause stenosis by callus formation or malalignment.

Lateral Stenosis

A fractured pedicle (Fig 15–6) may cause stenosis by callus formation or by fracture malalignment. Fracture of the facets may cause narrowing of the lateral recess by fracture malalignment (Fig 15–7,A,B).

Soft Tissue Lesions

Ruptured ligaments allow dislocation or luxation of the spine (Fig 15–8) and cause stenosis by displacement. A ruptured posterior longitudinal ligament may cause stenosis by osteophytes due to ligamentous avulsion. Ruptured posterior ligaments

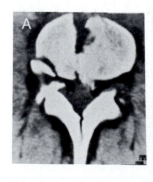
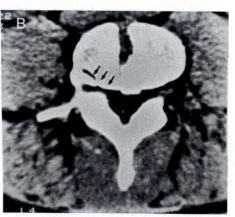

FIG 15–3.
A, acute injury to L4. Minimal osseous displacement. No neurologic deficit. Conservative treatment. **B,** posttraumatic lateral stenosis with typical radicular claudication pain due to lateral recess encroachment.

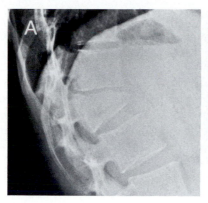
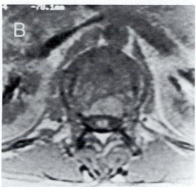
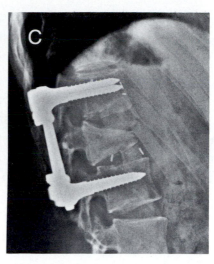

FIG 15–4.
A, posttraumatic kyphotic deformity after distraction-compression injury of T12 with intact posterior wall but grossly disrupted posterior ligaments and fractured anterior part of the vertebral body. **B,** MRI indicates concentric spinal stenosis due to a "bow string" effect of the spinal cord in the kyphotic area. **C,** postoperative correction by a combined procedure: anterior disc excision and posterior fixation with CD instrumentation.

and muscles may produce stenosis by increasing the kyphotic deformity (see Fig 15–4).

Disc Lesions

A ruptured annulus fibrosus may cause stenosis by a herniated disc due to trauma.[25]

DIAGNOSTIC PROCEDURES

Clinical Evaluation

The examination of an injured spine may provide first details about the kind of injury and the probability of spinal stenosis. These include:

1. Deformity and irregularity of the trunk position.
2. Neurologic evaluation: Neurologic deficits may indicate compression. Apart from motor and sensory deficits of the lower limbs, the evaluation of anal sphincter activity, bladder function, and sensory functions in the perineal area are important. Neurologic assessment using the Frankel et al.[13] classification have been proved to be useful.

In late posttraumatic stenosis, the classic clinical symptoms of neurogenic intermittent claudication may also be present. Symptoms are often not well described and may be constantly or intermittently present after physical effort. Pain might be less in the kyphotic posture or decrease in a lying position. Some patients will feel more pain when walking downhill than walking uphill, because the lumbar spine is flexed when doing the latter. Walking has to be stopped after a certain distance because of increasing leg pain. Relief is afforded by a bent-forward position or by sitting. If there is posttrau-

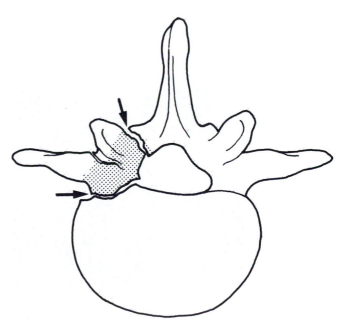

FIG 15–5.
Posterior stenosis caused by displaced fractured lamina.

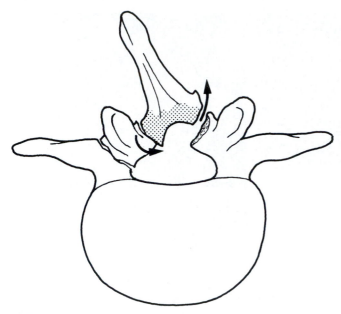

FIG 15–6.
Lateral fracture including pedicle and facets may produce stenosis of the lateral recess

matic kyphosis, with or without stenosis, the upright posture has to be compensated for by hyperlordosis in adjacent segments. Pain induced by overload of these facets might disguise the classic pain caused by the stenosis. Twenty-five percent of late pain in patients after conservatively treated thoracolumbar burst fractures was interpreted by Denis[7] as such posture-induced pain. The localization of pain might be vaguely defined and may have a radicular distribution or may present as low back pain with or without radiation distally.

Imaging

To evaluate spinal stenosis, imaging techniques are necessary. In the acutely injured patient, plain lateral and anteroposterior (AP) radiographs are made to evaluate gross deformities (without moving the patient to prevent further injury). If neurologic deficits are present, CT or magnetic resonance imaging (MRI) evaluation is performed as soon as medically possible to decide on further treatment strategy.

Plain Radiographs

Stenosis after acute injury is suspected in the presence of:

1. Fracture of the vertebral body, with severe kyphotic deformity (>30 degrees), and decreased body height.
2. Fractured posterior wall (retropulsed bony fragment) (Fig 15–9).
3. Dislocation of the facets.
4. Translational displacement.
5. Increased interpedicular distance.
6. Offset of the spinous process in the AP or lateral view.
7. Fracture of the facets (see Fig 15–7A,B).

Myelogram

A useful tool to determine the AP diameter of the spinal canal is the myelogram (Fig 15–10). Changes in flexion and extension can be studied in late posttraumatic cases. The lower limit of normal values is indicated as being 12 mm.[18] This value is probably high, as discussed in Chapters 2 and 10.

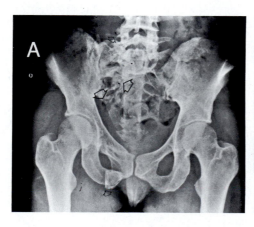
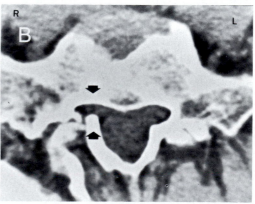

FIG 15–7.
A, pelvic ring fracture, 9 years after an automobile accident. The fracture involved the anterior and posterior part of the pelvis including the right lumbosacral joint and the trans- verse process of L5 *(arrows).* **B,** the fractured and displaced lumbosacral joint causes stenosis of the lateral recess with clinically manifest root claudication.

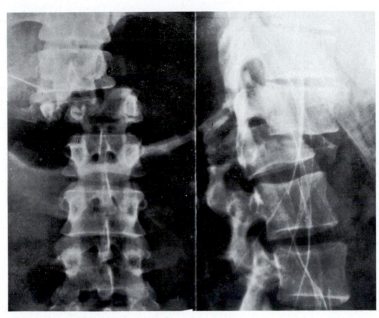

FIG 15–8.

Fracture dislocation of the spine. Conservatively treated rotational injury with dislocation of T12–L1 and complete paraplegia at the level of T12 due to compromised width of the spinal canal.

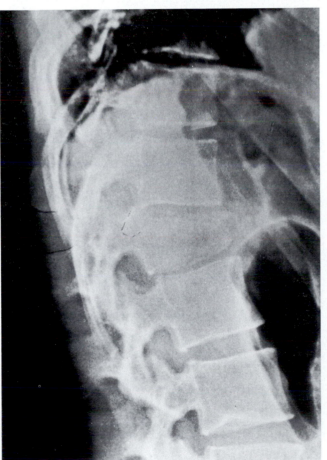

FIG 15–9.

Flexion-distraction fracture of the L1 vertebra. Note the encroachment on the spinal canal by the retropulsed fragment of the fractured posterior wall. Increased interspinous distance by distraction injury of the posterior ligaments.

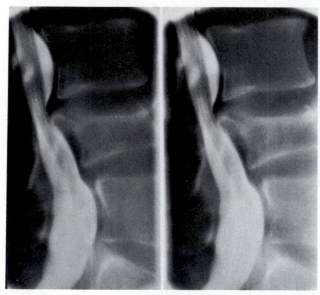

FIG 15–10.
Myelogram after conservatively treated fracture of L2 showing the postoperative stenosis caused by a posteriorly displaced fragment.

An AP diameter of 10 mm is more often considered to be the upper limit of absolute stenosis. A cross-sectional area is probably even more meaningful (see Chapters 2 and 10).

CT and MRI

CT scans and MRI are necessary for exact anatomic evaluation of the stenosis. Stenosis is present if narrowing of the spinal canal by bony structures or soft tissue is present in the central or lateral compartments (Fig 15–11); if the cross-sectional area of the dural sac is 100 mm^2 or less—Adams and Hutton[2] measured CT scans an⁻ stated that a cross-sectional area of the lumbar dural sac of 180 ± 50 mm^2

is normal (see Chapter 10); and if displacement with luxation of the facet joints is visible.

TREATMENT OF POSTTRAUMATIC STENOSIS

The goal of treatment is to eliminate compression and prevent recurrence of spinal stenosis and deformity. Therefore, decompression and stabilization is required.

Decompression

A generally accepted indication for immediate operative decompression after spinal injury is progressive neurologic deterioration with visible stenosis of the spinal canal. The indication for decompression in cases with neurologic deficit and confirmed stenosis is commonly accepted.[5, 26] Gertzbein et al.[15] emphasize the argument of the evolution of the neurologic symptoms and advocate decompression only in cases with 50% narrowing and neurologic deterioration. Operative decompression of the spinal canal without neurologic defects but with confirmed stenosis can be accomplished by indirect methods.[15, 21] that avoid manipulation inside the spinal canal.

In healed fractures with stenosis, malalignment with kyphotic deformity may aggravate the encroachment of the spinal canal.

Techniques

Anterior.—Since most traumatic stenosis is caused by posterior displacement of a fractured frag-

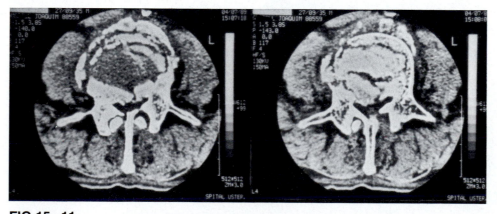

FIG 15–11.
Burst fracture of L4 with severe compromise of the spinal canal. The CT scan reveals the degree of encroachment, mainly due to retropulsation of the fractured vertebral wall.

ment of the posterior wall of the vertebral body into the spinal canal, an anterior approach for decompression seems appropriate. A transperitoneal approach for the lumbosacral junction is preferred, whereas for the rostral segments a retroperitoneal approach is chosen. A partial vertebrectomy of the posterior parts of the fractured vertebral body allows an extensive decompression by removal of the fractured fragments within the vertebral canal (Fig 15–12). A ventral decompression also may be useful in acute and chronic posttraumatic stenosis. In cases with posterior instability, anterior decompression and posterior stabilization is justified.

Posterior.—In acute vertebral fractures with retropulsed fragments, a posterior decompression may be successfully performed. After a laminectomy, the fragment may be pushed forward into the fractured vertebral body with a specially designed pestle. A posterolateral approach is useful for bone grafting and decompression of the spinal canal. After osteotomy of the transverse process, the lateral aspect of the pedicle is exposed. The spinal canal is entered laterally by removing the (fractured) pedicle. Under visual control, the canal may safely be cleared of bony fragments (Fig 15–13).

Laminectomy as an isolated procedure is rarely justified for decompression of a fracture of the lumbar spine. Laminectomy has no decompressing ef-

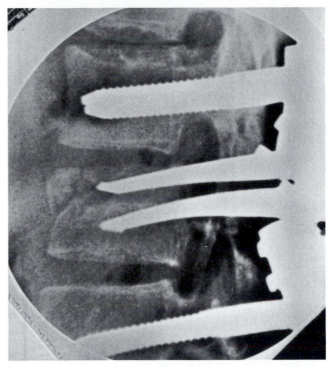

FIG 15–13.
Decompression and stabilization from a posterior approach (intraoperative view). Decompression of the spinal canal is performed by a posterolateral approach: The lamina and pedicle are removed and the spinal canal is freed from bony fragments under visual control. To restore the original height of the vertebral body, a distractor is inserted via an opening in the lateral vertebral wall. By distraction, the depressed end plate is pushed to its original position. The bone graft is inserted via the same approach. The reduction is maintained by transpedicular internal fixation.

fect in fractures,[23] increases instability, and enhances progression of the kyphosis.[19]

Indirect.—In fractures with an intact posterior longitudinal ligament, decompression of the spinal canal may be achieved by applying distraction.[1, 11, 12, 14] The lengthening of the posterior longitudinal ligament pushes the fragments ventrally with a mean improvement in canal compromise of approximately 30%.[12] With the same maneuver, the lateral recess and the foramen are widened by separating the facets.

Stabilization

Since the decompressing action requires removal of bone, the remaining stability should be a primary concern. Bone removal causes the anterior elements of the spine to fail under compressive forces and the

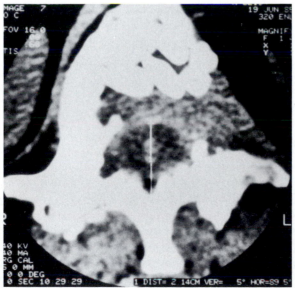

FIG 15–12.
Anterior decompression. A hemivertebrectomy was performed to restore the width of the spinal canal by removing the bone fragments. A bone graft (rib) has been placed anteriorly.

posterior elements to fail under tensile forces. Therefore, both anterior and posterior procedures should be accompanied by a stabilization: anteriorly by a compression-resistant system and posteriorly with a tension band. In addition, the fixation should take into account the instability caused by the injury. Some authors[15, 22] advocate a combined AP approach for unstable burst fractures. However, newly designed implants allow a single-stage procedure either from anterior[10, 19] or posterior[9, 12, 21] with reliable stability and satisfactory alignment. Therefore, it seems reasonable to choose the approach according to the need for decompression rather than on the basis of the instability.

Techniques

Anterior.—After decompression, a bone graft is needed to replace the vertebral body. In most unisegmental decompressions, a compression-resistant corticocancellous bone graft from the iliac crest is chosen. If more segments have to be replaced, a fibular strut graft might be useful. Internal fixation is advocated by several authors.[10, 19, 20]

Posterior.—Internal fixation to enhance stability in fracture treatment of the thoracolumbar and lumbar spine is generally accepted. Several implants are available. To achieve reduction, stability, and painless mobility with a minimum of fused segments, transpedicular fixation systems have proved to be superior to the longer fusing rod systems.[9, 20, 21]

PREVENTION OF POSTTRAUMATIC STENOSIS

Anatomic reduction and stabilization in injuries of the spine are the most effective ways to achieve neurologic decompression and prevent the development of posttraumatic spinal stenosis in the majority of cases. According to Weinstein et al.,[30] initial aggressive surgical treatment is not necessarily needed in stable fractures and acceptable long-term results may be obtained by conservative treatment. However, in their patients, postoperative immobilization ranged from immediate ambulation up to 3 months in a body cast, which seems unacceptable for most patients. Restoration of the anatomy and stability of a fractured spine, however, appears to be more consistent and satisfactory after surgical treatment.[9, 11, 19, 21, 22] Operative treatment of spinal fractures is also recommended to prevent pain and late neurologic complications. Denis et al.[8] reported 17% late neurologic symptoms in patients with conservatively treated unstable burst fractures who initially had no neurologic defects.

Several authors have found no apparent correlation between the amount of spinal canal obstruction and the neurologic symptoms[4, 5, 15, 17] Bradford and McBride,[5] however, found that the neurologic deficit correlated directly with the amount of bony stenosis and that recovery depended on the effectiveness of the decompression. This statement is in accordance with the findings of several other authors.[10, 22, 28] Therefore, if neurologic deficits are present, and CT or MRI demonstrates encroachment of the spinal canal, decompression is indicated. Self-remodeling of the narrowed spinal canal has been described.[30] Edwards and Levine[11] have shown that complete restoration of the compromised canal is not necessary. The degree of recovery from neurologic symptoms did not change with decompression in canals with width of 66% or more.

To prevent posttraumatic spinal stenosis, it is necessary to restore adequate stability in acute or chronic traumatic instabilities of the spine to prevent secondary dislocation of fragments or increasing kyphotic deformity with narrowing of the spinal canal. To prevent neurologic deficits by narrowing of the neural canal, a decompression of canals with less than 66% of the normal width is recommended.

LATE OUTCOME OF POSTTRAUMATIC STENOSIS

Untreated posttraumatic stenosis may cause mechanical or neurologic problems.

Neurologic

Syringomyelia occurs with an incidence of 0.3% to 2.3%, and may appear as early as 2 months[29] after the injury. Syringomyelia is characterized by pain and numbness. Motor deficit occurs later and less frequently, but when present is more disabling.[3, 29] In a few cases, other neurologic symptoms such as hyperhidrosis, spasticity, and impaired temperature sensation have been described;[3] therefore, any patient who presents with new neurologic defects after a spinal trauma should undergo investigation for syringomyelia. MRI is the investigative technique of choice, but a combination of myelography and CT scanning is also valuable. The therapeutic approach to syringomyelia remains controversial; also, neurologic recovery only improves to a minor degree after surgical decompression, but marked pain relief has been reported.[3] A syringosubarachnoid shunt[27] or syringoperitoneal shunt[24] left in place permanently has been advocated to drain the cyst.

Mechanical

The unbalanced load on the spine caused by the kyphotic deformity results in increased stress on facets adjacent to the fracture. This may cause a secondary painful syndrome and early degenerative changes. Pain also may develop by incongruency and joint deformation after fracture. In the anterior column, an injured disc sometimes leads to a painful collapsing segment.

REFERENCES

1. Aebi M, Etter C, Kehl T, et al: Stabilization of the lower thoracic and lumbar spine with internal spinal skeletal fixation system. *Spine* 1987; 12:544–551.
2. Adams MA, Hutton WC: Prolapsed intervertebral disc: A hyperflexion injury. *Spine* 1982; 7:184.
3. Anton HA, Schweigel JF: Posttraumatic syringomyelia: The British Columbia experience. *Spine* 1986; 11:865–868.
4. Atlas SW, Regenbogen V, Rogers LF, et al: The radiographic characterization of burst fractures of the spine. *AJR* 1986; 147:575–582.
5. Bradford DS, McBride GG: Surgical management of thoracolumbar spine fractures with incomplete neurologic deficits. *Clin Orthop* 1987; 218:201–216.
6. Dali BE, Stauffer ES: Neurologic injury and recovery patterns in burst fractures at the T12 or L1 motion segment. *Clin Orthop* 1988; 233:171–176.
7. Denis F: The three column spine and its significance in the classification of acute thoracolumbar spinal injuries *Spine* 1983; 8:817–831.
8. Denis F, Armstrong GWD, Searls K, et al: Acute thoracolumbar burst fractures in the absence of neurologic deficit. *Clin Orthop* 1984; 189:142–149.
9. Dick W, Kluger P, Magerl F, et al: A new device for internal fixation of thoracolumbar and lumbar spine fractures, the fixateur interne. *Paraplegia* 1985; 23:225–232.
10. Dunn HK: Anterior spine stabilization and decompression for thoracolumbar injuries. *Ortho Clin North Am* 1986; 17:113–119.
11. Edwards CC, Levine AM: Early rod sleeve stabilization of the injured thoracic and lumbar spine. *Orthop Clin North Am* 1986; 17:121–145.
12. Esses SI, Botsford DJ, Kostuik JP: Evaluation of surgical treatment for burst fractures. *Spine* 1990; 15:667–673.
13. Frankel HL, Hancock DO, Hyslpo G, et al: The value of postural reduction in initial management of closed injuries of the spine with paraplegia and tetraplegia. *Paraplegia* 1969; 7:179–192.
14. Fredrickson EB, Mann KA, Yuan HA, et al: Reduction of the intracanal fragment in experimental burst fractures. *Spine* 1988; 13:267–271.
15. Gertzbein SD, Court-Brown CM, Marks P, et al: The neurological outcome following surgery for spinal fracture. *Spine* 1988; 13:641–644.
16. Hashimoto T, Kaneda K, Abumi K: Relationship between traumatic spinal canal stenosis and neurologic deficits in thoracolumbar burst fractures. *Spine* 1988; 13:1268–1272.
17. Keene JS, Fischer SP, Vanderby R, et al: Significance of acute spinal posttraumatic bony encroachment of the neural canal. *Spine* 1989; 14:799–802.
18. Kirkaldy Willis WH, Paine KWE, Cauchoix J, et al: Lumbar spinal stenosis *Clin Orthop* 1974; 99:30.
19. Kostuik JP, Matsusaki H: Anterior stabilization, instrumentation and decompression for posttraumatic kyphosis. *Spine* 1989; 14:379–386.
20. Louis R: Spinal stability as defined by the three column spine concept. *Anat Clin* 1985; 7:33.
21. Magerl F: Stabilization of the lower thoracic and lumbar spine with external skeletal fixation. *Clin Orthop* 1984; 189:125–149.
22. McAfee PC, Yuan HA, Fredrickson BE, et al: The value of computed tomography in thoracolumbar fractures. An analysis of one hundred consecutive cases and a new classification. *J Bone Joint Surg [Am]* 1983; 65:461–473.
23. Morgan TH, Wharton GW, Austin GN: The results of laminectomy in patients with incomplete spinal cord injuries. *Paraplegia* 1971; 9:14.
24. Phillips TW, Kindt GW: Syringo-peritoneal shunt for syringomyelia: A preliminary report. *Surg Neurol* 1981; 16:462–466.
25. Pratt ES, Green DA, Spengler DM: Herniated intervertebral discs associated with unstable spinal injuries. *Spine* 1990; 15:662–666.
26. Richaud J, Bousquet P, Ealet G, et al: Récalibrage par voie postérolatérale des sténoses traumatiques récentes du rachis dorsal et lombaire. Modalités et résultats à propos de 31 observations. *Neurochirurgie* 1990; 36:27–38.
27. Tator C, Mesuro K, Rowed DW: Favorable results with syringo-subarachnoid shunts for treatment of syringomyelia. *J Neurosurg* 1982; 56:517–523.
28. Trafton PG, Boyd CA: Computed tomography of thoracic and lumbar spine injuries. *J Trauma* 1984; 24:506–515.
29. Vernon JD, Silver JR, Ohry A: Posttraumatic syringomyelia. *Paraplegia* 1982; 20:339–364.
30. Weinstein JN, Collato P, Lehmann TR: Thoracolumbar burst-fractures treated conservatively: A long term follow-up. *Spine* 1988; 13:33–38.

16

Cauda Equina Syndrome in Spinal Stenosis

Thomas W. McNeill, M.D.

Cauda equina syndrome may be defined as partial or complete loss of control of bowel or bladder and sexual function due to compression of the cauda equina in the lumbar spine. If the compression is at the lumbosacral junction, the only findings will be perineal numbness, pelvic floor paralysis, dysfunction of bowel and bladder, and loss of sexual function. If the compression of cauda equina takes place at a higher level in the lumbar spine, then partial or complete paralysis of the legs may also be present. The cauda equina syndrome is the most severe of the many nerve compression syndromes that occur in the lumbar spine. Any source of compression on the dural contents or nerve roots may produce partial or complete cauda equina syndrome. However, the commonest etiologic factors are massive disc herniation (often in a narrow canal) and severe spinal stenosis from any cause.

Cauda equina syndrome may present acutely with the onset of paralysis taking place within hours or days, or may present chronically with the onset being of indefinite duration often extending over months or years. The acute variety of cauda equina syndrome is most often caused by sudden massive disc herniation,[7] whereas the chronic variety of cauda equina syndrome most often is caused by spinal stenosis and may develop slowly over years as spinal stenosis gradually becomes more severe.

ANATOMY

The individual lumbar nerve roots originate in the lumbar enlargement of the spinal cord, located in the lower thoracic and upper lumbar regions of the adult spine. Distal to the lumbar enlargement is the conus medullaris which extends over the body of L1 and is approximately 2.5 cm in length.[5] The bundle of nerves extending distally is called the cauda equina (see Chapter 3). It consists of both lumbar and sacral nerves. The nerves of origin for the sacral parasympathetic outflow and for sacral sensory paths all originate in the conus medullaris.[5, 21] The lumbar nerves contain parasympathetic, sympathetic, somatic motor, and all sensory components. The autonomic nervous system is purely motor and is subdivided into parasympathetic and sympathetic components. The sensory component from the viscera is not part of the autonomic nervous system. Nonetheless, the two components—both sensory from (afferent) and motor to (efferent) the pelvic viscera—are essential for their normal function. These functions are those of micturition, defecation, and sexual response. The somatic motor nerves of the lumbosacral plexus control voluntary muscle function and reflex function of the striated muscles of the lower extremities, external sphincters, and pelvic floor. The visceral motor nerves (autonomic efferents) control the involuntary smooth muscle function of sexual organs, blood vessels, colon, rectum, and bladder.

The lumbar parasympathetic portion of the autonomic nervous system originates in preganglionic cells in the conus medullaris. These fibers descend distally along with the sacral nerve roots to synapse with a short postganglionic fiber which usually lies within the innervated organ. These parasympathetic nerve fibers collectively form the "presacral plexus." The innervated end organs are colon, rectum, genital organs, and bladder.

The lumbar sympathetic nerves originate in preganglionic cells in the thoracic spinal cord and upper lumbar cord. The postganglionic sympathetic neuron has its synapse with the preganglionic neuron in the paraspinal sympathetic chain or accessory ganglia, such as the celiac or superior mesenteric ganglia. In the pelvis, the sympathetic fibers also innervate rectum, colon, bladder, and sexual organs. Additionally, sympathetic fibers provide motor control for vessels in the limbs and piloerector muscles of hair.

The afferent (sensory) nerves ascend from viscera and sexual organs and are necessary to complete the reflex arc for normal functions such as micturition, defecation, and sexual response.

Sympathetic efferents, when stimulated, produce bladder relaxation and internal sphincter contraction. They also produce urethral smooth muscle sphincter contraction. Sympathetic efferent tone produces inhibition of peristalsis and inhibition of penile or clitorial erection. Nonetheless, sympathetic fibers mediate a significant portion of the motor component of orgasm and ejaculation. The parasympathetic outflow causes contraction of the smooth muscles of the bladder and relaxation of the internal sphincter. Parasympathetic efferent tone causes increase in peristalsis, relaxation of the internal rectal sphincter, and erection of penis and clitoris. Parasympathetic stimulation also is responsible for vaginal lubrication, and engorgement of the labia and vaginal wall.[10]

INTEGRATED PELVIC VISCERAL FUNCTION

Sexual function requires the integrated and complex reflex coordination of higher cortical centers, spinal cord centers, sympathetic and parasympathetic nervous systems, somatic efferents and afferents (Table 16–1). If any one of the components of this complex system is interrupted, the function may be altered. In the female, conception is possible even with complete absence of normal sexual responsiveness. In the male, on the other hand, the entire reflex arc must be present for ejaculation to be possible. The neural components of sexual responsiveness, excitation, and orgasm are essentially the same in both sexes. The presence of normal hormonal stimulation is also a necessary component for normal sexual responsiveness in both sexes.

The neural control of defecation and urination are very similar. Both are subject to voluntary control after infancy and both require an integrated spinal reflex which requires the intact connections of cortical function, spinal cord function, peripheral nerve function (both sensory and motor), and both parasympathetic and sympathetic function. When either the bladder or bowel is distended, an impulse normally originates in stretch receptors in the wall of either organ. This occurs when the bladder is distended to about 400 mL.[11] Control of bowel or blad-

TABLE 16–1.

Pelvic Visceral Neurologic Function*

Level	Micturition/Defecation	Sexual Response	Orgasm
Cortical, pons	Control by inhibition of reflex	Initiation of excitement phase	
Cord	Integration of reflex	Integration of reflex	
Sensory	Stretch receptor detection of bladder or rectal filling	Initially varied sensory input	Continued genital stimulation required
Motor, sympathetic	Internal sphincter contraction inhibits detrusor inhibits peristalsis	Inhibition prior to orgasm	Rhythmic, smooth muscle contraction; male—ejaculation
Motor, parasympathetic	Detrusor contraction peristalsis	Penile, clitoral, labial engorgement and lubrication, ejaculation	Contraction of vaginal, urethral, uterine muscle; male—ejaculation
Motor, somatic	Inhibition of external sphincter	Pelvic floor contraction	

*Adapted from Weinstein JN, Wiesel S (eds): *The Lumbar Spine.* Philadelphia, WB Saunders Co, 1990.

der function is dependent upon awareness of this feeling of distention. This awareness allows voluntary inhibition of micturition and defecation. Sympathetic efferent activity causes inhibition of peristalsis and bladder detrusor relaxation. Sympathetics also cause internal sphincter contraction. With the release of central inhibition, the complex reflex of micturition or defecation takes place without further central control being necessary.[10, 11, 21] Bilateral sympathectomy, if it includes the L1 ganglion, will result in significant sexual dysfunction.[22]

THE DENERVATED BLADDER

In instances in which there has been interruption of sacral nerves to the bladder or spinal cord injury, the bladder responses change with time. Initially, there is urinary retention present with bladder flaccidity and overflow incontinence. The bladder empties poorly and may become severely distended with severe retention. At the least, there are increased residual volumes. The bladder has a flat, filling curve on a cystometrogram.

Eventually, uninhibited parasympathetic activity to the bladder will result in detrusor spasm or hypertonicity, leading to a small hypertrophic bladder. There may be a dissociation between parasympathetic and sympathetic activity. If sympathetic activity remains, the internal sphincter may remain functional. This may result in high pressures and ureteral dilatation. Incontinence results from interruption of both the parasympathetic and sympathetic nerves.[11, 14]

CAUDA EQUINA SYNDROME

Chronic

The patient with spinal stenosis may present with symptoms of urinary incontinence or hesitancy or urgency of gradual onset. These symptoms may develop over a period of months or years. The symptoms may or may not be associated with the typical symptoms of pseudoclaudication, which are more easily recognized as being of spinal origin. The patient is usually middle-aged or older. Symptoms of sciatica and backache for many years are common. A history of specific injury is unusual. The gradual onset of symptoms is due to the slowly diminishing volume of the spinal canal in the stenotic patient. Symptoms of perianal or perineal pain are often associated with neurogenic bowel or bladder dysfunction caused by the gradual onset of spinal stenosis. These symptoms are often considered to be neurotic in nature, but have a significant physiologic basis if caused by stenosis and should warn the clinician of the possibility of this diagnosis. These patients have been recognized in the spine literature, and in 1986 were classified as "group II" in the series of patients of Kostuik et al.[9]

Acute

The acute variety of cauda equina syndrome may be caused by many different compressive lesions of the cauda equina. These include primary and metastatic tumors; infections, including pyogenic and granulomatous; fractures; disc herniations; and iatrogenic causes. By far, the greatest number of patients with acute cauda equina syndrome will be found to have massive disc herniations, often in a small spinal canal.[3, 8, 13, 15, 16] Relative to the number of disc herniations present at any individual lumbar level, cauda equina syndrome is more likely to occur with disc herniations in the upper lumbar spine. However, relative to the total number of cauda equina syndrome described, the majority are still due to lesions at L4–5 and L5–S1. This is because disc herniations at these levels are far more numerous than those in the upper lumbar spine. Lastly, the rare intrathecal disc herniation has a high probability of producing cauda equina syndrome.[1, 2, 7, 9, 12, 17, 20]

For purposes of classification three groups of acute cauda equina syndrome have been described.[19] Group I patients have an onset that is sudden without premonitory symptoms and without warning. Group II patients give a previous history of sciatica and back pain prior to the acute onset of urinary retention (pelvic visceral paralysis). Group III patients present with back pain and sciatica, either unilaterally or bilaterally, following which urinary retention develops but with a short interval. This third group of patients presenting with acute cauda equina syndrome may not consult a physician or emergency center immediately. Conversely, they may have been admitted to the hospital with uncontrollable pain in the back and legs and normal pelvic visceral function, only to develop paralysis while in the hospital. Patients may then be thought to have urinary retention because of narcotic medication or enforced bed rest, resulting in a missed diagnosis for days or weeks.

Recent Experimental Evidence

A better understanding of the pathogenesis and prognosis of cauda equina syndrome has been the source of active scientific inquiry recently. Some of the pathophysiologic differences between slow and rapid onset compression are discussed in Chapter 7. A rapid onset rate always results in more pronounced effects. Delamarter, Sherman, and Carr[6] won the Volvo Award for Spinal Research in 1991 for an animal model of an acute cauda equina syndrome. They tested the hypothesis that the recovery of symptoms is related to the duration of neural compression. (They had previously demonstrated that the vascular supply recovers, even after a duration of 3 months of compression.) They produced 75% constriction of the cauda equina in a series of dogs by placing a constricting band around the cauda. This degree of constriction was sufficient to produce hind leg paralysis, tail paralysis, and bowel or bladder paralysis in all dogs. Whether the constriction was released immediately, at 1 hour, 6 hours, 24 hours, or 1 week following compression, all dogs recovered neurologic function within 6 weeks. The immediately decompressed dogs recovered within 2 to 5 days. The 1-hour, 6-hour, and 24-hour compression periods resulted in paralysis for 5 to 7 days, and the 1-week compression resulted in persistence of the paralysis for 7 to 10 days with tail-wagging function diminished for 4 weeks. Return of bladder function also required 4 weeks. This study is of great importance since previous anecdotal evidence had suggested that decompression must be completed within a very short time of onset or recovery will not take place. Apparently we have more time than we thought we had in the past.

A second issue, which has important clinical implications, centers around the question of the nature and severity of injury to elements of the cauda equina depending upon whether or not the site of compression is in one area or two areas separated by some distance. Double-level cauda equina compression was produced experimentally[4,18] demonstrating that with one area of compression blood supply is altered only under the area of compression, whereas with double-level nerve compression, the blood supply is altered in the entire cauda equina between the two levels of compression. This, too, has important implications for treatment and may explain the clini-

cal observation that long-term results in treatment of the cauda equina syndrome caused by spinal stenosis appear better when several levels are decompressed rather than one level only. Obviously, the decompression should include all stenotic levels.

Physical Examination

Previous teaching described a cauda equina syndrome in its full-blown state as consisting of perianal numbness; urinary retention; constipation; unilateral sciatica of severe, unremitting nature; perineal numbness; and numbness in the soles of the feet. This full-blown syndrome is not present in a significant number of cases.[9] In acute cauda equina syndrome the findings in a full-blown case would always include numbness in the distribution of sacral roots (which would include buttocks, perineum, scrotum, labia, penis, and clitoris). Depending upon the level of the obstruction within the lumbar canal, these findings may also include various degrees of diminished sensation in the legs and feet. Numbness in the soles of the feet indicates sacral root involvement. A motor examination may reveal absence of the anal "wink" reflex, and bulbocavernosus reflex along with varying degrees of hyporeflexia and weakness in the lower extremities. Severe bladder paralysis may be present without leg pain symptoms,[14] and leg signs may be unilateral as well.[9] Examination of the abdomen may reveal bladder distention. In patients with cauda equina syndrome, it is common to find signs of the other common lumbar nerve compression syndromes. Depending on the level of the lesion, lower extremity reflexes and muscle strength may be altered. The bilateral straight leg raising test is often positive.

Physical findings in the chronic cauda equina syndrome may be much more subtle. Rectal tone may be diminished, and sensation may be altered in the perineum, but this is often much less dramatic than what is seen in acute cauda equina syndrome. Lower extremity neurologic findings may be entirely normal at rest and present only with provocative testing such as walking and spinal extension (see Chapter 17).

Investigations

In acute cauda equina syndrome the most easily obtained and simplest test for a clear view of the level and extent of abnormality remains the water-soluble myelogram. Computed tomography (CT) examination without previous myelography may give a false impression of a patent lumbar spinal canal. Magnetic resonance imaging (MRI) may well provide the same information as myelography, but often is not readily accessible or as easily obtained. Spinal abnormalities are not the only concern, however. It is of great value to the prognosis of these patients to obtain urodynamic studies. At the least, a postvoiding residual urine specimen will give a hint of the degree of bladder involvement.

In a chronic cauda equina syndrome, a thorough neurologic workup, complete neurologic assessment, and myelogram with a postmyelographic CT examination should be obtained. It is my personal belief that MRI is of less value in assessing these patients. The urologic assessment should ideally include an intravenous pyelogram, electrodiagnostic sphincter function assessment, urodynamic testing, and tests of renal function.

Treatment

The only available treatment for cauda equina syndrome remains complete surgical decompression of all the involved neural elements. In the past, this has been achieved by a variety of operative interventions. When a massive unilateral disc hernia is present, a one-sided laminectomy and discectomy was the most common treatment modality in the cases of Aho et al.[1] Where there is a significant degree of associated spinal stenosis, a bilateral laminectomy should be selected, because complete decompression is important.

In a chronic cauda equina syndrome a decompression should include all significant areas of stenosis including both central and lateral decompression where appropriate.

The scheduling of the surgical procedure should be considered to be urgent in an acute cauda equina syndrome. There is no evidence in the neurosurgical and orthopaedic case studies or experimental literature to indicate that there is a specific time requirement for decompression, but there is no reason to wait. In the material of Aho et al.[1] there was a suggestion that the quality of postoperative improvement was somewhat better if the surgery took place within 3 days of the onset of neurologic dysfunction. In the material of Kostuik et al.,[9] there was no correlation between the duration of preoperative symptoms and the final end result of surgery. The previously mentioned experimental work also suggests that the surgical treatment is urgent but not emer-

gent. The reason for this is that the neural elements of the cauda equina are capable of recovering from compressive injury, whereas the spinal cord is not. In chronic cauda equina syndrome, the decompression is not urgent and should be performed when medically prudent. A full workup should always be performed.

In acute cauda equina syndrome the patient seldom recovers completely and residual bladder dysfunction is the rule, rather than the exception, whatever the timing of the surgical decompression. The degree of dysfunction can only be accurately detected with urodynamic studies and sequential residual urine studies. If saddle anesthesia persists following decompression, then pelvic visceral function will remain severely disturbed. Bilateral sciatica is also considered to have a poor prognosis. Patients are not necessarily disabled by the urinary dysfunction, but tend to adjust by a variety of means including the Valsalva and Credé maneuvers. Rarely is intermittent catheterization required. Patients also adjust well to rectal and anal dysfunction using techniques which are easily learned and easily adapted to the disability.

In chronic cauda equina syndrome recovery is slow and incomplete. The patient should be told that it is hoped that the surgery will prevent further deterioration in function, and that improvement will probably be partial at best. This is extremely important to avoid disappointment postoperatively.

SUMMARY

Cauda equina syndrome is a pelvic, visceral dysfunction associated with compression of the cauda equina. The syndrome may include lower extremity involvement, either unilaterally or bilaterally. Cauda equina syndrome is either acute or chronic. In the acute variety the usual cause is massive disc herniation, often in a significantly stenotic canal. If disc herniation is proximal in the lumbar spine, cauda equina syndrome is relatively more likely, whereas with intrathecal herniation cauda equina syndrome is probable. Chronic cauda equina syndrome is secondary to slowly developing spinal stenosis and most often presents as bladder dysfunction. Perineal and rectal pains may be present, but other findings may be few or absent.

Decompression of acute cauda equina syndrome

is urgent but not emergent. Delay in diagnosis and delay in treatment, at least up to 3 days, does not affect the prognosis or eventual outcome of treatment even in the acute cauda equina syndrome. The standard recommended in previous texts, i.e., that acute cauda equina syndrome be dealt with as an emergency on the same day, is not substantiated by either reported clinical materials or experimental data. Further, this standard has not been met in any of the series presented in the literature to date. This does not mean that there is reason for unnecessary delay. In the chronic cauda equina syndrome decompression should be directed toward all of the elements of stenosis and should be done when medically expedient, after completion of a thorough medical workup.

REFERENCES

1. Aho AJ, Auranen A, Pesonen K: Analysis of cauda equina symptoms in patients with lumbar disc prolapse. *Acta Chir Scand* 1969; 135:413–420.
2. Anderson JT, Bradley WE: Neurogenic bladder dysfunction in protruded lumbar disk and after laminectomy. *Urology* 1976; 8:94–96.
3. Choudhury A, Taylor JC: Cauda equina syndrome in lumbar disc disease. *Acta Orthop Scand* 1980; 51:493–499.
4. Cornefjord M, Olmaker K, Takahasi K, et al: Impairment of nutritional transport at double level cauda equina compression. Presented at the International Society for the Study of the Lumbar Spine. Heidelberg, Germany, May 12–16, 1991.
5. Countee RW, Vijayanathan T, Martin BF, et al: The conus medularis: Physiological, anatomical and clinical considerations, in Camino M, O'Leary P (eds): *The Lumbar Spine.* New York, Raven Press, 1987, pp 171–182.
6. Delamarter RB, Sherman JE, Carr JB: Cauda equina syndrome: Neurologic recovery following immediate, early or late decompression. Presented at the International Society for the Study of the Lumbar Spine. Heidelberg, Germany, May 12–16, 1991.
7. Floman Y, Wiesel SW, Rothman RH: Cauda equina syndrome presenting as a herniated lumbar disc. *Clin Orthop* 1980; 147:234–237.
8. Jennett BW: A study of 25 cases of compression of the cauda equina by prolapsed intervertebral disc. *J Neurol Neurosurg Psychiatr* 1956; 19:109–116.
9. Kostuik JP, Harrington I, Alexander D, et al: Cauda equina syndrome and lumbar disc herniation. *J Bone Joint Surg [Am]* 1986; 68:386–391.
10. Lindsey DF, Holms JE: *Basic Human Neurophysiology.* New York, Elsevier Science Publishing Co, Inc, 1984, pp 269–307.
11. McGuire EJ: Neuromuscular dysfunction of the lower urinary tract, in Walsh PC, Gittes RF, Perlmutter AD, et al (eds): *Campbell's Urology.* Philadelphia, WB Saunders Co, 1986, pp 616–627.
12. Peyser E, Harari A: Intradural rupture of lumbar intervertebral disk. *Surg Neurol* 1977; 8:95–98.
13. Raaf J: Some observations regarding 905 patients operated upon for protruded lumbar intervertebral disc. *Am J Surg* 1959; 97:388–399.
14. Rosomoff HL, Johnston JDHJ, Gallo AE, et al: Cystometry as an adjunct in the evaluation of lumbar disc syndrome. *J Neurosurg* 1970; 33:67–74.
15. Scott PJ: Bladder paralysis in cauda equina lesion from disc prolapse. *J Bone Joint Surg [Br]* 1965; 47:224–235.
16. Shephard RH: Diagnosis and prognosis of cauda equina syndrome produced by protrusion of lumbar disc. *Br Med J* 1959; 2:1434–1439.
17. Spangfort EV: The lumbar disc herniation: A computer-aided analysis of 2,504 operations. *Acta Orthop Scand [Suppl]* 1972; 1–142.
18. Takahasi K, Olmaker K, Rydevik B, et al.: Double-level cauda equina compression: Continuous monitoring of intramural blood flow. Presented at the International Society for the Study of the Lumbar Spine. Heidelberg, Germany, May 12–16, 1991.
19. Tandon PN, Sankaran B: Cauda equina syndrome due to lumbar disc prolapse. *Indian J Orthop* 1967; 1:112–119.
20. Tay ECK, Chacha PB: Midline prolapse of a lumbar intervertebral disc with compression of the cauda equina. *J Bone Joint Surg [Br]* 1979; 41:43–46.
21. Walton J (ed): *Brain's Diseases of the Nervous System.* Oxford, Oxford University Press, 1985, pp 593–603.
22. Whitelaw GP, Smithwick RH: Some secondary effects of sympathectomy, with particular reference to disturbance of sexual function. *N Engl J Med* 1951; 245:121–130.

PART III

Diagnosis

17

History and Physical Examination in Spinal Stenosis

Gunnar B.J. Andersson, M.D., Ph.D.

Thomas W. McNeill, M.D.

The patient's description of his or her problem is the key to the clinical evaluation, and therefore requires careful attention. This is obviously the case in the spinal stenosis patient as well. The interview logically starts with the patient's present problem, and then proceeds to discuss previous spinal problems, the general medical condition of the patient, and any previous health problems. In addition, social and work-related factors need to be covered, at least superficially. The most important information is that related to the patient's pain. Pain intensity, its location and distribution; its relationship to activities; and response to rest or specific treatment are all important. Severity of pain is individual, and can be described in many different ways. It can be verbally recorded or recorded on a visual-analog scale. Since the intensity of pain can vary over the day, from day to day, or with activity, additional information may be required. The quality of pain is also important, as is information about the presence or absence of paresthesias and numbness, weakness, a rubbery feeling in the legs, and similar symptoms. The distribution of pain can be described verbally, but in our opinion is best illustrated on a pain drawing (Fig 17–1). The drawing has the advantages of providing a more complete description, it can be filled out while waiting, and it also can be used to screen for specific syndromes and psychological disturbances.

HISTORY OF PATIENTS WITH SPINAL STENOSIS

More variation exists in the presenting complaints of patients with spinal stenosis than in any of the other syndromes producing low back pain (Table 17–1). In fact, some patients refer to the presenting clinical symptoms as bizarre. Further, from the point of view of symptoms, spinal stenosis is not one entity. Rather there are four recognizable subsyndromes of "spinal stenosis": (1) neurogenic intermittent claudication (pseudoclaudication); (2) radicular pain (sciatica); (3) atypical leg pain, and (4), rarely, chronic cauda equina syndrome. Pseudoclaudication is the unique syndrome of spinal stenosis, but individual patients may present with almost any conceivable combination of the four complaints. Furthermore, an individual patient may have any one or several of these subsyndromes at different times during the course of the illness. Also, neurogenic intermittent claudication is not unique to lumbar spinal stenosis, but can occur with thoracic and cervical spinal stenosis as well.

An insidious onset of slowly progressing symptoms is common.[5] Often, the patients have had some complaints of low back pain for several years

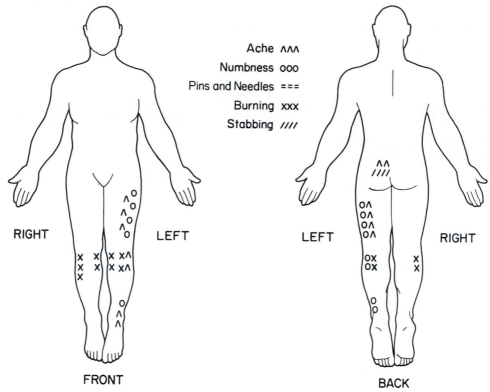

Ache ∧∧∧
Numbness ooo
Pins and Needles ===
Burning xxx
Stabbing ////

RIGHT   LEFT   LEFT   RIGHT

FRONT   BACK

FIG 17–1.
A pain drawing by a patient with spinal stenosis.

TABLE 17–1.

Characteristics of the Patient With Lumbar Spinal Stenosis*

Patient is more often older than 50 yr
Men are more frequently affected than women
Morning pain and stiffness
Sitting and squatting relieves the pain
Leaning forward relieves the pain
Extension aggravates the pain
Leg symptoms are often bilateral
Leg pain is more common than either weakness or paresthesias
Walking aggravates or produces the leg symptoms
Gradual onset of sphincter disturbance—slow and subtle
Symptoms of long duration and gradually increasing

*Adapted from Andersson GBJ, McNeill TW: *Lumbar Spinal Syndromes.* Vienna, Springer-Verlag, 1989, pp 100–108.

before seeking medical attention. The most common complaint is that of back pain,[4] but leg pain with or without nerve root deficit is not uncommon (Table 17–2). The lower back pain may be typical of degenerative spinal conditions with morning stiffness relieved by mild limbering-up exercises but aggravated by moderate walking; a "gelling phenomenon" with stiffness following any period of rest may be present. The pain is often mild or absent with sitting. Patients with neurogenic intermittent claudica-tion (spinal stenosis) and true claudication (arterio-sclerotic peripheral vascular disease, ASPVD) (Table 17–3) both experience leg pain with walking which is relieved by rest.[3] Both groups of patients are likely to be older than 50 years. Unfortunately, some pa-tients may have both pseudoclaudication and true claudication since both are relatively common. In pa-tients with pure pseudoclaudication the posture while walking is typically one of a flexed back. They will sometimes describe how they can walk for longer periods in a store, leaning forward supported on a shopping cart. Extension of the spine will often provoke symptoms while flexion will relieve them. Thus, many patients when experiencing pain while walking will stop and bend forward or squat to re-lieve their pain. The patients may be able to walk only a few hundred meters but may be able to ride a bicycle for kilometers. Peripheral vascular changes are absent and pulses are present; skin color is nor-mal; hair and nails are normal; skin temperature is normal; and signs of neuropathy are absent.

Riding a stationary bicycle for exercise will pro-voke symptoms in ASPVD but often not in spinal stenosis.[1] Further, the disappearance of symptoms with rest is often more rapid in vascular claudica-

TABLE 17–2.

Preoperative Signs and Symptoms of Patients Operated on by Verbiest for Lumbar Spinal Stenosis (N = 116)*

Signs and Symptoms	Types of Stenosis (%)†		
	Absolute (n = 49)	Mixed (n = 35)	Relative (n = 32)
Lumbago	67	69	78
Sciatica	10	11	47
Sciatica with motor deficit	57	49	47
Motor deficit, no sciatica	20	29	—
Pseudoclaudication only	12	11	—
Pseudoclaudication plus other symptoms	67	74	56

*Adapted from Verbiest H: Lumbar spinal stenosis: Morphology, classification and long-term results, in Weinstein JN, Wiesel S (eds): *The Lumbar Spine.* Philadelphia, WB Saunders Co, 1990, pp 546–589..

†Absolute = there is no reserve capacity in the relation between the volume of neural content and the capacity of the vertebral canal (midsagittal diameters ≤10 mm); Relative = the reserve capacity is very small (midsagittal diameters 10–13 mm); Mixed = areas of absolute and relative stenosis are present (midsagittal diameters in portions ≤10 mm, in other portions 10–13 mm).

TABLE 17–3.

Signs and Symptoms in Patients With True Claudication and Pseudoclaudication (Neurogenic Intermittent Claudication)*

Neurogenic Claudication	True Claudication
Leg pain with walking	Leg pain with walking
Relieved by rest (more slowly)	Relieved by rest (more rapidly)
Aggravated by lumbar extension	Not aggravated by lumbar extension
Relieved by spinal flexion	Not relieved by spinal flexion
Bicycle riding not provocative	Bicycle riding provocative
Peripheral pulses present	Peripheral pulses absent
Trophic changes absent	Trophic changes present
Peripheral neuropathy absent	Peripheral neuropathy may be present
Flexed posture with walking	Flexed posture absent

*Adapted from Andersson GBJ, McNeill TW: *Lumbar Spinal Syndromes.* Vienna, Springer-Verlag, 1989, pp 100–108.

tion; not infrequently there is an element of remaining pain and discomfort in the spinal stenosis patient. While walking in ASPVD can sometimes be resumed after a minute or less, it is not infrequent that the spinal stenosis patient rests for 10 to 20 minutes before resuming walking. Walking can also provoke paresthesias and weakness in the patient with stenosis, who may also experience "drop attacks" or a sudden tendency to fall while walking.

Paresthesias, weakness, and numbness, along with sciatic pain, are also common, but not consistent, complaints in patients with spinal stenosis.[2, 7] These symptoms are often typical of an individual lumbar nerve root and are referred to as "radiculopathy" (nerve root deficit) which is distinct from the symptoms of pseudoclaudication. Atypical leg pain occurs as well with a nonradicular distribution, vague localization, and inconsistencies in location and presentation.[6] A few patients will have groin, perianal, vulvar, or testicular pain, which may be associated with a chronic cauda equina syndrome.

PHYSICAL EXAMINATION

The physical examination of a patient with spinal stenosis should follow the same general principles as any spine examination. It will rarely be diagnostic, and not infrequently the findings are few. The examination can conveniently follow the routine described in Table 17–4, starting with the patient standing and then moving on to examining the patient sitting and finally lying down first on the back and then on the abdomen. The examination involves inspection, palpation, determination of range of motion (ROM), and a few neurologic tests.

Inspection

The patient should be barefoot at the time of examination and undressed such that the entire length of the spine can be observed. Inspection should include observation of the patient's gait, including the ability to stand on toes and heels. The surface of the back is observed for pigmented spots (café au lait), localized blisters (herpes zoster), and other abnormalities. The posture is then inspected not only from the back but also from the side and the front.

TABLE 17–4.

Segmental Innervation of the Lower Limb Musculature

Joints and Prime Movers	Cord Segments						
	L2	L3	L4	L5	S1	S2	S3
Knee							
Extensors	x	X	X				
Flexors			x	X	X	x	x
Ankle							
Extensors (dorsiflexors)			X	X	x		
Flexors (plantar flexors)				x	X	X	
Pretalar-subtalar joint							
Invertors			X	X	x		
Evertors				X	X	x	
Toes							
Extensors				X	X	x	
Flexors					X	X	x
Intrinsic foot muscles						X	x

X = principal cord segment.

Head position, lordosis, kyphosis, and scoliosis are evaluated. In patients with spinal stenosis, a kyphotic posture is quite common. Frequently the patient walks "hunched over" and may require a cane for balance. Scoliosis, when present, is often lumbar and not infrequently associated with radicular complaints.

Palpation

Palpation of the spine is done to detect muscle spasms which are uncommon in spinal stenosis, but would tend to make the paravertebral muscles firm and sometimes bulging. Local masses are uncommon but should be palpated for. Local tenderness is determined by palpation over the spinous processes, the muscles, and over the iliac crests and sacrum. Tenderness at the sciatic notch is also determined.

Range of Motion

Range of motion is determined with the patient standing and the examiner observing from the back. During the examination, the pattern of motion is also recorded and the patient is told to express whether or not pain occurs. We suggest starting the examination with the patient bending forward and then backward. This motion should first be done with the examiner just viewing the flexion-extension movement and then during simultaneous palpation which makes it easier to detect any olisthesis, which is often present in degenerative spinal stenosis. The examination is then continued with lateral bending and finally rotation. To isolate rotation to the lumbar spine, the pelvis should be stabilized either by the examiner's hands holding the iliac crests or by determining rotation with the patient sitting. Determination of the precise ROM of the lumbar spine is difficult and has led to the development of several different methods. Generally, in stenotic patients, ROM is not critical to the diagnosis and need not be quantified. What is important, however, is that these patients often have lost their ability to extend the spine beyond the upright posture, and that this movement is often painful.

Straight Leg Raising

With a patient sitting, straight leg raising (SLR) is tested as well as patellar and Achilles reflexes. The straight leg raise test involves the patient extending the leg while sitting on the examination couch. Patellar and Achilles reflexes as well as quadriceps strength are now tested. The patient is then asked to lie down on the back. In this position, the straight leg raise is repeated lifting one leg at a time from the examination table and the angle at which pain occurs recorded (Fig 17–2). The knee should be extended and it should be recorded whether pain occurs in the lower back or in the leg. To increase the stretch of the sciatic nerve, the ankle joint can be extended at the same time. A positive straight leg raise test should be distinguished from inability to extend the leg owing to hamstring muscle tightness. Raising of the unaffected leg in patients with sciatica can sometimes cause pain in the opposite leg. This is called a positive contralateral straight leg raise test. Examination for the presence of Lasègue's sign is another test performed to test for sciatic nerve in-

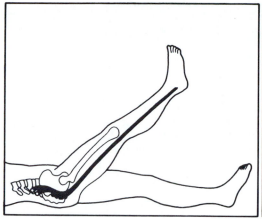
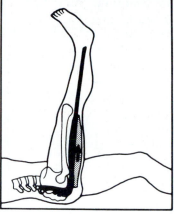

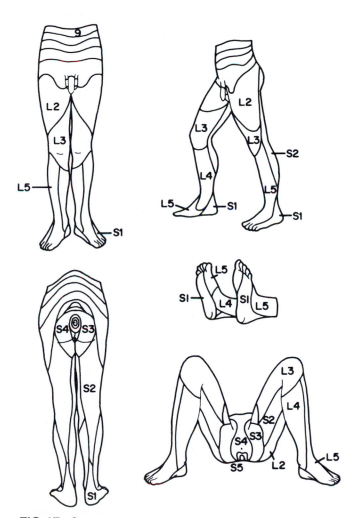

FIG 17–2.
Straight leg raise test. (*Note:* Many elderly patients with spinal stenosis have short, tight hamstring muscles preventing the leg from being raised fully.)

volvement. In this test, the hip and knee are both flexed 90 degrees. From that position, the knee joint is extended and the degree of extension at which pain occurs is recorded. SLR is often negative in patients with spinal stenosis, but can be dramatically positive.

NEUROLOGIC EXAMINATION

The neurologic examination in patients with suspect spinal stenosis involves testing for lower leg reflexes, motor function, and sensation. Most lower back disorders causing neurologic changes in the lower extremities either influence the patellar and Achilles reflexes or the strength of the extensor hallucis longus.

The patellar or quadriceps reflex is elicited when the patellar tendon is firmly tapped. It is the response of the quadriceps femoris muscle and requires an intact L4 spinal nerve. The Achilles or triceps surae reflex, also termed the *ankle jerk,* is elicited by firmly tapping the Achilles tendon. An absence of this reflex indicates S1 nerve root involvement. The triceps surae reflex can also be elicited by tapping under the plantar aspect of the foot, the plantar reflex. Sometimes the tibialis posterior reflex is elicited by tapping the tendon behind the medial malleolus, which results in an inversion of the foot. It is primarily a test of the L5 nerve root, but the tibialis posterior muscle is not exclusively innervated by L5. Brisk or weak reflexes should not be interpreted as abnormal, particularly if the reflexes are symmetric. Sometimes the reflex has to be reinforced by Jendrassik's maneuver in which the patient hooks the fingers of both hands together and pulls apart as the tendon is tapped.

FIG 17–3.
Dermatomes of the lower limbs. (Adapted from Wilson FC: *The Musculoskeletal System,* ed 2. Philadelphia, JB Lippincott Co, 1983, p 70.)

The most important motor function to determine is the extension power of the extensor hallucis longus. A reduction in extension power indicates involvement of the L5 nerve root. The test is done by asking the patient to extend both big toes and hold them firmly while pulling down on both toes at the same time. The extensor digitorum muscles (also innervated by L5) can be tested at the same time by pulling the whole foot downward. Plantar flexion strength, the loss of which would indicate S1 root involvement, and inversion-eversion strength can also be tested. The loss of eversion strength would primarily indicate S1 nerve root involvement, while the loss of inversion strength would indicate L4 root involvement. Quadriceps strength is determined by having the patient extend the lower leg against resistance. Note that few muscles are innervated by one nerve root only and, therefore, a weakness may go unnoticed. Conversely, an observed weakness may not implicate one specific nerve (see Table 17–4).

The neurologic examination should also include the Babinski test which is elicited by stimulating the plantar skin of the foot from the heel forward. When the toes flex, the response is negative. If the big toe extends, however, the test is positive, indicating an upper motor neuron lesion. The sensation of the lower legs is tested to determine whether specific dermatomes are affected or not (Figs 17–3 and 17–4). The vibratory sensation in the feet is almost always diminished in spinal stenosis. Atrophies are rare, but are, of course, recorded when present.

The neurologic examination is rarely helpful in confirming the diagnosis of spinal stenosis, but is helpful in excluding other causes for the patient's pain. Unequivocal radicular findings are present

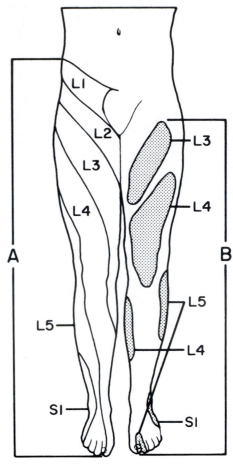

FIG 17–4.
Segmental dermatonal distribution on the left *(A)* and autonomous sensory zones on the right *(B)*.

TABLE 17–5.

Laterality of Permanent Radicular Disturbances (PRD) and Those Occurring During Periods of Pseudoclaudication (PC, Neurogenic Intermittent Claudication) (N = 195)*

Radicular Disturbances	PRD (%)	During PC (%)	No PC (%)
Bilateral identical (BI)	11.3	8.7	2.6
Bilateral unequal (BU)	31.7	12.3(BU)	16.3
		3.1(UL)	
Unilateral (UL)	46.7	26.2 (BI)	8.2
		1.0(BU)	
		11.3(UL)	
None at rest (10.3%)		8.2 (BI)	
		0.5(BU)	
		1.6(UL)	
Totals	89.7	72.9	27.1

*Adapted from Verbiest H: Lumar spinal stenosis: Morphology, classification and long-term results, in Weinstein JN, Wiesel S: *The Lumbar Spine*. Philadelphia, WB Saunders Co, 1990, pp 546–589.

only in a minority of cases. Sometimes having the patient walk for a while before the examination is helpful to the diagnosis. Neurologic signs such as weakness, numbness, reflex change, or SLR signs may be present only after exercise and disappear rapidly with rest. The patient's symptoms may also increase with walking (Table 17–5).

It must be remembered that patients with spinal stenosis typically are elderly, in whom reflexes may be depressed or absent and peripheral sensation impaired by poor circulation, diabetic neuropathy, and similar disorders. Palpation of pulses should be done routinely, and the gross temperature sense (cold, warm, etc.) of the feet should be recorded.

SUMMARY

Spinal stenosis is rarely a clinical diagnosis, yet clinical symptoms can be quite characteristic. Elderly patients with sciatica, neurogenic claudication, atypical leg pain, and chronic cauda equina symptoms should be investigated further with this diagnosis in mind. The clinical examination, while rarely specific, is useful primarily to exclude other possible causes for the above symptoms. The structural examinations discussed in Chapters 18 through 22 often confirm the clinical suspicion, while sometimes neurodiagnostic methods and studies of the lower extremity circulation are necessary to obtain the final diagnosis.

REFERENCES

1. Dyck P, Doyle TP: Bicycle test of Van Gelderen in the diagnosis of intermittent cauda equina compression syndrome: Case report. *J Neurosurg* 1977; 4:667–670.
2. Epstein JA, Epstein BS, Lavine LS: Nerve root compression associated with narrowing of the lumbar spinal canal. *J Neurol Neurosurg Psychiatry* 1962; 25:165–176.
3. Hawkes CH, Roberts GM: Neurogenic and vascular claudication. *J Neurol Sci* 1978; 38:337–345.
4. Porter RW, Hibbert C, Wellman P: Back ache and the lumbar spinal canal. *Spine* 1980; 5:99–105.
5. Spengler DM: Current concepts review. Degenerative stenosis of the lumbar spine. *J Bone Joint Surg [Am]* 1987; 69:305.
6. Van Akkerweeken PF: *Lateral Stenosis of the Lumbar Spine.* Utrecht, The Netherlands, Libertas, 1989.
7. Verbiest H: *Neurogenic Intermittent Claudication. With Special Reference to Stenosis of the Lumbar Vertebral Canal.* New York, North Holland/American Elsevier, 1976.

18

Plain Film Analysis of Spinal Stenosis

Jordan D. Rosenblum, M.D.
Tony Kim, M.D.
Sunjay Verma, M.D.
Ruth G. Ramsey, M.D.

With the widespread availability of computed tomography (CT) and magnetic resonance imaging (MRI), there has been an evolution in the radiologic imaging of spinal stenosis. The importance of plain radiographs of the spine has greatly diminished as these newer modalities have taken their place. There is still a role for plain films of the spine and in many cases they will still be the first imaging modality chosen. The ready availability and speed with which plain radiographs may be obtained make them ideal for the initial evaluation of spinal abnormalities, in directing further workup, and in many cases, avoiding costly additional studies. Radiographs of the spine serve a vital role in directing the course of further imaging to the appropriate level. In addition, the best imaging modality for further workup may be suggested by determining whether an abnormality is predominantly osseous or soft tissue. The goal of this chapter is to outline the routine radiologic views used in evaluating the spine, review the radiographic signs that may be identified, and briefly cover the different pathologic processes that may cause spinal stenosis.

The patient with symptoms suggesting spinal stenosis should first be evaluated with plain films of the region suggested by clinical symptoms. Analysis of these radiographs, in correlation with the clinical examination and history, will often suggest the most likely etiology, at least into the broad categories:

congenital, acquired, posttraumatic, neoplastic, or other less common causes. Not infrequently, more than one such cause may be suggested, such as a congenitally narrow canal that has been further compromised by degenerative changes or trauma. In general, spinal stenosis may be divided into three categories: central stenosis, foraminal stenosis, and stenosis of the lateral recesses. Central stenosis, in which there is narrowing of the vertebral canal, may be congenital or may occur with a herniated disc or posterior osteophyte. Foraminal stenosis may be seen with herniated discs, posterior osteophytes, degenerative changes of the facet joints, or any process that impinges on the neural foramen. The lateral recess lies just medial to the pedicle and is intimately related to the superior articulating facet. Because of this relationship, degenerative changes of the facet joints may cause stenosis of the lateral recess and compress the nerve root lying in the recess. Although this is not usually visible by plain films, the presence of degenerative changes of the facet joints in association with radicular pain should suggest the possibility of disease impinging on the lateral recess and prompt imaging by CT to more fully evaluate that region. In order to recognize such abnormalities the appropriate studies must be ordered and both the normal appearance and the appearance of possible abnormalities must be appreciated.

STANDARD VIEWS

Examination of the lumbar spine includes anteroposterior (AP), lateral, and 45-degree oblique views (Figs 18–1 through 18–4) as well as a lateral spot film of the sacrum centered on the L5–S1 disc space. If the sacrum is not well visualized on the AP film, a spot view of the sacrum in an AP projection should also be included. These may be supplemented by flexion and extension views when there is a clinical suspicion of instability, as in a postsurgical patient, post-trauma, or secondary to spondylolysis or spondylolisthesis.

PLAIN FILM ANALYSIS

The lumbar spine must be evaluated for congenital anomalies that may narrow the vertebral canal.

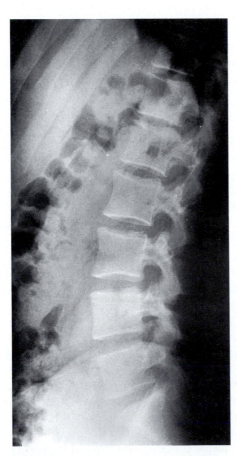

FIG 18–1.
Normal lateral view of the lumbar spine.

On the AP view the interpedicular distance should be identified. In the normal person it increases progressively from the L1 to the L5 level. Progressive narrowing of the interpedicular space is seen in congenital dysplasias such as achondroplasia with resultant narrowing of the vertebral canal. On the lateral view, short pedicles may indicate the presence of congenital stenosis. The number of lumbar-type vertebral bodies should also be noted and any variation from normal segmentation should be documented. Errors of segmentation may, at times, lead to confusion in interpreting CT scans or MRIs. Prior knowledge of such normal variation will eliminate any later confusion. Accurate identification of the level of an abnormality is necessary before any surgical correction may be attempted. On the lateral view, both the vertebral bodies as well as the disc space should be examined for possible degenerative change. The spinous processes and laminae should also be identified to indicate any previous surgical procedure involving the lumbar spine. Scalloping of the posterior aspect of the vertebral body suggests a congenital process such as achondroplasia, acromegaly, neurofibromatosis, mucopolysaccharidoses, or an acquired process such as a tumor within the vertebral canal causing pressure erosion.

Normal alignment of the lumbar spine should be present. Spondylolisthesis may cause impingement on the thecal sac and resulting compression of the nerve roots. Spondylytic spondylolisthesis is most common at the L5–S1 level (Figs 18–5 and 18–6), whereas degenerative spondylolisthesis is most common at L4–5. Spondylytic spondylolisthesis will produce nerve root impingement at the level of the defect while degenerative spondylolisthesis is more likely to produce constriction of the entire cauda equina (Fig 18–7). On the oblique views the neural foramen should be examined for encroachment by osteophytes arising from the interfacet joints or the posterior aspect of the vertebral body. The facet joints should be visualized and any widening or narrowing noted as well as any sclerosis of the facets that may indicate degenerative changes. The sacrum should be well visualized to rule out destructive lesions that may clinically mimic the symptoms of spinal stenosis at a higher level of the vertebral column. The overall bone density should be assessed for osteopenia indicating possible disuse or osteoporosis, realizing that this is an inexact method. Bony sclerosis, either focal or generalized, may indicate metastatic lesions, involvement by Paget's disease, or fluorosis, which may cause bony expansion and result in spinal stenosis.

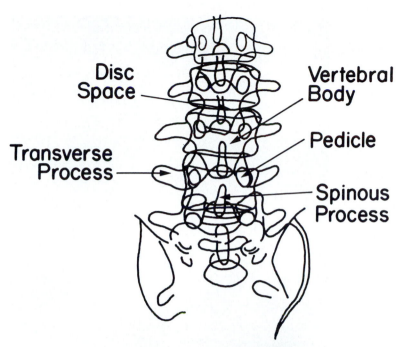

FIG 18–2.
Schematic drawing of the lumbar spine.

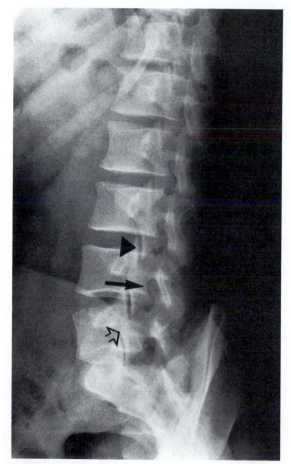

FIG 18–3.
Oblique view of the lumbar spine allows visualization of the neural foramen *(closed arrow)*, articulating facets *(arrowhead)*, and pars interarticularis region *(open arrow)*.

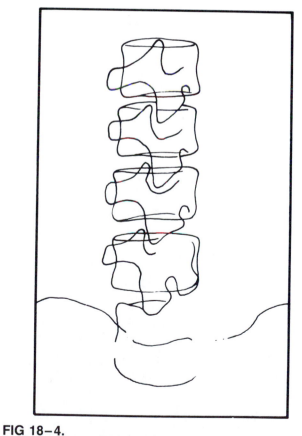

FIG 18–4.
Schematic drawing of the lumbar spine in the oblique projection demonstrates the relationship between the facet joints as well as the pars interarticularis region.

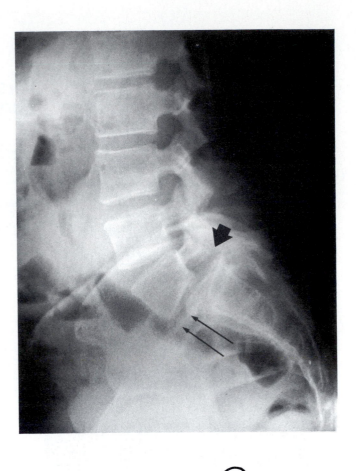

FIG 18–5.
Lateral view of the lumbosacral junction reveals a spondylolisthesis, or forward displacement of L5 on S1 *(long arrows).* There is also a spondylolysis seen *(short arrow)* as a gap in the pars interarticularis region.

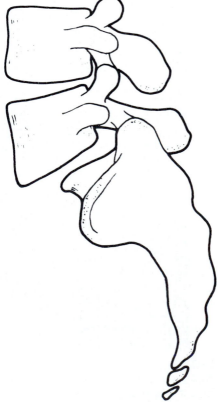

FIG 18–6.
Schematic drawing of the lumbosacral region demonstrating a spondylolisthesis of L5 on S1 comparable to that seen in Figure 18–11.

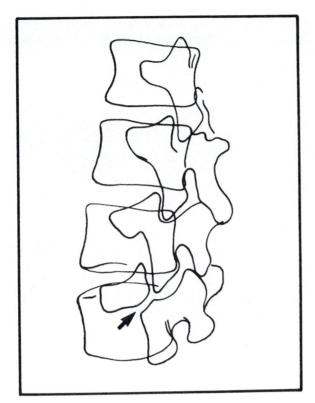

FIG 18–7.
Schematic drawing of a spondylolysis seen as a defect in the pars interarticularis.

OSTEOARTHRITIS

The most common cause of spinal stenosis seen by radiologists is due to osteoarthritis with degenerative changes of the spine. The pathologic and radiographic manifestations of spinal stenosis secondary to osteoarthritis are extremely varied. One of the most common signs is desiccation of the disc material with resultant loss of height of the disc space and the so-called vacuum disc phenomena of the intervertebral disc. There may also be extensive osteophyte formation from the vertebral body (Fig 18–8). The facet joints may show degenerative changes with either cystic degeneration, sclerosis, or productive new bone formation (see Fig 18–10). Inferior articular processes may enlarge so that they appear to meet in the midline. Vacuum phenomena may be seen in the facet joints. Degenerative changes of the facet joints may lead to either narrowing or widening of the joint space with resulting spondylolisthesis (so-called degenerative spondylolisthesis), even in the absence of a spondylolysis. This subluxation of one vertebral body on the next can cause signifi-

cant encroachment on the vertebral canal and is most commonly noted at the L4–5 level. In addition to causing constriction of the entire cauda equina as described earlier, the concomitant enlargement of the superior articular process of the level below may result in significant associated lateral recess stenosis. The vertebral canal may also be narrowed by hypertrophy of the ligamentum flavum which is frequently associated with hypertrophic changes of the facet joints and is strongly suggested by the presence of laminae which touch or even "shingle" with the superior lamina riding over the lamina below. Herniation of an intervertebral disc is one of the most common causes of acquired spinal stenosis; however, as it is not generally a plain film diagnosis, it will not be discussed further.

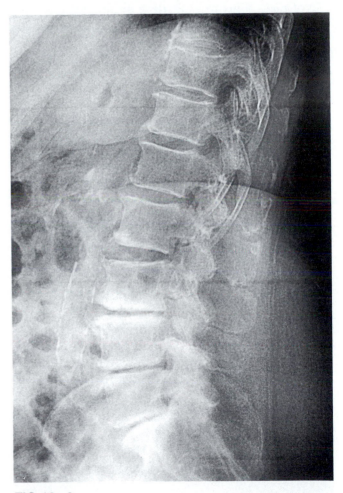

FIG 18–8.
Lateral view of the lumbar spine demonstrating marked degenerative changes with disc space narrowing and periarticular sclerosis.

TRAUMA

Spinal stenosis may also be a result of trauma to the spine. This may be evident on the plain film by the presence of bony fragments within the vertebral canal or by malalignment of the vertebral bodies with resulting impingement on the spinal canal (Figs 18–9 and 18–10). In other cases spinal stenosis may occur without plain film findings. This might be seen with a traumatic disc herniation or an epidural hematoma within the vertebral canal causing compression of the spinal canal contents. In these cases, plain films may be less helpful than CT or MRI but suspicion may be raised by identification of bony injury or soft tissue swelling. As noted previously, the role of plain films in evaluating trauma victims may be primarily to indicate levels of possible injury for evaluation by more specific means such as CT or MRI. Spinal stenosis may also result as a delayed consequence of traumatic injury. Malalignment of the vertebral bodies secondary to the injury can

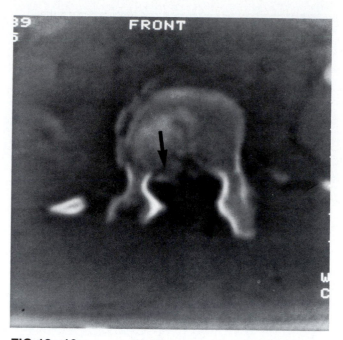

FIG 18–10.
CT of the L1 vertebral body in the same patient seen in Figure 18–9. Note the retropulsed fragments from the posterior vertebral body causing compromise of the spinal canal (arrow).

cause stenosis. In the lumbar spine this is most often seen with neglected burst fractures. Degenerative changes due to bony deformity or altered biomechanics may also result in late stenosis. In these cases, plain films may again suggest a possible narrowing of the canal which could then be evaluated by more specific means.

POSTOPERATIVE CHANGES

Postoperative changes constitute another significant cause of spinal stenosis. This is most commonly secondary to postoperative fibrosis and scar formation with resultant compression of the thecal sac or traction on the nerve roots. Although these findings require CT-myelography or MRI, plain films may suggest the diagnosis by revealing a history of previous surgery on the back which would then be examined by other imaging modalities. In the immediate postoperative period hematoma may sometimes cause compression of the spinal cord; however, this would not be visualized by plain films. This should not be a clinical problem as there would be little doubt as to the history of recent surgery.

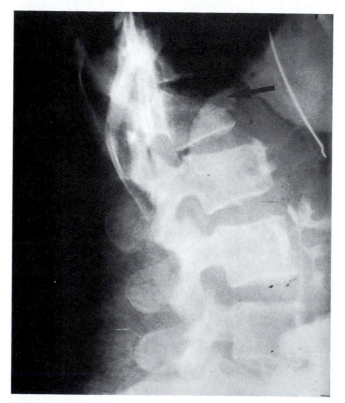

FIG 18–9.
Lumbar spine in a 30-year-old woman after a three-story fall. Note the loss of height of the L1 vertebral body anteriorly *(arrow).* Such injuries should be studied by CT or MRI to rule out compromise of the spinal canal.

NEOPLASTIC DISEASE

Spinal stenosis may also be due to neoplastic disease, either primary or metastatic. Metastatic disease, as elsewhere in the skeletal system, is overwhelmingly more common than primary malignancy. Any patient over the age of 45 to 50 years who presents with an acute onset of spinal stenosis type of symptoms must be suspected of having metastatic disease. Plain films should be the first imaging modality obtained and they frequently reveal evidence of metastases involving the spine. In males the most common metastatic lesions seen are the blastic metastases of prostate cancer or the lytic metastases of lung cancer, whereas in women lytic lesions due to metastases from breast or lung cancer would be the most common. The plain film findings with osteoblastic lesions include encroachment on

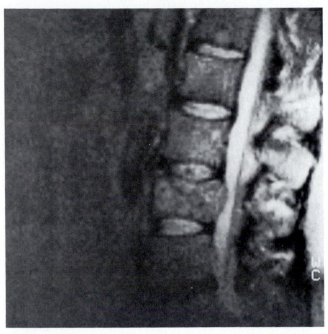

FIG 18–12.
T2-weighted sagittal MRI of the lumbar spine in the same patient seen in Figure 18–11. There is soft tissue extension posteriorly from the L3 vertebral body causing compression of the ventral aspect of the thecal sac.

the vertebral canal or neural foramen by metastatic lesions or secondary to collapse of the vertebral body. Lytic lesions may be seen as defects in the vertebral body or absent pedicles and there may be collapse of the vertebral body with resultant compression of the canal or neural foramen (Figs 18–11 and 18–12). Primary tumors of the spine are most commonly benign and include a wide variety of tumors including hemangioma, osteoblastoma, aneurysmal bone cyst, giant cell tumor, and chordoma. Less common primary malignancies of the spine include osteosarcoma or chondrosarcoma. Lymphoma of bone is a rare disease that uncommonly causes bony expansion; however, lymphomatous involvement in the paraspinal region, adjacent to the neural foramen, can extend into the foramen and cause compression of the nerve roots or the spinal cord. This might be seen on the plain film as a paraspinous mass in association with widening of the ipsilateral neural foramen. Further description of neoplastic disease involving the spine is beyond the scope of this chapter but the possibility of neoplasm should be considered in a patient presenting with spinal stenosis type of symptoms.

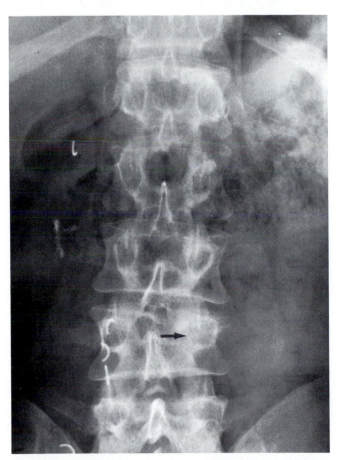

FIG 18–11.
AP view of the lumbar spine in a 34-year-old man with metastatic colon cancer. The patient complained of bilateral leg weakness. Note the loss of the left pedicle at L3 *(arrow)* as well as the depression of the superior end plate.

CONGENITAL STENOSIS

Congenital spinal stenosis may be secondary to a congenitally short pedicle, narrowing of the interpedicular distance, or congenital or acquired thickening of the lamina (see Chapter 12). Achondroplasia deserves particular note because of the frequent occurrence of spinal stenosis in patients with this disorder. Achondroplasia is the most common form of dwarfism and represents an abnormal development of enchondral bone. Plain film findings are diagnostic and in the spine include a normal spinal length but an increase in the ratio of disc space height to vertebral body height as well as posterior scalloping of the vertebral bodies. The interpedicular distance characteristically decreases from cranial to caudal in the lumbar region, while the pedicles are short and thick causing a decrease in the sagittal diameter of the cord. There is often an exaggerated lumbar lordosis with a horizontally oriented sacrum. Because of the congenitally narrow vertebral canal these patients are particularly susceptible to any additional compromise of the canal such as that due to degenerative change or trauma. Cord compression most commonly occurs in these patients in adulthood and usually occurs at the thoracolumbar or lumbar region.

Another uncommon cause of congenital spinal stenosis is a group of related metabolic disorders termed *mucopolysaccharidoses*. These disorders cause widespread abnormality of the skeletal system and nervous system as well as the visceral organs. One of the more common subtypes is Morquio's disease, or mucopolysaccharidosis type IV, which has been estimated to occur in 1 in 40,000 births. Radiologically the spine demonstrates universal platyspondyly or loss of height of all of the vertebral bodies with an anterior central beak which is almost pathognomonic of Morquio's disease. The L1 or L2 vertebral body is often hypoplastic and may be posteriorly displaced, causing stenosis of the vertebral canal.

OSSIFICATION OF THE POSTERIOR LONGITUDINAL LIGAMENT

A relatively uncommon cause of spinal stenosis is ossification of the posterior longitudinal ligament (OPLL). This is best seen on the lateral radiograph where there is a characteristic dense line of ossification running along the posterior spinal line. It is most common in the cervical spine followed by the thoracic and the lumbar spine. The ossified ligament may measure up to 5 mm in thickness and may cause significant impingement on the ventral aspect of the spinal cord.

INFECTION

Infection is another uncommon cause of spinal stenosis. Epidural abscess is a rare occurrence which can cause compression of the spinal cord. The plain film evaluation of an abscess causing compression is most often normal but may reveal a paraspinal mass with widening of the paraspinal line and possibly destruction of the adjacent vertebral body. An abscess of this type is usually secondary to osteomyelitis of the vertebral body. Infections initially involve the subchondral vertebral end plate or, less com-

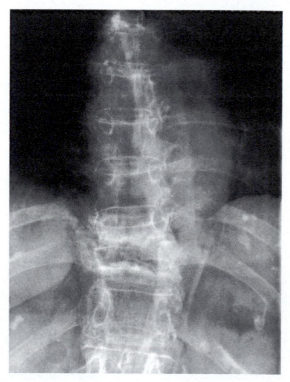

FIG 18–13.
AP view of the thoracolumbar junction in a patient with a known paraspinal tuberculous abscess. Note the loss of height of the T10 and T11 vertebral bodies, as well as the marked bony sclerosis. These findings suggest a relatively chronic destructive process.

may lead to spinal stenosis. The most common of these is osteoporosis. This is defined as normal bone mineralization with a deficiency of bony matrix. In routine radiologic practice the most common cause is postmenopausal osteoporosis. The plain film findings include diffuse osteopenia of the vertebral bodies with increased prominence of the vertebral trabecular pattern. There may be biconcave deformities of the vertebral end plates. Although not in itself a cause of spinal stenosis, osteoporosis may lead to compression fractures of the vertebral body with displacement of the posterior aspect of the vertebral body into the vertebral canal and resultant decreased volume of the spinal canal.

Fluorosis is a rare condition secondary to an increased uptake of fluoride-containing compounds. There is hypertrophic bone formation, particularly at the attachment of ligaments and on the plain film, and ossification of the ligaments as well as diffuse osteosclerosis of the bones is seen. The bones themselves become thickened and there is often extensive ossification of the intervertebral disc. The resultant bone thickening may cause compression of the nerve roots in the neural foramen.

PAGET'S DISEASE

Paget's disease affects patients of middle age and beyond with a male predominance of approximately 2 to 1. It is a disease of unknown etiology which may result in spinal stenosis by expansion of bone trabeculae which increases the size of the vertebral bodies. Paget's disease frequently begins with a lytic phase which progresses to a mixed lytic and osteoblastic phase and finally into an osteoblastic phase in which the characteristic pattern includes coarse thickened trabeculae and diffuse bony sclerosis. In the spine there is frequently marked sclerosis of the margins of the vertebral body giving the so-called picture frame appearance. The overall size of the vertebral body increases; hypertrophic new bone formation around the vertebral canal and neural foramen causes narrowing. In addition, the bone, although increased in density, is abnormally weak, thus increasing the risk of compression fractures which may lead to impingement of the spinal cord.

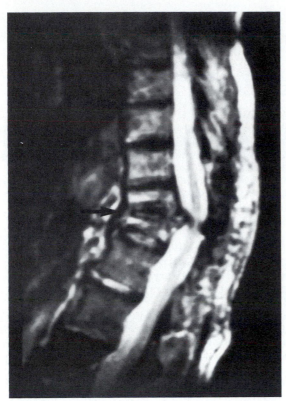

FIG 18–14.
T2-weighted sagittal MRI of the thoracolumbar region demonstrates collapse of the T10 and T11 bodies with resultant compression of the thecal sac and spinal stenosis. This is the same patient as seen in Figure 18–12.

monly, the adjacent disc material, and cause progressive vertebral body destruction and intervertebral disc destruction. This pattern of vertebral destruction with involvement of an intervening disc space is one means of differentiating infection from neoplastic disease, which characteristically spares the disc material. In the case of a tuberculous abscess (Pott's disease), the late stages may demonstrate a severe kyphosis secondary to vertebral body collapse (a gibbus deformity) (Figs 18–13 and 18–14). In this case the clinical symptoms would be helpful in making a diagnosis and the patient may have other evidence of tuberculosis including an abnormal chest film, an elevated white blood cell count, and fever.

METABOLIC DISEASE

Metabolic diseases provide an additional and somewhat varied category of disease states which

SUMMARY

MRI and CT scanning are clearly the modalities of choice for detailed evaluation of spinal lesions. Nevertheless, plain film analysis of spinal lesions remains the most efficient and inexpensive means of initial evaluation. Although frequently nonspecific, plain films may demonstrate the level of abnormality to be evaluated as well as often suggesting the nature of the disease process. In cases where the disease is predominantly osseous, such as posttraumatic injuries with a question of bony fragments within the spinal cord, or degenerative disease with neural impingement secondary to osteophytes, CT with or without myelography may be the imaging modality of choice. When plain films suggest the possibility of soft tissue abnormality but without bony abnormality such as tumor, abscess, hematoma, or posttraumatic injury, MRI with its multiple imaging planes may be more efficacious as a next step. In a patient with radicular symptoms but with normal radiographs of the spine, a diagnosis of a herniated nucleus pulposus would be high on the list of differential diagnoses, and although there remains some debate about the imaging modality of choice, the consensus seems to be rapidly shifting toward MRI as the next step. In cases of trauma with a low clinical index of suspicion for injury, plain films may be the only imaging modality necessary and thus obviate the additional cost and radiation exposure of the CT scan.

BIBLIOGRAPHY

1. Altman RD, Brown M, Gargano F: Low back pain in Paget's disease of the bone. *Clin Orthop* 1987; 217:152.
2. Atlas SW, Regenbogen V, Rodgers LF, et al: The radiologic characterization of burst fractures of the spine. *AJNR* 1986; 7:675–682.
3. Chester W, Chester EM: The vertebral column in acromegaly. *AJR* 1940; 44:552–557.
4. Daffner RH: *Imaging of Vertebral Trauma.* Rockville, Md, Aspen, 1988.
5. Edeikin J: *Roentgen Diagnosis of Diseases of Bone,* ed 3, vol 2. Baltimore, Williams & Wilkins Co, 1981.
6. Harsh GR, Sypert GW, Weinstein PR, et al: Cervical spine stenosis secondary to ossification of the posterior longitudinal ligament. *J Neurosurg* 1987; 67:349–357.
7. Hinck VC, Hopkins CE, Clark WM: Sagittal diameter of the lumbar spinal canal in children and adults. *Radiology* 1965; 85:929–937.
8. Kaplan PA, Orton DF, Asleson RJ: Osteoporosis with vertebral compression fractures, retropulsed fragments, and neurologic compromise. *Radiology* 1987; 165:533–535.
9. Ramsey RG: Neuroradiologic evaluation of spinal stenosis, in Margulis AR, Gooding CA (eds): *Diagnostic Radiology 1989.* Berkeley, Calif, University of California Press. 1989, pp 289–296.

19

Spinal Stenosis: Evaluation by Computed Tomography

Sunjay Verma, M.D.

Jordan D. Rosenblum, M.D.

Tony Kim, M.D.

Ruth G. Ramsey, M.D.

Spinal stenosis and some of its causes are discussed elsewhere in this book, with emphasis on radiologic evaluation by plain films (see Chapter 18) and myelography (see Chapter 22). The focus of this chapter is on computed tomography (CT) evaluation, and its relative benefits. The benefits of CT over plain films and conventional myelography are, in general, as follows:

The first advantage of CT, especially in evaluation of the spine, is that it can provide *apparent* greater resolution than plain films. This has become possible with the modern high resolution CT scanners. This increased resolution is brought about not by actually increasing the *spatial* resolution in comparison with plain films but by the increased ability of CT to appreciate density differences (i.e., by increasing the *density* resolution). Densities that on plain film appear simply the same are differentiated by CT. This is especially true in the water and soft tissue density ranges. Thus, by CT, the intervertebral disc has a different density and may be differentiated from ligament density. Ligament may be further differentiated from water density, which is the same as cerebrospinal fluid (CSF) density. This, added to densities that were already readily differentiated on plain films, dramatically enhances imaging potential.

The four basic densities on *plain film*, in order of decreasing density, are bone (calcification), soft tissue (which includes muscle, water, and ligament), fat, and air. With CT, *smaller quantities* of these can now be adequately differentiated. Thus, within the vertebral canal, the skeleton (which is bony density) is differentiated from the epidural fat surrounding the thecal sac, and this is further differentiated from the CSF (or water density) which is contained within the thecal sac. Thus an *apparent* increase in spatial resolution is achieved by an increase in density resolution.

Even further enhancement of the above effects may be achieved by introducing intrathecal contrast, and imaging on the appropriate window settings; this is known as the *CT myelogram*. This gives still another density level to the CSF within the thecal sac, which makes it easier to delineate borders of the thecal sac against soft tissue or disc. An added advantage, which may not be pertinent in the particular setting of spinal stenosis, but becomes important for evaluating intradural pathologic changes, is direct visualization of intrathecal contents as they are bathed by contrast material.

A second advantage of CT imaging is the ability to image in different planes, either directly or by multiplanar re-formation. Usually the spine is im-

245

aged in axial cross section, perpendicular to the vertebral canal. However, at the level of the discs, axial slices parallel to the plane of the disc are also obtained. Computer-generated reconstruction of the data into sagittal or coronal images is also possible, which facilitates visualization of alignment of vertebral bodies and other structures such as the atlantoaxial joint or the facet joints (Fig 19–1; see also Fig 19–6). Still another advantage is the ability to process data to obtain three-dimensional images, which has proved particularly helpful to referring physicians.

CT has the ability to choose a window to visualize a spectrum of densities. Depending upon the organs being visualized, imaging may be enhanced to highlight the focus of interest, by choosing the appropriate contrast and window settings. For evaluation of bony structures, a wide window setting is used. Evaluation of soft tissue structures requires more narrow window settings. For imaging of an organ that is relatively homogeneous in density, evaluation of subtle density differences may be further enhanced by narrower windows. This is useful for imaging of the spine, because bony structures may be visualized on one window, and the soft tissues within and around the spine may be visualized on another window setting.

For purposes of general evaluation, and especially to rule out disc disease in the lumbar level, the three lowermost intervertebral discs are covered. Axial slices at 5-mm contiguous intervals are used starting at the L3 level to cover the L3–4, L4–5, and L5–S1 discs. At our institution, we go back specifically at the disc levels and obtain oblique axial slices parallel to the plane of the disc at 3-mm contiguous intervals. If the CT examination is directed specifically for spinal stenosis, usually all five lumbar disc levels are imaged with similar CT protocol techniques as described above. For these evaluations, bony and soft tissue windows are obtained for every image.

BASIC DEFINITIONS

Simply stated, spinal stenosis is compression of neural tissue caused by narrowing of the *vertebral canal.* Stenosis may be classified anatomically as central or lateral stenosis (see Chapter 2). Margins of the *central canal* are formed anteriorly by the vertebral body and discs, posteriorly by the lamina and

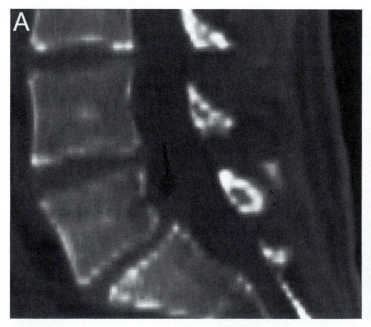 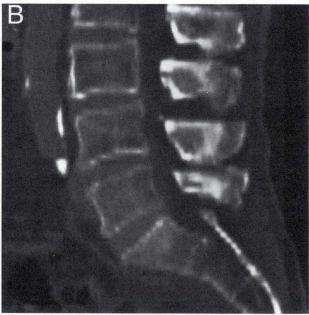

FIG 19–1.
Computer-generated reconstruction of data from contiguous axial images into sagittal images, on bone window settings. **A,** midline sagittal reformat image of the lumbosacral spine, demonstrating anterolisthesis of L5 on S1. Note disc pseudobulge *(black arrow).* **B,** midline sagittal reformat image of short pedicle syndrome. Note the severe decrease in AP diameter of the vertebral canal even though the pedicles themselves are not visualized on this particular image. They were evident on the appropriate paramidline sagittal reconstructions.

A

B

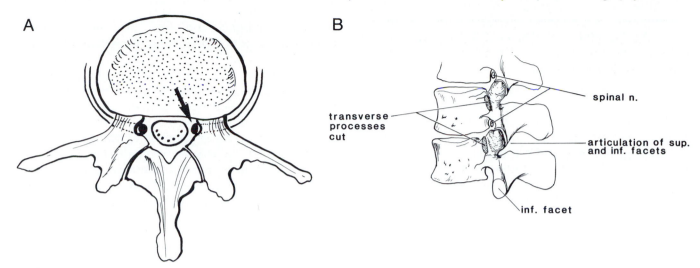

FIG 19–2.
A, diagram of a normal lumbar vertebra in the axial projection. Note the nerve root as it traverses the lateral recess *(arrow)*, and continues through the subarticular canal, underneath the pedicle, finally exiting via the neural foramen. **B,** diagram in the lateral view of the normal lumbar intervertebral foramen, which is the most lateral part of the subarticular canal. The transverse processes of the vertebral bodies have been cut to better illustrate the appearance of the interarticulating facets. Note the nerve root as it exits through the intervertebral neural foramen. The normal foramen measures 8 to 10 mm in height and 4 to 6 mm in its sagittal diameter. Also note that the nerve is situated in the upper half of the foramen above the intervertebral disc level. The nerve roots at this level are named for the vertebral body under whose pedicle they exit.

ligamentum flavum, and laterally by the pedicle and articular pillars (made up of superior and inferior facets and their articulations, the facet joints). The exit pathway of the nerve root is encircled by the most lateral aspect of the vertebral canal. This will be referred to as the *subarticular canal.* The lateral aspect of the subarticular canal is formed by the *neural foramen.* The most medial aspect of the subarticular canal is called the *lateral recess.* The borders of this *lateral recess* are formed anteriorly by the posterior vertebral body edge, laterally by the pedicle, and posteriorly by the superior and inferior articulating facets (Figs 19–2 and 19–3).

There are quantitative measurements that have been ascribed to spinal stenosis. An anteroposterior (AP) diameter of less than 11.5 mm, or a cross-sectional area of less than 1.45 cm^2 defines the upper limits of central spinal stenosis (see Fig 19–3). Recent information indicates that these measures may be quite generous, and often more stringent criteria are used. A lateral recess measurement of less than 3 mm is considered abnormally small and constitutes lateral spinal stenosis. Normal ligamentum flavum thickness varies according to the level in the spine, and is normally within 1.5 mm in the cervical and 4 mm in the lumbar regions.

The causes of spinal stenosis can be divided broadly into two categories on the basis of acquired or congenital disease. These entities have been covered in previous chapters and will be discussed here as they relate to CT diagnosis. Of course, combinations of acquired and asymptomatic congenital diseases may become superimposed to cause symptomatic spinal stenosis.

Degenerative disease is the most common acquired cause of spinal stenosis. This is covered next. Other forms of acquired disease which will be discussed are spondylolisthesis and spondylolysis, trauma, iatrogenic causes, and neoplasm. Congenital and developmental spinal stenosis are then discussed.

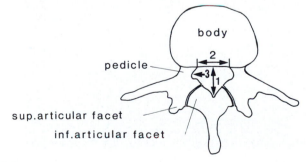

FIG 19–3.
Schematic diagram corresponding to Figure 19–2,A, illustrating various useful measurements to determine spinal stenosis. *(1)* AP or sagittal diameter. *(2)* Transverse or interpedicular diameter. *(3)* Lateral recess *(short arrow).*

ACQUIRED SPINAL STENOSIS

Degenerative Stenosis

The most commonly encountered cause of spinal stenosis is that caused by degenerative joint disease (DJD), also known as *osteoarthritis.* Just as DJD affects the rest of the skeleton, particularly in the interphalangeal, knee, and hip joints, so it affects the spine as well. The classic findings of DJD are those seen in the rest of the skeleton, and are discussed in Chapters 18 and 22. These too are the findings seen on CT, only with great sensitivity, owing to the better resolving power of CT.

The findings are (1) joint space narrowing at the intervertebral disc, and posterior intervertebral (facet) joint levels, (2) increased bony sclerosis (eburnation) due to reactive bone formation, or overgrowth in the form of osteophytes, and (3) consequent deformity.

DJD occurs most often in middle-aged and elderly patients, affecting most frequently the lower lumbar levels of L4–5 and L5–S1. CT examination readily demonstrates the presence of hypertrophic degenerative changes involving the margins of the vertebral bodies, as well as the posterior intervertebral (facet) joint spaces. Narrowing of the joint space and cystic degenerative changes are more easily appreciated on CT compared with plain films or magnetic resonance imaging (MRI). Hypertrophy of facet joints with marginal bone formation results in cupping of the superior articulating facet around the inferior facet.

It is these hypertrophic changes which frequently lead to subarticular stenosis, both at the lateral recess and beyond. This results in encroachment on the exiting nerve root and so-called lateral spinal stenosis. This is important because this leads to symptoms of radicular neuropathy (Fig 19–4).

Central stenosis refers to narrowing of the central vertebral canal (the "spinal canal") (see Kirkaldy-Willis and McIvor in the Bibliography). The presence of degenerative osteophytes at the back of the vertebral body is one of the most common causes. Another common cause of central stenosis is from *posterior elements,* or the shingling of one lamina under another. The posterior elements are made up of both bony and soft tissues at the posterior aspects of the vertebral canal. The bony structures include the facet joints, lamina, and spinous processes. The most important soft tissue structure of the posterior elements is the ligamentum flavum, which connects the laminae along the posterior lateral aspect of the vertebral canal. Degeneration of the intervertebral disc space results in subluxation of the facet joints. Hypertrophy, or shortening of the ligamenta flava, caused by shortening of the motion segment, and then hypertrophy of the articulating facets follow. This, in turn, can cause encroachment upon the ver-

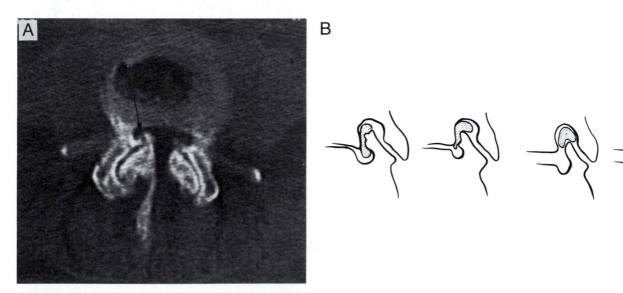

FIG 19–4.

A, axial scan of lumbar spine on bone windows. There is stenosis of both the right and left lateral recesses. It is more severe on the right side owing to osteophytes arising from the facets *(arrow).* Note the vacuum disc, which is another sign of degenerative joint disease (DJD). **B,** schematic illustration of progressive degeneration and encroachment upon the subarticular canal and neural foramen with DJD. The diagram on the *far right* is normal. Progressive DJD as facet degeneration and subluxation ensues is illustrated in the diagrams to the *left* (after Shapiro[12]).

A

B

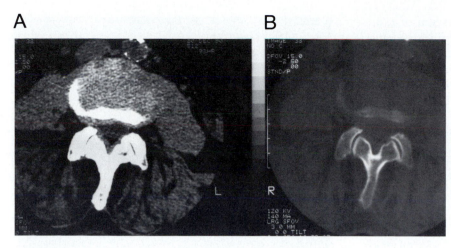

FIG 19–5.
A and **B,** soft tissue and bone windows at level of L3–4 intervertebral disc. There is minimal disc bulge. Note the epidural fat within the vertebral canal, the obliteration of which is often a useful indirect sign for spinal stenosis.

tebral canal and thus cause central spinal stenosis as well as lateral stenosis.

CT is exquisitely suited for detection of these changes. The classic CT finding of central spinal stenosis in the lumbar spine is a triangular appearance known as *trefoil*. This is the alteration of the shape of the lumbar canal from its normal oval configuration to a triangular appearance. It is caused by a circumferential reduction in the dural sac size from anterior encroachment at the posterior edge of the vertebral body, either by osteophytes or disc, and posterolateral encroachment on both sides by hypertrophied ligamenta flava. These direct signs are readily seen by CT owing to the density differences of the above stenosing components. This classic trefoil appearance on CT corresponds on myelography to what is classically referred to as "waisting" (see Chapter 22). A further indirect sign of spinal stenosis is the loss of the epidural fat which surrounds the thecal sac and exiting nerve roots. In fact, often it is this secondary sign that alerts the radiologist to the diagnosis of spinal stenosis at a particular level (Fig 19–5). Comparison with unaffected adjacent levels is useful.

Spondylolysis and Spondylolisthesis

Spondylolysis refers to a break in the pars interarticularis, usually at the L5–S1 level (see Chapter 14). It is usually bilateral, and may be associated with various degrees of spondylolisthesis. *Spondylolisthesis,* or simply olisthesis, is defined as slippage of one vertebra upon another. The olisthesis may be anterior (anterolisthesis) or, less commonly, posterior (posterolisthesis). The cause of spondylolisthesis is spondylolysis or degenerative disease (osteoarthritis) with degeneration of the discs, and subluxation of the interfacet joints, which results in displace-

ment of the vertebra (see Chapter 11). Thus, even though in most discussions of spinal stenosis, spondylolysis and spondylolisthesis are listed separately from degenerative or osteoarthritic spinal stenosis, they are in fact commonly associated with one another, since the disc often degenerates prematurely in spondylytic spondylolisthesis.

On axial imaging of CT, the appearance may be confusing to the uninitiated (Fig 19–6). Axial images of anterolisthesis demonstrate a band of disc material on the posterior aspect of the inferior end plate

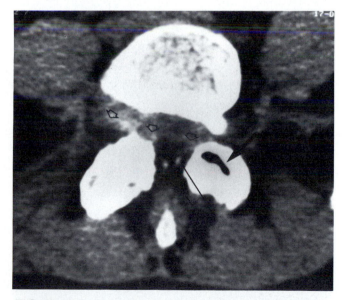

FIG 19–6.
Axial slice of lumbar spine using the soft tissue window technique, demonstrating a pseudobulge from spondylolisthesis *(open arrowheads)*. There is significant spinal stenosis. The thecal sac is poorly seen owing to circumferential compression. Note the bilateral ligamentum flavum calcification *(arrows)*. There is a vacuum facet on the left *(large arrow)*, and facet hypertrophy on the right.

of the superior vertebral body, reminiscent of a diffuse disc bulge. However, this is not due to a bulging disc, and so is called a *pseudobulge* sign. It is therefore often helpful to view the lateral tomogram, or reformat sagittal reconstructions to visualize the slippage of one vertebral body onto the other (see Fig 19–1,A).

Spondylolysis, which is the actual break in the pars interarticularis (which is the junction of the pedicle, superior articulating facet, and inferior articulating facet), is best seen by CT either in the sagittal or axial plane. Axial images will demonstrate the lysis at this level as an extralucent line across the region of the pedicle (Figs 19–7 and 19–8). For the purpose of identifying fractures, CT is superior to either the plain film or MRI. It is superior to plain films because of better resolution, as discussed earlier; it is superior to MRI for identification of bony anatomy and fractures because of its ability to give the detail of the bony structures as a positive density as compared with MRI in which calcium is demonstrated as a signal void (or *lack* of density).

Posttraumatic and Iatrogenic Causes of Spinal Stenosis

Late changes following fracture of the spine (posttraumatic) and following spinal surgery may result in spinal stenosis (see Chapter 13). Bony, soft tissue, or metal fixation devices introduced adjacent to the canal may result in exuberant new bone for-

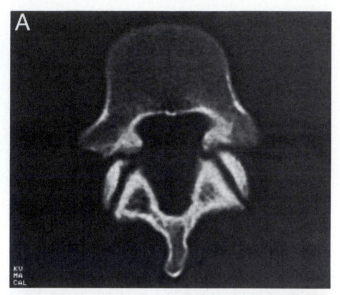

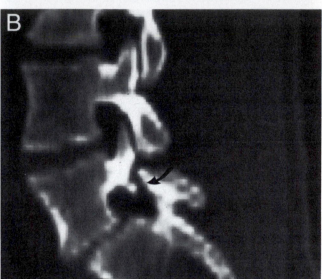

FIG 19–8.
A, another example of spondylolysis *(arrows)*. Note sclerosis around lysis denoting its chronic nature. **B,** computer-generated sagittal re-formation demonstrates a pars defect at the isthmus fracture *(arrow)*. Compare with normal level above.

mation during reparative attempts by the body. Instability, be it posttraumatic or postoperative, may lead to accelerated degenerative changes, which may contribute to spinal stenosis (Fig 19–9).

Postoperative Spinal Stenosis

After attempted surgical spinal fusion, overgrowth or migration of the fusion mass may constrict the spinal canal (Fig 19–10). Epidural scarring

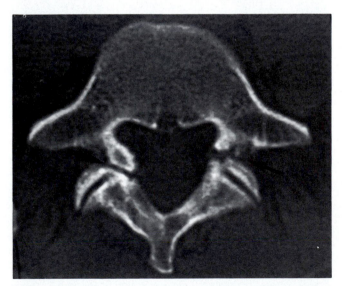

FIG 19–7.
Spondylolysis. There is an extralucent line across the region of the pedicles bilaterally that corresponds to the lysis *(arrows)*. Note bony fragmentation.

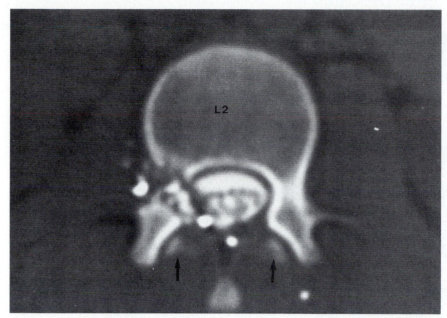

FIG 19–9.
Gunshot through the L2 vertebral body on the bone window setting. The trajectory is through the shattered right pedicle, through the vertebral canal, and into the posterior soft tissues. There is epidural mass effect upon the thecal sac. Note the bottom edges of the inferior facets of L1 *(arrows)*.

following laminectomy can also compromise the spinal canal. An epidural hematoma or abscess following surgery or trauma may likewise cause compromise of the vertebral canal, either acutely or subacutely.

Epidural Lipomatosis

An unusual cause of spinal stenosis is epidural lipomatosis, which usually occurs in the lumbar and

thoracic regions following prolonged corticosteroid therapy. This results in compression of the thecal sac by the excessive accumulation of epidural fat. Idiopathic cases have also been described. Hypertrophy of postlaminectomy fat grafts has been seen rarely.

Neoplastic Causes of Spinal Stenosis

Any extradural (epidural) mass that occurs in the spine is capable of causing spinal stenosis. These

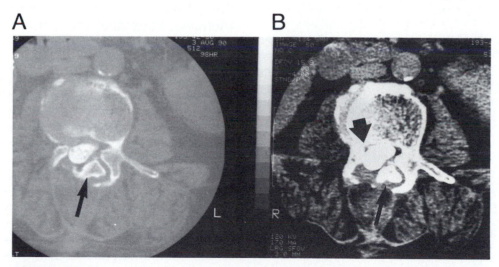

FIG 19–10.
A and **B,** postoperative lumbar spine visualized using bone window and soft tissue window techniques at two different levels 3 mm apart. There is both AP and transverse diameter stenosis. Migration of the bony mass *(long arrow)* is responsible for the majority of the stenosis. Post-laminectomy scar is evident by hyperdense soft tissue dorsal to the thecal sac, loss of vertebral canal fat, and later recess stenosis on the right *(short arrow)*.

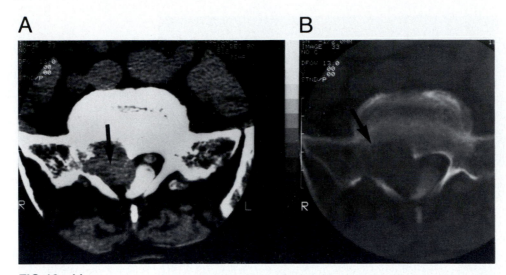

FIG 19–11.
A, B, soft tissue and bone windows of an axial slice at the L5–S1 level showing metastatic thyroid carcinoma. There is a lytic bony lesion in the right sacrum, with soft tissue epidural extension *(arrows).* There is compression of the thecal sac on the right, and the right nerve root cannot be visualized (compare with the left).

entities include benign or malignant primary bone tumors that involve the spine, including expansile lesions such as aneurysmal bone cyst, giant cell tumor, osteoblastoma, osteoid osteoma, chordoma, and sometimes hemangioma.

The most common neoplastic cause of stenosis is metastatic disease. Metastatic infiltration of the vertebral body, which often extends beyond its normal confines and commonly into the epidural space, is a cause of stenosis as well as pathologic fracture secondary to bony vertebral destruction by tumor. In the case of lymphoma, often there is epidural infiltration even without apparent bony changes. The extent of epidural infiltration and its effects on the thecal sac and neural elements are well seen by CT, especially after introduction of intrathecal contrast (Fig 19–11).

CONGENITAL AND DEVELOPMENTAL SPINAL STENOSIS

Congenital and developmental spinal stenosis may be divided into hereditary congenital disturbances, such as achondroplasia, hypochondroplasia (a related condition), Morquio's mucopolysaccharidosis, and short pedicle syndrome, and those caused by pathologic developmental or metabolic conditions. The latter include diffuse idiopathic skeletal hyperostosis (DISH), posterior longitudinal ligament calcification (CPLL), and, less commonly, ankylosing spondylitis, acromegaly, fluorosis, calcium pyrophosphate dehydrate crystal deposition disease (CPPD or pseudogout), and Paget's disease of bone. Some of the more common of these entities are described below.

Short Pedicle Syndrome (Developmental Stenosis, Idiopathic Stenosis)

This condition occurs when one or several segmental levels of the spinal canal become stenotic in the sagittal dimension as a result of abnormal development of the pedicles. Specifically, the pedicles are short and stocky (Fig 19–12). This in itself may result in acceptable spinal canal cross-sectional dimensions, but does not leave much room for additional compromise, as occurs with superimposed degenerative or other disease processes (see Figs 19–1,B and 19–12,C). In contrast to the short pedicles, the posterior elements may appear hypertrophic at the involved levels. Any additional hypertrophy of the ligamentum flavum or inferior and superior facets further compromises the canal. Therefore, even a minimally bulging disc, which in ordinary circumstances would have imperceptible effects, can now cause symptomatic compression of neural tissue. Although this is essentially a congenital condition, clinical presentation of this syndrome often occurs around middle age since that is when the superimposed degenerative disease process occurs.

A   B

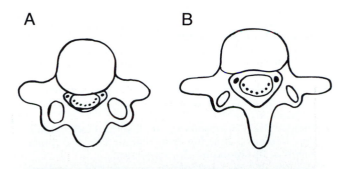

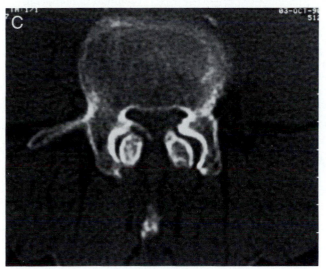

FIG 19–12.
A, B, schematic diagram illustrating the difference between the lumbar vertebra in **(A)** congenital stenosis and **(B)** in the normal spine. **B** illustrates congenital stenosis of the lumbar spinal canal with thick pedicles and laminae. Note encroachment upon the thecal sac and cauda equina (after Shapiro[12]). **C,** axial slice of the lumbar spine using the bone window technique, demonstrating the short pedicle syndrome. Note compromised AP diameter. Also note the "vertical" orientation of the facet articulation that is also commonly seen with this syndrome. (Incidentally, there is ligamentum flavum calcification on the right side.)

Achondroplasia

Achondroplasia, an autosomal dominant hereditary disease, is the most common form of dwarfism. It is a disorder of enchondral bone formation due to abnormal development in cartilage. This results in early closure of cartilaginous neurocentral synchondroses in the vertebrae, and the formation of short, squat pedicles; this in turn results in a generally small central canal. It usually involves all levels of the spine, and is characterized by not only a decreased AP diameter due to short pedicles but a decreased transverse diameter as well. The interpedicular distance (transverse diameter) decreases progressively in the lower lumbar region, which is

the opposite of normal. This is one of the hallmarks of the achondroplasia on the AP plain film. Other classic findings include lordosis, particularly at the lumbosacral junction, and kyphosis at the thoracolumbar junction. The foramen magnum may also be compromised.

Other Developmentally Acquired Stenoses

Certain metabolic conditions may be associated with spinal stenosis. Calcification and ossification of ligaments due to various conditions may result in compromise of the vertebral canal.

Diffuse Idiopathic Skeletal Hyperostosis

Probably the most common developmental condition is DISH. The cause of this syndrome is unknown, but results in enthesopathy in a systemic distribution with classic "whiskering" at the ligamentous and tendinous insertions. In the spine, there is calcification, most often along the anterior longitudinal ligament but which may extend circumferentially around the vertebral body and around the disc spaces. When involvement of the posterior longitudinal ligament from this process occurs, vertebral canal encroachment may follow. Isolated calcification of the posterior longitudinal ligament also is found to occur at the cervical level in Japanese patients.

Calcium Pyrophosphate Dehydrate Deposition Disease

Calcification and ossification of the ligamentum flavum is an unusual cause of central canal stenosis, particularly in the cervical and thoracic regions. This finding has been reported in patients with CPPD, inflammatory spinal arthritis, and also in patients with degenerative osteoarthritic stenosis.

SUMMARY

Spinal stenosis is a commonly encountered clinical problem. Degenerative osteoarthritis and its complications are the most common causes, but a number of less common causes include both congenital and acquired diseases. CT has greatly improved our ability to diagnose this important clinical entity. MRI has become increasingly important in recent years, and presumably will become the mainstay of clinical diagnosis in years to come, especially with further improvement in technology.

BIBLIOGRAPHY

1. Brant-Zawadzki M: Traumatic lesions of the spinal column, in Latchaw RE (ed): *Computed Tomography of the Head, Neck, and Spine.* St Louis, Mosby-Year Book, Inc, 1985, pp 693–705.

2. Dorwart RH, Vogler JB, Helms CA: Spinal stenosis. *Radiol Clin North Am* 1983; 21:301–325.

3. Helms CA, Vogler JB: Computed tomography of spinal stenosis and arthrosis, in Genant HK, Chafetz N, Helms CA (eds): *Computed Tomography of the Spine.* San Francisco, University of California Press, 1982, pp 187–220.

4. Heithoff KB: Pathogenesis and high resolution computed tomographic scanning of direct bony impingement syndromes of the lumbar spine, in Genant HK, Chafetz N, Helms CA (eds): *Computed Tomography of the Spine.* San Francisco, University of California Press, 1982, pp 227–244.

5. Kirkaldy-Willis WH, McIvor GWD: Editorial comment. Lumbar spinal stenosis. *Clin Orthop* 1976; 115:2–3.

6. Mall JC, Kaiser JA: Computed tomography of the postoperative spine, in Genant HK, Chafetz N, Helms CA (eds): *Computed Tomography of the Spine.* San Francisco, University of California Press, 1982, pp 245–252.

7. Meyer JD: Computed tomographic myelography in degenerative disc disease and spinal stenosis. CT evaluation of the postoperative spine, in Latchaw RE (ed): *Computed Tomography of the Head, Neck, and Spine,* ed 2. St Louis, Mosby-Year Book, Inc, 1990, pp 619–657.

8. Mikhael MA, Ciric I, Tarkington JA, et al: Neuroradiologic evaluation of lateral recess syndrome. *Radiology* 1981; 140:97–107.

9. Peyster RG. Spinal stenosis, in Taveras J (ed): *Radiology: Diagnosis, Imaging, Intervention,* vols 1–3. Philadelphia, JB Lippincott Co, 1986–1988.

10. Ramsey RG: Neuroradiologic evaluation of spinal stenosis, in Marqulis AR, Gooding CA (eds): *Diagnostic Radiology.* San Francisco, University of California Press, 1989, pp 331–338.

11. Resnick D: Degenerative diseases of the vertebral column. *Radiology* 1985; 156:3–14.

12. Shapiro R: *Myelography.* St Louis, Mosby-Year Book, Inc, 1984, pp 497–539.

13. Taylor S: CT of the normal and abnormal spine, in Latchaw RE (ed): *Computed Tomography of the Head, Neck, and Spine.* St Louis, Mosby-Year Book, Inc, 1985, pp 595–616.

14. Wynne-Davies R, Walsh WK, Gormley J: Achondroplasia and hypochondroplasia—clinical variation and spinal stenosis. *J Bone Joint Surg [Br]* 1981; 63:508–515.

20

Magnetic Resonance Imaging in Lumbar Spinal Stenosis

Charles N. Aprill, M.D.
Russell Bodin, R.T.

Magnetic resonance imaging (MRI) has emerged as an important modality for the evaluation of lumbar spine disorders. In the mid-1980s, the development of high-resolution surface coils resulted in a marked improvement in the visualization of the lumbar spine. This development made MRI a practical option for the detection of lumbar disc disease.[26] There have been few controlled prospective studies to evaluate the diagnostic efficacy of MRI.[20] However, a prospective study by Modic et al. confirmed that technically adequate MRI was equivalent to myelography and computed tomography (CT) scanning, individually or in combination, in the diagnosis of lumbar canal stenosis.[70]

MRI technology is in rapid evolution. In the last 5 to 10 years, there have been improvements in all of the basic components of MRI systems. Although the *magnets* have not changed appreciably, improved methods of protecting and shimming the magnets have resulted in greater homogenicity of magnetic fields. Methods of reducing the sound from *radiofrequency transmitters* have improved patient acceptance with resulting decreased patient motion. Continuing development of better *receiving coils* has resulted in a steady improvement in resolution. Stronger *gradient coils* allow more precise spatial localization. Improved *computer* electronics and the development of new software have maintained or improved the signal-to-noise ratio while allowing for thinner sections. Even the method of transferring the image data to film has improved, resulting in hard copies of sharper quality. As a result, any statements about the application of MRI to a specific condition will be outdated by the time they are published.

New and faster imaging techniques are emerging. These provide high contrast between the cerebrospinal fluid (CSF) and surrounding tissues in much less time than standard sequences currently employed. Postprocessing of these data result in images similar to conventional contrast myelography.[44, 45] There is no end in sight as ultrafast scanning is on the horizon.[17] Any of these techniques and techniques not yet developed may prove to be of great value in assessing the stenotic lumbar spine.

A formal explanation of MRI is beyond the scope of this chapter. There are adequate texts detailing the imaging process[15] and its specific application to the spine.[68] However, some background information is required for the clinician to make sense of the image data.

"T-ING OFF"

The use of the letter T as it pertains to MRI is often a source of confusion. Magnetic field strength is measured in units of T (tesla). This particular unit was adopted in 1956, the centennial of Nikola Tesla's birth.[51] Systems in clinical use operate at low-(0.1–0.3 T), mid-(0.4–0.6 T), or high-(0.7–1.5 T) field strength. There are advantages and disadvantages to each. Adequate evaluation of the lumbar spine can be accomplished with mid- or high-field strength systems.[52]

In the clinical MRI situation, protons (hydrogen nuclei) are being excited by radiofrequency pulses. In any given tissue, there are both physical and chemical relationships at the nuclear level which govern how the protons will respond. Excited protons return to the equilibrium state by a process called relaxation. For each tissue, there are definable, independent relaxation time constants. T1 is the longitudinal and T2 the transverse relaxation time. The MRI signal, basic for image formation, is dependent on the T1 and T2 characteristics of tissues in the survey area. Other factors, such as the number of protons (proton density) and the relative position (static or flowing) of protons, influence the image.[13] To assess the T1 and T2 characteristics of tissues, a variety of imaging techniques are available. Spin echo (SE) pulse sequences are probably the most commonly employed in clinical practice. A series of radiofrequency pulses are generated at various time intervals. The SE sequence is defined by the TR (time to repetition of radiofrequency pulse) and TE (time to the echo). By using various TR-TE combinations, the relative contributions of T1 and T2 may be assessed as contrast on the resulting images.[12]

Many of the images in this chapter were acquired on a system operating at 0.6 T. The T1-weighted images were generated employing SE pulse sequences with short TR (400–800 ms) and short TE (20–40 ms).

IMAGING PROTOCOLS

Modern MRI is complex. Published strategies[55] and protocols[47] for imaging of the lumbar spine agree that the use of high-resolution surface coils is mandatory. The acquisition of data with T1 and T2 contrast is recommended and, as a general rule, section thickness should be kept in the range of 4 to 5 mm. Imaging in the sagittal and axial planes is standard.

The routine use of inversion recovery (IR), gradient echo (GE),[106] and more exotic sequences, as well as imaging in coronal or oblique planes, remain moot issues. The development of multiangle, variable interval scanning techniques[86] has tempted some

to return to a shortened "gap" technique for axial imaging. Efforts to reduce scan time may be motivated by the desire to limit patient motion and the need to maintain high throughput. Tailoring the scan technique to a specific clinical situation is ideal[69]; however the nature and specific relationships of discoverable pathologic changes cannot be known *a priori* in most instances.

At present, there really is no consensus standard as to what constitutes an adequate MRI examination of the lumbar spine. The number and type of pulse sequences, number of imaging planes, and number of sections for planes, as well as thickness of sections, are all arbitrary within certain limits. Decisions regarding parameters are based on patient tolerance and the available time for scanning. These are determined in part by the skill, interest, and philosophy of the technical staff and imaging physicians at each scanning facility. Demands on systems for large numbers of studies may necessitate fixed time allotments and concise protocols. Patient condition and ability to cooperate directly affect the time required for scanning and resultant image quality.

Motion, whatever its source, remains the primary cause of image degradation.[28] Techniques for suppression of physiologic motion, such as that associated with CSF pulsation[90] and abdominal movement and vascular pulsation[25, 35, 57, 76] are helpful in minimizing artifacts.

Voluntary or involuntary patient motion can be minimized by keeping scan times as short as possible, educating the patient on the importance of remaining still, and making the scan as comfortable as possible. However, many factors are beyond the control of the imager. An unconscious, sedated, or sleeping patient may lie still, but these patients often move inadvertently. Anxious, and psychologically or physically distressed patients may not be able to lie still for sequences requiring 5 to 15 minutes. As a result, in clinical practice, scans employing a wide variety of techniques are presented for diagnostic evaluation.

One of the authors (C.N.A.) has reviewed lumbar spine scans acquired in 1990 in which the protocol produced only 25 images (9 sagittal sections SE T1 images, 5-mm thickness; 5 sagittal gradient echo images, 7-mm thickness; and 11 axial images 5-mm thickness employing multiangle variable interval scanning techniques through the disc spaces). These studies can be obtained in approximately 30 minutes and, as such, are attractive. However, they may not be adequate for the complete evaluation of lumbar spine disorders.

SPACES AND CONTENTS

Stenosis refers to narrowing or constriction. The proper object of study in the evaluation of stenosis is available space. The space within the spinal column may be conveniently divided into a vertebral (central) and multiple intervertebral (root) canals. These canals serve as conduits for traverse of neural and vascular structures. The larger vertebral or central canal extends through the lumbar spine as a continuous longitudinal space of tubular configuration. The osteoligamentous margins are the posterior surfaces of vertebral bodies and discs, and the posterior longitudinal ligament in front, and the anterior surfaces of laminae and ligamentum flavum in back. The vertebral pedicles form an interrupted lateral margin.[24] The central canal is generally round in cross section at upper and mid-lumbar levels, becoming more triangular in configuration at lower lumbar levels. Occasionally, an exaggerated triangular trefoil configuration is seen at the lower levels, most commonly at L5.[30] The dominant contents of the central canal are the thecal sac, the internal vertebral venous plexus, and varying amounts of epidural fat. The thecal sac is generally seen as round in cross section. Its posterolateral margins lie in close proximity to the laminae and ligamentum flavum. Its anterior margin approximates the middle of the vertebral bodies and intervertebral discs. The anterior thecal sac is in intimate contact with the posterior longitudinal ligament in the midline. Commonly, a membrane between the two (plica medianus dorsalis) divides the anterior epidural space into left and right compartments.[46, 62] The most prominent components of the internal venous plexus are the paired anterior internal vertebral veins. These veins course in the longitudinal axis of the lumbar spine and lie in the anterolateral aspect of the epidural space.[5] The space surrounding the neural and vascular structures is filled with fat. Prominent accumulations regularly occur in the midline posterior to the thecal sac and in the anterolateral aspects of the epidural space.

Between the pedicles, the lateral wall of the central canal is deficient. Paired lateral fenestrations occur at each segment. These intervertebral canals or foramina are known by many names.[8] They have been referred to as the "radicular canals,"[104] "nerve root canals,"[10, 21] and more recently "root canals."[85] Each root canal is an osteoligamentous tunnel which may be divided into three zones: entrance zone, midzone, and exit zone.

The infundibular *entrance zone* (lateral recess) has no medial wall and is continuous with the central canal. Its lateral wall is a groove on the medial aspect of each pedicle. Anteriorly it is bounded by the back of the vertebral body, while posteriorly it is covered by the vertebral laminae and anteromedial edge of the inferior articular process that projects from the laminae. The entrance zones accommodate the dural root sleeves. These lateral extension of the thecal sac are visualized on prone and oblique myelography.[92, 98]

The tubular *midzone* (pedicle zone) is bounded above and below by the pedicles of the suprajacent and subjacent vertebrae. The anterior boundary is formed by the posterior surface of the vertebra above, the intervertebral disc, and the uppermost portion of the vertebra below. The posterior margin is formed by the capsular portion of the ligamentum flavum above and the anterior surface of the superior articular process of the vertebra below. The midzone accommodates the dorsal root ganglion and ventral roots. This space is recognizable at epidurography.[31, 59] Traversing the midzone with the neural structures are several prominent venous channels. These are true radicular veins.[38] They connect the ascending lumbar veins of the external vertebral plexus with the anterior internal vertebral veins of the internal venous plexus.

The planar *exit zone* (foramen proper) is defined by the lateral margin of the intervertebral pedicle. This hiatus has been compared to "a doorway at the end of a passage."[22]

For descriptive purposes, the margins of the various spaces will be defined in the coronal plane as depicted in Figure 20–1. The lateral margin of the central canal corresponds to the lateral border of the thecal sac between the dural root sleeves. This correlates generally with the position of the main trunks of the anterior internal vertebral veins. The midzone of the root canals is defined by the medial and lateral margins of the vertebral pedicles. The entrance zone of the root canals is the area between the central canal and the midzone. The exit zone of the root canals is defined by the lateral margin of the pedicles.

THE CONTAINER

The vertebral bodies, their posterior arches, and the soft tissue linkages at each motion segment form

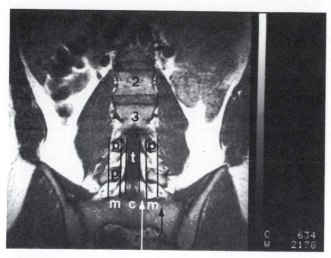

FIG 20–1.
Coronal section of the lumbar spine. Image demonstrates the central and root canals at the level of the L4–5 and L5–S1 segments in the coronal plane. The limits of the central canal *(c)* may be defined by the lateral margin of the thecal sac. The limits of the *midzone* of the root canal *(m)* are defined by the medial and lateral margins of the vertebral pedicle *(p)*. The space between these two zones *(white arrow)* is the *entrance zone* of the root canal. The *exit zone* is defined by the lateral margin of the pedicles. The space immediately lateral to the *exit zone (black arrow)* is referred to as extraforaminal.

the boundaries of the central and root canals. As such, they may be thought of as the walls of a container. The sectional anatomy of the lumbar spine as defined by cryoplaning techniques has been described by Rauschning.[84] The sectional anatomy as defined by MRI in three planes has been detailed in atlas form.[1] The structural elements of the lumbar spine are particularly well suited to MRI employing SE T1-weighted pulse sequences.

The cortical bone of vertebral bodies, laminae, and articular processes produces very little signal and therefore appears dark or black. Ligamentous tissues such as the outer annulus and longitudinal ligaments also produce little signal. At bony-ligamentous interfaces, the ability to discriminate bone and soft tissue may be lost. The marrow space displays a mottled intermediate signal owing to its mix of cancellous bone, marrow elements, and varying amounts of fat.

The epidural and perineural spaces are filled with fat which displays high signal intensity. Against this background, the neural and vascular structures with their intermediate signal intensities are conspicuous.

The CSF in the thecal sac is seen as intermediate to low signal intensity, appearing relatively gray. Contained intrathecal rootlets and the most prominent extrathecal neural structures, the dorsal root ganglia, display intermediate signal intensity slightly brighter than the CSF.

Vascular structures in the epidural and perineural spaces vary in signal intensity depending on their size, and the direction and speed of blood flow within the vessels. For the most part, unenhanced veins have intermediate signal, similar or slightly lower than neural tissues.

SAGITTAL PLANE

Sagittal images should extend from one margin of the vertebral column to the other so as to include the full width of the root canals. A minimum of 9 images at 5-mm section thickness (assuming a 20%, 1-mm interslice gap) is required to cover this area. If thinner sections are employed, the number necessary to cover the distance increases, i.e., 11 images at 4 mm, 15 images at 3 mm. Midline sagittal sections (Fig 20–2) demonstrate the largest anteroposte-

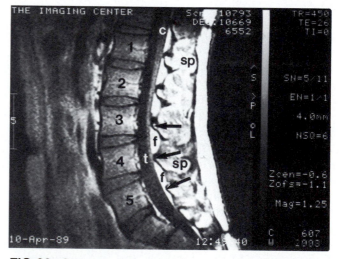

FIG 20–2.
Sagittal MRI SE T1, 4-mm thickness. The midline section is defined by the spinous processes *(sp)*. Accumulations of fat *(f)* are interposed between the bases of the processes posterior to the thecal sac *(t)*. Small amounts of fat and numerous epidural vessels can be seen in the anterior epidural space between the vertebral bodies and thecal sac. The conus medullaris *(c)* terminates near the thoracolumbar junction. The midline sagittal diameter of the central canal is determined by the distance from the posterior vertebral body to the base of the spinous processes *(arrows)*.

rior dimension of the central canal. The posterior vertebral margins are slightly scalloped producing a shallow concavity which is filled by epidural fat and elements of the anterior epidural venous plexus. The disc margins project just beyond the adjacent vertebral end plates. This is the normal appearance of the intervertebral disc and does not represent a pathologic "bulge." The normal intervertebral disc is larger than the adjacent vertebral end plates.

The bases of the spinous processes form the posterior bony limits of the central canal. Accumulations of fat are almost constantly present interposed between these processes. The fat is compliant, but can act as a mass deforming the thecal sac in some instances.[48]

The spinal cord terminates at the focal enlargement of the conus medullaris. This termination is at or near the thoracolumbar junction. The position may vary slightly in normal individuals. It is often difficult to distinguish the conus from the proximal cauda equina. This junctional area should be visualized on all MRI scans of the lumbar spine.

Sections just medial to the pedicle (Fig 20–3) demonstrate the entrance zone of the root canal. The discovertebral margins are a particularly important area, as disc protrusion or bony ridge formation compromising the space lie in this region. The low-signal-intensity ligamentum flavum extends from the anterior surface of the superior lamina to the su-

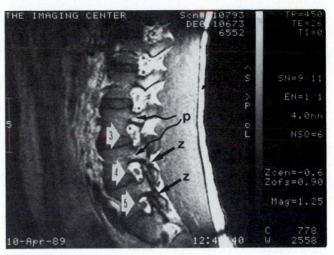

FIG 20–4.
Sagittal MRI SE T1, 4-mm thickness. Parasagittal section through the vertebral pedicles. Section defines the *midzone* of the root canals. Epidural fat fills the canal surrounding the segmental neural elements and associated radicular vessels (*3, 4, 5 white arrows*). The prominent structure in the *midzone* is the dorsal root ganglion of each segmental nerve. The smaller structures commonly seen in the intervertebral canal represent radicular veins. The posterior wall of the canal is formed by the facet joint complex (*z arrows*). The superior and inferior margins are formed by the pedicles (*p*) of the vertebrae above and below. The inverted teardrop configuration of the root canal is appreciated in the sagittal plane.

perior tip of the lamina below. The space is occupied by the segmental dural root sleeves. Each sleeve contains CSF, and the dorsal and ventral rootlets which will form the segmental nerve. These neural elements are seen as discrete structures of intermediate signal intensity within the bright epidural fat.

Sections through the vertebral pedicle (Fig 20–4) demonstrate the midzone of the root canal. The configuration of the root canal on sagittal images is that of an inverted teardrop. There is ample perineural fat surrounding the neural and vascular elements within this canal. The size and shape of the canal are not fixed. Changes occur in both flexion and extension. The overall area is reduced in extension and rotation of the motion segment.[34, 102]

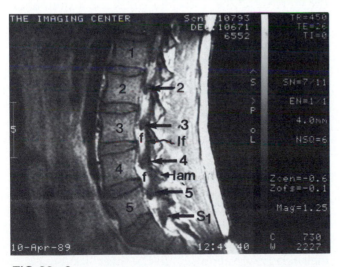

FIG 20–3.
Sagittal MRI SE T1, 4-mm thickness. Parasagittal section just medial to the spinous pedicle. This section defines the *entrance zone* of the root canals. Epidural fat (*f*) is interposed between the segmental dural root sleeves (*2, 3, 4, 5, S₁ arrows*). The *entrance zone* is bounded by the vertebral body and intervertebral disc anteriorly and the lamina (*lam*) and ligamentum flavum (*lf*) posteriorly.

AXIAL PLANE

Axial sections should be sequential to include all of the spine in the survey area. Studies with sections

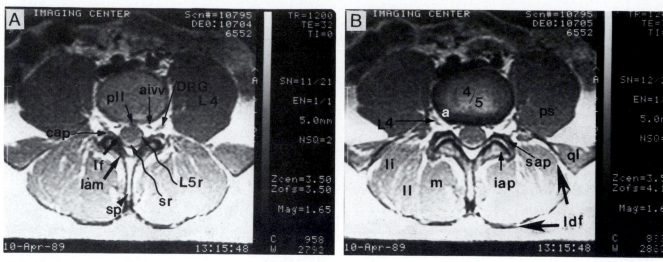

FIG 20−5.
Axial MRI SE T1, 5-mm section thickness. **A,** section through the lower body and inferior end plate of L4. The central portion of the posterior longitudinal ligament *(p11)* is seen in the midline between the vertebral body and the anterior margin of the thecal sac. The anterior internal vertebral veins *(aivv)* lie in the anterolateral aspect of the central canal. The dorsal root ganglion *(DRG)* of L4 is seen in the *midzone* of the root canal. The ganglion occupies the upper third of the canal. The superior capsular ligament *(cap)* of the L4−5 facet joint is the lateral extension of the ligamentum flavum *(lf)*. The L4 laminae *(lam)* join at the base of the spinous process *(sp)*. The isolated intrathecal rootlets of L5 *(L5r)* are seen at the anterolateral margin of the thecal sac. The sacral rootlets *(sr)* of the cauda equina lie near its dorsal margin. **B,** section through the L4−5 intervertebral disc *(4/5)*. The anterior ramus of L4 *(L4)* is usually separated from the posterolateral disc annulus *(a)* by a strip of epidural fat. *iap* = inferior articular process of L4; *sap* = superior articular process of L5. Note the symmetric size and orientation of articular processes. The psoas *(ps)* and quadratus lumborum *(ql)* muscles lie anterior to the deep layer of lumbodorsal fascia *(ldf)*. The lumbar iliocostalis *(li)*, longissimus *(ll)*, and multifidus *(m)* muscles are invested by the superficial and deep layers of the lumbodorsal fascia.

limited to the disc spaces do not properly address the central canal at the level of the pedicle and result in incomplete assessment of posterior arch structures.

The use of longer repetition times (TR 1,000–1,200 ms) allows a sufficient number of images at 4-mm section thickness to survey the lower three lumbar motion segments in the transverse plane.

Sections through the lower vertebral body and end plate and intervertebral disc (Fig 20−5A,B) demonstrate the central canal and both root canals of a given segment. The vertebral and disc margins should be smooth and regular. The posterior arch is continuous across the back of the canals. The relative size and orientation of articular processes is best demonstrated in this plane of view. Pathologic changes arising from the vertebral end plates, disc, or facet joints,[3, 6] and adversely affecting either the central or root canals, are readily recognized on the axial sections. Several sequential sections are required to evaluate a root canal fully.

The size and configuration of the central canal are best demonstrated on axial sections through the midbody (Fig 20−6,A). At the midbody-midpedicle level, the osteoligamentous margins of the central

canal are complete. Developmental and acquired abnormalities of the spine which alter the size or shape of the central canal are easily appreciated (see Fig 20−6,A). The L5−S1 segment has anatomic features which differentiate it from the other motion segments in the lumbar spine, prompting Rauschning to refer to this as the "totaliter aliter L5/S1 segment."[85] The pedicles are larger and the ligamentous support more extensive than at other levels.[61] The root canals are longer.[46] As a result, more sections must be reviewed to understand the relationships of the dorsal ganglia, radicular vessels, and structural elements (Fig 20−6B,C,D).

The intrathecal rootlets are organized in a very definable pattern.[105] Segmental elements can often be identified at the lower lumbar levels based on their relative position within the thecal sac.

CORONAL PLANE

Posterior coronal images provide information about paraspinous muscles and posterior elements

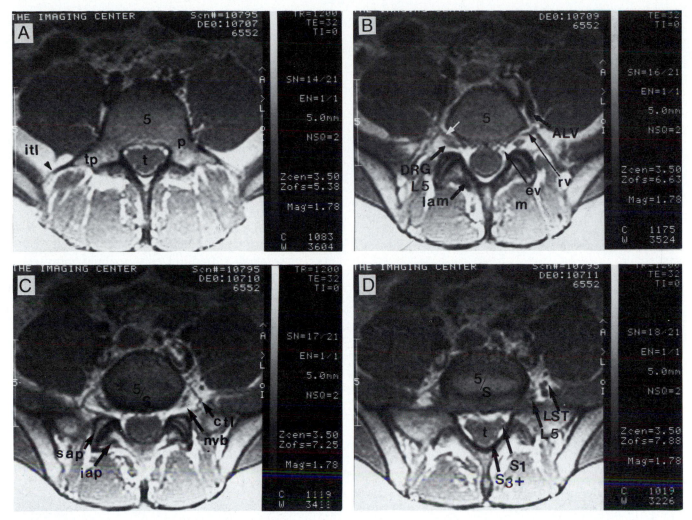

FIG 20–6.
Axial MRI SE T1, 5-mm thickness. **A,** section through the midbody of L5. Stout pedicles *(p)* and thick, short transverse processes *(tp)* characterize the lowest lumbar vertebra. The ileotransverse ligament *(itl)* is prominent and stabilizes this segment. *t* = thecal sac. **B,** section through the upper one-half L5–S1 root canal, and the lower body–posteroinferior end plate of L5. The epidural venous plexus *(ev)* communicates with the ascending lumbar vein *(ALV)* of the external plexus by way of radicular veins *(rv)* at each segment. At times, the dorsal ganglia *(DRG)* and radicular veins *(white arrow)* lie in juxtaposition, as seen on the right, simulating enlargement of the ganglion. *lam* = lamina; *m* = multifidus muscle. **C,** section through the lower half of the L5–S1 root canal. The canal is bounded in front by the posterolateral disc annulus and in back by the L5–S1 facet joint complex *(iap L4, sap L5).* Note the articular surfaces and articular cartilage of the facet joints. The neurovascular bundle *(nvb)* includes the anterior ramus of L5 and its accompanying radicular veins. In the distal root canal, these structures lie in close proximity to the corporotransverse ligament *(ctl).* This is one of the unique features of the L5–S1 motion segment. **D,** section through the upper sacral canal. The thecal sac *(t)* is completely surrounded by bone. The intrathecal rootlets of S1 can be identified within the S1 dural root sleeve *(S₁).* A conglomerate of lower sacral rootlets *(S₃₊)* can be identified more posteriorly. In this image, the interposed S2 rootlets are recognizable. The anterior ramus of L5 *(L5)* is extraforaminal at this level. Elements of the lumbosacral trunk *(LST)* and associated vessel lie anterior to the sacral ala and medial to the iliopsoas musculature.

(Fig 20–7). More anterior coronal sections demonstrate the root canals. The oblique course of the segmental neural elements and the position of the dorsal ganglion[19] are nicely displayed in this plane of view (Fig 20–8,A). The special relationships of the L5 segmental nerve to its long osteoligamentous tunnel are particularly well shown (Fig 20–8,B). A major advantage of MRI over CT scanning is the ability to directly acquire data in any plane. Coronal imaging was useful in planning acquisition in spine deformities (Fig 20–9).[4]

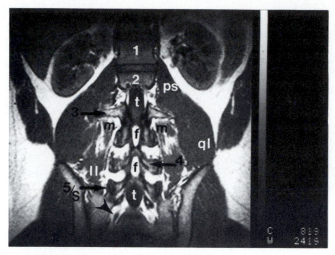

FIG 20–7.
Coronal MRI SE T1, 4-mm thickness. Section through posterior elements of the midlumbar spine. The L1 and upper L2 vertebral bodies are demonstrated. The right transverse process of L3 is usually the largest in the lumbar spine. The laminae (L4) curve upward to meet at the base of the spinous process. The L5–S1 facet joint is labeled *(5/S)*. The joints at all three motion segments are visualized. The thecal sac *(t)* is identified at both the upper and lower ends of the lumbar spine. Because of the lumbar lordosis, fat *(f)* in the posterior epidural space is interposed. The dorsal ganglion of S1 *(arrowhead)* can be identified in the mid-S1 root canal. Psoas *(ps)*, quadratus lumborum *(ql)*, lumbar longissimus *(ll)*, and multifidus *(m)* muscles can all be recognized on coronal sections through the posterior elements.

ADDITIONAL SEQUENCES

A variety of tissues are available for imaging in the lumbar spine. Routine examination should include SE T2-weighted images. The T2-weighted image is quite sensitive to the relative hydration of the intervertebral disc[67] (Fig 20–10,A). By employing a multiecho technique, additional "proton density" images are generated during the same acquisition. The SE proton density images are useful in the evaluation of articular cartilage and ligamentous structures.[43] In our practice, routine lumbar survey also includes sagittal GE images. Acquisition time is less than SE T2 images. The resulting "myelogram effect" may make extradural abnormalities more conspicuous (Fig 20–11A,B,C). This technique has other advantages, including fat suppression for evaluation of marrow space abnormalities.[11, 106]

A complete lumbar survey consists of SE T1 sequences in the sagittal, axial, and coronal planes and supplementary sagittal SE proton density, SE T2-weighted, and GE sequences. Such a series requires 70 to 80 images of 4- to 5-mm section thickness. This is adequate for imaging most lumbar disorders and requires 45 to 90 minutes of acquisition time. Special conditions may warrant additional sections employing different and perhaps specific parameters (plane of imaging, pulse sequence, section thickness, con-

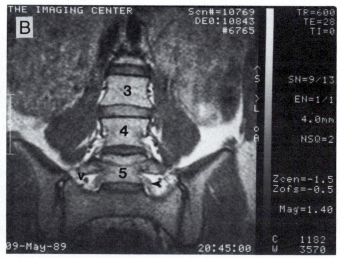

FIG 20–8.
Coronal MRI SE T1, 4-mm sections. **A,** section through the "midzone" of root canals at lower two motion segments. The oblique course of segmental neural elements is graphically demonstrated in the coronal plane. Note the position of the dorsal ganglia *(arrowheads)* of the right L4 and L5 nerve, beneath the pedicles. The dural root sleeve of the left L5 nerve traverses the entrance zone *(arrow)* just medial to the pedicle. An ample amount of perineural fat surrounds the neural elements. **B,** section just anterior to **A.** The left L5 dorsal ganglion and nerve *(arrowhead)* traverse a long root canal as they course anteriorly and inferiorly over the sacral ala. The nerve lies below the large pedicle and transverse process of L5. It is immediately lateral to the inferior L5 end plate and posterolateral-lateral margin of the L5–S1 disc. In this long canal, the nerve is susceptible to compression at a number of points. Note the large vein *(v)* lying adjacent to the right L5 nerve.

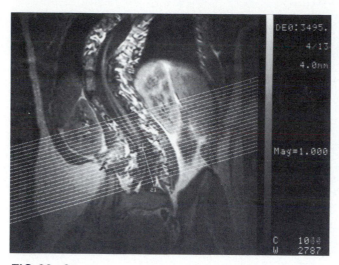

FIG 20–9.
Coronal MRI SE T1, 4-mm thickness. Midcoronal section for localization. A 20-year-old woman with moderately severe dorsal dextroscoliosis secondary to diastematomyelia. Localizer lines are for planning the plane of acquisition (oblique transverse).

trast enhancement, etc.). Clinical circumstances may dictate deletion of some of the basic sequences.

STENOSIS

Classification of stenosis has been discussed (see Chapter 2). Spinal stenosis is the result of a variety of pathologic processes. It is seen throughout life, oc-

curring as a congenital phenomenon and in association with the final stages of spinal maturation.

Severe congenital stenosis is known to occur in certain genetic conditions with hereditary transmission. Achondroplasia is the paradigm of this type of stenosis. Defective bone formation occurs at the growth plate of long bones resulting in reduced length. In the vertebral column, the defect in bone formation occurs at the pedicles resulting in abnormally short and thickened pedicles. The result is markedly reduced sagittal and transverse diameters of the central canal and contraction of the root canal.[78]

Severe narrowing of the central and root canals occurs as a result of advanced spondylosis and the associated osteoarthritis of the facet joints in the elderly. The pathoanatomy of spondylotic stenosis has been the subject of several anatomic studies.[21, 56, 94] MRI can demonstrate the degenerative changes associated with advanced spondylosis. Loss of nuclear signal on SE T2-weighted images reflects degradation of the nucleus.[67] Alteration of marrow space signal is associated with chronic disc degeneration.[71] Sagittal sections document the loss of disc height, formation of osteophytic ridges, subluxation, hyperostosis, and hypertrophy of articular processes, and resulting compromise of available space (Fig 20–12).

The central canal may be small by development without obvious associated disease. Both genetic[81] and environmental[18] factors have been implicated. In the developmentally small central canal, there is associated reduction in the size of the root canals.[79] Although not primarily symptomatic, small size of spinal spaces is of significance as it predisposes to symptomatology with lesser degrees of pathologic

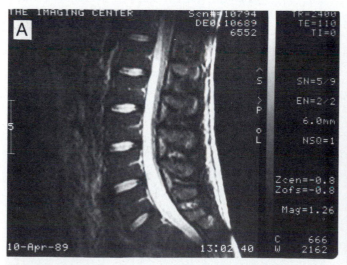

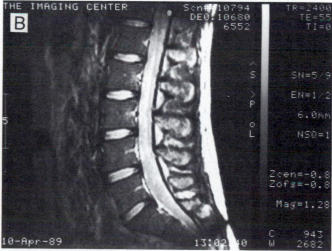

FIG 20–10.
Sagittal MRI SE multiecho sequence. **A,** midsagittal section T2-weighted (TR 2,400 ms, TE 110 ms). **B,** sagittal midline section proton density image (TR 2,400 ms, TE 55 ms).

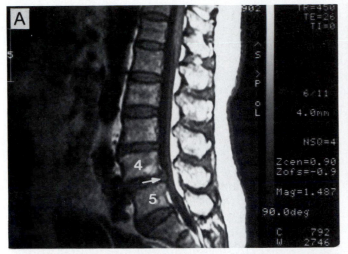

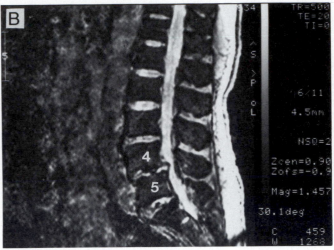

FIG 20–11.

A 72-year-old woman with back pain and left lower extremity pain, weakness, and altered sensation. **A,** sagittal MRI SE T1, 4-mm thickness. Midline section. Moderate-sized disc herniation (prolapse) at L4–5 *(arrow)*. **B,** sagittal MRI gradient echo, 4.5-mm thickness. Midline section. Bright signal from CSF and intervertebral disc renders L4–5 disc prolapse and resulting pathologic impression on thecal sac more conspicuous. **C,** axial MRI SE T1, 5-mm thickness. Section through L4–5 interspace. Disc prolapse *(thick white arrow)* projects into central canal deforming the thecal sac. The lesion is more prominent to the left of the midline obliterating the epidural fat in the left anterior epidural space. Note the normal complement of fat posterior to the thecal sac. Moderately advanced facet joint arthropathy bilaterally is characterized by hypertrophy and sclerosis *(black arrows)*.

derangement.[56] Anatomic studies to determine the dimensions of the "normal canal" have concentrated on the midsagittal diameter.[29, 50] It is generally accepted that a midsagittal diameter in excess of 12.5 mm is normal. Diameters of less than 12 mm are pathologic. Verbiest has further classified the patho-

logically small canal into "relative narrowing" in which the midsagittal diameters range from 10 to 12 mm, and "absolute narrowing" in which the midsagittal diameter is less than 10 mm.[103] Properly performed CT scanning provides very accurate measurements of the midsagittal diameter of the central

FIG 20–12.

Sagittal MRI SE T1, 4-mm thickness. Parasagittal section just medial to the pedicle. Section is through the entrance zone of the L4–5 and L5–S1 root canals. Advanced spondylotic pathologic changes at L4–5. The disc space is markedly narrowed and fat has infiltrated the subchondral marrow space of adjacent vertebrae *(bright signal)*. Osteophytic ridges project from the end plates *(short arrow)*. Collapse of the disc space has resulted in upward subluxation of the L5 superior articular process *(long arrow)*. The tip of the process lies just below the dorsal ganglion of L4. Similar changes, though less advanced, are occurring at L5–S1.

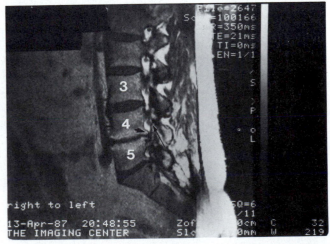

canal.[33, 58] As such, the axial CT scan has been considered the gold standard for evaluation of the size of the central canal. Improvement in the quality of axial MRI, however, threatens the primacy of CT in this regard (Fig 20–13).

Experimental studies on human cadavers have shown that the minimal space required for the cauda equina and thecal sac at the L3 level is 77 ± 13 mm^2. This represents approximately 45% of the normal cross-sectional area of the thecal sac at the L3 level. This appears to be a critical size, as further constriction of the thecal sac results in a marked increase in pressure among the nerve roots of the cauda equina.[95, 97] This value correlates well with the cross-sectional area of the thecal sac as determined by CT scanning in patients with symptoms of spinal stenosis.[9, 96]

POSTERIOR ARCH

Pathologic changes in the ligamentum flavum can produce severe thecal compression (Fig 20–14).[100] The ligamentum flavum differs from the anterior and posterior longitudinal ligaments and the disc annulus. It is composed of a disproportionately large amount of elastic tissue by comparison with other spinal ligaments. This may account for the shortening and thickening of the ligamentum flavum in certain conditions.[83] The anterior and posterior longitudinal ligaments as well as the outer annulus contain a higher content of type I collagen. This difference in tissue characteristics may account for the higher signal intensity noted on MRI of the ligamentum flavum.[43]

The multiplanar (orthogonal) capabilities of MRI make it ideal for evaluating the lumbar facet joints.[60] A variety of pathologic conditions involving the facet joints may adversely affect the central and root canal. Overgrowth of degenerative facet joints resulting in radicular symptoms was described 30 years ago.[32] Alterations in the configuration of the root canal by hypertrophied and hyperostotic articular processes are nicely demonstrated in the sagittal plane (Fig 20–15). The size of the root canal varies depending on posture. The area of the canal is smallest in extension.[75] Anatomic studies[102] and dy-

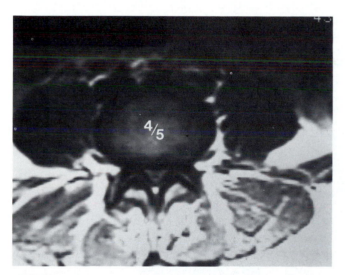

FIG 20–13.
Axial MRI SE T1, 5-mm thickness. Section through L4–5 disc. "Idiopathic" stenosis in a 25-year-old woman being evaluated for nonspecific low back pain following a minor injury. Disc contour is normal. The size of the articular processes is not unusual. The ligamentum flavum is not thickened. A small collection of fat is identified in the posterior epidural space. The central canal is extremely small. The thecal sac is markedly contracted and triangular in configuration. Elements of the distal cauda equina are seen as focal areas of intermediate signal at the periphery of the thecal sac. There is a minimal amount of CSF seen as a zone of low signal (dark) in the center of the thecal sac.

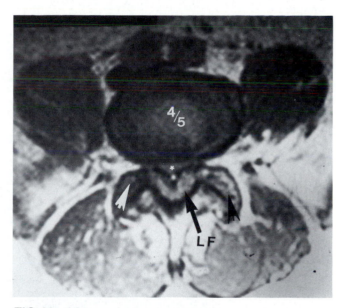

FIG 20–14.
Axial MRI SE T1, 5-mm thickness. Section through the L4–5 motion segment. Severe central stenosis is secondary to massive hypertrophy of the ligamentum flavum (black arrow LF). Note the relatively bright signal intensity of the ligamentum flavum compared with the outer annulus of the intervertebral disc. The thecal sac (*) is markedly compressed. There is underlying pathologic change of both facet joints. Low signal reflects sclerosis of the superior articular process of L5 on the right (white arrowhead). There is irregular "pitting" of the articular surface of the superior articular process of L5 on the left (black arrowhead).

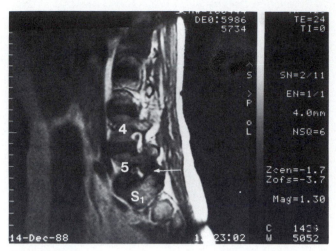

FIG 20-15.
Sagittal MRI SE T1, 4-mm thickness. Section through mid-zone of right-sided root canals. Note the normal size and configuration of the L4−5 root canal with ample perineural fat. The dorsal ganglion of L4 is unremarkable. Contrast with the L5−S1 root canal. The smaller amount of fat reflects reduction in available space. The L5 dorsal ganglion can be identified and is not obviously compressed. Articular processes of L5−S1 (arrow) are enlarged. Low signal from the articular processes reflects bony sclerosis. Isolated enlargement of the posterior joint complex results in lateral stenosis.

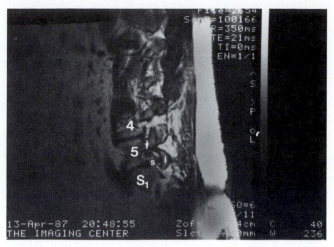

FIG 20-16.
Sagittal MRI SE T1, 4-mm thickness. Section through mid- and exit zones of L5−S1 root canal. There is marked narrowing of the L4−5 and L5−S1 disc spaces. Despite the narrowing, the L4−5 root canal is not compromised. Note the relative position of the inferior articular process of L5 (i) and the superior articular process of S1 (s). The superior subluxation of the S1 process impinges on the L5 dorsal ganglion (arrow). Subluxation without degenerative change of the articular processes has resulted in lateral stenosis.

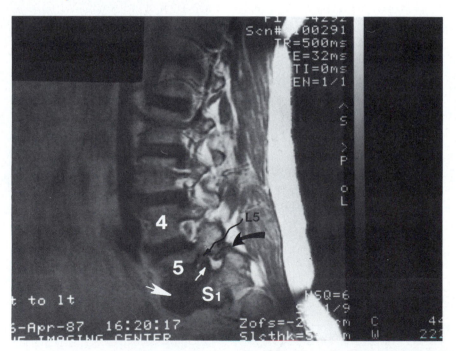

FIG 20-17.
Sagittal MRI SE T1, 4-mm thickness. Section through the midzone of the root canal. A 54-year-old man with lytic-type spondylolysis of the L5 pars interarticularis (curved black arrow). Note severe degeneration of the intervertebral disc with marked narrowing of the interspace and large anterior spondylophytic ridge (large white arrow). A smaller ridge has formed on the posterolateral aspect of the inferior L5 end plate (small white arrow). Vertical narrowing of the radicular canal is the result of deformity associated with spondylolysis. Disc space narrowing has further reduced the height of the root canal. The two factors acting in concert markedly compromise the space available in the midzone. The L5 dorsal ganglion (wavy black arrow) is deformed.

namic CT-myelogram studies[77] demonstrate impingement of neural elements by hypertrophied articular structures during extension or torsion of the spine. The dorsal ganglion is extremely sensitive to mechanical pressure.[49] Studies suggest the dorsal root ganglion plays an important role in the mediation of low back pain.[107] MRI can demonstrate subluxation of the superior articular process (Fig 20–16). The development of dynamic MRI techniques may allow a more definitive noninvasive method of evaluating dynamic stenosis.

Lytic spondylolysis and associated spondylolisthesis is a relatively common lesion but is an uncommon source of symptomatic neural compression.[27] MRI accurately depicts the defect in the pars interarticularis.[53] Neural tissues do not slide during motion of the spine but rather adapt by passive deformation.[14] Additional compressive force from a second

lesion may be sufficient to result in generation of symptoms (Fig 20–17).

It is not only the magnitude but the rate and direction of pressure that determines changes in nerve structure and function.[91] Imaging in multiple planes may be necessary to define the minimal compression sufficient to account for the symptoms (Fig 20–18).[40]

DEGENERATIVE SPONDYLOLISTHESIS

As an entity, degenerative spondylolisthesis[64] warrants special consideration. This lesion is a common cause of symptomatic spinal stenosis. The pathoanatomy involves both the anterior and poste-

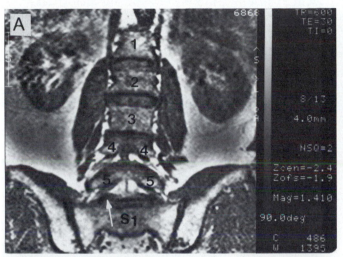

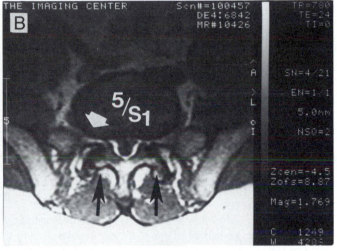

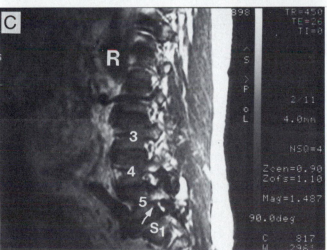

FIG 20–18.
A 67-year-old man presented with back and leg pain, weakness, and altered sensation in the lower extremities, greater on the left than on the right. **A,** coronal MRI SE T1, 5-mm thickness. Section through the midzone of the L4–5 and L5–S1 root canal. Disc degeneration with narrowing of the interspace results in approximation of the pedicles. Focal degenerative bulge (protrusion) *(arrow)* further compromises the available space for the right L5 segmental nerve. Coronal sections suggest a mid to upper lumbar list to the left. **B,** axial MRI SE T1, 5-mm thickness. Section through the L5–S1 interspace showing bilateral L5–S1 facet joint arthropathy *(black arrows).* There is narrowing of the joint spaces, sclerosis of the articular surfaces, and forward subluxation of the inferior articular processes of L5. The disc annulus bulges around its circumference with slight focal prominence (protrusion) at the right posterolateral margin *(white arrow).* **C,** sagittal MRI SE T1, 4-mm thickness. Parasagittal section through the midzone of the root canal. The disc annulus protrudes slightly, entrapping the L5 nerve beneath the pedicle *(arrow).* There is ample fat in the posterior aspect of the root canal. The nerve is fixed in this anterior position by transforaminal ligaments (Grab).

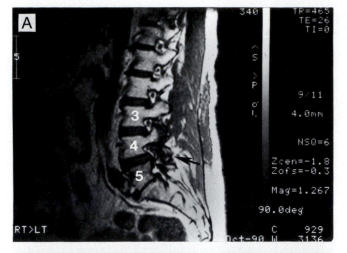

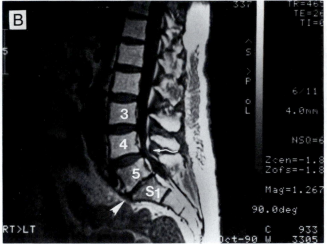

FIG 20–19.

A 65-year-old man presented with back and bilateral leg pain and altered sensation in the lower extremities. **A,** sagittal MR SE T1, 4-mm thickness. Section through the midzone of the root canals. There is marked arthropathy of the L4–5 facet joint complex. Hypertrophy of the superior articular process of L5 and the capsular ligament of the L4–5 joint *(arrow)* act in concert to narrow the root canal at the midzone. Space for neural and vascular elements is reduced significantly when compared with adjacent normal levels. **B,** sagittal MR SE T1, 4-mm thickness. Midsagittal section shows isolated disc resorption at L5–S1 *(arrowhead)*, slight forward slip of L4 on L5 (mild olisthesis), and slight posterior annular bulge (protrusion) of the L4–5 disc. Focal central canal narrowing and the thecal deformity are secondary to the mass effect of the intact posterior arch *(wavy white arrow)*. Compression is due to the forward displacement of laminae and ligamentum flavum in this case of degenerative spondylolisthesis.

rior column, results in central and lateral stenosis, and requires understanding of the biomechanics of instability.

Problems related to symptomatic degenerative spondylolisthesis generally occur in subjects over 50 years of age. The lesion predominates in women and usually occurs at the L4–5 motion segment. There are a number of predisposing factors.

Anatomic studies on skeletons of subjects over 40 years of age consistently revealed deterioration of the interspinous ligaments between L4 and L5.[87] Clinical-radiologic studies of patients with degenerative spondylolisthesis have documented a peculiar alignment of the articular processes at L4–5.[93] These combined factors render the L4–5 segment vulnerable to shear forces in the z-axis.

Conditions which favor increased stability at L5–S1 induce greater stresses across the L4–5 segment. These include developmental factors such as sacralization of L5[88] or a deep-seated L5 vertebra with large transverse processes,[63] and acquired conditions such as disc space narrowing at L5–S1 secondary to isolated disc resorption or prior surgery.[36]

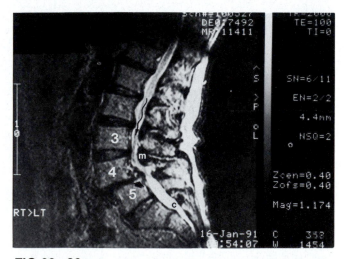

FIG 20–20.

Sagittal MRI SE T2, 4.4-mm thickness. Midsagittal section. A 69-year-old woman presented with moderately severe back pain, bilateral leg pain, weakness, and altered sensation. There was grade II spondylolisthesis with a forward shift of L4 on L5 and marked degeneration and disc space narrowing at the L4–5 disc. The central canal is severely narrowed. The thecal sac is compressed between the intact posterior arch of L4 *(m)* and the posterosuperior margin of the L5 vertebral body *(thick black arrow)*. The severity of the stenosis may be indicated by the absence of CSF pulsation artifact below the stenotic site. The CSF in the lower lumbar cistern *(c)* is bright with no obvious pulsation artifact. Contrast this with the motion artifacts in the CSF column above the level of the stenosis *(wavy arrow)*.

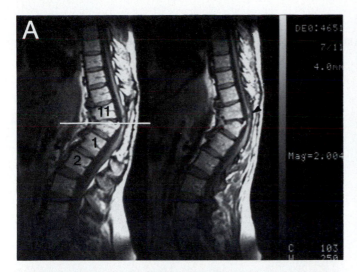

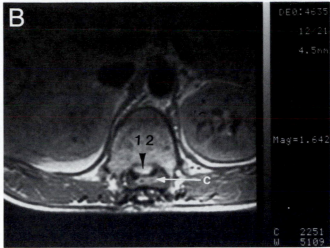

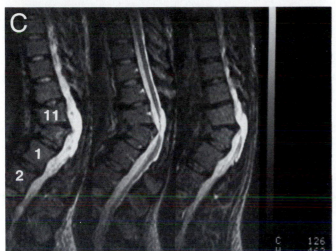

FIG 20–21.
A 30-year-old woman 10 years post–thoracolumbar burst fracture and posterior decompression. **A,** sagittal MR SE T1, 4-mm thickness. Section through the central spinal canal. Anterior wedge compression fracture of T12 results in gibbus deformity. There is "retropulsion" of the posterosuperior corner of T12 into the central canal. Small cysts have developed within the distal cord *(arrowhead)*. The *white line* denotes plane of section **(B)**. **B,** axial MR SE T1, 4.5-mm thickness. Section through the upper third of the T12 vertebral body. Retropulsed bone fragment *(arrowhead)* projects into the central canal. The posterior arch has been previously resected (original decompression). The spinal cord *(c, white arrow)* is seen as a flattened oval structure of intermediate signal. Small zones of low signal represent cystic cavities within the cord substance. **C,** sagittal SE T2, 4.5-mm thickness, motion suppression technique. T2 contrast graphically demonstrates CSF column. Sections document "adequate" decompression of the posterior canal. The thoracic cord is more clearly delineated on this image sequence and the degree of focal atrophy of the cord is better appreciated.

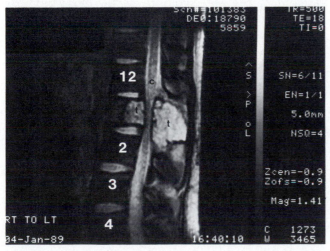

FIG 20–22.
Sagittal MRI gradient echo (GE), 5-mm thickness. Midsagittal section of a 14-year-old boy with a known aneurysmal bone cyst of the L1 vertebral body. Tumor *(t)* involves the posterior half of the L1 body and extends in a circumferential fashion to involve the entire posterior arch of L1. Expansion of the bony mass results in narrowing of the central spinal canal. c = spinal cord. Stenosis is occurring at the junction of the distal conus and proximal cauda equina. Note the absence of CSF at the site of maximum narrowing. A variety of pulse sequences were employed in this study. This GE sequence provided the best delineation of tumor margins.

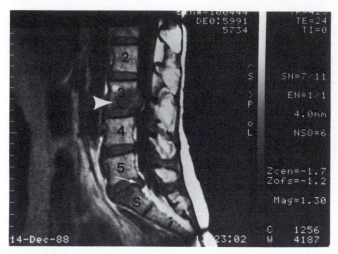

FIG 20–23.
Sagittal MRI SE T1, 4-mm thickness. Midsagittal section. A 56-year-old woman complained of severe back pain radiating into the left buttock, thigh, and leg. The L5–S1 disc is abnormal. Note herniation, specifically posteroinferior prolapse *(small white arrow)*. There is an abnormal marrow space signal from the L3 vertebral body *(large white arrowhead)*. The intermediate to low signal irregularly distributed through the posteroinferior body replaces the normal fatty marrow. Ill-defined expansion of the posterior vertebral body acts as a mass in the epidural space. Diagnosis: metastatic malignancy, primary bronchogenic carcinoma, unsuspected prior to MRI.

Thus several factors acting in concert predispose the L4–5 motion segment to this condition.

Degenerative spondylolisthesis can result in significant narrowing of both root canals and the central canal. Narrowing of the root canals is the result of osteoarthritic changes in the facet joints, resulting subluxation, and vertebral olisthesis (Fig 20–19,A). Disc degeneration with resultant narrowing and bulging (protrusion) of the disc annulus may not be significant (Fig 20–19,B).

The central canal is also narrowed by hypertrophy of the articular processes. Anterolisthesis rarely progresses beyond grade I. However, as the degree of slip increases, the central canal is severely compromised (Fig 20–20). The intact posterior arch follows the superior vertebral body as it slips forward and compresses the thecal sac against the posterior margin of the vertebral body below. CSF pulsation artifacts are common on T2-weighted images even in the lumbar spine. The absence of such artifacts below the site of constriction may be a reflection of the severity of stenosis.[89]

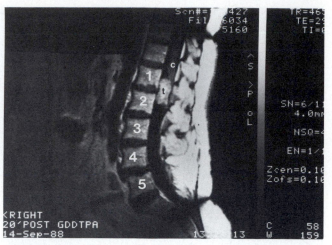

FIG 20–24.
Sagittal MR SE T1, 4-mm thickness. Midsagittal section. A 72-year-old woman presented with back pain (day and night) and progressive weakness in both lower extremities. The presumptive diagnosis: "cauda equina syndrome secondary to spinal stenosis." Image was obtained 20 minutes after intravenous injection of gadolinium DTPA (pentetic acid). The anterior vertebral column is generally well-preserved. There is no evidence of spondylosis on midline section. The sagittal diameter of the central canal is normal. A moderately large enhancing oval tumor mass *(t)* lies immediately posterior to the L1–2 interspace. This intradural-extramedullary lesion displaces the distal conus *(c)* and compresses the elements of the proximal cauda equina. Diagnosis: benign schwannoma.

NONDEGENERATIVE STENOSIS

Narrowing (stenosis) of the central and root canals may result from trauma. Compression and burst fractures are common at the thoracolumbar junction. In the acute phase, MRI is effective in localizing the lesion and defining the degree of neural compression.[7] Follow-up studies may be employed to evaluate the efficacy of surgical decompression, the presence of residual impingement by extradural mass, as well as the status of neural elements (Fig 20–21A,B,C). MRI is sensitive to the spectrum of changes occurring with progressive myelopathy from myelomalacia[82] to syrinx formation.[39]

Tumors arising in the bony elements of the spine may give rise to compressive symptoms. Benign tumors causing stenosis are rare.[64, 65] Reports of assessment of such tumors by MRI are also rare.[72, 109] MRI provides a noninvasive method of detecting the lesion, defining the extent of bone and soft tissue involvement, and assessing the degree of

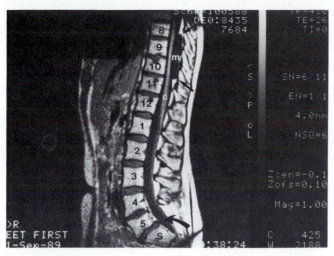

FIG 20–25.
Sagittal MR SE T1, 4-mm thickness. Midline section of a 20-year-old woman with known lytic-type spondylolysis of L5 with first-degree spondylolisthesis. She had chronic back pain, weakness, and altered sensation in both lower extremities. There was a previous workup with *lumbar* myelography and postmyelographic CT scanning. Note first-degree spondylolisthesis of L5 on S1 *(curved black arrow)*. Conus *(c)* terminates at the thoracolumbar junction. Note Schmorl-type end-plate lesions at lower thoracic segments. Mass *(m)* in the posterior epidural space extends from the level of mid-T8 to inferior T10 *(straight black arrows)*. Resonance characteristics on T1 and T2 scans indicate a cyst. The lesion deforms the thecal sac, and displaces and compresses the cord. Diagnosis: benign extradural arachnoid cyst.

stenosis and resulting neural compression (Fig 20–22).[65, 73]

Metastatic involvement of the vertebral column is far more common. MRI is capable of detecting metastases at a very early stage.[2] Malignancy may be totally unsuspected (Fig 20–23). Comparative studies suggest that MRI is an attractive alternative to myelography in the study of cord compression secondary to metastatic disease.[16]

Primary neurogenic tumors (intradural-extramedullary) can produce compression of the cauda equina. The resulting symptoms may suggest spinal stenosis, particularly in the elderly patient (Fig 20–24). Intradural tumors and stenosis may coexist.[66] These lesions are readily diagnosed by MRI.[23] The addition of gadolinium enhancement aids in the characterization of lesions.[101]

A variety of benign cystic lesions may compress the thecal sac.[41] MRI has been shown to be effective in detecting and characterizing these abnormalities.[99] Because of its large field-of-view capability and the absence of ionizing radiation, MRI can be

employed to survey multiple segments of the spine when there is suspicion of an occult compressive lesion (Fig 20–25).[42]

Outcome studies evaluating surgery for spinal stenosis have generally relied on myelography and myelography-CT for diagnosis.[37, 54, 74] In his monograph on lumbar spinal stenosis, Postacchini speaks to the diagnostic value of MRI in stenosis.[80] However, he devotes only one page to the subject. Such is the case of a powerful diagnostic tool in rapid evolution.

Experience with MRI since 1986 has convinced imagers and clinicians of the value of this modality in the assessment of lumbar spinal stenosis.

REFERENCES

1. Aprill C: Lumbar spine, in El-Khoury G, Bergman R, Montgomery W (eds): *Sectional Anatomy by MRI/CT*. New York, Churchill Livingstone Inc, 1990, pp 466–500.
2. Avrahami E, et al: Early MR demonstration of spinal metastasis in patients with normal radiographs and CT and radionuclide bone scans. *J Comput Assist Tomogr* 1989; 13:598–602.
3. Azzam C: Midline lumbar ganglion/synovial cyst mimicking an epidural tumor: Case report and a review of pathogenesis. *Neurosurgery* 1988; 23:232–234.
4. Barnes P, et al: MRI in infants and children with spinal dysraphism *AJR* 1986; 147:339–346.
5. Batson O: The vertebral venous system. *AJR* 1957; 78:195–220.
6. Baum J, Hanley E: Intraspinal synovial cysts simulating spinal stenosis. *Spine* 1986; 11:487–489.
7. Blumenkopf B, Juneau P: Magnetic resonance imaging (MRI) of thoracolumbar fractures. *J Spinal Disord* 1988; 1:144–150.
8. Bogduk N, Twomey L: *Clinical Anatomy of the Lumbar Spine*. Melbourne, Churchill Livingstone, 1987.
9. Bolender N, Schönström N, Spengler D: Role of computed tomography and myelography in the diagnosis of central spinal stenosis. *J Bone Joint Surg [Am]* 1985; 67:240–246.
10. Bose K, Balasubramanian P: Nerve root canals of the lumbar spine. *Spine* 1984; 9:16–18.
11. Bradley W: When should GRASS be used? *Radiology* 1988; 169:574–575.
12. Bradley W, Tsuruda J: MR sequence parameter optimization: An algorithmic approach. *AJR* 1987; 149:815–823.
13. Breger R, et al: T1 and T2 measurements on a 1.5 T. commercial MR imager. *Radiology* 1989; 171:273–276.
14. Brieg A: *Biomechanics of the Central Nervous System*. St Louis, Mosby-Year Book, Inc, 1960.
15. Bushong F: Magnetic resonance imaging: Physical and biological principles, St Louis, Mosby-Year Book, Inc, 1988.
16. Carmody R, et al: Spinal cord compression due to

metastatic disease: Diagnosis with MR imaging vs. myelography. *Radiology* 1989; 173:225–229.

17. Chien D, Edelman R: Ultrafast imaging using gradient echoes. *Magn Reson Q* 1991; 7:31–56.

18. Clark G, Panjabi M, Wetzel F: Can infant malnutrition cause adult vertebral stenosis? *Spine* 1985; 10:165–170.

19. Cohen M, et al: Cauda equina anatomy II: Extrathecal nerve roots and dorsal root ganglia. *Spine* 1990; 15:1248–1251.

20. Cooper L, et al: The poor quality of early evaluation of magnetic resonance imaging. *JAMA* 1988; 259:3277–3280.

21. Crock H: Isolated lumbar disc resorption as a cause of nerve root canal stenosis. *Clin Orthop* 1976; 115:109.

22. Crock H: Normal and pathological anatomy of the lumbar nerve root canals. *J Bone Joint Surg [Br]* 1981; 63:847.

23. Dillon W, et al: Intradural spinal cord lesions: Gadolinium DTPA enhanced MR imaging. *Radiology* 1989; 170:229–237.

24. Dommisse G: Morphological aspects of the lumbar spine and lumbosacral region. *Orthop Clin North Am* 1975; 6:163–175.

25. Edelman RR, et al: Frodo pulse sequences: A new means of eliminating motion, flow and wraparound artifacts. *Radiology* 1988; 166:231–236.

26. Edelman RR, et al: High resolution surface-coil imaging of lumbar disc disease. *AJR* 1985; 144:1123–1129.

27. Edelsen J, Nathan H: Nerve root compression in spondylolysis and spondylolisthesis. *J Bone Joint Surg [Br]* 1986; 68:596–599.

28. Ehman R, et al: Influence of physiologic motion on the appearance of tissue and MR images. *Radiology* 1986; 159:777–782.

29. Eisenstein S: The morphometry and pathological anatomy of the lumbar spine in South African Negroes and Caucasoids with specific reference to spinal stenosis. *J Bone Joint Surg [Br]* 1977; 59:173–180.

30. Eisenstein S: The trefoil configuration of the lumbar vertebral canal. A study of South African skeletal material. *J Bone Joint Surg [Br]* 1980; 62:73–76.

31. Emery I, Hamilton G: Epidurography using metrizamide: An outpatient examination. *Clin Radiol* 1980; 31:643–649.

32. Epstein J, Epstein B, Levine L: Nerve root compression associated with narrowing of the lumbar spinal canal. *J Neurol Neurosurg Psychiatry* 1962; 25:125.

33. Eubanks B, Cann C, Brant-Zawadzki M: CT measurement of the diameter of the spinal and other bony canals: Effects of section angle and thickness. *Radiology* 1985; 157:243–246.

34. Farfan H: Effect of torsion on the intervertebral joints. *Can J Surg* 1969; 12:336.

35. Feimlee J, Ehman R: Spatial presaturation: A method for suppressing flow artifacts and improving depiction of vascular anatomy and MR imaging. *Radiology* 1987; 164:559–564.

36. Frymoyer J, et al: A comparison of radiographic findings in fusion and non-fusion patients ten or more years following lumbar disc surgery. *Spine* 1979; 4:435.

37. Garfin S, et al: Laminectomy: A review of the Pennsylvania Hospital experience. *J Spinal Disord* 1988; 1:116–133.

38. Gargano F, Meyer J, Sheldon J: Transfemoral ascending lumbar catheterization of the epidural veins in lumbar disc disease. *Radiology* 1974; 111:329–336.

39. Gebarski S, et al: Post-traumatic progressive myelopathy. *Radiology* 1985; 157:379–385.

40. Golub B, Silverman B: Transforaminal ligaments of the lumbar spine. *J Bone Joint Surg [Am]* 1969; 51:947–956.

41. Goyal R, et al: Intraspinal cysts: A classification and literature review. *Spine* 1987; 12:209–213.

42. Gray L, Djang W, Friedman A: MR imaging of thoracic extradural arachnoid cysts. *J Comput Assist Tomogr* 1988; 12:646–648.

43. Grenier K, et al: Normal and degenerative posterior spinal structures: MR imaging. *Radiology* 1987; 165:517–525.

44. Haacke EM, Lenz G: Improving image quality in the presence of motion by using rephasing gradients. *AJR* 1987; 148:1251–1258.

45. Haacke EM, et al: Steady state free precession imaging in the presence of motion: An application for improved visualization of the cerebrospinal fluid. *Radiology* 1990; 175:545–552.

46. Hasue M, et al: Anatomic study of the interrelation between lumbosacral nerve roots and their surrounding tissues. *Spine* 1983; 8:50–58.

47. Herzog R: Magnetic resonance imaging of the spine, in Frymoyer J (ed): *The Adult Spine—Principles and Practices.* New York, Raven Press, 1991, pp 457–510.

48. Herzog R, et al: The importance of posterior epidural fat pad in lumbar central canal stenosis. *Spine* 1991; 16(suppl):227–233.

49. Howe J, Loeser J, Calvin W: Mechanosensitivity of dorsal root ganglia and chronically injured axons: A physiological basis for the radicular pain of nerve root compression. *Pain* 1977; 3:25–41.

50. Huizinga H, Heiden J, Vinken P: The human lumbar vertebral canal. A biometric study. *Proc Kon Med Akad Wet C* 1952; 55–22.

51. Hurwitz R: Eccentric inventor Nikola Tesla: Father of today's MR technology. *Diagnostic Imaging* November 1988, pp 413–414.

52. Jack C, et al: Field strength in neuroimaging: Comparison of 0.5 T. and 1.5 T. *J Comput Assist Tomogr* 1990; 14:505.

53. Johnson D, et al: MR imaging of the pars interarticularis. *AJNR* 1988; 9:1215–1220.

54. Johnsson K, Willner S, Petterson H: Analysis of operated cases with lumbar spinal stenosis. *Acta Orthop Scand* 1981; 52:427–433.

55. Kaiser M, Ramos L: *MRI of the Spine: A Guide to Clinical Applications.* New York, Thieme Medical Publishers, Inc, 1990.

56. Kirkaldy-Willis W, et al: Pathology and pathogenesis of lumbar spondylosis and stenosis. *Spine* 1978; 3:319–328.

57. Kneeland J, Hyde J: High resolution MR imaging with local coils. *Radiology* 1989; 171:1–7.

58. Lancourt J, Glenn W, Wiltse L: Multiplanar computerized tomography in the normal spine and in the

diagnosis of spinal stenosis: A gross anatomic-computerized tomographic correlation. *Spine* 1979; 4:379–390.

59. Lewit K, Sereghy T: Lumbar peridurography with special regard to the anatomy of the lumbar peridural space. *Neuroradiology* 1974; 8:233–240.

60. Liu S, et al: Synovial cyst of the lumbosacral spine: Diagnosis by MR imaging. *AJR* 1990; 154:163–166.

61. Luk K, Ho C, Leong J: The iliolumbar ligament: A study of its anatomy, development and clinical significance. *J Bone Joint Surg [Br]* 1986; 68:197–200.

62. Luyendijk W, van Voorthusen A: Contrast examination of the spinal epidural space. *Acta Radiol* 1966; 5:1051–1066.

63. MacGibbon B, Farfan H: A radiologic survey of various configurations of the lumbar spine. *Spine* 1979; 4:258.

64. Macnab I: Spondylolisthesis with an intact neural arch. The so-called pseudospondylolisthesis. *J Bone Joint Surg [Br]* 1950; 32:325.

65. Masaryk T: Spine tumors, in Modic M, Masaryk T, Ross J (eds): *Magnetic Resonance Imaging of the Spine.* St Louis, Mosby-Year Book, Inc, 1989, pp 220–231.

66. McGuire R, Brown N, Green B: Intradural spinal tumors and spinal stenosis. *Spine* 1987; 12:1062–1066.

67. Modic M: Magnetic resonance imaging of intervertebral disc disease: Clinical and pulse sequence considerations. *Radiology* 1984; 152:103–111.

68. Modic M, Masaryk T, Ross J (eds): *Magnetic Resonance Imaging of the Spine.* St Louis, Mosby-Year Book, Inc, 1989.

69. Modic M, Ross J: Magnetic resonance in the evaluation of low back pain. *Orthop Clin North Am* 1991; 22:283–301.

70. Modic M, et al: Lumbar herniated disc disease and canal stenosis: Prospective evaluation by surface coil MR, CT, and myelography. *AJR* 1986; 147:757–765.

71. Modic M, et al: Degenerative disc disease: Assessment of changes in vertebral body marrow with MR imaging. *Radiology* 1988; 166:193–199.

72. Moriwaka F, et al: Myelopathy due to osteochondroma: MR and CT studies. *J Comput Assist Tomogr* 1990; 14:128–130.

73. Nosrat O, et al: Aneurysmal bone cyst of the spine. *J Neurosurg* 1985; 63:685–690.

74. Paine K: Results of decompression for lumbar spinal stenosis. *Clin Orthop* 1976; 115:96–100.

75. Panjabi M, Takata K, Goel V: Kinematics of the lumbar intervertebral foramen. *Spine* 1983; 8:348–357.

76. Pattany P, et al: Motion artifact suppression technique (MAST) for MR imaging. *J Comput Assist Tomogr* 1987; 11:369–377.

77. Penning L, Wilmink J: Posture-dependent bilateral compression of L4 and L5 nerve roots in facet hypertrophy: A dynamic CT-myelographic study. *Spine* 1987; 12:488–500.

78. Ponseti I: Skeletal growth and achondroplasia. *J Bone Joint Surg [Am]* 1970; 52:701.

79. Porter R, Pavitt D: The vertebral canal I. Nutrition and development: An archeological study. *Spine* 1987; 12:901–906.

80. Postacchini F: *Lumbar Spinal Stenosis.* New York, Springer-Verlag, 1989, p 171.

81. Postacchini F, Massobrio M, Fero L: Familial lumbar stenosis. *J Bone Joint Surg [Am]* 1985; 67:321–323.

82. Ramanauskas W, et al: MR imaging of compressive myelomalacia. *J Comput Assist Tomogr* 1989; 13:399–404.

83. Ramsey R: The anatomy of the ligamenta flava. *Clin Orthop* 1966; 44:129–166.

84. Rauschning W: Detailed sectional anatomy of the lumbar spine, in Rothman S, Glenn W (eds): *Multiplanar CT of the Spine.* Baltimore, University Park Press, 1985, pp 33–85.

85. Rauschning W: Normal and pathologic anatomy of the lumbar root canals. *Spine* 1987; 12:1008–1019.

86. Reicher M, et al: Multiple-angle, variable interval, nonorthogonal MRI. *AJR* 1986; 147:363–366.

87. Rissanen P: Comparison of pathologic changes in intervertebral disc and interspinous ligament of the lower part of the lumbar spine in the light of autopsy findings. *Acta Orthop Scand* 1964; 34:54.

88. Rosenberg N: Degenerative spondylolisthesis. Predisposing factors. *J Bone Joint Surg [Am]* 1975; 57:467.

89. Rubin J, Enzmann D: Imaging of spinal CSF pulsation by 2-DFT MR: Significance during clinical imaging. *AJR* 1987; 148:973–982.

90. Rubin J, Wright A, Enzmann D: Lumbar spine: Motion compensation for cerebrospinal fluid on MR imaging. *Radiology* 1988; 167:225–231.

91. Rydevik B, Brown M, Lundborg G: Pathoanatomy and pathophysiology of nerve root compression. *Spine* 1984; 9:7–15.

92. Sackett J, et al: Metrizamide—CSF contrast medium. Analysis of clinical application in 215 patients. *Radiology* 1977; 123:779–782.

93. Sato K, et al: The configuration of the laminas and facet joints in degenerative spondylolisthesis: A clinicoradiologic study. *Spine* 1989; 14:1265–1271.

94. Schneck C: The anatomy of lumbar spondylosis. *Clin Orthop* 1985; 193:20.

95. Schönström N, et al: Pressure changes within the cauda equina following constriction of the dural sac. *Spine* 1984; 9:604–607.

96. Schönström N, Bolender N, Spengler D: The pathomorphology of spinal stenosis as seen on CT scans of the lumbar spine. *Spine* 1985; 10:806–811.

97. Schönström N, Hansson T: Pressure changes following constriction of the cauda equina. An experimental study in situ. *Spine* 1988; 13:385–388.

98. Skalpe I, Amundsen P: Lumbar radiculography with metrizamide, *Radiology* 1975; 115:91–95.

99. Sklar E: Acquired spinal subarachnoid cysts: Evaluation with MR, CT-myelography, and intraoperative sonography. *AJR* 1989; 153:1057–1064.

100. Stollman A, et al: Radiologic imaging of symptomatic ligamentum flavum thickening with and without ossification. *AJNR* 1987; 8:991–994.

101. Sze G, et al: Gadolinium DTPA in the evaluation of intradural extramedullary spinal disease. *AJNR* 1988; 9:153–163.

102. Tajima N, Kawano K: Cryomicrotomy of the lumbar spine. *Spine* 1986; 11:376.

103. Verbiest H: Pathomorphologic aspects of develop-

mental lumbar stenosis. *Orthop Clin North Am* 1975; 6:177–196.

104. Vital J: Anatomy of the lumbar radicular canal. *Anat Clin* 1983; 5:141–151.

105. Wall E, et al: Cauda equina anatomy I: Intrathecal nerve root organization. *Spine* 1990; 15:1244–1247.

106. Watanabe A, et al: Gradient echo MR imaging of the lumbar spine: Comparison with spin echo technique. *J Comput Assist Tomogr* 1990; 14:410.

107. Weinstein J: Mechanism of spinal pain: The dorsal root ganglion and its role as a mediator of low back pain. *Spine* 1986; 11:999–1001.

108. Weinstein J: Differential diagnosis and surgical treatment of primary benign and malignant neoplasms, in Frymoyer J (ed): *The Adult Spine—Principles and Practice,* New York, Raven Press, 1991.

109. Yuh W, et al: Lumbar epidural chordoma: MR findings. *J Comput Assist Tomogr* 1989; 13:508–510.

21

Computed Tomography–Discography In Spinal Stenosis

Charles N. Aprill, M.D.

Stenosis implies compromise of available space. The use of the term *spinal stenosis* usually implies pathologic changes involving bony elements. However, any tissue which narrows the central or root canals may be considered a source of spinal stenosis. In this context, pathologic changes altering the configuration of the intervertebral disc and resulting in a mass effect warrants consideration in this book.

MASS EFFECTS

A number of terms are used to describe disc disease producing mass effects. Generally, any distortion of disc contour with extension beyond the usual confines may be considered a "rupture."[28] If the annular fibers are intact, then the term *bulge* (protrusion) is appropriate. This condition may be generalized (circumferential), as occurs in spondylotic degeneration with narrowing of the interspace. It may be limited to a smaller area of the disc circumference (focal), as occurs in the torsion injury described by Farfan.[13]

Theoretically, as disruption of annular fibers occurs, nuclear material can be displaced. Disc "herniation" is the result of such annular disruption and nuclear displacement. Herniation may be divided into three categories: prolapse, extrusion, and sequestration. Prolapse occurs when material from the nuclear region extends through the fibers of an incomplete annular rent. The outermost "capsular fibers" of the annulus remain intact restraining the disc material. Extrusion occurs when the capsular fibers of the annulus are disrupted and disc material is no longer constrained. Sequestration occurs when extruded material migrates away from the site of annular disruption. Such a classification is based on criteria established by Macnab,[28] Masaryk et al.,[29] and others.[7, 42] The differences in these lesions have potential therapeutic implications.

Unenhanced computed tomography (CT) provides excellent visualization of disc contour, and distortions of that contour are apparent.[17, 53] Williams et al.[52] pointed out that CT defines the disc margin but does not fully delineate the severity of pathologic changes occurring within the disc substance. Primary disc lesions cause unusual densities at the annular margin,[9, 54] but the differentiation of disc "bulge" or "herniation" can be difficult. Fries et al.[16] suggested that the size of the mass effect could be a criterion for the diagnosis of disc extrusion.

Magnetic resonance imaging (MRI) evolved from a useful alternative to myelography and CT in the evaluation of disc disease[10, 31] to the most accurate, noninvasive method of identifying and characterizing disc abnormalities[29, 32] (Fig 21–1). However, noninvasive imaging modalities may not completely characterize pathologic disc changes in all instances. Foraminal herniations may be missed by CT myelography.[26] In a cadaver study comparing MRI and dis-

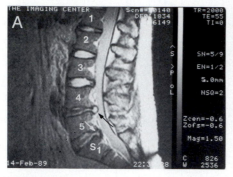
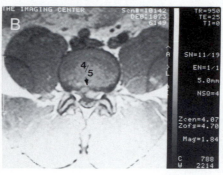
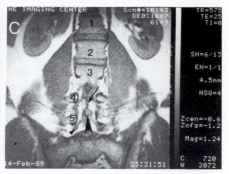

FIG 21–1.

A 45-year-old man with severe back pain and progressive weakness and pain in both lower extremities. **A,** sagittal MRI, spin-echo (SE) proton-density image. Midline section. Moderately large disc herniation (specifically, prolapse) at L4–5. The posterior disc "capsule" appears to be intact *(black arrow)*. The prolapsed disc material has higher signal intensity than the parent disc. Note nuclear degradation of both the L4–5 and L5–S1 discs (decreased signal). There is a posterior "bulge" (protrusion) or "herniation" (prolapse) at L5–S1 *(white arrow)*. **B,** axial MRI, SE T1-weighted im- age. Section through the L4–5 intervertebral disc. The disc lesion *(arrow)* is central in location but extends more to the left of the midline. There is gross deformity of the thecal sac. Note the large central canal. **C,** coronal MRI SE T1-weighted image. Section through anterior epidural space at lower two motion segments. The lesion at L4–5 is seen as a round mass within the central canal near the midline *(large arrowhead)*. Note the relationship to the posterior longitudinal ligament *(black arrow)* and the L5 nerve on the right *(small arrowhead)*.

cography with cryomicrotome sections, MRI was sensitive to only two thirds of the radial fissures demonstrated by discography.[55]

DISCOGRAPHY

Any discussion of CT-discography must first address the topic of discography. Discography is an invasive test providing direct information about disc morphology. Opponents of discography call attention to the work of Earl Holt published a quarter of a century ago.[20] In his conclusions, Holt alludes to the fact that improvement of contrast agents and techniques might render discography more useful as a diagnostic test. Indeed, this is the case. The use of Holt's paper as a scientific standard has been challenged.[40] The work has been repeated with strict attention to the shortcomings of the original study. As far as pain response is concerned, discography performed with modern contrast agents, by skilled practitioners employing standardized techniques, has a low false-positive rate.[51]

Despite difficulty in interpreting the images, there is little doubt as to the accuracy of discography in defining the pathoanatomy of the disc. In a classic radiologic-anatomic study, Pierre Erlacher[12] demonstrated that the dispersal of contrast material within the disc, as seen on radiographs, correlated exactly with the dispersal of vital stains seen on anatomic sections. The recent elegant studies of Rosenbaum and Yu have confirmed the accuracy of injection techniques in depicting internal disc architecture.[37] These authors compared CT-discography using radiographic contrast agents with MRI-discography employing paramagnetic contrast material (gadopentate dimeglumine). Cryomicrotome sections stained with organic dyes served as a reference standard. Radial and circumferential tears, as well as separations within the annular fibers, were accurately imaged.

Postacchini,[35] in his monograph on spinal stenosis, indicates that discography is a useful tool in the evaluation of those patients in whom the cause of compression of neural structures is unclear. In some cases of radiculopathy, he recommends discography to define the role of the disc in the neural compression syndrome. Disc bulge (protrusion) or herniation (prolapse or extrusion) are more common in symptomatic radiculopathy than in pure bony stenosis. In cases of cauda equina compression, he suggests discography to differentiate between a large disc lesion causing primary compression and a smaller disc lesion producing compression in a "pathologically narrow lumbar canal."[35]

I[6] have not employed discography in the evaluation of patients with known spinal stenosis. vanharanta et al. pointed out the value of discography with CT-discography in clinical practice for diagnosis of low back pain without neural impingement signs.[48] This is the most common indication for discography and CT-discography (Fig 21–2).

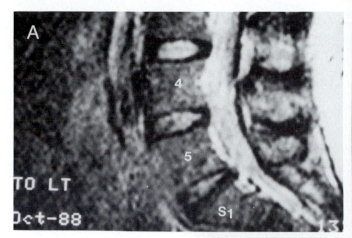

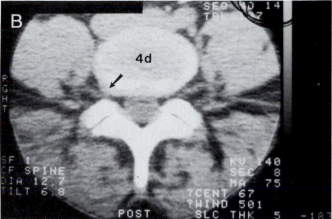

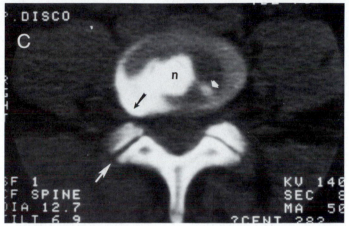

FIG 21–2.
A 42-year-old woman with back pain, predominantly right-sided, radiating into the right buttock and thigh. The patient's complaints also include right leg weakness and altered sensation. **A,** sagittal MRI SE T2-weighted image. Midline section. MRI was interpreted as "grossly normal." The patient's body build (5'2", 170 lb) was thought to result in less than optimal image quality. There is no obvious pathologic change at L4–5. **B,** axial CT through the L4–5 intervertebral disc. Note the asymmetric prominence of the right posterolateral disc margin *(arrow).* **C,** axial CT through the L4–5 disc approximately 1 hour post–disc injection. Contrast fills the well-organized nuclear zone *(n).* A needle track is evident on the left *(small white arrow).* Contrast material extends to the right posterolateral annular margin by way of a wide posterolateral fissure. This probably represents coalescense of several concentric fissures. A small focal protrusion or prolapse projects into the midzone of the right L4–5 root canal *(black arrow).* Compare this with **B.** Note asymmetry of facet joint widths with the right being wider than the left *(white arrow).* This might reflect pathologic facet distraction implying a coexisting injury in the posterior column.

Posterior protrusion or herniation may be the cause of significant neurologic symptoms, particularly if onset is sudden. Acute symptoms are more common in younger patients, but posterior protrusions are more common in subjects over 30 years of age. The older patients seem to have greater disc degeneration but are less often acutely symptomatic from fixed protrusion.[49] Disc abnormalities exerting pressure on neural elements may not be fixed. The morbid anatomy related to intermittent neural compression (dynamic stenosis) may not be fully demonstrated by static CT or MRI. In this regard, myelography is superior.[41] Still, myelography lacks sensitivity in the central canal at the L5–S1 level and in the evaluation of root canal stenosis.

CT-DISCOGRAPHY

The biomechanical forces acting on the spine in flexion[19, 44] may be duplicated by intradiscal injections. The pathoanatomic changes of gradual disc prolapse[2] may be demonstrated on postinjection axial CT scans. The importance of contrast dispersal as seen in the axial plane was reported by Quinnell and Stockdale in their study of artifacts associated with disc injection.[36] The value of axial plane imaging in discography was documented in a cadaver study by Videman et al.[50] These authors found that the axial image was important in 25% of cases, demonstrating findings not recognizable on frontal and lateral radiographs. These findings included the width and location of fissures, protrusions, and prolapses. A detailed classification of annular degeneration and disruption has emerged from this work.[38] This classification has been utilized in the study of disc deterioration and back pain.[45–47]

The first clinical report of CT-discography in 1984 addressed the use of the technique in defining lateral herniations resulting in compromise of the root canal (lateral stenosis)[4] (Fig 21–3). Troisier and Cypel[43] believe that discography is an important factor in deciding between surgery and chemonucleolysis in patients with symptoms of neural compression. Edwards et al.[11] found CT-discography to be of prognostic value in a similar group of patients undergoing chemonucleolysis. Contrast staining of the disc herniation was the critical factor (Fig 21–4).

Contrast material mixes slowly with the nuclear matrix by diffusion.[1] In vitro studies have shown differential absorption of water-soluble contrast material by discal and peridiscal tissues. Nuclear material has an affinity for contrast agents employed in discography. Annular tissue does not absorb the

contrast; there is little staining of fat; and scar tissue absorbs only a small amount by comparison with nuclear material.[21]

CT-discography has been shown to demonstrate lateral herniations[25] and recurrent disc herniations following surgery.[18] In a large comparative study evaluating the efficacy of diagnostic studies including myelography, CT, CT-myelography, and CT-discography, Jackson et al.[22] found CT-discography to be the most accurate method for anatomic definition of disc herniations. The procedure is extremely sensitive to foraminal herniations and very specific for recurrent postoperative herniations (Fig 21–5).

The technique for lumbar discography has been discussed in detail elsewhere.[6, 27, 39] CT scanning following discography is a specialized examination and should not be performed employing the same protocols used for routine CT of the lumbar spine. The purpose of postinjection CT is to define the dispersal pattern of contrast material within the disc. Gantry angulation to approximate the angle of the disc is more important following disc injection than in routine scanning. Sections 5 mm thick with overlap (3- or 4-mm table increments) provide the best detail. The images should be photographed at window-center settings designed to optimize the differentiation of contrast material and bone. This is different from the routine soft tissue and bone detail window-center settings employed in routine scanning. It is only necessary to study the disc space

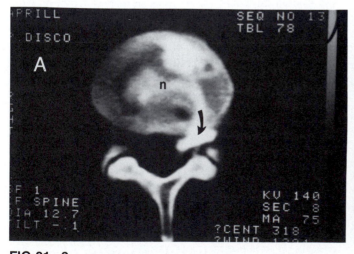

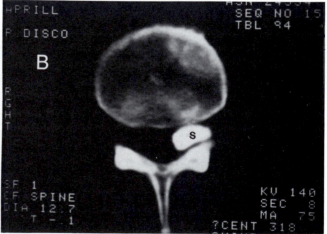

FIG 21–3.
A 45-year-old man with back pain and severe left leg pain and weakness. Prior unenhanced CT scan demonstrated a mass lesion in the left L4–5 root canal. Differential diagnosis included "disc herniation vs. primary neurogenic tumor." **A,** axial CT through the lower half of the L4–5 intervertebral disc, approximately 1 hour post–disc injection. Contrast fills a moderately disorganized nuclear zone *(n)* and extends through a left posterolateral radial fissure into the L4–5 root canal *(arrow).* **B,** section 6 mm cephalad to **A.** Contrast material is seen as a discrete collection filling the mid- or entrance zone of the left L4–5 root canal. This contrast material defines an extruded, sequestered disc fragment(s).

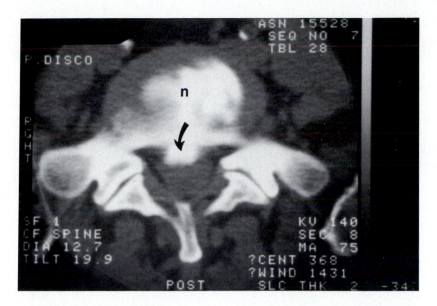

FIG 21–4.

A 46-year-old man with back pain. Prior myelogram reported as negative, myelography-CT as demonstrating "disc bulge, no frank herniation." Axial CT, 1 hour post–disc injection at L5–S1. There is satisfactory opacification of the nuclear zone *(n)*. Contrast extends into a moderate-sized disc herniation (prolapse) central or right paracentral in location *(arrow)*.

(end plate to end plate) in most instances so only three or four sections are required at each level. In my practice, only those discs associated with pathologic pain response are studied by CT, regardless of their appearance on nucleogram. Obviously, if the technique is to be employed for the evaluation of mass effects in stenosis, then all levels studied by discography should be evaluated by CT-discography.

Needle tracks should not be confused with pathologic disruptions of the disc annulus.[30] Small-gauge

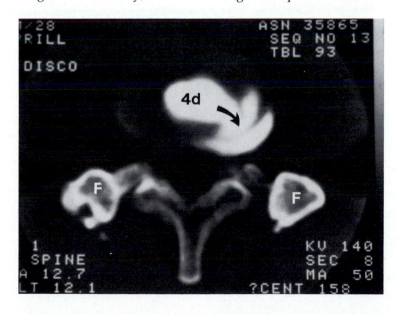

FIG 21–5.

A 32-year-old woman with persisting back and left leg pain following an apparently successful posterolateral-intertransverse fusion. Axial CT through the L4–5 intervertebral disc, 1 hour post–disc injection. Note mature-appearing fusion masses *(F)*. Contrast material defines the well-organized nuclear zone *(4d)* and a series of concentric inner and outer annular fissures *(arrow)* extending to the left posterolateral disc annulus. The outer disc margin projects into the midzone of the left L4–5 root canal producing lateral stenosis. Is this lesion a large focal bulge (protrusion) or a disc herniation (prolapse)?

needles (nos. 22 and 25) do not produce large tracks. However, as a precaution, it is advisable to perform disc puncture from the side opposite the dominant symptoms.

An important use of CT-discography is documentation of proper nuclear injection and, conversely, the recognition of erroneous, extranuclear annular injections.[36] In a recent paper concerning the relevance of discography combined with CT scanning,[5] the authors concluded the study was superfluous in light of modern imaging. They demonstrate a figure which shows an annular injection at L5–S1, apparently unrecognized.[5, P482] Were the authors more aware of the proper technique and utilization of postinjection CT for documentation, their conclusions might be different.

Discography is a safe procedure[34] when performed by a trained, skilled practitioner. It is not without its risks. The major complications of infection and neural injury have been detailed elsewhere.[6] The work of Fraser et al.[14, 15] regarding discitis following discography makes a compelling case for considering all such postprocedure incidents as infectious in origin.

Modern discography should be performed employing an extrapedicular approach, if possible. Such an approach eliminates the problem of postprocedure headache and other complications associated with lumbar puncture. However, the extrapedicular approach places the extrathecal neural elements at risk.[23, 24, 33] Modern techniques are effective in addressing this problem. However, the physician with special training (anesthesiologists with pain management training; neurosurgeons, orthopaedists, and physical medicine specialists with formal spine training; and radiologists with neuroradiologic training) is not necessarily versed in the performance of this specialized technique. Diagnostic disc puncture should not be performed without sufficient training to ensure it can be completed safely.

Disc injections in the stenotic patient pose special problems. The injection of fluid into the intervertebral disc stiffens the spine,[3] increases disc height, and reduces disc bulge.[8] While intradiscal injections do not pose a great risk of disc disruption, Jayson et al.[23] did report bursting of grossly abnormal discs at sites of posterior and posterolateral degeneration. The patients being evaluated for stenosis are likely to be older with more advanced spondylotic pathology. Postacchini[35] addresses this issue by recommending slow injection of contrast material to avoid a sudden rise in intradiscal pressure and potential increased neural compression. The fact that many such degenerated discs have an incompetent nuclear envelope may obviate this caution.

CONCLUSION

In conclusion, discography (with CT-discography) is a useful technique in selecting patients for chemonucleolysis and perhaps percutaneous discectomy. It has value in differentiating between recurrent disc herniation and postoperative scar. Insofar as these considerations may be applied to the stenotic patient, CT-discography is useful. However, the role of CT-discography in the evaluation of spinal stenosis patients is relatively small. As high-quality MRI becomes more readily available, it is likely to limit the use of invasive techniques even for these indications.

Discography remains the sole method for associating pain response and specific pathoanatomy in patients with primary axial pain, without definitive neural compression, and in whom imaging studies are indeterminate. CT-discography is a vital part of the discographic procedure documenting proper nuclear injection and defining pathologic dispersal.

REFERENCES

1. Adams M, Dolan P, Hutton W: The stages of disc degeneration as revealed by discograms. *J Bone Joint Surg [Br]* 1986; 63:36.
2. Adams M, Hutton W: Gradual disc prolapse. *Spine* 1985; 10:524.
3. Andersson G, Schultz A: Effects of fluid injection on mechanical properties of the intervertebral disc. *J Biomechanics* 1979; 12:453.
4. Angtuaco E, Holder JC, Boop WC, et al: Computed tomographic discography in the evaluation of extreme lateral disc herniation. *Neurosurgery* 1984; 14:350–351.
5. Antti-Poika I, Soini J, Tallroth K: Clinical relevance of discography combined with CT scanning. A study of 100 patients. *J Bone Joint Surg [Br]* 1990; 72:480–485.
6. Aprill C: Diagnostic disc injection, in Frymoyer JW (ed): *The Adult Spine: Principles and Practice* New York, Raven Press, 1991, pp 420–442.
7. Bosacco S, Berman A: Surgical management of lumbar disc disease. *Radiol Clin North Am* 1983; 21:377–393.
8. Brinckmann N, Horst M: The influence of vertebral body fracture, intradiscal injection and partial discectomy on the radial bulge and height of the intervertebral discs. *Spine* 1985; 10:138.
9. Dillon W, et al: Computed tomography in differential

diagnosis of the extruded lumbar disc. *J Comput Assist Tomogr* 1983· 7:969–975.

10. Edelman R: High resolution surface coil imaging of lumbar disc disease. *AJNR* 1985; 6:479–485.

11. Edwards W, Orme T, Orr-Edwards G: CT/discography: Prognostic value in the selection of patients for chemonucleolysis. *Spine* 1987; 12:792–795.

12. Erlacher P: Nucleography. *J Bone Joint Surg [Br]* 1952; 34:204–210.

13. Farfan H: Effect of torsion on the intervertebral joints. *Can J Surg* 1969; 12:336.

14. Fraser R, Osti O, Vernon-Roberts B: Discitis after discography: Incidence and pathological findings. *J Bone Joint Surg [Br]* 1987; 69:26.

15. Fraser R, Osti O, Vernon-Roberts B: Discitis following discography: An experimental study. *J Bone Joint Surg [Br]* 1987; 69:31.

16. Fries J, *et al*: Computed tomography of herniated and extruded nucleus pulposus. *J Comput Assist Tomogr* 1982; 6:874–887.

17. Godersky J, Erickson D, Seljeskog E: Extreme lateral disc herniation: Diagnosis by computed tomographic scanning. *Neurosurgery* 1984; 14:549–552.

18. Grenier N, Vilal JM, Grezelle JF, et al: CT-discography in the evaluation of the postoperative spine. Preliminary results. *Neuroradiology* 1988; 30:232–238.

19. Hickey D, Hukins D: Relation between the structure of the annulus fibrosis and the function and failure of the intervertebral disc. *Spine* 1980; 5:106.

20. Holt E: The question of lumbar discography. *J Bone Joint Surg [Am]* 1968; 50:720–726.

21. Jackson R, Glah J: Foraminal and extraforaminal lumbar disc herniation: Diagnosis and treatment. *Spine* 1987; 12:577–585.

22. Jackson R, Cain DE, Jacobs RR, et al: The neuroradiographic diagnosis of lumbar herniated nucleus pulposus I: A comparison of computed tomography, myelography, CT-myelography, discography, and CT-discography. *Spine* 1989; 14:1356–1361.

23. Jayson M, Herbert C, Bark SJ: Intervertebral disc: Nuclear morphology and bursting pressures. *Ann Rheum Dis* 1973; 32:308–315.

24. Konings J, Veldhuizen A: Topographic anatomical aspects of lumbar disc puncture. *Spine* 1988; 13:958–961.

25. Kornberg M: Extreme lateral lumbar disc herniations. Clinical syndrome and computed tomography recognition. *Spine* 1987; 12:586–589.

26. Kurobane Y, Takahashi T, Tajima T, et al: Extraforaminal disc herniation. *Spine* 1986; 11:260–268.

27. Laredo J, et al: Technique of lumbar chemonucleolysis, in Bard M, Laredo J (eds): *Interventional Radiology in Bone and Joint*. Vienna, Springer-Verlag, 1988, pp 101–122.

28. Macnab I: *Backache*. Baltimore, William & Wilkins Co, 1977, pp 91–96.

29. Masaryk T, Ross JS, Modic MT, et al: High resolution MR imaging of sequestered lumbar intervertebral discs. *AJNR* 1988; 9:351–358.

30. McCutcheon M, Thompson W: CT scanning of lumbar discography. A useful diagnostic adjunct. *Spine* 1986; 11:257–259.

31. Modic M, Masaryk T, Boumphrey F, et al: Lumbar herniated disc disease in canal stenosis: Prospective evaluation by surface coil MR, CT, and myelography. *AJNR* 1986; 7:709–711.

32. Osborn A, Hood RS, Sherry RG, et al: CT/MR spectrum of far lateral and anterior lumbosacral disc herniations. *AJNR* 1988; 4:775–778.

33. Patsiaouras T, Bulshrode C, Cook P, et al: Percutaneous nucleotomy: An anatomic study of the risk of root injury. *Spine* 1991; 16:39–42.

34. Piepgras U, Kammerer V, Huber G: Comparison between myelography and discography for lumbar prolapsed intervertebral discs. *Rontgenblatter* 1976; 29:193–200.

35. Postacchini F: Lumbar spinal stenosis, Wein, New York, 1989, Springer-Verlag pp. 148–154.

36. Quinnell R, Stockdale H: An investigation of artifacts in lumbar discography. *Br J Radiol* 1980; 53:831–839.

37. Rosenbaum A, Yu S: MR/discography: A comparison of CT/discography and cryomicrotomes. Part II: Clinical applications XIV. Symposium Neuroradiologicum. Proceedings, London, 1990. *Neuroradiology*, in press.

38. Sachs B, Vanharanta H, Spivey MA, et al: Dallas discogram description. A new classification of CT-discography in low back disorders. *Spine* 1987; 12:287–294.

39. Sachs B, Vanharanta H, Spivey MA, et al: Techniques for lumbar discography and computed tomography/discography in clinical practice. *Orthop Rev* 1990; 19:775–778.

40. Simmons J, et al: A re-assessment of Holt's data on "The question of lumbar discography." *Clin Orthop* 1988; 237:120–124.

41. Sortland O, Magnaes B, Hauge T: Functional myelography with metrizamide in the diagnosis of lumbar stenosis. *Acta Radiol Suppl (Stockh)* 1977; 355:42–54.

42. Teplick J, Haskin M: CT and lumbar disc herniation. *Radiol Clin North Am* 1983; 21:259–288.

43. Troisier G, Cypel D: Discography: An element of decision. Surgery versus chemonucleolysis. *Clin Orthop* 1986; 206:70–78.

44. Twomey L, Taylor J: Flexion creep deformation and hysteresis in the lumbar vertebral column. *Spine* 1982; 7:116.

45. Vanharanta H, Sachs BL, Spivey MA, et al: The relationship of pain provocation to lumbar disc deterioration as seen by CT/discography. *Spine* 1987; 12:295–298.

46. Vanharanta H, Sachs BL, Spivey MA, et al: A comparison of CT/discography pain response in radiographic disc height. *Spine* 1988; 13:321–324.

47. Vanharanta H, Guyer RD, Ohnmeiss DO, et al: Disc deterioration in low back syndromes. A prospective multicenter discography study. *Spine* 1988; 13:1349–1351.

48. Vanharanta H, Sachs BL, Ohnmeiss DO., et al: Pain provocation and disc deterioration by age. A CT/discography study in low back pain population. *Spine* 1989; 14:420–423.

49. Vernon-Roberts B: Disc pathology and disease states, in Ghosh P (ed): *The Biology of the Intervertebral Disc*, vol 2. Boca Ratan, Fla, CRC Press, 1988, pp 73–119.

50. Videman T, Malamivaara A, Mooney V: The value of the axial view in assessing discograms. An experimental study with cadavers. *Spine* 1987; 12:299–304.
51. Walsh T, et al: The question of lumbar discography revisited: A controlled prospective study of normal volunteers to determine the false-positive rate. *J Bone Joint Surg [Am]* 1990; 72:1081–1088.
52. Williams A, Haughton V, Meyer G, et al: Computed tomographic appearance of the bulging annulus. *Radiology* 1982; 142:403–408.
53. Williams A, Haughton V, Daniels DL, et al: CT recognition of lateral lumbar disc herniation. *AJNR* 1982; 3:211–213.
54. Williams A, Haughton V, Daniels DL, et al: Differential CT diagnosis of extruded nucleus pulposus. *Radiology* 1983; 148:141–148.
55. Yu S, Selher LA, Ho PS, et al: Comparison of MR and discography in detecting radial tears of the annulus: A post-mortem study. *AJNR* 1989; 10:1077–1081.

22

Myelographic Evaluation of Spinal Stenosis

Tony Kim, M.D.

Sunday Verman, M.D.

Jordan D. Rosenblum, M.D.

Ruth G. Ramsey, M.D.

Myelographic examination of the lumbar spine remains an important and frequently requested diagnostic procedure in the evaluation of spinal stenosis. Beginning with an introduction to the biological properties of myelographic contrast media, this chapter then focuses upon the most common indication for myelography: acquired spinal stenosis due to degeneration of the intervertebral disc and to the resulting spondylosis and disc herniation. Myelographic technique, normal anatomy, and pathology are presented. Less common causes of spinal stenosis, such as congenital, traumatic, neoplastic, infectious, and metabolic processes, are discussed briefly.

CONTRAST MEDIA

Water-soluble, nonionic, iodinated contrast media are the current media of choice for myelography. Water-soluble contrast media have several advantages over iophendylate (Pantopaque), an oil-based contrast agent which is now rarely, if ever, used. Any oil-based contrast medium which remains in the subarachnoid space also degrades future magnetic resonance (MR) examinations by producing areas of increased signal intensity that may obscure pathologic changes. The lower density and viscosity of water-soluble media compared to oil-based media produce superior resolution of fine intraarachnoid structures and permit greater filling of the nerve root sleeves. Complete absorption into the bloodstream eliminates the need for removal by the myelographer following the study. Nonionic contrast media compared to ionic media containing the same iodine concentration do not produce the same salt-forming radicals, therefore resulting in lower osmolality. This property produces lower central nervous system (CNS) toxicity and allows nonionic contrast agents to be used safely throughout the cerebrospinal fluid (CSF) space.

The first widely used, water-soluble, nonionic contrast agent was metrizamide (Amipaque), which is representative of the biological behavior of the other agents in this class of media. Since 1985 metrizamide has been replaced by iohexol (Omnipaque) and iopamidol (Isovue), both nonionic, water-soluble contrast media, which are less neurotoxic. Absorption of iohexol into the bloodstream from CSF occurs through arachnoid villi and granulations which project into venous sinuses. These arachnoid proliferations are predominantly located along the superior sagittal sinus and near the origins of the spinal nerve root sleeves. The absorption of contrast media probably occurs at the arachnoid villi and granulations closest to the injection site.

The biological half-life of iohexol in CSF is approximately 4 hours after a lumbar injection, and 90% is excreted in the urine by 24 hours. The blood level of contrast rises within 1 hour and peaks after 4 hours. Elimination of contrast from the bloodstream is primarily renal, and therefore adequate renal function and hydration are important factors for a safe examination. Approximately 4% of the iohexol is recovered from the feces at 48 hours. A total dose of over 3 g of iodine should be avoided.

The possibility of an anaphylactoid or cardiovascular reaction should always be considered with parental administration of an iodinated contrast agent. Appropriate personnel, medication, and equipment should therefore be available to treat any reaction. Patients with known iodine allergies should, of course, never be injected.

Neurotoxic effects of iohexol are due to cerebral cortical, meningeal, or radicular irritation. The symptoms include headache, convulsions, radicular pain, dizziness, nausea, vomiting, and meningeal signs. Phenothiazine derivatives and other drugs which lower the seizure threshold, e.g., monoamine oxidase inhibitors, tricyclic antidepressants, analeptics, antihistamines, CNS stimulants, and some antifungal drugs, should be avoided for 48 hours before and 24 hours after myelography. The frequency of major adverse reaction to iohexol is approximately 0.02%.

LUMBAR EXAMINATION

Technique

Sedation prior to the myelogram procedure is not routinely required but 5 to 10 mg of diazepam (Valium) by intramuscular injection is usually effective for the anxious patient, and may also reduce the risk of convulsions. The patient is placed prone on a fluoroscopy table with a pillow under the abdomen to reduce the normal lordotic curve of the lumbar spine. After sterile preparation of the skin and injection of local anesthetic, a 22-gauge spinal needle is introduced into the subarachnoid space at the L2–3 or L3–4 intervertebral levels. The pillow should sufficiently reduce the normal lumbar lordosis so that no angulation of the needle is required in order to avoid the posterior spinous processes. Occasionally a midline approach is ineffective because of severe degenerative changes or a heavily calcified posterior spinal ligament, and a paramedian approach is required to avoid these obstacles. When the needle tip

is in the subarachnoid space the CSF should flow freely. Poor flow may indicate a subdural position or severe spinal stenosis. A small test dose of contrast may be injected to determine the location of the needle tip.

When the needle is in the subarachnoid space, approximately 15 mL (180 mg/mL of iodine) of water-soluble nonionic contrast is introduced. A smaller amount is injected if severe stenosis is present. Prone frontal, prone oblique, and lateral films are then obtained with the head of the table elevated approximately 60 degrees to keep the contrast media within the lumbosacral subarachnoid space. Fully upright and occasionally forceful extension views may be necessary to demonstrate an abnormal disc.

The lumbosacral subarachnoid space is voluminous, accounting for nearly 40% of the total subarachnoid capacity. The nerve roots form the lateral margins of the contrast column as they travel obliquely and caudally to exit the vertebral canal through the intervertebral foramina. As the nerve root exits the thecal sac it carries for a short distance into the intervertebral foramen a triangular sleeve of dura and arachnoid. This contrast-filled nerve root sleeve, with the nerve root seen as a thin linear lucency, is best demonstrated on oblique views. The apex of the nerve root sleeve is the point of exit of the nerve root from the thecal sac. The nerve root courses along the medial and inferior surface of the pedicle from which it takes its number. At the level of the pedicle, the nerve root travels through a fat-filled space which is bound anteriorly by the vertebral body, laterally by the pedicle, and posterolaterally by the facets. This space is the lateral recess (Fig 22–1). The L4 nerve root exits through the L4–5 intervertebral foramen just inferior to the L4 pedicle and superior to the L4–5 disc. The dorsal and ventral roots join to form the spinal nerve just distal to the dorsal ganglion and within the intervertebral foramen; the ganglion is located just below the pedicle.

Spondylosis

The term *spondylosis* as it is used here refers to stenosis of the vertebral canal caused by degenerative changes of the spine including vertebral and facet osteophytes, ligamentous hypertrophy, and posterior bulging of the disc without disc herniation. These degenerative changes are the most common causes of spinal stenosis. The intervertebral disc consists of a nucleus pulposus surrounded by a fi-

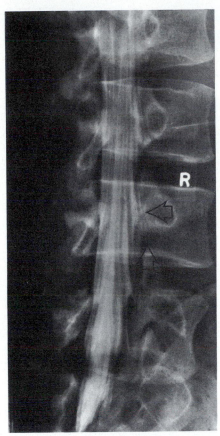

FIG 22–1.
Normal oblique view. The nerve roots appear as thin, linear lucencies within the contrast-filled lumbosacral thecal sac. The *horizontal arrow* points to the lateral recess. The *vertical arrow* points to the intervertebral foramen.

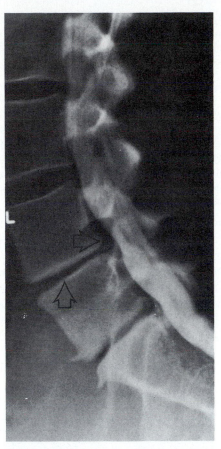

FIG 22–2.
Gaseous degeneration of disc. The *vertical arrow* points to gas in the narrowed L4–5 intervertebral space. Gas is also seen at the narrowed L5–S1 level. The horizontal arrow points to posterior bulging disc material and small end-plate osteophytes. Note the smooth defect along the ventral contrast column.

brous capsule, the annulus fibrosus. By the fourth and fifth decades of life the once soft nucleus has degenerated into fibrous tissue. This process is accompanied by decreasing water content. Severely desiccated discs may demonstrate a central lucency on radiographs which represents gas that has diffused into a partial vacuum within the degenerated disc. As discussed in Chapter 11, degeneration leads to formation of osteophytes along the vertebral end plates which project into the vertebral canal and to formation of osteophytes at the facet joints which project into the intervertebral foramina and lateral recesses (Fig 22–2). Fibrous and fatty infiltration of the ligamenta flava produce thickening. Narrowing of the disc space also causes buckling and thickening of the ligamenta flava resulting in further stenosis of the vertebral canal.

Posterior bulging of the intervertebral disc is usually diffuse and symmetric. Posterior bulging is most common at the cervical and lumbar levels be-

cause the lordotic configuration of the spine at these levels brings the greatest weight-bearing load on the posterior margins of the vertebrae. The bulging disc and marginal intervertebral osteophytes located anteriorly in combination with the hypertrophied ligamenta flava and facet osteophytes located posteriorly act as a vise upon the spinal cord and nerve roots. The problem can be aggravated by the presence of a congenitally small vertebral canal produced by short pedicles with or without associated narrowing of the interpedicular distance.

Increased intervertebral mobility due to laxity of the degenerated motion segment can also lead to spondylolisthesis. Usually in spondylolisthesis the superior vertebral body is subluxated anteriorly relative to the more inferior vertebra. The vertebral body and facet subluxation results in spinal stenosis due to compression of the thecal sac between the superior end plate of the lower, more posterior vertebral body and the posterior elements of the upper, more anterior vertebral body. Overlapping of the facets results in narrowing of the intervertebral foramina (Fig 22–3).

The myelographic appearance of spondylosis is that of a smooth, circumferential narrowing of the contrast column at the intervertebral level caused by anterior and bilateral posterolateral extradural defects. The overall appearance is that of a belt fastened too tightly around the contrast column (Fig 22–4). The nerve roots are displaced anteromedially and the nerve root sleeves may not fill with contrast. Occasionally the vertebral stenosis caused by spondylosis may be sufficiently severe to delay or obstruct passage of contrast (Fig 22–5). Postmyelogram computed tomography (CT) is usually performed for detailed evaluation and frequently begins at the L1–2 level and extends to the sacrum. The myelo-

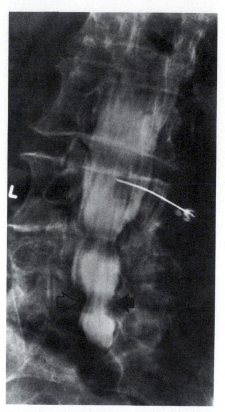

FIG 22–4.
Bulging disc and facet hypertrophy. Oblique view of lumbosacral spine demonstrates an anterior epidural defect *(open arrow)*, which represents bulging disc material, and a posterior defect *(solid arrow)*, which represents bony and ligamentous hypertrophy of the facets.

gram often provides good information on which levels to scan.

Disc Herniation

As the disc ages, fissures form in the annulus fibrosus which allow the nucleus pulposus to herniate and to project into the vertebral canal and intervertebral foramina. Disc herniations in the lumbosacral spine are primarily located posterolaterally. This results in compression of the spinal nerve roots which lie in the cranial half of the foramina, just beneath the pedicle. Posterior central herniations are less common and anterior herniations are rare. The most commonly affected levels in the lumbar spine are at the L4–5 and L5–S1 disc spaces. These two levels account for over 90% of solitary disc herniations with herniation at the L4–5 level slightly more frequent. Higher levels of herniation are more common with advancing age, and may therefore be present in the stenotic age group. Radiographic signs of multi-

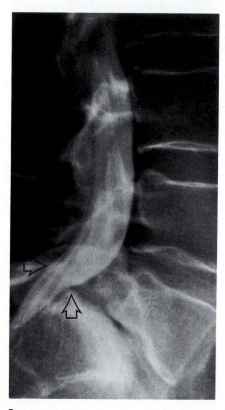

FIG 22–3.
Spondylolisthesis with stenosis. Spondylolisthesis at the L5–S1 level demonstrates mild compression of the thecal sac between the posterior margin of the S1 end plate *(vertical arrow)* and the posterior processes of L5 *(horizontal arrow)*. Spondylolysis is present, resulting in less severe stenosis than would be seen if the posterior process of L5 were pulled anteriorly with the subluxated L5 vertebral body.

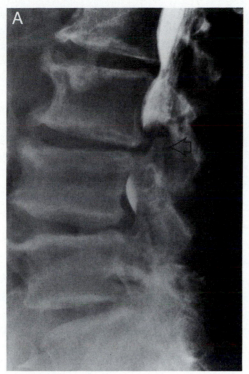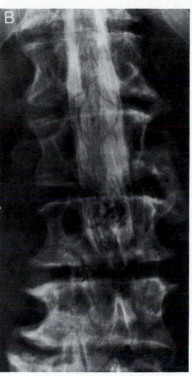

FIG 22–5.
Spondylosis and spinal stenosis. **A,** lateral view demonstrates obstruction of contrast flow past severe spinal stenosis at the L3–4 level *(arrow).* A small amount of contrast is seen caudal to the stenosis. **B,** the frontal view demonstrates the typical bilateral tapered appearance of spinal stenosis due to spondylosis *(arrow).* Note the cluster of dilated veins cranial to the L3–4 stenosis.

ple herniations are present approximately 15% of the time. Since only one of the herniations may produce symptoms, clinical correlation is necessary (see Chapter 17).

The myelographic appearance of a symptomatic disc herniation can vary widely, depending on its size, location, and the diameter of the vertebral canal. A central disc herniation into a capacious vertebral canal must be large in order to cause symptoms, whereas a small disc herniation or posterior bulging into a narrowed canal can result in spinal stenosis and produce severe symptoms. Similarly a small disc herniation into the confined space of a lateral recess or intervertebral foramen may be symptomatic.

The characteristic myelographic appearance of a herniated lumbar disc is a sharply defined indentation at an intervertebral space along the anterolateral surface of the contrast column. The extradural defect can extend slightly above or below the vertebral interspace and is seen best on the lateral or oblique projections. Disc herniation characteristically displaces nerve roots posteriorly with occasional thick-

ening of the nerve root. The nerve root sleeve may not fill with contrast (Fig 22–6). If the herniated disc material breaks off into the vertebral canal, the disc fragment may migrate anywhere although it more commonly travels craniad. It can be located between intervertebral levels and may compress two nerve roots. Disc herniation can usually be differentiated from a posterior bulging disc with an intact annulus because a bulging disc typically produces a bilateral, symmetric, and rounder defect which does not extend superior or inferior to the vertebral interspace.

A normal myelogram does not completely exclude the possibility of disc herniation because contrast in the nerve root sleeve rarely extends into the intervertebral foramen beyond the margin of the pedicle, and a far-lateral disc herniation may compress a nerve root without deforming the contrast column. A postmyelogram CT scan will demonstrate a herniated disc in this location.

Focal, anterolateral, extradural defects in the contrast column may represent lesions other than a herniated disc. These lesions include tumor, bone fragments, arachnoiditis, scarring, abscess, and he-

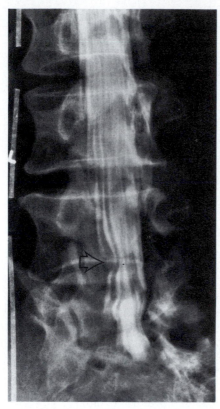

FIG 22–6.
Spondylosis and spinal stenosis. Oblique view shows an anterolateral, epidural defect in the contrast column at the L4–5 level with thickening and medial displacement of the L5 nerve root *(arrow)*.

matoma. Although their myelographic appearances may be indistinguishable from herniated disc, a history of trauma, multiple myelograms, spinal surgery infection, or malignancy elsewhere usually points to the correct diagnosis. The defect in the contrast column caused by a malignancy is usually not confined to the intervertebral disc level and is more lobulated and more extensive than that caused by a herniated disc.

NONDEGENERATIVE SPINAL STENOSIS

Processes other than degenerative changes of the vertebrae can produce spinal stenosis. These nondegenerative processes include congenital stenosis, trauma, surgery, infection, neoplasm, and idiopathic or metabolic causes. All produce symptoms proportional to their degree of cauda equina and nerve root compression. The common myelographic appearance of all of these processes is focal or diffuse indentation or obstruction of the contrast column. If the flow of contrast is completely obstructed, a cervical or lumbar puncture may be necessary to introduce contrast past the level of obstruction in order to outline the configuration and extent of the obstructing lesion. Unlike the defects seen with disc herniation and spondylosis the thecal deformity may not be located at an intervertebral level. The deformities are usually associated with readily apparent bone abnormalities.

Congenital Stenosis

The most common cause of congenital stenosis is idiopathic shortening of the pedicles which results in a generalized narrowing of the anteroposterior diameter of the bony vertebral canal (see Chapter 12). This process in itself rarely produces symptoms but it can significantly aggravate the spinal stenosis caused by otherwise common degenerative hypertrophic bony and ligamentous changes. Another cause of generalized spinal stenosis is achondroplasia. A defect in enchondral bone formation produces short vertebral bodies with wide end plates. The combination of periosteal bone formation creating thick pedicles and laminae and the premature closure of synchondroses involved with neural arch development act together to cause narrowing of the anteroposterior and interpedicular diameters of the vertebral canal (Fig 22–7). This produces a triangular or trefoil configuration of the canal when viewed axially. As degenerative changes appear, which in a normal patient would be insignificant, severe spinal stenosis can occur, predominantly in the lower lumbar region.

Other causes of congenital spinal stenosis include hypochondroplasias and Morquio's mucopolysaccharidosis.

Trauma

Vertebral body fractures can result in displacement of bone fragments into the vertebral canal or intervertebral foramina. Subluxation of the vertebral bodies due to transverse fractures, ligamentous injuries, or spondylolysis can also compromise the vertebral canal. These gross findings are readily seen on plain films of the spine and can explain symptoms referable to that level. A hematoma will probably not appear on plain films; a myelogram may demon-

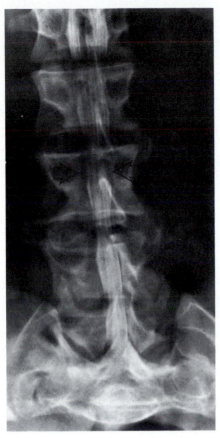

FIG 22–7.
Lumbar myelogram of an achondroplastic dwarf illustrates the typical narrowed interpedicular distance *(arrow)*. The anteroposterior diameter of the vertebral canal is also narrowed. This makes the patient particularly vulnerable to relatively mild degenerative changes that result in spinal stenosis.

strate a rounded, focal, or diffuse defect along the contrast column. MR is the examination of choice for evaluation of a hematoma.

Iatrogenic

Surgery can cause spinal stenosis due to bone fragments or foreign bodies left within the vertebral canal. Bony overgrowth and accelerated degenerative changes can also occur after spinal fusion. Compression of the thecal sac by postoperative hematoma or scarring which cannot be seen on plain films may be demonstrated by myelography, postmyelogram CT, and MR.

Infection

Infection typically involves the intervertebral disc space and the two adjacent vertebral bodies.

Narrowing of the vertebral interspace, cortical erosion, or vertebral body collapse may be demonstrated by plain films, but the determination of associated soft tissue spread and severity of spinal stenosis is better made with myelography and best made with MR. If a large epidural defect that extends over several vertebral levels is seen on myelogram or MR, tuberculosis or fungal infection should be suspected. Invasion of the epidural space by sterile inflammatory tissue can be seen in Pott's disease of the spine.

Neoplasm

Spinal stenosis due to metastatic infiltration of the vertebrae is much more common than stenosis caused by primary bone tumors such as osteoblastoma, aneurysmal bone cyst, or giant cell tumor. Although expansion or collapse of the vertebral body may be evident on plain films, myelography can be useful to demonstrate the extent and severity of soft tissue invasion into the vertebral canal, particularly prior to radiation therapy. However, MR has essentially replaced myelography for evaluation of metastatic disease.

Idiopathic and Metabolic

Diffuse bony expansion involving the vertebrae can compromise the vertebral canal. The bone changes are easily demonstrated by plain films, and myelography is usually not required unless complications such as vertebral body collapse occur. These processes include Paget's disease, acromegaly, fluorosis, and epidural lipomatosis which may be idiopathic or associated with steroid therapy or Cushing's disease.

BIBLIOGRAPHY

Compere EL, Keyes DC: Roentgenological studies of the intervertebral disc: A discussion of the embryology, anatomy, physiology, clinical and experimental pathology. *AJR* 1933; 29:774–797.

Coventry MB, Ghormley RK, Kernohan JW: The intervertebral disc: Its microscopic anatomy and pathology. *J Bone Joint Surg* 1945; 27:233–247.

Crock HV: Normal and pathological anatomy of the lumbar spinal nerve root canals. *J Bone Joint Surg [Am]* 1981; 63:487–490.

Dorwart RH, Vogler JB, Helms CA: Spinal stenosis. *Radiol Clin North Am* 1983; 21:301–325.

Kido DK, Gromey DG, Pavese AM, et al: Human spinal arachnoid villi and granulations. *Neuroradiology* 1976; 11:221–228.

Mikhael MA, Ciric I, Tarkington JA, et al: Neuroradiological evaluation of lateral recess syndrome. *Radiology* 1981; 140:97–107.

Nowicki BH, Yu S, Reinartz JR, et al: Effect of axial loading on neural foramina and nerve roots in the lumbar spine. *Radiology* 1990; 176:433–437.

Resnick D: Degenerative diseases of the vertebral column. *Radiology* 1985; 156:3–14.

Robertson HJ, Smith RD: Cervical myelography: Survey of modes of practice and major complications. *Radiology* 1990; 174:79–83.

Russell EJ: Cervical disc disease. *Radiology* 1990; 177:313–325.

Shapiro R: *Myelography,* ed 4. St Louis, Mosby-Year Book, Inc, 1984.

Yu S, Haughton VM, Sether LA, et al: Annulus fibrosus in bulging intervertebral discs. *Radiology* 1988; 169:761–763.

23

The Neurodiagnostic Evaluation of Spinal Stenosis

Scott Haldeman, M.D., Ph.D. F.R.C.S.

Definitions and classifications of spinal stenosis generally include two points: (1) narrowing of the osseoligamentous spinal canals which (2) causes compression of neural structure.[42] By definition the morphologic shape or size of the canal is less important than the presence of neurologic compromise. It is only when the narrowing of the canal reaches the point where it encroaches on the nervous system that spinal stenosis can be considered significant. The multiple imaging techniques used to define the shape and size of the central canal and neural foramina must therefore be considered second-level tests after it has been determined that there is neural compromise.

The topic which is not addressed in this chapter is that of so-called nonsymptomatic spinal stenosis. This term implies that morphologic encroachment on the dural space or neural canals may have some significance in the absence of clinically documentable neural disturbance. Since by far the majority of the diagnoses of spinal stenosis and virtually all treatment is on symptomatic patients, the term *spinal stenosis,* as used in this chapter, refers to a pathologic narrowing of the neural canals of sufficient magnitude to cause symptoms or clinical findings on examination and testing.

NEUROLOGIC CONSEQUENCES OF SPINAL STENOSIS

The neurologic presentation of spinal stenosis follows five potential patterns depending upon the location and extent of the stenosis. Each of these patterns has well-defined neurologic findings on clinical examination and require specific electrodiagnostic testing for confirmation (see Table 23–1).

Spinal Pain

Spinal pain can occur with or without radiation into the extremities and in its simplest form is not associated with fixed neurologic deficits. In the early stages of this presentation it may not be possible to differentiate the pain from that associated with spinal lesions such as intervertebral disc disease or facet degeneration. In these situations the diagnosis of spinal stenosis is commonly made after an imaging study. Such a diagnosis must always be questioned. There is very little evidence that spinal stenosis per se is a painful lesion at rest unless it causes one of the four patterns listed below. Pain is more likely to be due to discogenic, facet, or soft tissue disturbances which often are part of the stenotic process (in spondylitic or acquired stenosis). Furthermore, pain may be totally unrelated to the stenosis and may be coincidental with congenital stenosis, spondylolisthesis, or even preexisting acquired stenosis.

The clinical neurologic examination of these patients does not differ from that of other patients with back pain. By definition, neurologic and neurophysiologic testing in these patients will be within normal limits. The examination is geared toward localizing the source of pain rather than assuming that the observed stenosis is the correct diagnosis. If the source of pain makes up a component of the stenotic lesion, as in facet degeneration and hypertrophy or disc herniation, then appropriate management of these problems can be instituted.

TABLE 23–1.

The Neurologic Consequences of Spinal Stenosis*

Symptoms	Neurologic Examination	Neurologic Testing
Localized back pain	History No neural deficits	None or normal
Neurogenic claudication	History ? Deficits after walking	? H, F, SER before/after walking
Radiculopathy	Radicular neurologic deficits	EMG, H, F, DSER
Cauda equina syndrome	Bilateral LMN deficits, saddle anesthesia, BCR	PER, BCR, CMG, NPT
Myelopathy	UMN deficits	SER, CMG, CMER

*H = H reflex; F = F response; EMG = electromyography; SER = somatosensory evoked response; DSER = dermatomal SER; PER = pudendal evoked response; BCR = bulbocavernosus reflex; CMG = cystometrogram; CMER = cortical motor evoked responses; NPT = nocturnal penile tumescence; LMN = lower motor neuron; UMN = upper motor neuron.

Neurogenic Claudication

The symptoms referred to as *intermittent neurogenic claudication* are those which are most commonly associated with the diagnosis of spinal stenosis. Verbiest[51–53] presents three criteria for this diagnosis: (1) neurologic symptoms and pain in the lower extremities that impedes walking; (2) the ability to resume walking after 10 to 20 minutes; and (3) in the presence of permanent deficits the symptoms of neurogenic claudication must exceed the area of involvement of the permanent deficits. A discussion of the physiologic basis of this process, i.e., increased lordosis vs. changes in blood supply in the standing position, may be found elsewhere in this book.

Intermittent neurogenic claudication is clinically the most characteristic of any of the presentations of spinal stenosis. Verbiest[51, 53] notes that its presentation is influenced by the length of the morbid history and the length of the area of stenosis. He noted that these symptoms could be found in all patients with a morbid history of between 4 and 10 years.

The neurologic evaluation of these patients consists of establishing a history and then attempting to document neurogenic changes which come on with walking and are relieved by rest. This requires the clinical and electrodiagnostic examination of a patient both at rest and after the precipitation of symptoms by walking. Clinical changes in straight leg raising as well as motor, sensory and reflex findings are looked for. Electrodiagnostic testing has been used in an attempt to document changes in somatosensory evoked responses, H reflexes, or, more recently, cortical motor evoked responses before and after walking. Studies utilizing these tests to document neurogenic claudication have met with mixed results.

Radiculopathy

Stenosis of the intervertebral foramina and the lateral recesses may cause entrapment of the nerve root and permanent radicular neurologic changes. The processes which result in stenotic changes commonly encompass extended areas of the spine. Unlike classic unilateral disc herniation, the radicular deficits in stenosis may therefore be at multiple levels and present bilaterally. The degree of deficit can vary greatly, however, from side to side and at different levels. At times a single-level unilateral deficit may be the presenting or primary finding in spinal stenosis, making the clinical differentiation from disc herniation very difficult.

The clinical, neurologic, and electrodiagnostic studies in this situation do not vary from those used in the investigation of any other cause of radiculopathy. The primary points which must be kept in mind are the higher incidence of bilateral or multiple-level nerve root deficits and the spreading of radicular deficits on walking.

Cauda Equina Syndrome

Stenosis of the lumbosacral central canal can reach such a degree of severity as to cause compression of the cauda equina and the development of cauda equina syndrome. This can occur slowly over years and present with gradual but progressive symptoms. Alternatively, it can present as a sudden decompensation of the cauda equina with rapid onset of symptoms.

The classic presentation of cauda equina syndrome includes the development of bilateral leg pain, weakness, and sensory changes, perianal or saddle anesthesia, bladder and bowel incontinence, and impotence or orgasmic dysfunction. The extent of these changes is dependent upon the level of the compromise; higher cauda equina compression can cause paraplegia whereas lower cauda equina syndrome may present primarily as bowel and bladder symptoms.

There should be very little difficulty in diagnosing the patient with acute, bilateral cauda equina syndrome after a basic neurologic history and examination. The diagnosis of a more gradually developing, unilateral and especially lower cauda equina syndrome affecting primarily bowel, bladder, and sexual function, on the other hand, may require a very accurate clinical examination and the use of sophisticated electrodiagnostic and neurophysiologic tests which evaluate the sacral nerve roots.

Myelopathy

Central canal stenosis in the thoracic and cervical spine can result in compression of the spinal cord and the development of a true myelopathy. As in the case of cauda equina syndrome, this can occur slowly over years, especially in the presence of spondylosis. Alternatively, myelopathy can come on rapidly as a decompensation of the compromised spinal cord. The latter situation classically occurs following trauma or some other cause of inflammation which results in swelling within a preexisting stenotic canal.

The clinical presentation is dependent upon the level of the myelopathy, the severity of the myelopathy, and the acuteness of its onset. Acute complete paraplegia is rarely associated with spinal stenosis unless there is superimposed trauma. The more common situation is a slowly progressive paraplegia with concomitant gait and balance disturbances, predilection weakness in the lower extremities, and variable degrees of sensory loss (unilateral, bilateral, or Brown-Séquard). This is associated with bladder retention and overflow incontinence, disturbance of voluntary bowel function, and impotence or anorgasmia.

The clinical neurologic examination in the early phases of myelopathy caused by stenosis requires a more thorough history than usual, a skilled physical examination, and time in order to elicit subtle signs of weakness and balance disturbance as well as bladder, bowel, and sexual changes which may not be obvious in a routine examination of a patient with spinal pain. These signs may then have to be defined and differentiated from lesions other than stenosis. This may require advanced imaging studies as well as the use of somatosensory evoked potentials, cortical evoked potentials, cystometry, and studies of bowel and sexual functions.

CLINICAL NEUROPHYSIOLOGIC TESTS

The basic clinical examination of a patient suspected of having spinal stenosis is discussed in Chapter 17. In this chapter, those laboratory tests which help define the neurologic deficits associated with spinal stenosis are discussed. The primary goal of such tests is to confirm or clarify the clinical examination findings and to look for subtle neurologic deficits which may be difficult to elicit on examination. The latter may be due to pain or poor patient cooperation which can result in confusing or inconclusive clinical findings.

The clinical neurophysiologic investigation includes electrodiagnostic studies which look directly at the conduction of a nerve, and neuromuscular function, as well as neurophysiologic tests that look at bowel, bladder, and sexual function. The goal of the neurodiagnostic evaluation is to differentiate between spinal pain without deficits, intermittent neurogenic claudication, radiculopathy, cauda equina syndrome, and myelopathy. Many of these tests can also give information as to severity, chronicity, and level of the deficits caused by a stenotic lesion.

The first electrodiagnostic method for detecting lumbar radiculopathy to be incorporated into clinical practice was needle electromyography (EMG). As early as 1950 Shea and colleagues[46] confirmed the presence of denervation potentials in muscles affected by lesions which compress nerve roots. The correlation of EMG findings with intervertebral disc lesions was soon confirmed.[55] It became evident, however, that EMG by itself would not provide the type of differentiation between peripheral, radicular, and spinal cord lesions that was required for an accurate diagnosis. The demonstration in man of the F response by Magladery and McDougal in 1950[37] and the further investigation of the H reflex by Schenck in 1951[43] provided the tools to look directly at conduction through the nerve root. At the same time increased interest and utilization of nerve conduction techniques for the diagnosis of peripheral entrapment or metabolic neuropathies allowed for the differentiation between proximal and distal neurologic lesions.

The past decade has seen the widespread use of

somatosensory evoked responses to look specifically at spinal cord lesions and sensory radicular deficits. These tests allow for the differentiation of lesions affecting the peripheral and central components of the sensory neuraxis. Techniques have been developed so that each dermatome innervated by a single nerve root can be studied, making the test more specific. Techniques for stimulating lower sacral nerve roots have also been developed, allowing for the diagnosis of spinal lesions affecting bowel and bladder function. More recently, the ability to cortically evoke motor responses in peripheral muscles is being studied to further evaluate spinal cord and radicular function.

This has led to a situation where the skilled electrodiagnostician has, at his or her command, a large battery of tests which allow for the evaluation and differentiation of each of the potential levels of neurologic deficit associated with spinal stenosis. The major tests which are commonly used to investigate such neurologic deficits and to differentiate them from other neurologic lesions are shown in Figure 23–1.

The utilization and interpretation of these tests require a reasonable knowledge of spinal and peripheral nerve anatomy, as well as an understanding of the advantages and disadvantages of each of the tests. It is often necessary to use a battery of tests to determine whether a nerve root lesion exists, whether it is acute or chronic, its exact level, and whether it is primarily motor, sensory, or both. Each nerve root has a sensory, central, and motor component. Unfortunately, the different nerve roots combine and separate in the lumbar and sacral plexuses and there is a fair amount of overlap and variation in the innervation of muscles by different nerve roots. For this reason no single test can determine the presence of all nerve root lesions. Figure 23–2 illustrates how lumbosacral radiculopathy can be investigated using a battery of tests.

Spinal cord and cauda equina lesions require specific tests of sacral nerve function using bulbocavernosus and pudendal evoked potentials as well as direct testing of bowel, bladder, and sexual function.

Electromyography

The needle EMG is the most widely used and probably the most sensitive method available for de-

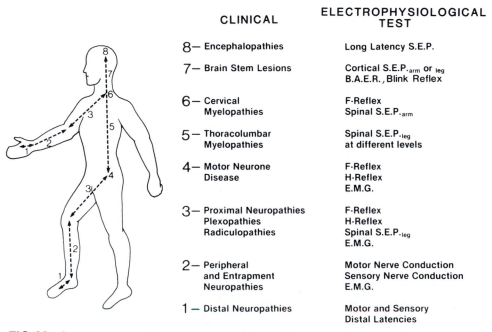

CLINICAL

8 — Encephalopathies

7 — Brain Stem Lesions

6 — Cervical
Myelopathies

5 — Thoracolumbar
Myelopathies

4 — Motor Neurone
Disease

3 — Proximal Neuropathies
Plexopathies
Radiculopathies

2 — Peripheral
and Entrapment
Neuropathies

1 — Distal Neuropathies

ELECTROPHYSIOLOGICAL TEST

Long Latency S.E.P.

Cortical S.E.P.$_{arm}$ or $_{leg}$
B.A.E.R., Blink Reflex

F-Reflex
Spinal S.E.P.$_{arm}$

Spinal S.E.P.$_{leg}$
at different levels

F-Reflex
H-Reflex
E.M.G.

F-Reflex
H-Reflex
Spinal S.E.P.$_{leg}$
E.M.G.

Motor Nerve Conduction
Sensory Nerve Conduction
E.M.G.

Motor and Sensory
Distal Latencies

FIG 23–1.
Electrodiagnostic evaluation of the somatic neuraxis. The localization of potential lesions and the more common electrodiagnostic tests which can be used to differentiate between various causes of neurologic symptoms in the extremities. *S.E.P.* = somatosensory evoked potential; *B.A.E.R.* = brainstem auditory evoked potential.

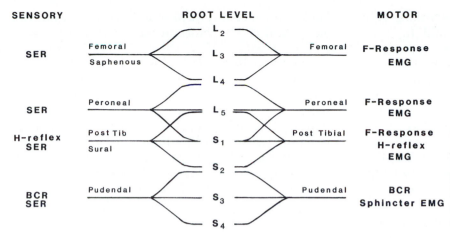

FIG 23–2.
Electrodiagnostic testing procedures for lumbosacral nerve root function. *SER* = somatosensory evoked responses; *BCR* = bulbocavernosus reflex; *Post Tib* = posterior tibial nerve. (From Haldeman, S: *Spine* 1984; 9–1. Used by permission.)

termining the presence of a peripheral motor nerve or root injury. It is also a test which can determine whether denervation is acute or chronic, and with which some degree of quantitization is possible. It has the primary disadvantages of being dependent on the skill and experience of the person performing the test, of being unable to measure sensory deficits, and of requiring a few weeks after onset of the radiculopathy before becoming unequivocally positive.

Technical Considerations.—EMG is performed by inserting either a bipolar or a monopolar needle electrode into the belly of a muscle and measuring electrical activity generated in the muscle under different circumstances. The electrical activity is observed on the monitor of one of the many commercially available EMG instruments. It is now possible for modern equipment to store EMG signals and to analyze the amplitude, morphology, and duration of potentials and then to print specific potentials on command. This has helped, but not eliminated, some of the subjective problems of EMG interpretation.

Muscle activity is observed under four circumstances. First, on insertion of the needle the muscle reacts with a short burst of electrical potentials (the insertional activity). When the needle stops moving and the muscle is relaxed, a second reading is taken. Normally, there is no activity in this resting state. Third, the patient is asked to contract the muscle very lightly so that one or two isolated motor units may be assessed for amplitude, morphology, and duration. Finally, the patient is asked to contract the muscle maximally. During this stage the recruitment of muscle motor units occurs with increasing amount of activity until the entire screen is filled with potentials. This is the so-called interference pattern and is a crude assessment of the contraction ability of the muscle.

Precautions.—EMG is a relatively benign procedure with very few major complications. It is, however, an uncomfortable test and therefore should be ordered only if some change in diagnosis or approach to the patient is expected to result from its use. The only potential complications are associated with bleeding and infection. Bleeding disorders are the primary contraindications for the routine use of EMG. Patients on anticoagulants or with a bleeding disorder should be assessed before EMG is performed by using bleeding and prothrombin times and perhaps a platelet count. Unless the bleeding disorder is severe, however, it is still possible to perform needle EMG on isolated muscles with increased care and maintaining hemostatic procedures longer than usual. A brief bacteremia can also occur following EMG even with the use of sterile needles. In the immunosuppressed patient or in the presence of cardiac valvular disease, the patient must be observed after an EMG for signs of infection, even though prophylactic antibiotics are not generally recommended.[48]

Acute Denervation.—Signs of acute denervation are the most dramatic and convincing of the abnormalities which can occur in patients with radiculopathy. The denervation potentials occur as a result of the muscle membrane losing its neuronal control and becoming more sensitive to irritation. The muscle membrane then begins generating potentials at rest. These potentials, known as fibrillations, positive sharp waves, and fasciculations, can be seen on the EMG oscilloscope with the muscle at rest. This denervation phenomenon also leads to increased or prolonged insertional potentials. If the denervation is severe, the muscle may also show diminished recruitment and interference patterns. Unfortunately, the denervation potentials do not appear until 10 to

14 days after the nerve is injured, thus making very early EMG testing useful only in establishing baseline muscle activity. The time it takes for denervation to be completed is dependent on the length of the nerve from the lesion to the muscles being tested. The paraspinal muscles are affected first, followed by the proximal extremity muscle at 3 to 4 weeks. It can take up to 6 weeks for distal extremity muscles to show signs of denervation.[11] Increased insertional potentials can occur slightly earlier than active denervation potentials but are much more difficult to interpret and often cannot be separated from poor relaxation or muscle spasm. For this reason increased insertional potentials alone should not be considered a reliable indication of denervation.

Chronic Denervation.—Approximately 10 to 12 weeks following acute denervation, nerves begin to sprout to innervate adjacent muscles which have been deprived of their nerve supply. This results in motor unit potentials with much longer duration, polyphasia, and higher amplitude (Fig 23–3). This is due to the fact that a single nerve fiber will be activating a larger number of muscle fibers than are seen under normal circumstances. These polyphasic potentials are relatively easy to distinguish from normal motor unit potentials provided the examiner is familiar with the variation in duration and morphology of motor units in different muscles. As more and more neuronal elements drop out, the recruitment pattern and the ability of the muscle to generate an interference pattern will diminish. This corre-

lates in a crude way with muscle weakness but can also be affected by effort on the part of the patient.

Interpretation.—The ability to determine the level of a suspected radiculopathy depends on the selection of muscles sampled. There is no uniform or recognized correct number or group of muscles which should be sampled. As a basic rule of thumb, two muscles from each of the major nerves or nerve roots where a lesion is suspected should be tested, one being proximal, the other more distal. Paraspinal muscles are the first to show denervation changes. These muscles are also the only ones innervated by the posterior primary division of the nerve root and, therefore, in posterior primary lesions may be the only muscle where EMG abnormalities are noted.[16, 18, 29] Only deep paraspinal muscles show reasonable segmented innervation and can be used for segmental localization.[40] Superficial paraspinal muscles, on the other hand, show considerable segmental overlap.[22, 31] L4 radiculopathies are primarily noted in the quadriceps femoris muscles. L5 radiculopathies show EMG abnormalities in the tibialis anterior, tibialis posterior, and gluteus medius, whereas S1 radiculopathies commonly express themselves as abnormalities in the gastrocnemius and gluteus maximus. There is a fair amount of overlap in the innervation of these muscles so that denervation in one muscle alone without similar changes in other muscles makes accurate localization to a specific nerve root difficult.

The correlation of EMG with spinal lesions has

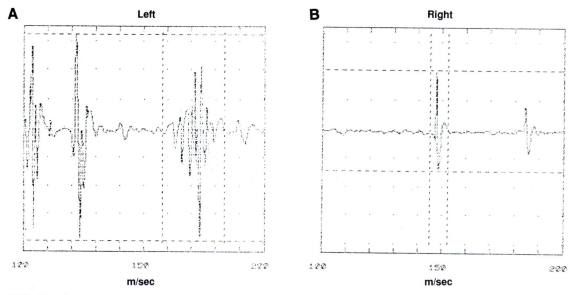

FIG 23–3.
A and **B**, polyphasic motor unit potentials from the left gastrocnemius muscle of a 55-year-old man with a well-defined chronic S1 radiculopathy. Normal motor unit potentials are noted in **B**.

been quite variable. Lane and co-workers[35] demonstrated a correlation with disc herniation determined by either myelography or surgery to be as high as 85%. Other laboratories, however, have tended to show a somewhat lower correlation. Knutsson[34] reported a 77% correlation, while Hoover et al.[27] had only a 60% correlation and Fisher et al.[17] had a 70% correlation. The correlation with spinal stenosis has been in the same order of magnitude, with Jacobson[28] finding 77% of patients with this diagnosis having abnormal EMGs. Seppalainen et al.,[45] on the other hand, found EMG abnormalities in 36 out of 37 patients with surgical spinal stenosis. Positive EMGs have also been found in the presence of a normal myelogram and it has been postulated that the radiculopathies seen in these situations are caused by lateral entrapment of the nerve root.[35, 49] Getty[20] found that EMG was of assistance in identifying nerve root involvement in 70% of patients with leg pain and bony encroachment of the lateral recesses.

Spinal Reflex Studies

The ability to test conduction through a nerve root has a number of advantages. Reflex studies reflect disturbances within the spinal cord as well as the peripheral nerve and, in the case of the H reflex and the bulbocavernosus reflex, are influenced by sensory as well as motor nerve root injuries. They also have the advantage of not requiring the insertion of needles and are, for the most part, better tolerated by patients.

The disadvantages of these tests include the fact that they cannot differentiate between acute and chronic changes, they offer very little in the way of quantitation, and, with the possible exception of the H reflex, are not felt to be as sensitive as EMG. Despite these shortcomings it is often very useful to perform these studies which may be the only means of demonstrating a radicular lesion.

The H Reflex.—The observation that the deep tendon reflexes responsible for the ankle jerk could be slowed or eliminated as a result of lumbosacral root compression was made by Malcolm in 1951.[38] At the same time Schenk[43] and Magladery and McDougal[37] began to study the H reflex in detail and relate it to the clinical ankle jerk. It soon became evident that the H reflex could be utilized to document radicular lesions.

The H reflex, named after Hoffman who demonstrated its presence in animals in 1922,[26] is obtained by placing a surface electrode over the midcalf and recording the electrical response generated during contraction of the soleus muscle on stimulation of the posterior tibial nerve in the popliteal fossa (Fig 23–4). When performing this test, stimulation of the posterior tibial nerve causes a direct, early, or M (muscle) response, which appears on the monitor. This is due to orthodromic stimulation of the motor nerve. Approximately 23 to 32 ms later a second

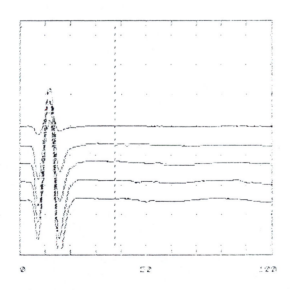

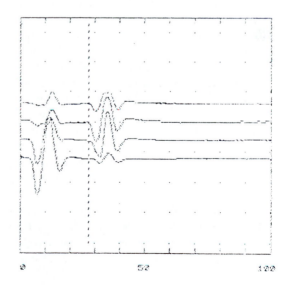

Left H Reflex   **Right H Reflex**

FIG 23–4.
H reflex studies in a 55-year-old man with a well-defined left-sided radiculopathy (same patient as in Fig 23–3). The right side demonstrates a normal H reflex response.

contraction of the soleus is generated and the electrical potential of this reflex can be recorded. This later, or H reflex has specific characteristics in that it varies in amplitude depending on the stimulus intensity. Initially, the amplitude of the H reflex increases as the stimulus intensity increases. It reaches a maximum intensity (H_{max}) after which it diminishes with further increases in stimulus intensity (Fig 23–4, right).

The H reflex has been demonstrated to follow a monosynaptic reflex pathway primarily through the S1 nerve root and has both motor and sensory components traveling in nerve fibers of large diameter. In theory, the H reflex should be elicitable in any muscle which can generate a tendon reflex. In practice, in the adult population, study of the H reflex is limited to the soleus muscle.

The H reflex has been demonstrated to reflect the Achilles tendon reflex extremely well and there is a high correlation between absent H reflexes and S1 radiculopathies.[5, 6, 8, 44] Some authors are of the opinion that there is a 100% correlation with S1 radiculopathies,[5, 6] while others have found a slightly lesser correlation.[2, 17] Of interest is the observation that H reflexes are not commonly abnormal in L5 radiculopathies even though the ankle jerk is innervated partially by L5 fibers.[5, 6] This allows for a fairly clear method of distinguishing S1 from L5 root lesions.

The H reflex is usually performed bilaterally and the response in the symptomatic leg compared with the response in the asymptomatic leg. Normal latencies of this response vary with age, height, and leg length and can be greatly influenced by any peripheral neuropathic process. The normal latencies which have been published vary slightly from laboratory to laboratory. Eisen and Hoirch[11] noted a normal latency of 28.5 ± 2 ms with an upper limit of normal at 33.5 ms. Kimura[33] noted a normal latency of 29.5 ± 2.4 ms with an upper limit of 34 ms. A side-to-side latency difference of 1.5 ms has been considered abnormal when strict technical criteria are used. A side-to-side difference of 2.5 to 3.0 ms should be considered definitely abnormal. Somewhat lesser agreement exists as to the importance of diminished amplitude. Nonetheless a 50% reduction of H_{max} amplitude on the symptomatic side compared with the asymptomatic side may reflect early S1 radicular changes.[11]

The F Wave Response.—F waves were first described by Magladery and McDougal in 1950[37] and named after the fact that they were initially recorded from the small muscles of the foot. Since then, these late responses have been recorded from most muscles where a twitch response can be obtained on supramaximal stimulation of a motor nerve. This response appears to involve purely motor nerve pathways and can occur following section of the sensory nerve root.[19, 39] It is now assumed to occur as a result of the antidromic stimulation of anterior horn cells in the spinal cord by some form of recurrent interneuron, or alternatively by direct dendritic tree excitation.[16, 39] The orthodromic responses elicited in this manner result in the late response recorded over the muscle. This response, therefore, allows for the measurement of conduction within the motor or anterior nerve root.

The F response shows an average amplitude of 1% of the M response.[12] It is variable in morphology and amplitude, and its latency can vary up to 7 ms (Fig 23–5, right). For this reason it is necessary to elicit 10 to 20 responses for every nerve tested and to be sure that the shortest latency of these responses is the one that is recorded. The normal latency varies with the height or leg length of the subject being tested, and it is therefore necessary to compare the symptomatic with the asymptomatic side. Under normal circumstances the side-to-side latency difference should not exceed 2 ms,[11] although many laboratories prefer a 3-ms difference to be present before considering an F response abnormal. It is essential, however, that sufficient responses be recorded to ensure that the shortest response has been obtained before the F response is declared abnormal by these criteria. The F response has an advantage over EMG in that it becomes abnormal immediately after an injury has occurred. This means that the F response may be the only means of detecting a motor radiculopathy in the first 3 to 4 weeks before needle EMG abnormalities become evident. It has been estimated that changes in the F response may be the only electrodiagnostic abnormality in up to 15% of patients with radiculopathy. F response abnormalities have been reported to exist in up to 85% of myelographically confirmed cases of disc herniation.[13] F responses, however, are normal in purely sensory radiculopathies and do not differentiate between acute and chronic radiculopathies.

Bulbocavernosus Reflex.—Commonly utilized F responses and H reflexes are not able to measure conduction within the lower sacral nerve roots, cauda equina, and conus medullaris. In order to study these structures it is necessary to electrically elicit and measure the bulbocavernosus reflex. This

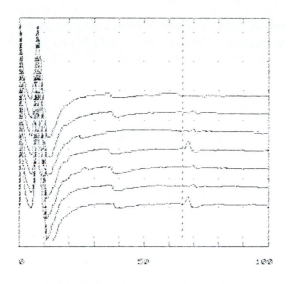
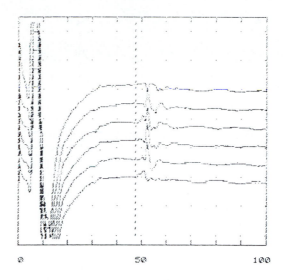

Left Posterior Tibial F response

Right Posterior Tibial F response

FIG 23–5.
F response from the posterior tibial nerve of a 55-year-old man with a well-defined left-sided radiculopathy (same patient as in Fig 23–3). The right side shows a normal F response.

reflex measures conduction within the pudendal nerve through its branches, the dorsal nerve of the penis or the clitoral nerves, which are sufficiently close to the surface for direct stimulation. This can be accomplished either bilaterally or unilaterally and a response is elicited over the pelvic floor muscle at a fixed latency of 28 to 42 ms.[9, 24, 25] Figure 23–6 illustrates the nature of this response and its presumed pathway.

Bulbocavernosus reflex abnormalities have been studied in patients with peripheral neuropathies and major cauda equina lesions.[24, 25, 47] Examples of unilateral abnormalities in cauda equina lesions have been noted (see Fig 23–7), but there has not, as yet, been any published large series of cases which demonstrate the sensitivity of this test in isolated sacral nerve root lesions.

Peripheral Nerve Conduction Studies

Motor and sensory nerve conduction studies do not measure radicular or spinal cord function directly. Nonetheless it is often necessary to carry out such studies in order to reach an accurate diagnosis of neurologic deficits in the extremities. These studies become important under specific circumstances. For example, the documentation of a generalized peripheral neuropathy can be very important in the differential diagnosis of neurologic findings in the lower extremities which may be confused with gait, reflex, and bladder changes associated with spinal

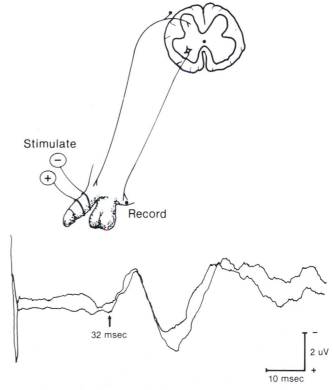

FIG 23–6.
The bulbocavernosus reflex response. Upper figure illustrates the location of stimulation and recording electrodes. The lower figure shows a typical response. (From Haldeman, S: *Spine* 1984; 9–1. Used by permission.)

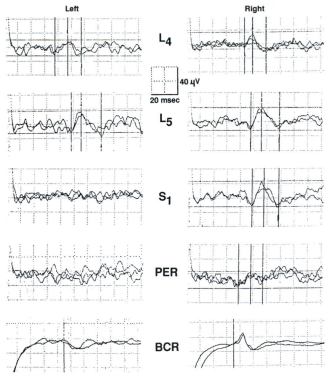

FIG 23-7.
Evoked potentials from the L4, L5, and S1 dermatomes, pudendal evoked potentials *(PER)*, and bulbocavernosus reflex *(BCR)*, from a 55-year-old man with unilateral cauda equina (polyradicular) syndrome affecting the S1-4 nerve roots. The L4 and L5 nerve roots are spared.

lesions. Peripheral neuropathies can cause abnormal reflex, motor, and sensory changes as well as abnormally prolonged F responses and H reflexes. When the neuropathy is severe, distal muscles may also demonstrate signs of denervation. The only way to confirm the presence of a peripheral neuropathy and, in many instances, explain specific clinical and electrodiagnostic findings is by performing routine nerve conduction studies.

Peripheral entrapment syndromes and direct nerve injuries can also be distinguished from radiculopathies by means of nerve conduction studies. For example, peroneal entrapment at the fibular head, causing weakness in dorsiflexion of the foot, may be difficult to distinguish from an L5 radiculopathy in the absence of specific nerve conduction studies. Tarsal tunnel syndrome may result in numbness in the foot similar to that caused by more proximal lesions and require plantar nerve conduction latencies for an adequate diagnosis.

Sensory nerve conduction in peripheral nerves also adds to the understanding of the nature of a sensory radiculopathy. Subjective sensory changes can occur as a result of either preganglionic or postganglionic radicular injury which can be differentiated using sensory conduction studies. Peripheral sensory nerve conduction studies would be normal in preganglionic lesions and abnormal in postganglionic lesions. For this reason it is becoming increasingly popular to measure peripheral sensory nerve conduction and somatosensory evoked responses at the same time.

Somatosensory Evoked Responses

The inability to detect purely sensory radiculopathies has been one of the major shortcomings of EMG and F response studies. H reflexes have been of some value for S1 sensory radiculopathies but of no value for other spinal nerve roots. The introduction of somatosensory evoked potentials has helped to correct this deficiency. Somatosensory evoked responses, in addition, allow for the evaluation of central pathways within the spinal cord and brain.

These responses can be recorded over the spine at virtually any level and over the scalp in the midline at the central electroencephalographic recording site. When evoked responses are recorded simultaneously over the T12 or L1 spinous processes and over the scalp, the differentiation between peripheral and central conduction times or velocities is possible. Because these responses have a very small amplitude it is necessary to utilize computer averaging of 200 to 500 responses in order to obtain a clean, well-defined recording with clearly marked and reproducible positive and negative peaks. The spinal evoked potential is typically a triphasic response with a prominent negative peak. This response has been postulated to be generated within the conus medullaris and the entering nerve roots.[10, 15, 41] The cortical evoked potential is a complex wave form with an initial positive peak which is felt to reflect potentials within the thalamocortical pathways.[7, 30] The central conduction time, which measures conduction within the dorsal column and brainstem pathways, is obtained by subtracting the latency of the spinal evoked response from the latency of the cortical evoked responses.

It is possible to stimulate a wide variety of lower extremity nerves and structures and elicit a somatosensory evoked response. Large mixed nerves, such as the peroneal and posterior tibial, were used in the initial research and are still the primary nerves used for studying spinal cord dorsal column function. Although it is very easy to obtain evoked responses on stimulation of these nerves, there is a disadvantage in that these are mixed nerves originating from more than one nerve root level. For this reason, the mixed nerve evoked response is commonly normal in single-level radiculopathies. Stimulation of pure sensory nerves, such as the saphenous, superficial peroneal, and sural nerves, is one method of reducing this disadvantage and increasing sensitivity. Another means of defining a specific nerve root is to stimulate areas of skin that are generally accepted as having a single dermatomal innervation. These dermatomal evoked responses are somewhat more difficult to obtain and are strongly influenced by any form of peripheral neuropathic process. Nonetheless, when comparisons are made between symptomatic and asymptomatic extremities, these responses hold the promise of defining a specific level of sensory radiculopathy (see Fig 23–7).

The recording of cortical responses on stimulation of the pudendal nerve, which carries fibers from the S2, S3, and S4 nerve roots, can be utilized to document suspected cauda equina or spinal cord lesions (see Fig 23–7). These tests are of particular value in cases of bowel, bladder, or sexual dysfunction.[24, 25]

Cortical Motor Evoked Responses

The development of a clinically useful magnetic stimulator by Barker et al. in 1985[1] has led to the investigation of cortically evoked motor responses in peripheral muscles as a means of studying spinal cord and nerve root injuries. This test is performed by discharging a stored electrical charge through a coil applied to the scalp, thus causing a magnetic field which penetrates the scalp to stimulate cortical neurons and dendrites. Recording is performed by means of surface electrodes over specific muscle groups in the upper or lower extremities. Eisen and Shtybel[14] have demonstrated abnormalities in these cortical evoked responses in patients with a number of neurologic diseases including myelopathies and plexopathies. In multiple sclerosis this test appears to be more sensitive than somatosensory evoked potentials which raises the possibility of increasing the neurodiagnostic sensitivity in other spinal cord or peripheral nerve lesions. This has been confirmed by Maertens de Noordhaut et al.[36] in a series of patients with cervical spondylosis or disc herniation in whom myelopathy was suspected or confirmed. They found a close correlation between clinical findings, radiologic studies, and motor evoked potential abnormalities. Furthermore, 22% of patients with cervical symptomatology without radiologic cord compression had abnormal findings which inferred that this test may measure root compression.

The possibility that cortical motor evoked potentials may be of value in patients with spinal stenosis has been raised by Wehling and Schulitz.[54] They report that these responses became abnormal after walking in patients with neurogenic claudication. This observation, however, will require further investigation before the usefulness of this test is determined in these patients.

Neurovisceral Studies

The potentially most serious and debilitating symptoms of both cauda equina syndrome and spinal cord stenosis is the disruption of neurogenic control of bowel and bladder and, to a lesser degree, sexual dysfunction. There are, however, many metabolic, psychological, and infectious causes of bladder, bowel, and sexual function abnormalities which, in patients with spinal stenosis, must be differentiated from neurogenic disturbances. Neurovisceral studies are used to document abnormalities in these organs and, when taken together with electrodiagnostic and clinical tests, offer some indication as to the cause of the symptoms.

Cystometry.—The measurement of pressure changes within the bladder during infusion of water or carbon dioxide remains the most widely used test for the diagnosis of a neurogenic bladder. The infusion of water or CO_2 as well as the measurement of bladder pressure is achieved by means of a catheter inserted into the bladder through the urethra. The normal response is a slow increase in pressure within the bladder until a critical volume is reached, at which point the patient gets the feeling of fullness. With further filling there is a reflex contraction of the bladder which increases the pressure and causes the urge to void. The normal person is then able to voluntarily suppress the urge to void and reduce the bladder pressure temporarily.

In the presence of a spinal cord lesion there is a disturbance in the normal connections between the brain and the reflex centers within the sacral spinal cord which serve the bladder. This results in loss of central inhibition to these centers. The cystometrogram reflects these changes by demonstrating a hyperactive bladder with a small filling volume and the inability to suppress reflex contractions voluntarily.

Cauda equina lesions, on the other hand, result in the inability of the bladder to contract. This results in a bladder with a very large capacity and an inability to generate reflex contractions. Continuous monitoring of bladder and urethral pressure may give additional information on the micturition reflex, but this is not widely used.[3, 4]

Colonometry.—The testing of bowel function in patients with spinal lesions has not gotten much attention in the literature. It is, however, possible to measure changes in bowel compliance in the same manner that cystometry measures bladder compliance. By measuring bowel pressure upon the infusion of tap water, it is possible to differentiate normal from hyperreflexic and hyporeflexic colonic contractions. It has been demonstrated that spinal cord injuries can cause colonic hyperreflexia whereas peripheral neuropathies (and presumably cauda equina lesions) can cause hyporeflexia in the colon.[21, 23]

Penile Tumescence.—Impotence and anorgasmia are common following spinal cord and cauda equina injuries. The primary testing procedure in male patients is the measurement of nocturnal penile tumescence (NPT) and rigidity.[32, 50] Loop strain gauges are placed around the base and tip of the penis in order to measure changes in penile diameter and firmness while the patient is asleep. Monitoring may be necessary for more than one night to ensure that rapid eye movement (REM) sleep, which is associated with NPT, has occurred. There are portable NPT measurement instruments available. However, the simultaneous recording of EEG and eye movement makes for a more accurate test.

CONCLUSION

The neurologic diagnosis of the mechanism of symptom production in patients with spinal stenosis requires an accurate history and physical examination together with the judicious use of electrophysiologic and neurophysiologic testing procedures. It should be possible, in most patients, through this process to determine whether spinal stenosis observed on imaging studies is responsible for pain, neurogenic claudication, radiculopathy, cauda equina syndrome, or myelopathy.

REFERENCES

1. Barker AT, Jalinous R, Freeston IL: Non-invasive magnetic stimulation of the human motor cortex. *Lancet* 1985; 1:1106–1107.
2. Baylan SP, Yu J, Grant AE: H reflex latency in relation to ankle jerk electromyographic, myelographic, and surgical findings in back pain patients. *Electromyogr Clin Neurophysiol* 1981; 21:201–210.
3. Bhatia NN, Bradley WE, Haldeman S, et al: Continuous monitoring of bladder and urethral pressure, a new technique. *Urology* 1981; 18:207–210.
4. Bhatia NN, Bradley WE, Haldeman S, et al: Continuous ambulatory urodynamic monitoring. *Br J Urol* 1982; 54:357–359.
5. Braddom RL, Johnson EW: Standardization of H reflex and diagnostic use in S1 radiculopathy. *Arch Phys Med Rehabil* 1976; 55:161–166.
6. Braddom RL, Johnson EW: H reflex: Review and classification with suggested clinical uses. *Arch Phys Med Rehabil* 1976; 55:412–417.
7. Cracco RQ: Spinal evoked response: Peripheral nerve stimulation in man. *Electroencephalogr Clin Neurophysiol* 1973; 35:379–386.
8. Deschuytere J, Rosselle N: Diagnostic use of monosynaptic reflexes in L5 and S1 root compression, in Desmedt JE (ed): *New Developments in Electromyography and Clinical Neurophysiology*. Basel, Karger, 1973, pp 360–366.
9. Dick HC, Bradley WE, Scott FB, et al: Pudendal sexual reflexes: Electrophysiologic investigations. *Urology* 1974; 3:376–379.
10. Dimitrijevic MR, Larsson LE, Lehmkuhl D, et al: Evoked spinal cord and nerve root potentials in humans using a noninvasive recording technique. *Electroencephalogr Clin Neurophysiol* 1978; 45:331–340.
11. Eisen A, Hoirch M: The electrodiagnostic evaluation of spinal root lesion. *Spine* 1983; 8:98–106.
12. Eisen A, Odusote K: Amplitude of the F-wave: A potential means of documenting spasticity. *Neurology* 1979; 29:1306–1309.
13. Eisen A, Schamer D, Melmed C: An electrophysiological method for examining lumbosacral root compression. *Can J Neurol Sci* 1977; 2:117–122.
14. Eisen A, Shtybel W: Experience with transcranial magnetic stimulation. *Muscle Nerve* 1990; 13:995–1011.
15. Feldman MH, Cracco RQ, Farmer P, et al: Spinal evoked potential in the monkey. *Ann Neurol* 1980; 7:238–244.
16. Fisher MA: *Physiology and Clinical Use of the F Response*. Minimonograph no. 13. Rochester, NY, American Association of Electromyography and Electrodiagnosis, 1980.
17. Fisher MA, Shivde AJ, Teixera C, et al: Clinical and electrophysiological appraisal of the significance of radicular injury in back pain. *J Neurol Neurosurg Psychiatry* 1978; 41:303–306.
18. Fisher MA, Shivde AJ, Teixera C, et al: The F-response—a clinically useful physiological parameter for the evaluation of a radicular injury. *Electromyogr Clin Neurophysiol* 1979; 19:65–75.
19. Gassell MM, Wisandanger M: Recurrent and reflex discharges in plantar muscles of the cat. *Acta Physiol Scand* 1965; 66:138–142.
20. Getty CJM: "Bony sciatica": The value of thermography, electromyography, and water-soluble myelography, in Spencer CW III (ed): *Clinics in Sports Medicine, vol 5: Injuries to the Spine*. Philadelphia, WB Saunders Co, 1986, pp 327–351.
21. Glick ME, Meshkinpour H, Haldeman S, et al: Co-

lonic dysfunction in patients with thoracic spinal cord injury. *Gastroenterology* 1984; 86:287–294.

22. Gough JG, Koepke GH: Electromyographic determination of motor root levels in erector spinae muscles. *Arch Phys Med Rehabil* 1966; 47:9–11.

23. Haldeman S, Bradley WE, Bhatia NN, et al: Neurologic evaluation of bladder, bowel and sexual disturbances in diabetic men, in Goto Y, Horiuchi A, Kogure K (eds): *Diabetic Neuropathy: Proceedings of the International Symposium on Diabetic Neuropathy and Its Treatment, Tokyo, September 1981.* Amsterdam, Excerpta Medica, 1982, pp 298–301.

24. Haldeman S, Bradley W, Bhatia N, et al: Pudendal evoked responses in neurologic disease. *Neurology* 1982; 32:A67.

25. Haldeman S, Bradley WE, Bhatia NN, et al: Pudendal evoked responses. *Arch Neurol* 1982; 39:280–283.

26. Hoffman P: Untersuchungen über die Eigenreflexe (Sehnerreflexe) menschlicher Muskeln. Berlin, Springer, 1922.

27. Hoover BB, Caldwell JW, Krusen EM, et al: Value of polyphasic potentials in diagnosis of lumbar root lesions. *Arch Phys Med Rehabil* 1970; 51:546.

28. Jacobson RE: Lumbar stenosis. An electromyographic evaluation. *Clin Orthop* 1976; 115:68–71.

29. Johnson EW, Melvin JL: Value of electromyography in lumbar radiculopathy. *Arch Phys Med Rehabil* 1971; 52:239–243.

30. Jones SJ, Small DG: Spinal and subcortical evoked potentials following stimulation of the posterior tibial nerve in man. *Electroencephalogr Clin Neurophysiol* 1978; 44:299–306.

31. Jonsson B: Morphology, innervation, and electromyographic study of the erector spinae. *Arch Phys Med Rehabil* 1969; 50:638–641.

32. Karacan I, Solis PJ, Williams RL: The role of the sleep laboratory in the diagnosis of and treatment of impotence, in Williams RL, Karacan I, Frazier SH (eds): *Sleep Disorders: Diagnosis and Treatment.* New York, John Wiley & Sons, 1978.

33. Kimura J: *Electrodiagnosis in Diseases of Nerve and Muscle: Principles and Practice.* Philadelphia, FA Davis Co, 1983.

34. Knutsson B: Comparative value of electromyographic, myelographic, and clinical-neurological examination in diagnosis of lumbar root compression syndrome. *Acta Orthop Scand [Suppl]* 1961; 49:1–135.

35. Lane MD, Tamhankar MN, Demopoulos JT: Discogenic radiculopathy. Use of electromyography in multidisciplinary management. *NY State J Med* 1978; 32–36.

36. Maertens de Noorthout A, Remache JM, Pepin JL, et al: Magnetic stimulation of the motor cortex in cervical spondylosis. *Neurology* 1991; 41:75–80.

37. Magladery JW, McDougal DB: Electrophysiological studies of nerve and reflex activity in normal man. Identification of certain reflexes in electromyogram and conduction velocity of peripheral nerve fibers. *Bull Johns Hopkins Hosp* 1950; 86:265–290.

38. Malcolm DS: A method of measuring reflex times applied in sciatica and other conditions due to nerve root compression. *J Neurol Neurosurg Psychiatry* 1951; 14:15–24.

39. McLoed JG, Wary SH: An experimental study of the F wave in the baboon. *J Neurol Neurosurg Psychiatry* 1966; 29:196–200.

40. Pedersen HE, Blunck CJF, Gardner E: The anatomy of lumbosacral posterior rami and meningeal branches of spinal nerves (sinu-vertebral nerves). *J Bone Joint Surg [Am]* 1956; 38:277–291.

41. Phillips LH, Daube JR: Lumbosacral spinal evoked potentials in humans. *Neurology* 1980; 30:1175–1183.

42. Postacchini F: Lumbar spinal stenosis. Classification and treatment, in JW Weinstein, SW Weisel (eds): *The Lumbar Spine.* Philadelphia, WB Saunders Co, 1990, pp 594–611.

43. Schenck E: Untersuchungen über die Hemmungsphase nach einem 2-Neuronen-(Eigen) Reflex beim Menschen. *Pflugers Arch* 1951; 253:286–300.

44. Schuchmann JA: H reflex latency in radiculopathy. *Arch Phys Med Rehabil* 1978; 59:185–187.

45. Seppalainen AM, Alaranta H, Saini J: Electromyography in the diagnosis of lumbar spinal stenosis. *Electromyogr Clin Neurophysiol* 1981; 21:55–66.

46. Shea P, Woods W, Werden D: Electromyography in diagnosis of nerve root compression syndrome. *Arch Neurol Psychiatry* 1950; 64:93–104.

47. Siroky MB, Sax DS, Krane RS: Sacral signal tracing: The electrophysiology of the bulbocavernosus reflex. *J Urol* 1979; 122:661–664.

48. Skaggs H: *Guidelines in EMG. Professional Standards Committee.* Rochester, NY, American Association of Electromyography and Electrodiagnosis, 1979.

49. Tonzola RF, Ackil AA, Shahani BT, et al: Usefulness of electrophysiological studies in the diagnosis of lumbosacral root disease. *Ann Neurol* 1981; 9:305–308.

50. Torrens MJ: Neurologic and neurosurgical disorder associated with impotence, in Krane RJ, Siroky MB, Goldstein I (eds): *Male Sexual Dysfunction.* Boston, Little, Brown & Co, 1983, pp 32–48.

51. Verbiest H: Neurogenic intermittent claudication. Lesions of the spinal cord and cauda equina, stenosis of the vertebral canal, narrowing of intervertebral foramina and entrapment of peripheral nerves, in Vinken PJ, Bruyn GW (eds): *Handbook of Clinical Neurology,* vol 20, pt 2. New York, North Holland/Elsevier, 1976, pp 611–807.

52. Verbiest H: Stenosis of the lumbar vertebral canal and sciatica. *Neurosurg Rev* 1980; 3:75–89.

53. Verbiest H: Lumbar spinal stenosis. Morphology, classification and long-term results, in Weinstein JW, Wiesel SW (eds): *The Lumbar Spine.* Philadelphia, WB Saunders Co, 1990, pp 546–589.

54. Wehling P, Schulitz KP: The role of motor evoked potentials in the diagnosis of lumbosacral radiculopathies, in *Proceedings of the International Society for the Study of the Lumbar Spine,* Boston, June 13–17, 1990, p 26.

55. Wise CS, Ardizzone I: Electromyography in the intervertebral disc protrusions. *Arch Phys Med Rehabil* 1954; 35:442–446.

24

Radionuclide Studies in Spinal Stenosis

Amjad Ali, M.D.
Andrew S. Rosenson, M.D.
Ernest W. Fordham, M.D.

Radionuclide studies (bone scintigraphy, gallium citrate, and indium 111 leukocyte scans) play an important role in the evaluation of patients with a variety of orthopaedic disorders.[10] Evaluation of the skeleton as a source of pain is an important indication for skeletal imaging, particularly in patients who have signs and symptoms that do not point to a specific diagnosis or who have normal or inconclusive laboratory and radiographic studies.[34, 36] The bone scan is extremely sensitive for detection of skeletal abnormalities. It is a screening test that allows evaluation of both the axial and appendicular skeleton. It can effectively demonstrate whether a bone or joint is responsible for the patient's symptom. The etiology of the disease process can be identified if the pattern of involvement is sufficiently characteristic to permit recognition.[6] If not, a positive bone scan still pinpoints the involved bone or joint, and more specific laboratory and radiographic evaluation of the lesion can be undertaken.[67]Ga and ^{111}In leukocyte studies are very useful in evaluating patients with suspected bone or soft tissue infection. [111]In leukocyte studies, however, are considered more sensitive and specific than ^{67}Ga scans in patients with acute infections.[32, 36] Before we look at the roles of these scans in the management of patients with spinal canal stenosis, let us briefly review the basic concepts and technical considerations which are important in understanding and interpreting these studies.

BONE SCINTIGRAPHY

The available bone-seeking pharmaceuticals are analogs of calcium, the hydroxyl(OH) group, or phosphates. Sodium flouride (F18), which replaces a hydroxyl group to form fluroapatite, was a popular bone scanning agent in the late 1960s and early 1970s. The images were obtained with rectilinear scanners. The image quality represented considerable improvement over those obtained with the calcium analogs strontium 85 and strontium 87m.[7] However, modern high resolution gamma camera detectors do not have sodium iodide crystals thick enough to efficiently interact with high energy photons (511 keV) of NaF F18. Technetium 99m emits low energy (140 keV) photons which interact efficiently with the thin crystal available in most gamma cameras. Condensed phosphates and diphosphonates are easily tagged with ^{99m}Tc. At present, technetium-labeled diphosphonate, particularly methylene diphosphonate (MDP) and hydroxymethylene diphosphonate (HMDP), are the radiopharmaceuticals of choice for bone imaging. These agents localize in bone mineral matrix by a poorly understood mechanism of "chemisorption." The blood supply to the bone and rate of bone turnover are considered two of the most important factors in determining the amount of radiopharmaceutical uptake in any given bone (normal or abnormal).[36] The usual scanning dose of ^{99m}Tc-labeled phosphonates is 20 to 25 mCi in the adult. The pediatric dose is calculated according to body weight, with a minimum of 2.5 mCi. About 50% of the injected radiopharmaceutical localizes in bone; the rest is rapidly cleared from the blood pool, mainly through the kidneys, in the first few hours. Images of excellent quality with a good target-to-nontarget ratio can be obtained at 2 to 4 hours post-injection in most patients with normal cardiac and renal function. In patients with congestive heart failure or renal insufficiency, images should be delayed for an additional 2 to 3 hours to achieve a better target-to-nontarget ratio. The images are obtained in a total body format in the anteroposterior projection using gamma cameras with a large field or extrawide field of view. Recent im-

provements and advances in instrumentation have contributed to the superior quality of bone images. Spot images of selected regions or suspicious lesions should be taken using high resolution or a pinhole collimator at appropriate angles to obtain better detail and pinpoint anatomic localization of the lesion(s).

The introduction of single photon emission computed tomography (SPECT) has added a new dimension to bone imaging (Figs 24–1 through 24–7).[3] A rotating gamma camera acquires multiple images in a 360-degree orbit around the patient. These projection data are backprojected, and transaxial, coronal, and sagittal images are then reconstructed using sophisticated computer programs and algorithms, similar to those used for computed tomography (CT)

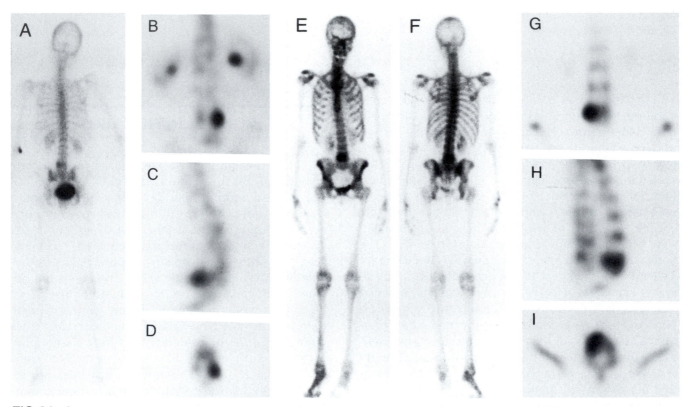

FIG 24–1.
These cases, involving patients with low back pain and right-sided lesions at L5–S1, demonstrate the anatomic information available with SPECT imaging. The small lesion seen on the posterior planar scan **(A)** of the first patient is positioned at the expected position of the posterior facet. This is convincingly confirmed by selected coronal **(B)**, sagittal **(C)**, and axial **(D)** tomographic planes generated by SPECT imaging. This type of degenerative abnormality is probably the most common lesion seen in patients with low back pain. Anterior **(E)** and posterior **(F)** planar whole-body sweeps of the second patient demonstrate a fairly striking (if less than sharply defined) productive, degenerative lesion involving the right side of L5; equal visualization on both views indicates that this lesion probably involves the vertebral body rather than the posterior elements. Coronal **(G)**, sagittal **(H)** and, particularly, axial **(I)** tomographic cuts generated by SPECT imaging clearly place the lesion along the lateral margin of the vertebral body. The intensity of this lesion indicates that the degenerative process responsible for the lesion and the patient's pain is currently in a very active phase. Note that the generalized osseous flush involving the entire right lower extremity implies, in addition, encroachment on nerves to produce this neurogenically elicited arterial response.

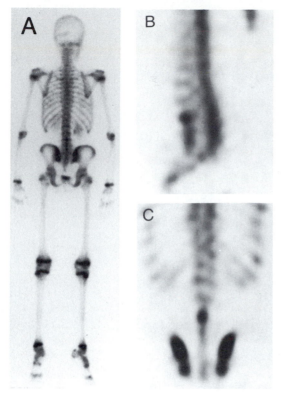

FIG 24–2.
This case, involving a 12-year-old boy with debilitating low back pain, sharply demonstrates the enhancement of both anatomic detail and increased contrast inherent to SPECT imaging. The posterior planar whole-body sweep **(A)** is normal. In retrospect one can just appreciate slight enhancement of the spinous process of L3. Note the striking definition and precise placement of the lesion in the base of the spinous process of L3 on selected sagittal **(B)** and coronal **(C)** tomographic planes. This lesion proved to be an osteoid osteoma, inapparent on plain radiographs and even difficult to appreciate on CT.

scans. These multiplanar tomographic images offer greater image contrast and more information when compared with the planar images. The anatomic location of the lesion within the bone can be more accurately determined. For example, with respect to spine pathology, the lesion can be localized to the vertebral body, neural arches, or spinous process (Figs 24–1 and 24–2). Several studies have shown improved sensitivity of skeletal SPECT over planar scintigraphy in evaluating pathologic changes in the temporomandibular joint, vertebral column, hip joints, and knee joints. However, because of the time required for acquisition and processing of SPECT data, it is neither possible nor practical to examine the whole body with this technique. It is, therefore, appropriate to limit this technique to sites that are symptomatic or suspicious on planar scintigraphy. It should also be noted that bone scanning does not compete with anatomic studies of x-ray tomography, CT, and magnetic resonance imaging (MRI), but plays a complementary role.

Radiation Dosimetry

The urinary bladder is the critical organ for intravenously administered ^{99m}Tc-labeled diphosphonate. Hydration of the patient and frequent voiding significantly reduce the radiation dose to the bladder and gonads. With frequent voiding, the radiation dose to the bladder is about 130 mrad/mCi. The ovarian and testicular radiation dose is estimated to be 12 mrad/mCi and 8 mrad/mCi, respectively. The total whole-body exposure is less than 500 mrad in adults. It is 49 mrad/mCi in a 1-year-old child and 21 mrad/mCi at age 10.[2] There is no evidence of any adverse biological effects from administration of bone-seeking radiopharmaceuticals in the commonly employed doses. Rare reports of allergic reactions to these radiopharmaceuticals have been mentioned in the literature.

GALLIUM SCAN

Gallium scans can be used as an adjunct to bone scintigraphy in the detection of ongoing infection. ^{67}Ga localization in inflammatory lesions is mediated in some way through the action of neutrophilic leukocytes. ^{67}Ga accumulation in a lesion is enhanced by increased blood supply and the "leaky" endothelium usually associated with an inflammatory process.[13] Tsan et al. have shown that ^{67}Ga may also be taken up directly by many microorganisms.[38] Serum transferrin, lactoferrin, and lysozymes also play variable roles in uptake of ^{67}Ga by the lesions. The usual dose of ^{67}Ga for detection of inflammatory lesions in adults is 3 to 5 mCi. The pediatric dose is 30 to 50 μCi/kg body weight. The patients are imaged in a total body format in the anteroposterior projection using a large field-of-view gamma camera fitted with a medium energy collimator. Spot images of the suspicious areas should be obtained in appropriate projections. The imaging is usually done at 48 to 72 hours post-^{67}Ga injection. Some amount of injected ^{67}Ga is normally excreted by the gastrointestinal tract. Use of laxatives, enemas, or serial abdominal imaging is considered

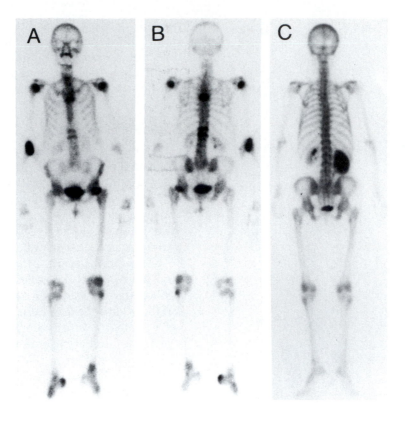

FIG 24–3.

Low back pain can originate from disease unrelated to the lumbar spine and associated structures. Radiographs had already demonstrated the vertebral compression at T6, T12, and L1 seen on anterior **(A)** and posterior **(B)** planar whole-body scans of this arthritic patient who had fallen several weeks previously. Clinical concern for additional disease, inapparent radiographically, aroused by low back pain not satisfactorily explained by the higher lesions, called for the bone scan which clearly demonstrates the left femoral neck fracture. This is not an uncommon experience in the nuclear medicine laboratory. Renal disease is also a common source of low back pain as demonstrated by the posterior whole-body sweep **(C)** showing a normal skeleton but a striking hydronephrosis of the right kidney. In a 25-year experience we have collected over a thousand cases of clinically unsuspected renal disease producing low back pain which led to skeletal scintigraphy.

helpful in differentiating mobile bowel activity from stationary activity in an inflammatory or neoplastic process in the abdomen. Scanning as early as 6 to 8 hours post-^{67}Ga injection can detect lesions, if target-to-nontarget ratios are high enough. However, most lesions are far better imaged at 48 or 72 hours. Renal activity persisting beyond 24 hours postinjection is indicative of renal disease such as pyelonephritis, tubular necrosis, abscess, etc. Evaluation of infection in injured (fracture, postsurgical) bone may be aided by comparing the relative uptake intensities and spatial distribution of ^{67}Ga and bone-seeking ^{99m}Tc-diphosphonate. The diagnosis of osteomyelitis is usually made if ^{67}Ga uptake in the lesion has a different distribution pattern or is of equal or greater relative intensity than the lesion seen on the ^{99m}Tc diphosphonate scan.[14] It should be noted that ^{67}Ga is a nonspecific disease finder since it localizes in septic and sterile inflammatory tissues, as well as in neoplasm.

Radiation Dosimetry

The total body radiation dose is calculated at 0.26 rad/mCi. The gastrointestinal tract is the critical organ. The large intestine receives about 0.9 rad/mCi. The radiation dose to ovaries is about 0.28 rad/mCi and to testicles, 0.24 rad/mCi.[12]

INDIUM LEUKOCYTE SCANS

Leukocytes accumulate at sites of infection and inflammation in the body and play an important role

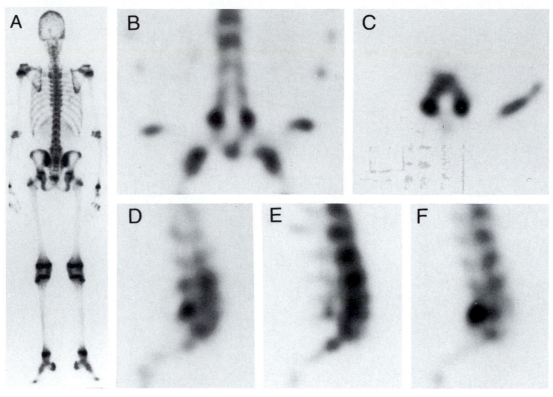

FIG 24–4.
Despite the lack of clear-cut lesions on the posterior whole-body planar sweep **(A)** of this young man with severe low back pain, bilateral disease at L–5 should be suspected because of the abrupt change in character in the posterolateral configuration of L–5 as compared with the segments above. Symmetric, paired lesions, lateral to the "cold hole" of the spinal canal are distinctly defined by the contrast-enhancing quality of SPECT imaging on coronal **(B)** and axial **(C)** images. The dual nature of the abnormality is also clearly defined on the sagittal planes: lesions are seen on two lateral planes **(D and F)** flanking the midline plane **(E)** through vertebrae proper which are free of lesions. The site of the lesions corresponds nicely with radiographically demonstrable spondylolysis; the activity seen scintigraphically implies an active reparative response by bone, which, in turn, implies current stress involving bone—stress that is probably responsible for the symptom of pain.

in the body defense mechanism by their chemotactic, phagocytic, and microbial destructive functions. After a small amount of leukocytes are labeled with gamma-emitting radioisotopes and reinjected, their distribution in the body can be imaged by a gamma camera. Increased accumulation of these leukocytes will be found at sites of active inflammation and infection. Several isotopes can be used to label leukocytes. At present, ^{111}In oxine is the most widely used radiopharmaceutical for leukocyte labeling. About 40 to 50 mL of the patient's blood is drawn in a syringe containing a small amount of anticoagulant. The white blood cells are separated from other blood components and labeled with 500 µCi of ^{111}In oxine and reinjected into the patient intravenously.[20] Total body images are obtained in the anterior and posterior projection at 4 and 24 hours postinjection using a large field-of-view gamma camera fitted with a medium energy collimator. Spot images of suspicious lesions are obtained in appropriate projections. Focal or diffusely increased uptake is noted at sites of infection and inflammation. The intensity of the uptake is proportional to the activity of the inflammatory process. The sensitivity, specificity, and overall accuracy of the test for detecting acute osteomyelitis is reported to be above 85% to 90% in various series.[11] The specificity is slightly lower as ^{111}In also accumulates in sterile inflammatory lesions and necrotic regions of tumors.[21] Several studies have shown ^{111}In leukocyte studies to be superior to sequential ^{99m}Tc diphosphonate and ^{67}Ga scanning in the diagnosis of acute and chronic osteomyelitis.[11, 24] If clinical suspicion of osteomyelitis is fairly high and if bone scans are negative, then in-

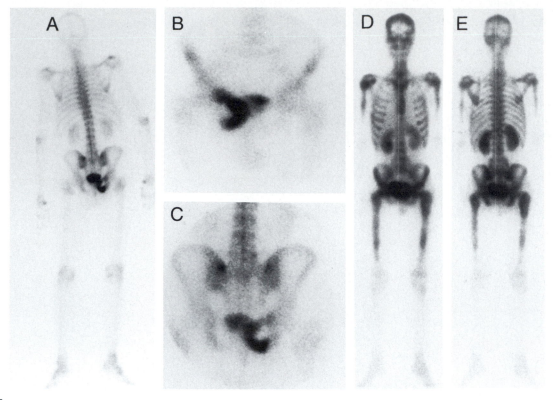

FIG 24–5.
Unsuspected metastatic tumor is not uncommonly responsible for pain, particularly low back pain. Low back pain, rather than symptoms related to pubic bones, brought this patient with unsuspected prostatic cancer to skeletal scintigraphy. Local pelvic disease, in this case **(A–C)** limited to the right pubis and ischium, is typical of regional prostatic metastases. Additional spot scintigrams **(B,** anterior; **C,** posterior) with bladder emptied following the standard whole-body planar sweep **(A)** demonstrate the lesion to advantage and confirm the second lesion in the superior aspect of the left sacroiliac joint. Note the subtle focal asymmetry in the lateral aspect of L5 on the posterior spot film **(C)** which may herald the appearance of yet another lesion. Even more striking are the anterior **(D)** and posterior **(E)** whole-body sweeps of a 24-year-old man with low back pain following an automobile accident. Persistence of the pain resulted in studies leading to removal of a low lumbar "disc" which did not alleviate the pain. After several months of unremitting pain the bone scan was obtained. Strikingly increased uptake is present throughout the entire axial skeleton and the proximal portions of the humeri and, particularly, the femora in a pattern pathognomonic for diffuse, coalescing metastatic tumor. Extensive radiography demonstrated abnormality only in the greater trochanter of the left femur with permeative changes. Biopsy yielded Ewing's sarcoma. Note the widening of the lower lumbar segments typical of fusion. Note also the subtle flush involving the left lower extremity, implying neurologic disturbance.

dium leukocyte scanning should always be considered. [111]In studies are also superior to gallium scans in evaluating possible infection at sites of recent surgery.

Radiation Dosimetry

The radiation exposure is high but acceptable in specific clinical situations. The spleen is the critical organ and receives about 6 to 18 rad/mCi. The whole-body absorbed radiation dose is about 0.5 rad/mCi.[20]

RADIONUCLIDE STUDIES IN MANAGEMENT OF SPINAL STENOSIS

There are many causes of spinal stenosis ranging from the congenital lesion in a newborn to degenerative diseases of older people. Similarly, patients' presenting complaints may include a wide spectrum of symptoms. Most patients have pain, radiculopathies, or muscle weakness. The clinical diagnosis can

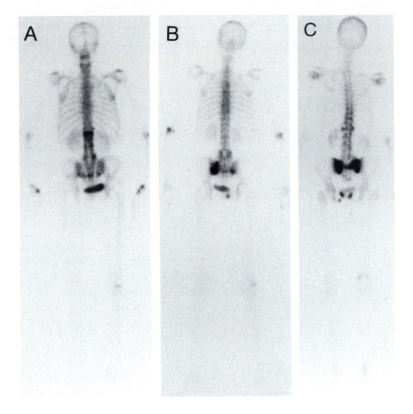

FIG 24–6.
Next to a bone infarct, the significant lesion most commonly missed radiographically, but which is clearly demonstrable by skeletal scintigraphy, is the sacral fracture. Patient **A** has cause enough for low back pain: a compression fracture at L1 and paired lesions at L3, L4, and L5–S1 which are typical of degenerative disease at the posterior facets (additional paired degenerative disease can be seen at two levels in the cervical spine). The row of lesions across the free border of the sacrum is pathognomonic of sacral fracture, typically painful while sitting down. Patient **B,** with the widened appearance of lower lumbar segments typical of fusion, and with uncomplicated hip prostheses, demonstrates a less-than-typical pelvic fracture. The left sacroiliac (SI) joint separation, in conjunction with lesions through the opposite obturator foramen, satisfy the requirement that a ring be broken in at least two places. The smaller lesion at the lower margin of the opposite (right) SI joint raises the question of another sacral free border fracture. Patient **C** demonstrates the classic H-shaped fracture involving both SI joints and across the fixed portion of the sacrum which is particularly painful with any weight-bearing. The scan also identifies lesions involving both obturator foramina, implying multiple fractures through the pelvic ring.

be difficult to establish and the differential diagnosis can be extensive. Once the diagnosis is suspected, high resolution imaging techniques are necessary to document the narrowing of the spinal canal and lateral recesses and the impingement on neural tissue. Radionuclide bone scans, which are extremely sensitive in demonstrating metabolic changes of a focal or diffuse nature in many skeletal disorders, do not have resolution sufficient to document anatomic narrowing of the canal or lateral recess. Even on SPECT images, which provide enough detail to identify the spinal canal in transverse and sagittal sections, one cannot appreciate changes in the dimension of the spinal canal to make a diagnosis of spinal canal stenosis with any degree of confidence. Moreover, any "hot" lesion in the posterior aspect of the vertebral body or along the neural arches will give a false impression of narrowing of the canal, as the scintigraphically hot lesion appears larger than it really is. There is, therefore, no role for bone imaging, planar scintigraphy, or SPECT in establishing the anatomic diagnosis of spinal canal stenosis. CT, MRI, and myelograms are considered the studies of choice in the initial workup and documentation of the diagnosis. These modalities are discussed in Chapters 19 through 22.

What is the role, then, of the bone scan in the management of patients with spinal stenosis? It is quite possible that in some patients with a presumptive or even confirmed diagnosis of spinal canal ste-

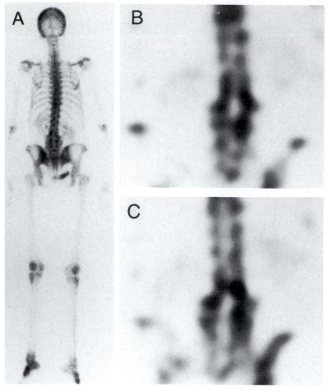

FIG 24–7.
The posterior planar whole-body sweep **(A)** of this patient with recurrent pain postlaminectomy clearly demonstrates the loss of spinous processes related to laminectomy and the apparent widening of the spinal column related to fusion. However, no focus for explaining the patient's pain was found until SPECT imaging was performed. Coronal planes **(B,C)** demonstrate extensive changes along the fusion, pinpointing, at the upper margin on the left side, a more focally intense lesion at the site of pseudarthrosis.

nosis, low back pain or referred pain in the lower extremity may be the result of some other disease process. In view of the age group of patients affected with spinal canal stenosis, it is important to rule out other causes of low back pain such as renal disease, vascular insufficiency, osteomyelitis, fracture, metastatic disease, and reflex sympathetic dystrophy.[23] Bone scintigraphy can be very helpful and cost-effective in evaluating some of these possibilities. Radionuclide bone scans can be very helpful in verifying the clinical significance of questionable vertebral or discovertebral abnormalities on plain radiographs. The bone scan will be positive if the questionable lesion seen on the plain film is metabolically active, which may explain the patient's symptoms. For example, radiographs of the lumbar spine show defects in the pars interarticularis in patients with spondylolysis and spondy-

lolisthesis. These defects usually appear normal on bone scintigraphy in asymptomatic patients. However, if spondylolysis or spondylolisthesis is producing low back pain as the result of recent injury or continued bone stress, the bone scan will demonstrate focal increased uptake at these defects (Fig 24–4).[4, 5] In patients with unstable and painful spondylolysis, the bone scan will also disclose focal increased uptake on the contralateral side of the pars defect owing to stress on that side of the vertebra.

Metastatic Disease

Bone scans are extremely sensitive in evaluating the possibility of bony metastasis. Less than 5% of bone scans are normal with radiographically apparent metastatic disease, while 10% to 40% of patients with skeletal metastasis have normal radiographs in the face of an abnormal bone scan.[31, 36] Metastatic disease produces a fairly typical pattern of randomly distributed focal lesions in the axial and peripheral skeleton which are easily recognized on total body or spot bone scintigraphy (Fig 24–5). Moreover, metastatic disease is still high in the differential diagnosis if a solitary focal lesions is noted in the axial skeleton, particularly the vertebral body or neural arch of the spine. Further evaluation of such lesions is then undertaken by CT, MRI, or bone biopsy. The exact location of the lesion can be marked on the skin under the gamma camera or the lesion can be stained with methylene blue under gamma camera monitoring to be followed by open biopsy of the marked bone.[17]

Paget's Disease

In some patients with Paget's disease of bone, structural deformities of the involved vertebra can cause narrowing of the spinal canal and may produce a variety of neurologic syndromes due to mechanical impingement and ischemia of nervous tissue caused by the diversion of blood into hyperemic areas of involved bone.[39] Involvement of bones most likely to cause nerve impingement (base of the skull, sacrum) is seen better on the bone scan than on the radiograph. Surgical decompression will be necessary in catastrophic and rapidly developing cases. Recent reports indicate successful treatment of Paget's disease and reversal of neurologic symptoms (pain, muscle weakness, etc.), if high-dose calcitonin therapy is started in the "premyeloneuropathic" or early stages of the neurologic syndrome.[3] A baseline bone scan in such cases would show mono- or poly-ostotic distribution of the disease. The intensity of the lesion would demonstrate the activity of the disease process. Changes in the intensity of the lesions on the serial bone scans, along with other biochemical parameters, would provide objective evidence of the true status of disease activity and the effectiveness of medical therapy.[35]

Osteomyelitis

If there is a suspicion of osteomyelitis of the spine or sacroiliac joint causing low back pain in a patient with spinal canal stenosis, then radionuclide studies provide useful clinical information. It is well known that plain radiographs are relatively insensitive in detecting the early changes of osteomyelitis.[25, 26, 36] ^{99m}Tc diphosphonate bone scans have been reported to be positive as early as 2 days after onset of the disease. The sensitivity of bone scans for detecting osteomyelitis in a nonviolated bone is about 90%.[36] The scans are also helpful in detecting unsuspected secondary sites of disease which occur in about 20% of patients with hematogenous spread of disease.[14] A positive ^{67}Ga scan increases the specificity of a bone scan finding and may increase the sensitivity slightly. Even higher sensitivity and specificity has been reported with the use of ^{111}In leukocyte studies in patients with osteomyelitis.[24, 26, 32, 36] The recommended approach is that a workup begin with plain radiographs of suspected bone and ^{99m}Tc bone scans. If the diagnosis is not clear, then a ^{67}Ga or ^{111}In leukocyte study, or both, should be performed. Negative bone and ^{67}Ga or ^{111}In leukocyte scans would effectively exclude the possibility of acute osteomyelitis.[16, 36] The combination of bone and ^{67}Ga scans may not be very helpful in confirming the diagnosis of acute osteomyelitis in a spine recently operated on (laminectomy with or without fusion). Increased uptake of these agents is present in the immediate postoperative phase owing to the healing process. However, certain patterns of uptake may favor the diagnosis of osteomyelitis. These include greater intensity, or different spatial distribution, of ^{67}Ga in the lesion when compared with the lesion seen on the ^{99m}Tc MDP bone scan. In patients with recent bone trauma, ^{111}In leukocyte studies are reported to be more sensitive than ^{67}Ga scans in evaluating the possibility of osteomyelitis in patients with existing bone trauma.[36]

Disc space infection often presents a difficult diagnostic problem in the differential diagnosis of low back pain, including patients presenting with steno-sis-type symptoms. The radiographic features of disc space infections are distinctive and fairly specific but may not appear for 2 to 8 weeks after onset of symptoms.[1] A study from the Mayo Clinic has reported ^{67}Ga scanning to be a useful noninvasive test in establishing the diagnosis of disc space infection in suspect clinical situations. They reported that ^{67}Ga scans become positive very early in the disease and carry a sensitivity of 89%, a specificity of 85%, and an accuracy of 86%.[1]

Degenerative Joint Disease

Skeletal imaging is not essential in the evaluation of patients with spinal canal stenosis secondary to degenerative joint disease. Longstanding disease showing extensive osteophytes and bridging of the disc spaces on radiographs may produce very little change on the bone scan. When positive, bone scans demonstrate low-grade unilateral or bilateral focal uptake at the posterior facet joints. The details, of course, are better seen on SPECT studies. However, unilateral uptake causes problems in the differential diagnosis, particularly in patients suspected to have malignancy. Since intensity of uptake usually reflects activity of the disease, a total body bone scan is an easy way of pictorially documenting the extent and relative severity of disease in the spine and extremities. In selected patients, serial bone scanning at appropriate intervals can be very helpful in long-term follow-up of the disease and in evaluating the effect of therapy.[8]

Fractures

Fractures of the spine, pelvic bone, or femoral neck may present difficulty in the differential diagnosis of low back pain in some patients with spinal canal stenosis, particularly those with coexisting osteoporosis which can produce fractures with minimal or no trauma (see Fig 24–3). It has been demonstrated that sacral fracture sometimes produces neurologic damage due to compression of nerve roots.[2, 29] Compression of the S1–2 nerve roots may produce symptoms of radiculopathy which may be difficult to distinguish clinically from herniation of the L5–S1 intervertebral disc. Evaluating the possibility of a recent fracture of the spine or pelvic bones in patients with spinal canal stenosis is another situation in which radionuclide studies can be very helpful, if radiographs are inconclusive (Fig 24–6). Several recent studies have indicated that stress fractures may not be evident on plain radiographs for about 10 to 12 days after the injury.[19, 36] Similarly, insufficiency fractures also present difficulty in diagnosis, as some of these fractures are negative on the radiograph and in some cases, changes are so subtle on the plain films that diagnosis of fracture cannot be established with any degree of confidence.[29, 33] Matin[19] has shown that 95% of the fractures in patients under the age of 65 years show increased activity on bone scintigraphy at the fracture site within 3 days of injury. It may take about 7 to 10 days for a fracture to show up on bone scans in patients above the age of 65 years.[19] A negative bone scan (at 7–10 days) would effectively exclude the possibility of a recent fracture. Stress fractures of the spine, pelvic bones, or femoral neck demonstrate focal areas of increased activity at the fracture site. Fatigue fractures of the sacrum present a characteristic H-shaped area of increased uptake on the bone scan with horizontal uptake across the mid- or lower portion of the sacrum and vertical increased activity in one or both alae of the sacrum.[29, 33] According to some authors, this pattern is so diagnostic of a traumatic lesion of the sacrum that further workup to confirm the diagnosis, such as tomography, CT scan, etc., may not be necessary.[29, 33] The pattern is easily differentiated from metastatic disease of the sacrum which usually presents with multiple randomly distributed focal areas of increased uptake. Insufficiency fractures of pelvic bone usually show vertical lesions through the pubic rami and sacroiliac joints. As these fractures heal, the bone scan gradually returns to normal in several months, unless there is some complication.

Painful Pseudarthrosis

Laminectomy, with or without spinal fusion, is a commonly performed surgical procedure for relief of pain in patients with spinal canal stenosis. The success rates of these procedures are reported in Chapters 27 and 33. Persistent back pain postoperatively or a "failed back syndrome" is, unfortunately, seen in some patients.[9, 18, 27] Several diagnostic procedures such as plain radiographs, tomograms, CT scans, and myelograms are done to determine the cause of persistent back pain.

Pseudarthrosis of a "fused" segment is believed to be a common cause of "failed back syndrome." It is very difficult to establish the diagnosis of painful pseudarthrosis using only clinical and radiographic criteria.[30, 37] Surgical exploration is considered the most reliable method of confirming this diagnosis.[22] Chronic stress at the bony margins of the pseudar-

throsis produces an osteoblastic response. This results in increased uptake of bone-seeking radiopharmaceutical. However, these lesions are difficult to appreciate on conventional planar bone scintigraphy owing to superimposition of radioactivity from the spine and surrounding spinal fusion mass. These lesions are easily detected on multiplanar SPECT images, in which superimposition of activity from adjacent planes is not a major problem (Fig 24–7). Recent studies have suggested that SPECT imaging of the spine can be very helpful in the postoperative evaluation of symptomatic patients.[22, 37] Slizofski et al. have reported bone scintigraphy to have a sensitivity of 78% and specificity of 83% in detecting sites of painful pseudarthrosis.[37] However, there are certain limitations: focal increased uptake may be present at sites of painless pseudarthrosis and the bone scans may not be very helpful in the first 6 months after surgery, since considerable increased uptake is usually noted at laminectomy and fusion sites during the healing phase.

Renal Abnormalities

Renal disease such as hydronephrosis, pyleonephritis, tumor, etc. can produce back pain. On some occasions, these processes may cause difficulty in the differential diagnosis of patients with suspected or confirmed spinal canal stenosis. Excretory urography, ultrasound, and CT examination of the abdomen are routinely employed in the workup of renal lesions. Radionuclide renal imaging with various radiopharmaceuticals provides functional information such as the status of renal perfusion, the glomerular filtration rate, the effective renal plasma flow rate, and quantitation of differential renal anatomic methods, and is very helpful in the medical and surgical management of various renal diseases.[15] Radionuclide diuretic renography using technetium TC 99m pentetate (DTPA) or iodine 131– or iodine 123– labeled o-iodohippurate is considered a very sensitive noninvasive test to differentiate a dilated renal collecting system from an obstructed one.[28]

About 50% or more of the bone-seeking radiopharmaceutical is normally excreted by the kidneys. This provides an opportunity to study renal anatomy and function on bone scintigraphy. Space-occupying lesions of kidneys and abnormalities of collecting systems are frequently detected on bone scans. Some of these are totally unsuspected clinically and often account for the symptom (usually back pain) which brought about the bone imaging procedure. This, then, can help direct other appropriate laboratory and radiographic studies to confirm and establish the diagnosis of kidney disease.

CONCLUSIONS

Radionuclide imaging procedures have little or no direct role in the evaluation of spinal stenosis per se. However, these procedures are quite useful and may even be the procedures of choice for evaluating certain conditions which may mimic, add to, or confuse the signs and symptoms of spinal stenosis. Radionuclide imaging can also be very helpful in the evaluation of postsurgical complications.

REFERENCES

1. Bruschwein DA, Brown ML, McLeod RA: Gallium scintigraphy in the evaluation of disc-space infections: Concise communication. *J Nucl Med* 1980; 21:925–927.
2. Byrnes DP, Russo GL, Ducker TB, et al: Sacrum fractures and neurological damage. *J Neurosurg* 1977; 47:459–462.
3. Collier BD, Hellman RS, Krasnow AZ: Bone SPECT. *Semin Nucl Med* 1987; 17:247–266.
4. Collier BD, Johnson RP, Carrera GF, et al: Painful spondylolysis or spondylolisthesis studied by radiography and single photon emission computed tomography. *Radiology* 1985; 154:207–211.
5. Elliot S, Hutson MA, Wastie ML: Bone scintigraphy in the assessment of spondylolysis in patients attending a sports injury clinic. *Clin Radiol* 1988; 39:269–272.
6. Fordham EW, Ali A, Turner DA, et al: The interpretive approach: Pattern recognition, in Fordham EW, et al (eds): *Atlas of Total Body Radionuclide Imaging*, vol 1. New York, Harper & Row, 1982, pp 12–13.
7. Fordham, EW, Ali A, Turner DA, et al: Methodology and instrumentation, in Fordham EW, et al (eds): *Atlas of Total Body Radionuclide Imaging*, vol 1. New York, Harper & Row, 1982, pp 17–40.
8. Fordham EW, Ali A, Turner DA, et al: Joint disease, in Fordham EW, et al (eds): *Atlas of Total Body Radionuclide Imaging*, vol 1. New York, Harper & Row, 1982, p 427.
9. Frymoyer JW, Hanley E, Howe J, et al: Disc excision and spine fusion in management of lumbar disc disease. A minimum ten-year followup. *Spine* 1978; 3:1–11.
10. Galasko CSB, Weber DA (eds): *Radionuclide Scintigraphy in Orthopaedics*. Edinburgh, Churchill Livingstone, 1984.
11. Gupta NC, Prezio JA: Radionuclide imaging in osteomyelitis. *Semin Nucl Med* 1988; 18:287–299.
12. Hoffer PB: Imaging technique, in Hoffer PB, Bekerman C, Henkin RE (eds): *Gallium-67 Imaging*. New York, John Wiley & Sons, 1976, pp 9–11.
13. Hoffer PB: Mechanism of localization, in Hoffer PB, Bekerman C, Henkin RE (eds): *Gallium-67 Imaging*. New York, John Wiley & Sons, 1978, pp 3–8.
14. Hoffer PB, Neuman RD: Gallium and infection, in Gottschalk A, Hoffer PB, Potchen EJ (eds): *Diagnostic Nuclear Medicine*, vol 2. Baltimore, Williams & Wilkins Co, 1988, pp 1111–1124.
15. Kim EE, Pjura GA, Lowry PA, et al: Principles of radionuclide studies of the genitourinary system, in Gottschalk A, Hoffer PB, Potchen EJ (eds): *Diagnostic Nuclear Medicine*, vol 2. Baltimore, Williams & Wilkins Co, 1988, pp 927–939.
16. Lewin JS, Rosenfield NS, Hoffer PB: Acute osteomyelitis in children: Combined Tc-99m and gallium-67 imaging. *Radiology* 1986; 158:795–804.
17. Little AG, DeMeester JR, Kirchner PT, et al: Guided biopsies of abnormalities on nuclear bone scans. *J Thorac Cardiovasc Surg* 1983; 85:396–403.
18. Lusins JO, Danielski EF, Goldsmith SJ: Bone SPECT in patients with persistent back pain after lumbar spine surgery. *J Nucl Med* 1989; 30:490–496.
19. Matin P: The appearance of bone scan following fractures including immediate and long-term studies. *J Nucl Med* 1979; 20:1227–1231.
20. McAfee JC, Subramanium G, Gagne G: Technique of leukocyte harvesting and labeling: Problems and perspectives. *Semin Nucl Med* 1984; 14:83–117.
21. McDougall IR, Baumert JE, Lantieri RL: Evaluation of In-111 leukocyte whole body scanning. *AJR* 1979; 133:849–854.
22. McMaster MJ: Stability of the scoliotic spine after fusion. *J Bone Joint Surg [Br]* 1980; 62:59–64.
23. Mcnab I, McCulloch J: *Backache*, ed 2. New York, Williams & Wilkins Co, 1990, pp 363–391.
24. Merkel KD, Brown ML, Dewanjee MK, et al: Comparison of indium labeled leukocyte imaging with sequential technetium-gallium scanning in the diagnosis of low grade musculoskeletal sepsis. *J Bone Joint Surg [Am]* 1985; 67:465–467.
25. Nelson HT, Taylor A: Bone scanning in the diagnosis of acute osteomyelitis. *Eur J Nucl Med* 1980; 5:267–269.
26. O'Mara RE: Benign bone disease, in Gottschalk A, Hoffer PB, Potchen EJ (eds): *Diagnostic Nuclear Medicine*, vol 2. Baltimore, Williams & Wilkins Co, 1988, pp 1058–1070.
27. Phesant HC, Dyck P: Failed lumbar disc surgery. *Clin Orthop* 1982; 164:93–109.
28. Pjura GA, Lowry PA, Kim EE: Radionuclide imaging of the upper urinary tract, in Gottschak A, Hoffer PB, Potchen EJ (eds): *Diagnostic Nuclear Medicine*, vol 2. Baltimore, Williams & Wilkins Co, 1988, pp 940–966.
29. Reis T: Detection of osteoporotic sacral fractures with radionuclides . *Radiology* 1983; 146:783–785.
30. Rothman RH, Booth R: Failures of spinal fusion: Cause, assessment, treatment. *Orthop Clin North Am* 1975; 6:299–301.
31. Schaffer DL, Pedegrass HP: Comparison of enzyme, clinical, radiographic and radionuclide methods of detecting bone metastasis from carcinoma of the prostrate. *Radiology* 1976; 121:431–434.

32. Schauwecker DS, Park HM, Mock BH, et al: Evaluation of complicating osteomyelitis with Tc-99m MDP, In-111 granulocytes, Ga-67 citrate. *J Nucl Med* 1984; 25:849–853.
33. Schneider R, Yacovone J, Ghelman B: Unsuspected sacral fractures: Detection by radionuclide bone scanning. *AJR* 1985; 144:337–341.
34. Schutte HE, Park WM: The diagnostic value of bone scintigraphy in patients with low back pain. *Skeletal Radiol* 1983; 10:1–4.
35. Serafini AN: Paget's disease of bone. *Semin Nucl Med* 1976; 6:47–58.
36. Silberstein EB, Brown ML, Rosenthal L, et al: Skeletal nuclear medicine, in Siegel BA, Kirchner PT (eds): *Nuclear Medicine Self Study*, Program 1. New York, Society of Nuclear Medicine, Inc, 1988, pp 93–125.
37. Slizofski WJ, Collier BD, Flatley TJ: Painful pseudoarthrosis following lumbar spine fusion: Detection by combined SPECT and planar bone scintigraphy. *Skeletal Radiol* 1987; 16:136–141.
38. Tsan MF, Chen WY, Scheffel U: Mechanism of gallium localization in inflammatory lesions. *J Nucl Med* 1977; 18:619.
39. Weisz GM: Paget's disease. *Spine* 1983; 8:192.

25

Peripheral Vascular Studies

Giacomo A. DeLaria, M.D.

The introduction of noninvasive techniques to evaluate patients suspected of having peripheral vascular disease revolutionized the practice of vascular surgery.[20] Subjective assessment of skin color and pulse were replaced with objective data. Standard chart recordings were readily reproducible and available for easy comparison. Improvements after vascular reconstruction were documented and the timing of secondary interventions to correct for the disease progression became more certain.[1] Today, the techniques of noninvasive vascular diagnosis are well established and laboratories are found in most hospitals. In the majority of institutions vascular surgeons direct the laboratories, but others are directed by either radiologists or medical specialists. There is some variation in both data collection and interpretation. Therefore, correct use of this information requires a sound understanding of these techniques and their limitations. More important, no data, no matter how well presented, can be used clinically unless there is a clear understanding of the underlying vascular conditions responsible for the abnormalities identified in these tests.

VASCULAR PATHOLOGY

Peripheral vascular disease is best understood if divided into four categories (Table 25–1). The first is proximal or inflow disease involving the aorta and its main iliac branches. The most profound example of this is total aortic occlusion (Fig 25–1), or Ler-iche's syndrome. Impotence, buttock and thigh claudication, along with absent femoral pulses, characterize the syndrome. Male patients in the fifth and sixth decades, most of whom smoke and are hypertensive, typify this group.[4] Symptoms are usually significant but the likelihood of either limb loss or gangrene is low and less than 6%.[12] On the other hand, patients under 40 years of age with aortoiliac disease are at significant increased risk for premature death from either myocardial infarction or stroke.[22]

The second group of patients exhibit a normal femoral pulse but weak or absent pedal pulses. Obstruction is usually in the superficial femoral artery at the level of Hunter's canal. These patients have significant calf claudication but little else. Risk of tissue loss is low and cessation of cigarette smoking and an exercise program may be all that is necessary as treatment.[26]

Diabetic patients and the very elderly exhibit the third arterial disease pattern: tibioperoneal obstruction. Nonhealing ulcers, infected toes, and rest pain are characteristic of this patient. Claudication is unusual. Treatment almost always requires either distal tibial bypass or extensive endovascular manipulation.[30] Often primary amputation is all that is possible.[9]

The final group includes those patients with combined disease. Here the risks of either limb loss or gangrene are high. Clinical management of these patients is difficult and requires the judgment of an experienced vascular surgeon and almost certainly contrast angiography.

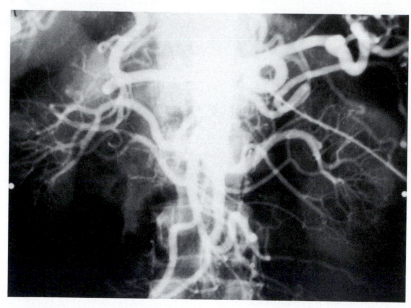

FIG 25–1.
Translumbar aortogram of a 56-year-old patient with total occlusion of the aorta. The primary complaint is thigh clau- dication. Rest pain is not present and there is no evidence of tissue compromise.

TABLE 25–1.
Vascular Pathology

Obstruction Category	Symptom	Amputation Risk*
Inflow disease		
Aortoiliac	Thigh claudication	–
Outflow disease		
Superficial femoral	Calf claudication	±
Tibioperoneal	Calf claudication and rest pain	+ +
Combined level	Rest pain and gangrene	+ + +

*– = low; ± = low to moderate; + + = often needed; + + + = high.

PHYSICAL DIAGNOSIS

Although the noninvasive laboratory is the best resource for the objective physiologic data required to confirm a patient's vascular diagnosis, its avail- ability does not in any way preclude the need for a complete physical examination. The examination be- gins with blood pressure assessment. Hypertension is very common in peripheral vascular patients. Comparison of blood pressures between arms is use- ful to evaluate the possibility of subclavian artery stenosis. Carotid, subclavian, brachial, and radial pulses are palpated in the upper extremity and com- pared with the femoral, popliteal, posterior tibial, and dorsalis pedis pulses in the legs. Pulses are best graded as being normal, reduced, or absent. More elaborate classifications are often misleading and im- ply a system of accurate quantification which in most hands does not exist. Pulses which are absent usually indicate severe vascular disease. However, certain anatomic variants such as congenital ab- sence of the dorsalis pedis artery can be identi- fied in 10% of normal patients.[18] In addition to pulse palpation, the vessel itself can be character- ized as firm, calcified, or aneurysmal. Aneurysm of the abdominal aorta must be excluded by either physical examination or abdominal ultrasound in the obese, difficult-to-examine patient. Ausculta- tion for bruits is especially important over the femoral arteries. A normal pulse in association with a bruit can indicate proximal obstructive dis- ease which can become hemodynamically signifi- cant after exercise. On the other hand, bruits can also arise from small branch arteries and be of no clinical importance. Other physical characteristics such as skin color, temperature, hair and nail growth, and the presence of digital ulcerations or gangrene must of course be recorded. However, these findings will often be absent in all but a few patients with claudication as their primary com- plaint. Tissue loss or ulceration rarely occurs in this group unless the underlying vascular disease is complicated by other systemic processes such as severe diabetes, collagen-vascular disease, chronic trauma, or infection.

DOPPLER VELOCITIES AND SEGMENTAL PRESSURES

Doppler ultrasound remains the basic tool in noninvasive vascular diagnosis. Introduced into clinical medicine by Satomura in 1959, this technique achieved wide acceptance through the efforts of Strandness and his colleagues at the University of Washington.[27, 29] Doppler ultrasound is based on the principle first described by Christian Johann Doppler in the early 19th century. The so-called Doppler shift is the audible change in frequency which occurs when a transmitted sound is reflected back from a moving object. The perceived frequency increases when the object is approaching a sound source and decreases when the object is moving away. The shift in frequency is proportional to the speed of the moving object and this mathematical relationship can be used to calculate velocity. Doppler ultrasound, when applied to flowing arterial blood, reflects those changes which occur from peak systolic forward flow through diastolic reverse flow. It should be emphasized, however, that blood velocity and not flow is being measured. Flow itself can only be determined when both blood velocity and volume are known (mL/min). High blood velocity does not necessarily equal high flow. Central blood velocity through a tight arterial stenosis can be very high although blood volume flow is low. In contrast, blood velocity in the venous system is low although actual blood flow in the large-capacity venous vessels is high. As will be described, spectral analysis of the Doppler signal is particularly helpful in this differentiation.

The continuous wave Doppler is a simple, reliable, and readily available device. Examples are found in all vascular laboratories, and in most emergency rooms and intensive care units.[28] It is useful in two important ways. First, Doppler signals obtained over individual arteries can either be heard or recorded on a strip chart. As illustrated in Figure 25–2, these signals can be classified as being triphasic, biphasic, monophasic, or absent. A triphasic signal describes the normal blood velocity profile in the peripheral artery. With mild to moderate obstruction, diastolic reversed flow is lost and the signal becomes biphasic. A monophasic signal indicates severe obstruction, and the absence of a signal confirms no flow. Absence of Doppler sound is highly significant and was associated in one report with a 74% likelihood of limb loss despite aggressive surgical intervention.[7] Although direct Doppler arterial evaluation is a handy tool for rapid estimates of blood flow, the information obtained is influenced by not only the angle of insonnation but also operator experience. At either extreme, excellent triphasic signal or absent sound, information is reliable. Between these two points the definition of disease is less secure. It must be emphasized that Doppler signals by themselves do not confirm blood flow. A common pitfall is the interpretation of a signal transmitted along an acutely thrombosed artery as evidence of flow when in fact no blood flow is present. Therefore, in order to improve the diagnostic accuracy of Doppler evaluation, the concepts of segmental pressure and the ankle-brachial index were developed.[32, 33]

Blood pressure in the leg or foot is certainly related to blood flow. However, Korotkoff's sounds as heard at the elbow are not present in the limbs. The systolic pressures in the legs can, however, be measured accurately by using the first appearance of a Doppler signal beyond a gradually deflating occlusive pneumatic cuff (Fig 25–3). Cuffs can be placed at three levels: thigh, calf, and ankle. The systolic pressure can be measured beyond each. As seen in Figure 25–4, segmental pressures at each level should be equal to a simultaneously measured brachial pressure. A patient with isolated iliac occlusion would be expected to have a reduced thigh pressure but no additional decreases at either the calf or ankle. Obstruction at the popliteal level would manifest as a segmental pressure decrease beyond the knee. In isolated tibioperoneal obstruction the first segmental pressure drop would be at the ankle.

Segmental pressures are certainly valuable and are the mainstay of vascular diagnosis. However, interpretation is not always clear-cut. For example, segmental pressure alone cannot reliably differentiate between a proximal iliac or femoral occlusion and a low femoral occlusion. In both conditions, the

ARTERIAL DOPPER TRACING

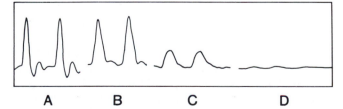

A B C D

FIG 25–2.
Examples of Doppler wave form tracings associated with varying degrees of arterial obstruction. **A,** normal triphasic signal. **B,** mild obstruction, biphasic signal. **C,** severe obstruction, monophasic signal. **D,** no flow.

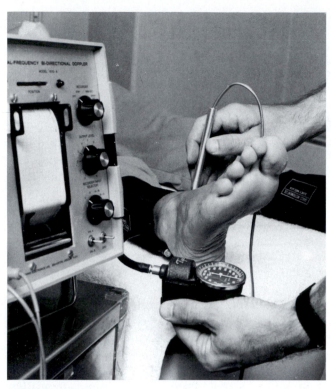

FIG 25–3.
Accurate determination of ankle pressure requires a tight-fitting cuff placed just above the malleoli. Doppler signals can be recorded over either the posterior tibial or dorsalis pedis arteries. Using this technique only the systolic pressure can be accurately determined.

thigh cuff cannot be positioned high enough to differentiate between the two. Both produce equivalent reductions in thigh pressure. Obviously, palpation of a normal femoral pulse or the recording of a triphasic Doppler signal over the femoral artery would help in this differentiation by excluding a proximal iliac or high femoral arterial occlusion. In elderly or diabetic patients with calcified and rigid blood vessels, segmental pressures by themselves can be misleading. Accurate pressure measurements require arterial occlusion and elimination of the Doppler signal. In this patient group, arteries cannot be compressed and above-normal segmental pressures are measured in circumstances in which blood flow is actually at ischemic levels. Again, patient examination along with close inspection of Doppler tracings in which only a depressed or monophasic signal is recorded will aid significantly in this differential. Finally, measurements obtained at rest can underestimate the extent of vascular disease. Segmental pressures that are normal at rest can decrease significantly after exercise. By using pharmacologic maneuvers stress gradients can be obtained without

exercise. Drugs such as tolazoline (Priscoline) or papaverine produce arterial vasodilation, thereby increasing the volume flow demands into a limb. If a hemodynamically significant stenosis is present there will be a drop in pressure beyond the stenosis. These techniques are both accurate and useful. However, they require an intraarterial injection and can be complicated by profound systemic hypotension. For this reason their use is limited to laboratories with special interests in these techniques.[8]

In most circumstances dynamic gradients are best elicited using an exercise treadmill (Fig 25–5). After stabilization, baseline segmental pressures are measured. The patient is walked on a treadmill until either claudication occurs or a defined test sequence has been completed. Immediately after exercise, the segmental measurements are repeated and compared to the data obtained at rest. A decrease greater than 10% to 15% in any measurement is significant and indicates a proximal stenosis which is hemodynamically significant. The time required for segmental pressures to return to normal is also important and correlates well with the degree of arterial stenosis.[24] The exercise test is perhaps most useful when used to distinguish neurogenic from vasculogenic claudication. The only requirement is that the patient be able to walk on the treadmill.

ANKLE-BRACHIAL INDEX

Even though Doppler techniques measure segmental limb pressures with great accuracy, early investigators recognized that the wide variety of normal pressures obtained among patients made a specific number difficult to interpret. For that reason, it was suggested that normalization of the ankle pressure to the brachial systolic pressure would be helpful. The usefulness of this index is now well established and in most cases the values obtained correlate well with ischemic disease. As seen in Table 25–2, a normal ankle-brachial index is somewhere between 0.8 and 1.0. Patients with claudication are usually above 0.5 and severe ischemia is not present above 0.3. Although the ankle-brachial index is a useful clinical tool it shares diagnostic pitfalls with segmental pressure measurements. Indices obtained at rest can be higher than those measured after exercise. Diabetic and elderly patients with calcified arteries have falsely elevated ankle-brachial indices, sometimes greater than 1.5 to 2.0, numbers that do

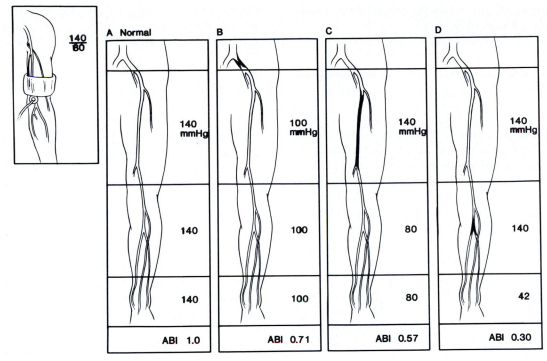

FIG 25–4.

In the absence of arterial obstruction, segmental pressures at three levels equal the brachial arterial pressure **(A)**. Iliac obstruction **(B)** results in equal reduction in segmental pressures in the leg. When only the superficial femoral artery is obstructed, the thigh pressure can be normal **(C)**. In isolated tibioperoneal obstruction **(D)** only the ankle pressure is reduced. When combined disease is present the greatest pressure reduction is always at the ankle. *ABI* = ankle-brachial index.

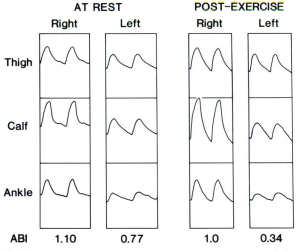

FIG 25–5.

Treadmill exercise test on a 49-year-old patient with isolated left superficial femoral occlusion. Pulse volume recordings (PVRs) and segmental pressures demonstrate a pressure reduction on the left. After exercise, the ankle-brachial index *(ABI)* decreases by 56%. There is a concomitant reduction in the pulse volume tracing. On the right, the normal leg, PVRs increase in response to exercise and the ABI drops slightly.

TABLE 25–2.

Ankle-Brachial Index

0.8–1.0	Normal or mild symptoms
0.5–0.8	Claudication
0.2–0.5	Severe claudication or rest pain
<0.2	Ischemia with tissue loss

not indicate an excess of arterial perfusion and actually defy interpretation. It must also be emphasized that although an ankle-brachial index less than 0.2 is certainly indicative of ischemia, one cannot with certainty predict the possibility of either tissue loss or the need for amputation.[23] Additional tests, including in most circumstances contrast angiography, must be obtained. Regardless, the ankle-brachial index is an important test and its reliability has been confirmed in many studies. There is little interobserver or intrapatient variability. Any change which is measured to be greater than 10% to 14% is usually significant.[13] Finally, it must be recognized that an abnormal ankle-brachial index is an indicator of a severe systemic disease. In one report, the 6-year mortality in a group of patients with ankle-brachial indices less than 0.3 was 64%.[11]

PULSE VOLUME RECORDING

As previously mentioned, Doppler wave forms are an excellent indicator of blood flow velocity. A clear triphasic signal confirms normal flow. However, Doppler signals can be difficult to obtain in certain limbs and success is very dependent on the expertise of the vascular technologist. Also, simultaneous Doppler signals at different levels are not possible with one technician. Comparisons between limbs over time, particularly after exercise, can be influenced by the measurement sequence.

Pulse volume recording (PVR) is a technique which can supplement information obtained using Doppler and segmental pressures to improve diagnostic reliability. The basic technique uses air-filled pressure cuffs placed simultaneously on both limbs at thigh, calf, and ankle levels. Each cuff is filled to approximately 50 mm Hg to fit snugly. The changes in limb volume which occur during arterial pulsations are reflected by air displaced in the cuff. This information is processed and the signal output can be recorded on a moving strip chart.[6] As seen in Figure 25–6, a normal PVR is almost indistinguishable from an intraarterial tracing. There are both systolic and diastolic peaks and a dicrotic notch. The normal reversed flow, as demonstrated by Doppler tracings, is not measured using air plethysmography and PVR. As systolic flow decreases the pulse volume tracing becomes more rounded, then flattens and disappears. Correlations of the PVR with segmental pressures can often help differentiate high femoral or iliac obstructions from superficial femoral occlusions. In patients with high femoral obstructions both the thigh PVR and segmental pressure will be decreased. When arterial obstruction is at the level of the superficial femoral artery, then segmental thigh pressure is decreased but thigh pulse volume is normal (Fig 25–7). PVRs in patients with arteriovenous fistulas are also remarkable. Systolic inflow into large-capacity venous systems results in extreme alterations of limb volume which are confirmed by the plethysmographic cuffs. PVR is also useful in the evaluation of patients with rigid arteries. In this group, as previously mentioned, segmen-

NORMAL

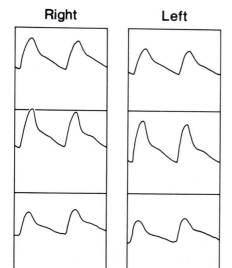

FIG 25–6.
Normal pulse volume recordings obtained in both legs at thigh, calf, and ankle levels. The phleborheographic tracing is almost indistinguishable from an intraarterial pressure recording.

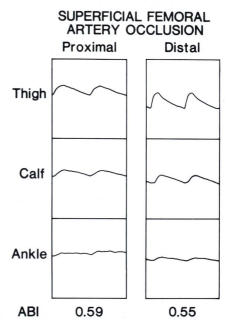

FIG 25–7.
Pulse volume recordings and ankle-brachial indices *(ABI)* obtained from limbs of two patients with proximal *(left)* and distal *(right)* superficial femoral artery occlusion. *Left,* the rounded thigh pulse volume recording in association with decreased ankle pressure indicates a high superficial femoral arterial occlusion probably at the origin. *Right,* the thigh pulse volume tracing is normal despite a comparable reduction in ankle pressure.

tal pressures are falsely elevated. Depressed pulse volume signals confirm reduced flow.

In general, PVR is an important component of arterial evaluation in patients with lower extremity vascular disease. It is versatile, simultaneous, and can be easily obtained at rest and after treadmill exercise. Good tracings require both accurate cuff placement and inflation. Interpretation is difficult in obese patients unless large-sized cuffs are available. Pulse volume changes are blunted in patients with concomitant venous obstructive disease. Normal segmental pressures and triphasic Doppler tracings at the ankle will exclude arterial disease in this patient group. Otherwise, PVR is an extremely valuable diagnostic method which provides clinical information that is both readily available and reliable.

PULSED DOPPLER, DUPLEX SCANNING, AND DOPPLER SPECTRAL ANALYSIS

All previous discussions of Doppler technology have been limited to the less sophisticated but certainly more commonly available continuous wave devices. In this instrument the probe contains at its tip not only a transmitting but a receiving crystal. Tissue penetration is a function of transmitted frequency which in most instruments varies between 5 and 20 MHz. The lower the frequency in megahertz the greater the depth of tissue penetration. The technologist has only to aim his probe in the anatomic location of a blood vessel to obtain a signal. Continuous wave Doppler receives signals from the entire blood vessel. Adjacent blood vessels, especially veins, can contaminate the signal and make analysis difficult. The observer cannot be sure if he is near to or distant from a region of arterial stenosis. In an effort to control for these variables the pulsed Doppler was developed.

The pulsed Doppler probe differs from a continuous wave device by having a signal crystal at its tip which is capable of both transmitting and receiving signals. The crystal transmits and receives according to the frequency of the opening and closing of a timed gate. The timing of this shutter influences the level from which the Doppler signal is received. At reduced shutter frequencies the depth is greater. The signal travels farther before its reflection is received. Therefore, the operator can, by adjusting the

frequency, define the level of interest. Also, since the sampling volume of a pulsed Doppler is less, there is little overlap and competing signals from adjacent vessels are eliminated. On the other hand, the small sampling size makes it very important to know the exact location of the blood vessel. What branch are you in and what is the anatomic relationship between possible arterial stenoses and the sampling site? To obtain this information a duplex scanner is required.

Simply put, duplex scanning is the technique which combines real-time ultrasound imaging with pulsed Doppler. Using an ultrasound probe a vessel is located and defined. The stored image graphically portrays the blood vessel and its wall thickness. It also defines stenoses and areas of calcification. Using this image for direction, along with a cursor on a video display terminal, the pulsed Doppler signal is positioned in the blood vessel. Analysis of the Doppler signal and its relationship to any arterial irregularity allows for exact diagnosis of not only the location of the stenosis but also its severity.[2]

The final step in this process is the analysis of the Doppler wave form. By breaking up the analog signal into its individual frequencies, more information is obtained then just triphasic vs. monophasic. As seen in Figure 25–8, the peak velocity, the amount of spectral broadening, and the diastolic component are all related to the degree of stenosis. When no signal is present and an ultrasound image confirms the location of the Doppler within a blood vessel, then vessel occlusion is confirmed. (Fig 25–9)

Although the duplex scan has its optimal use in the evaluation of the carotid artery, it has become increasingly important in the evaluation of lower extremity arterial disease. Its particular value lies in the assessment of the aortoiliac system. As previously mentioned, both segmental pressure measurement and also PVR are least accurate in the differentiation between high superficial femoral artery occlusion and common femoral or iliac disease. The duplex scan allows accurate imaging of both the external iliac and femoral arteries. Ultrasound will define the location of a stenosis and spectral analysis of the signal will characterize its severity. A normal triphasic pulsed Doppler signal, which includes diastolic reverse flow but no evidence of increased velocity or spectral broadening, essentially excludes the possibility of proximal aortoiliac obstructive disease.

More careful analysis of Doppler signals can provide information regarding pressure gradients across an arterial stenosis. A modification of the Bernoulli

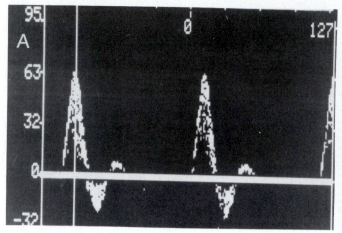
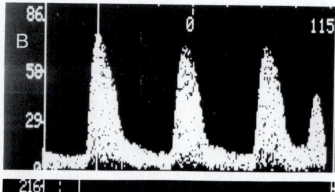
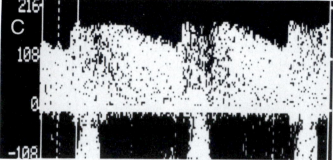

FIG 25–8.
Spectral analysis of pulsed Doppler signals obtained from the common femoral artery in three patients. **A,** normal tracing. Peak arterial systolic velocity is sharp and well defined. Diastolic reversed flow is present. A spectral window is seen within the systolic component. **B,** moderate stenosis. Peak velocity increases. Spectral broadening with loss of spectral window is present. Diastolic reversed flow is absent. **C,** severe stenosis. Velocity is greater than 100 cm/sec. There is marked spectral broadening. Systolic and diastolic flow cannot be distinguished.

equation which has been successfully applied to the measurement of aortic valve stenosis is used.[14] In this equation the pressure gradient (P) is calculated using the maximal Doppler velocity $(V)_{max}$

$$P = V^2_{max}$$

Comparison of calculated pressures against direct arterial measurement has, in at least one report, confirmed an excellent correlation ($r = .9$).[15] However, these calculations are more accurate at high or low gradients than at midrange. The addition of color flow process to spectral analysis provides even more information and has a reported 94% accuracy as compared with arteriography.[5] At present, the process requires expensive computer software and for this reason it is not as yet generally available.

COMPUTED TOMOGRAPHY SCANNING

Advances in radiologic techniques have raised the possibility of arterial diagnosis without the requirement for intraarterial contrast. Computed tomography (CT)-scanning has certainly proved itself valuable in the assessment of both aortic aneurysms and dissections.[16] CT scans are displayed as cross sections usually advanced in 1-cm segments. Many arterial stenoses are isolated and could be overlooked in this process. When CT scanning was compared with aortography in patients with aortoiliac disease, it was found to be superior only in those patients with severe calcification and unexpected aneurysms. Stenoses, particularly in the iliac arteries, were missed by the CT scan. This was particularly the case in patients with elongated and tortuous iliac arteries.[17] Therefore, CT scanning remains valuable in the evaluation of patients with arterial aneurysms but as yet has not proved useful in patients with isolated peripheral vascular obstructive disease.

MAGNETIC RESONANCE IMAGING

Magnetic resonance imaging (MRI) holds great promise for the noninvasive evaluation of patients with peripheral vascular disease.[21] Once techniques in imaging have been refined it will be possible to not only define anatomy and significant stenoses but also tissue function at the cellular level.

At present, MRI is an excellent technique to as-

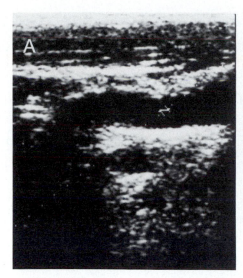
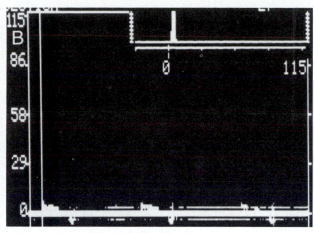

FIG 25–9.

A, duplex scan of the common femoral artery clearly outlines the vessel wall. The marking cursor is seen within the vessel. **B,** simultaneous Doppler tracing indicates no signal, which confirms total occlusion.

sess vascular anatomy. Images are produced which are equal to those seen with CT scanning. Both cross-sectional and sagittal sectional views are possible. More importantly, blood vessel flow in both arteries and veins is defined without the need for infusion of a contrast agent. On the other hand, MRI cannot as yet define arterial stenosis with accuracy as compared to arteriography and in this regard suffers the same faults as CT scanning.[31]

MRI can also be used to measure blood flow. Protons in blood passing through magnetic fields generate signals. The number of protons increases with flow and therefore will induce an appropriate signal change. At present, two techniques for blood flow measurement are being investigated. These two techniques are the "time of flight system" and "phase alteration." Neither technique has yet gained clinical ascendancy. Both methods have been used in arterial phantoms and clinical situations. Flow signals are similar to and correlate well with Doppler ultrasound.[10, 19, 25] MRI has several advantages over ultrasound. Flow can be measured in more than one dimension and there is no possible flow alteration caused by probe compression. Also, the number of access sites available for blood flow measurement are much greater with MRI than with ultrasound. On the other hand, ultrasound is far less expensive and results are immediate and do not require complex computer analysis.

Perhaps the most exciting possibility using MRI is ^{31}P magnetic resonance spectroscopy. Phosphorus is present in all tissue high-energy compounds and with metabolism inorganic phosphates are split from adenosine triphosphate to form adenosine diphosphate. This reaction can be monitored with MRI spectroscopy. Patients with ischemic limbs before and after exercise demonstrate deficiencies in another high-enery compound, creatine phosphate. Recovery time after exercise and also the improvement after vascular reconstruction can be monitored by measuring the amount of inorganic phosphate released from these compounds.[3]

Although MRI has at present limited application in vascular surgery, the development of small and perhaps less expensive devices could make it the preferred technique for noninvasive evaluation of patients with peripheral vascular disease both before and after reconstruction. For this to come about, cost and reliability must be improved and a clear superiority over presently available techniques, continuous wave Doppler and the duplex scanner, must be demonstrated.

CONCLUSIONS AND RECOMMENDATIONS

The differentiation between a neurogenic or vasculogenic etiology for claudication can be difficult in some patients. However, the number of patients in this category is small. Patients with leg cramps and absent pulses are usually referred to a vascular surgeon. In most circumstances, he or she will only consider the diagnosis of spinal stenosis in those patients with symptoms which are not supported by findings on either physical examination or in the noninvasive vascular laboratory.

The spine specialist examining a nonsmoking patient with no historical evidence of atherosclerotic vascular disease and an entirely normal peripheral vascular examination can pursue the treatment indicated for spinal stenosis or complicating musculoskeletal abnormalities. Patients older than 40 years, those with risk factors associated with vascular disease, and the difficult-to-examine or uncooperative patient, will require a baseline noninvasive arterial evaluation. This should include Doppler wave form analysis, segmental pressures, and calculation of the ankle-brachial index. PVRs at three levels and duplex scans of the aortoiliac system are useful, if available. Dynamic exercise testing is only necessary for those patients with abnormal vascular evaluation and musculoskeletal abnormalities insufficiently severe to explain a patient's complaints. Patients who demonstrate significant (>15%) change in segmental pressures or PVRs after exercise will in most circumstances require a complete vascular evaluation including angiography. The final decision regarding surgical treatment of a vascular abnormality will be made as regards both the severity of vascular obstruction and its relationship to the patient's complaints. The rare patient with both spinal stenosis and peripheral vascular disease could require separate treatment for both conditions to successfully alleviate symptoms. The more severe of the two diseases will of course be treated first.

In sum, both vascular and spine specialists must recognize the possibility that symptoms of spinal stenosis and arterial obstruction can be confused. A satisfactory history and physical examination will in most patients resolve this differential diagnosis. When a differentiation is unclear, appropriate testing in a vascular laboratory will provide sufficient information regarding vascular disease. Only rare patients will require contrast angiography to resolve the diagnosis. In the future, one test, MRI, has the potential to both diagnoses and direct treatment of both conditions, spinal stenosis and arterial obstructive disease.

REFERENCES

1. Bandyk DF, et al: Hemodynamics of vein graft stenosis. *J Vasc Surg* 1988; 8:688.
2. Barnes RW: New vascular diagnostic techniques. *J Vasc Surg* 1985; 2:340.
3. Berkowitz HD: Magnetic resonance diagnostic techniques. *J Vasc Surg* 1989; 9:394.
4. Corson JD, Brewster DC, Darling RC: The surgical management of infrarenal aortic occlusion. *Surg Gynecol Obstet* 1982; 155:369.
5. Cossman DV, et al: Comparison of contrast arteriography to arterial mapping with color-flow duplex imaging in the lower extremities. *J Vasc Surg* 1989; 10:522.
6. Darling RC, et al: Quantitative segmental pulse volume recorder: A clinical tool. *Surgery* 1972; 72:873.
7. Felix WR, Siegel B, Gunther L: The significance for morbidity and mortality of Doppler-absent pedal pulses. *J Vasc Surg* 1987; 5:849.
8. Flanigan DP, et al: Aortofemoral or femoropopliteal revascularization? A prospective evaluation of the papaverine test. *J Vasc Surg* 1984; 1:215.
9. Gregg RO: Bypass or amputation? Concomitant review of bypass arterial grafting and major amputations. *Am J Surg* 1985; 149:397.
10. Henriksen O, Stahlberg F, Thomsen C: In vivo evaluation of femoral blood flow measured with magnetic resonance. *Acta Radiol* 1989; 30:153.
11. Howell MA, et al: Relationship of severity of lower limb peripheral vascular disease to mortality and morbidity: A six-year follow-up study. *J Vasc Surg* 1989; 9:691.
12. Imparato AM, et al: Intermittent claudication: Its natural course. *Surgery* 1975; 78:795.
13. Johnston KW, Hosang MY, Andrews DF: Reproducibility of noninvasive vascular laboratory measurements of peripheral circulation. *J Vasc Surg* 1987; 6:147.
14. Kohler TR, et al: Assessment of pressure gradient by Doppler ultrasound: Experimental and clinical observations. *J Vasc Surg* 1987; 6:460.
15. Langsfeld M, et al: The use of deep duplex scanning to predict hemodynamically significant aortoiliac stenoses. *J Vasc Surg* 1988; 7:395.
16. Larson EM, Albrechtsson V, Christenson JT: Computed tomography versus aortography for preoperative evaluation of abdominal aortic aneurysm. *Acta Radiol* 1981; 25:95.
17. Limpert JD, Vogelzand RL, Yao, JST: Computed tomography of aortoiliac atherosclerosis. *J Vasc Surg* 1987; 5:814.
18. Lippert H, Reinhard P: *Arterial Variations in Man.* Munich, JF Bergmann Verlag, 1985.
19. Maier SE, et al: Human abdominal aorta: Comparative measurements of blood flow with MR imaging and multigated Doppler US[1]. *Radiology* 1989; 171:488.
20. Marinelli MR, et al: Non-invasive testing and clinical evaluation of arterial disease, A prospective study. *JAMA* 1979; 241:2031.
21. Mills CM, Brant-Zawadzki M, Crooks LE: Nucler magnetic resonance: Principles of blood flow imaging. *AJR* 1984; 142:165.
22. Najafi H, et al: Aortoiliac reconstruction in patients 32 to 45 years of age. *Arch Surg* 1970; 101:780.
23. Nicholas GG, Myers JL, DeMuth WE: The role of vascular laboratory criteria in the selection of patients for lower extremity amputation. *Ann Surg* 1982; 195:469.
24. Ouriel K, et al: A critical evaluation of stress testing

in the diagnosis of peripheral vascular disease. *Surgery* 1982; 91:686.

25. Podolak MJ, et al: Evaluation of flow through simulated vascular stenoses with gradient echo magnetic resonance imaging. *Invest Radiol* 1989; 24:184.

26. Quick CRG, Cotton LT: The measured effect of stopping smoking on intermittent claudication. *Br J Surg* 1982; 69(suppl):524.

27. Satomura S: Study of flow patterns in peripheral arteries by ultrasonics. *J Acoust Sci Jpn* 1959; 15:151.

28. Shoor PM, Fronek A, Bernstein EF: Quantitative transcutaneous arterial velocity measurements with doppler flowmeters. *Arch Surg* 1979; 114:922.

29. Strandness DE Jr, et al: Ultrasonic flow detection. A useful technique in the evaluation of peripheral vascular disease. *Am J Surg* 1967; 113:31.

30. Veith FJ, et al: Progress in limb salvage by reconstructive vascular surgery combined with new or improved adjunctive procedures. *Am Surg* 1981; 194:386.

31. Wesbey GE, et al: Peripheral vascular disease: Correlation of MR imaging and angiography. *Radiology* 1985; 156:733.

32. Winsor T: Influence of arterial disease on the systolic blood pressure gradients of the extremity. *Am J Med Sci* 1950; 220:117.

33. Yao JST, Hobbs JT, Irvine WT: Ankle systolic pressure measurements in arterial diseases affecting the lower extremities. *Br J Surg* 1969; 56:676.

PART IV

Treatment

26

Conservative Treatment of Spinal Stenosis: The Cornerstone

Sam W. Wiesel, M.D.
Scott D. Boden, M.D.

The number of patients with symptomatic lumbar spinal stenosis is increasing as the population ages. Otherwise healthy, elderly people may be handicapped by low back pain or leg pain secondary to mechanical pressure on the neural elements from advancing degenerative disease. Although the ultimate therapy for these patients is surgical decompression, the majority can be treated nonoperatively. The purpose of this chapter is to review the treatment goals and to discuss a number of nonoperative therapeutic modalities with emphasis on efficacy and indications.

TREATMENT GOALS

The primary aim is to return the patient to maximal function with the minimal amount of discomfort in the shortest period of time. Once the diagnosis of spinal stenosis has been established (see Section III) and more ominous causes of back pain have been ruled out, patients must first be educated to fully understand that a mild level of pain is not dangerous. In fact, mild discomfort can be a normal sequela of aging secondary to the usual degenerative processes which occur at the intervertebral discs, facet joints, and ligamentam flavam. This educative step is extremely important. It clarifies the benign origin of pain, and may help patients to adjust psychologically to their pain. Many patients, once they realize that their discomfort is not a sign of a serious underlying disorder, can function quite well. Patients with mild pain must be encouraged to return to as many activities as they can tolerate.

The goal of conservative therapy is to decrease the patient's symptoms. The treatment should be safe, effective, and at an acceptable cost. Each physician should have a logical sequence of therapeutic modalities in mind and understand the advantages and disadvantages of each type of treatment. Surgical intervention should only be considered after a reasonable and adequate trial of conservative care. The underlying pathologic changes in the shape of the spinal canal, intervertebral joint degeneration, and bony encroachment cannot be influenced by conservative measures. However, inflammation, which may contribute to a patient's pain, can usually be reduced and may lead to acceptable symptomatic relief.

CONSERVATIVE TREATMENT MODALITIES

There are many different nonoperative treatments available for the patient with spinal stenosis. Ideally, each therapy should pose a low risk to the patient, be based on physiologic principles with proven effectiveness in clinical trials, and be affordable. Unfortunately, most of the conservative therapeutic modalities have not been validated through properly controlled clinical trials. Many therapies are supported by conflicting claims of efficacy and some are based on empiricism and tradition. Few clinical trials are scientifically valid because of the difficulty in performing prospective double-blind studies in this field.

In this chapter we present the rationale behind the use of some of the more common therapeutic measures. First, each treatment modality is described, followed by the available scientific evidence for or against its use.

Bed Rest and Controlled Physical Activity

The traditional treatment of low back pain of any type has always included some degree of decreased physical activity. The advice in the past has ranged from complete bed rest to simply limiting a patient's physical activity. The amount of rest prescribed varies for each patient: these patients should not be fully mobilized until reasonably comfortable.

The type of abnormality will determine the duration of rest required. Most patients with acute back strain will need only 2 to 7 days of rest before they can ambulate. However, a patient with an acute disc may require up to 2 weeks. Patients with spinal stenosis have different requirements for rest depending on the radiculopathy component of their problem.

Complete bed rest for a long period (more than 2 weeks) has a deleterious effect on the body in general and should be avoided, and closely monitored when implemented. This holds especially true for the older population who constitute the majority of patients with symptomatic spinal stenosis. As the discomfort eases, each patient should be strongly encouraged to increase his or her general level of activity. The patient should be followed carefully and not allowed complete mobility until subjective signs, such as a list or paravertebral muscle spasms, disappear. The patient's physical activity is tailored to increase movement without incurring a return of symptoms.

The reason to decrease the physical activity of a stenotic patient is to allow any inflammatory reaction to subside. This can result in symptomatic relief which may or may not be permanent.

There have been no definitive studies of the effectiveness of bed rest or controlled physical activity in the treatment of spinal stenosis. Biomechanically, it has been demonstrated that the supine position significantly reduces the pressure on the intervertebral discs, compared with the sitting or standing positions.[36, 37] Assuming that increased load pressure on the structures in the low back increases symptoms, bed rest is a rational approach.

Clinically, bed rest has been compared with ambulation for the treatment of various degrees of low back strain.[46] Patients treated with strict bed rest experienced less pain and had a faster return to work than those required to remain ambulatory. In another randomized study, it was concluded that 2 days of bed rest was as effective as 7 days in low back pain patients with no neurologic deficit.[12] This investigation, however, was conducted with a highly selected group of patients—predominantly indigent patients from a primary care clinic setting and excluding compensation cases.

From the available evidence, controlled physical activity appears to be an effective conservative treatment for low back pain. However, the optional duration of bed rest remains in question. Two to 7 days is reasonable for acute problems, with the severity of symptoms at presentation and the response to rest serving as the guiding factors. Older patients (spinal stenosis) should be encouraged to resume as much activity as possible once the acute pain has disappeared.

Drug Therapy

The judicious use of medication is an important adjunct in the treatment of spinal stenosis. There are three main categories of drugs in common use: anti-inflammatory agents, analgesics, and muscle relaxants.

Anti-inflammatory agents are used because of the theoretical consideration that inflammation within the affected tissues is a major cause of pain in spinal stenosis. The leg pain that these patients experience is due not only to the mechanical pressure but also to the inflammation around the involved nerve roots.[31] If the inflammatory component can be dispelled, the patient's pain usually will subside.

There are a variety of nonsteroidal anti-inflammatory agents available. Based on several scientific studies, no one of these appears to be superior to the others.[25, 44, 46] It should be noted that these studies looked at the various agents in combination with bed rest. A double-blind, placebo-controlled trial of piroxicam (Feldene) showed that a greater amount of pain relief in the group treated with anti-inflammatory drugs was evident only during the first few days of back pain; however, after 2 weeks, more of the untreated group had returned to work.[2] Anti-inflammatory drugs should be considered only an adjunct and not as a primary treatment.

Oral corticosteroids are excellent anti-inflammatory agents and may be administered for a short time with rapidly tapering doses.[43] Unfortunately, the infrequent occurrence of avascular necrosis in the hip joints is an important complication which must be carefully explained to the patient.[15] The effects of oral steroids in spinal stenosis have not yet been studied in a prospective, double-blind trial.

Our preference is to begin the patient on adequate doses of aspirin, which is effective and inexpensive. One must be sure that the patient has no history of ulcers and understands the importance of obtaining a good blood level, i.e., of taking the medication at regular intervals and at the prescribed dosage. If the response is not satisfactory, nonsteroidal anti-inflammatory drugs, such as naproxen (Naprosyn), ibuprofen (Motrin, Nuprin, Advil), or indomethacin (Indocin), can be tried. Most patients will get significant relief from one of these agents. Again, all anti-inflammatory medications are utilized in conjunction with controlled physical activity to relieve pain; they do not replace adequate rest. Occasionally, after an initial recovery, a patient will experience intermittent recurrent attacks or complain of chronic low backache; in some instances these patients will be helped by a maintenance dose of an anti-inflammatory drug.

The most common side effects of nonsteroidal anti-inflammatory drugs are gastrointestinal and renal.[22, 24, 27] Aspirin and other nonsteroidal agents have been associated with acute gastrointestinal bleeding. A small number of patients have developed reversible renal failure from decreased renal prostaglandin production, and less frequently, an idiosyncratic interstitial nephritis. Other toxic effects of nonsteroidal drugs are neurologic, hepatic, or hematologic.[8] Phenylbutazone is associated with a rare and severe bone marrow toxicity, and should rarely be used. Gastrointestinal effects may be minimized by taking the medication after meals, adding histamine receptor blocking agents or antacids, and by reducing alcohol, caffeine, and tobacco consumption. In addition, geriatric patients may require decreased dosage owing to poor metabolism and by-product clearance.

Analgesic medication is very important during the acute phase of low back pain which often accompanies spinal stenosis.[46] The ideal is to keep the patient comfortable while resting. Most of the anti-inflammatory agents also have some analgesic properties. In more severe cases, most patients will respond to the addition of 30 to 60 mg of codeine. If stronger medication is necessary, which is extremely

rare, it is our opinion that the patient should be admitted to the hospital and given parental narcotics as required. As the pain decreases, nonnarcotic analgesics may substitute for the more potent drugs.

The biggest mistake seen is treatment with very strong narcotics, such as meperidine (Demerol) or oxycodone (a component of Percodan and Tylox), on an outpatient basis. Many of these patients become addicted to the medication. In other cases, patients try to short-cut the controlled physical activities and use analgesic medication instead. This, of course, will not work and when the patient tries to stop medication, the back pain returns.

Analgesic medication must be prescribed with great care for the low back pain patient. The treating physician must maintain control of the patient's drug use at all times; there are too many instances of patients taking undue advantage of the situation. Finally, narcotics have no place in the treatment regimen of patients with chronic low back problems.

Muscle relaxants are not routinely recommended for the treatment of spinal stenosis. Any existing muscle spasm is, in most cases, secondary to a primary problem. If pain can be controlled, the muscle spasm will usually subside.

Occasionally, however, muscle spasms will be so severe that some type of treatment is required. Carisoprodol (Soma), methocarbamol (Robaxin), or cyclobenzaprine (Flexeril) are drugs recommended to be taken in conjunction with an anti-inflammatory agent.[3] Although baclofen was shown to be somewhat effective in the relief of pain, the relatively high frequency of adverse reactions is prohibitive.[10] Most patients will experience a sedative effect from muscle relaxants. Other side effects include headache, nausea, dry mouth, dizziness, and blurred vision. Diazepam (Valium) should be discouraged since it is actually a physiologic depressant and depression is often an integral feature of the back pain syndromes.[34] Administration of diazepam to a depressed patient only increases his or her problems. If anxiety is prominent and a sedative is needed, phenobarbital will alleviate the symptoms. In patients with chronic low back pain without objective physical findings, antidepressant therapy may help alleviate some complaints.[1, 39] Clinical studies have shown the tricyclic antidepressants amitriptyline, imipramine, and doxepin to yield superior pain relief compared with placebo.[45]

In summary, drug therapy for low back pain should be viewed as an adjunct to adequately controlled physical activity. Anti-inflammatory medications should be the primary agent employed. Analgesic medications should be used selectively in a controlled environment and not for extended periods. Muscle relaxants are generally not recommended and if used should be carefully monitored.

Trigger Point Therapy

Trigger point therapy is indicated for nonradiating low back pain when an area of maximal tenderness can be identified. This procedure involves the injection of steroids and a local anesthetic (e.g., lidocaine) in an area of maximal tenderness in the low back. The precise mechanism of action is not clear, but may be related to modulation of peripheral nerve stimulation as it affects the afferent input perceived as pain.

Although anecdotal reports claim effectiveness for this technique, it has not been well studied in the setting of spinal stenosis. A prospective randomized double-blind evaluation of trigger point injection in 51 acute low back pain patients was conducted by Garvey et al.[19] Although not statistically significant, their data suggested that the medication is not the critical factor, since the patients treated with acupuncture had a greater rate of improvement in symptoms (61%) than the patients injected with lidocaine (Xylocaine) alone (40%) or with steroids (45%). Their intended control group received a coolant spray followed by pressure from a plastic needle guard, and had the highest rate of improvement (66%) and the greatest average subjective decrease in pain. Unfortunately, no patients were randomized to a "watch and wait" control group to evaluate for the placebo effect. Trigger point therapy is easy to perform, has a negligible risk, and may help certain patients. When patients with spinal stenosis have primary back pain that is not controlled by oral medication, a trigger point injection is certainly worth a trial. Further controlled research is required to delineate the true value of this modality.

Epidural Steroids

Epidural steroid injections are indicated for severe lumbar radiculopathy, and generally not for nonradiating low back pain. This treatment method has traditionally been viewed as a form of therapy intermediate between conservative and surgical management. It is a more aggressive attempt at pain relief after conservative therapy has failed, yet avoids the disadvantages of surgery. The rationale for epidural steroid injections is that lumbar radiculopathy involves a significant inflammatory component, evoked by chemical or mechanical irritation or an autoimmune response, which should be amenable to treatment with corticosteroid drugs in the early stages.[3]

Unfortunately, few studies have systematically and accurately studied the efficacy of this treatment modality.[30] Poorly controlled, nonrandomized investigations have yielded controversial results with rates of success ranging from 25% to 75%.[5, 40] Another problem is that some studies have attempted to compare the efficacy of epidural steroids with epidural saline injection, while others have compared their results with a true placebo (i.e., intraspinous ligament injection).[16] It is unclear whether the steroids themselves have a clinical effect, or if just the mechanical violation of the epidural space is important.[42] Cuckler et al. concluded that the addition of steroids to epidural injections of procaine (Novocain) worked no better than procaine alone in relieving symptoms.[6] Problems with this particular study were that the authors did not compare their results with those with no epidural injection. Further, the timing of the assessment of efficacy—24 hours after injection—was probably too soon to see beneficial effects in many patients.

Despite the lack of well-designed investigations, upon review of the literature certain trends seem to be evident. Epidural steroids appear to be more beneficial for acute rather than chronic radiculopathy, especially when no neurologic deficit is present. Improvement may not be noted until 3 to 6 days after injection and may be only temporary. No neurotoxicity has been reported in humans or animal models; complications stem from the technique of epidural injection and are rare.[5] Suppression of the plasma cortisol concentration may occur up to 3 weeks following the injection.[4]

We maintain that epidural steroids may be helpful in relieving the irritative component of radicular pain in 40% of patients. Until controlled investigations indicate otherwise, this treatment is worth trying in patients who have failed 6 weeks of conservative management in an effort to avoid a major invasive procedure.

Spinal Manipulation

Spinal manipulation is another popular nonoperative modality for the treatment of low back pain. In the United States, it is somewhat controversial because it is performed mostly by chiropractors. The principle involved is that any malalignment of the spinal structures can be corrected by some form of manipulation; the assumption is that the malalignment is the cause of the patient's pain. A study by the National Institute of Neurological and Communicative Disorders and Stroke concluded that there is "no statistical proof for or against either the efficacy of this spinal manipulation therapy or the pathophysiological foundation, from which it is derived."[41]

There have been several clinical randomized trials of the efficacy of manipulation. A few studies demonstrated that patients felt some immediate relief of pain but had no long-term benefits.[14, 20, 23] In a study which randomized 54 subjects to spinal manipulation or spinal mobilization, there was no difference in benefit perceived between the two treatment modalities.[21] However, those subjects who had suffered from backache for 2 to 4 weeks prior to treatment had more rapid improvement if they were subjected to spinal manipulation; this difference in response was not noted in the group with less than 2 weeks of symptoms prior to treatment.

The efficacy of spinal manipulation has not been scientifically proved or disproved.[7] Most previous studies have flaws: (1) the entry criteria are too broad, too narrow, or undefined; (2) there is poor uniformity or standardization in the manipulative techniques used by multiple manipulators; (3) measurements of outcome vary from return to work (affected by other factors) to subjective questionnaires; (4) invalid control maneuvers do not account for the personal contact of manipulation (placebo effect). It is reported[3, 10] that some patients have short periods of symptomatic relief after manipulation but must return for repeat sessions to maintain it, which increases the cost of treatment. In spinal stenosis, it should be appreciated that many patients also may have underlying systemic diseases, and if they are manipulated they may be harmed. A contraindication to manipulation is tumor or significant osteopenia. At present manipulation is not indicated for the routine treatment of spinal stenosis. There is no adequate scientific evidence to justify its routine use and it may result in serious complications.[9, 18]

Braces and Corsets

External support of the lumbar spine with a corset or a brace may be helpful for some patients with spinal stenosis. As the acute symptoms subside, a properly fitted corset or brace will aid the patient to regain mobility.[35] As recovery progresses, the brace should be abandoned in favor of an exercise program. However, many patients with spinal stenosis do not tolerate exercise very well and these patients can be maintained quite adequately with the use of a

brace. The young patient should rely on a brace only to hasten his or her return to ambulation. In theory, strong, flexible lumbar and abdominal muscles function as an excellent "internal brace" because they are adjacent to the structures (vertebrae) that they are supporting.

There are no convincing data supporting benefits from lumbar corsets and braces; these devices may in fact cause increased movements of the lumbar spine.[17] One study showed some relief of symptoms with a rigid plastic lordosis-reversing brace in patients with spondylolisthesis or spinal stenosis, but showed no benefit in chronic low back pain of unknown etiology.[47]

Despite the paucity of clinical data, there are two types of patient for whom the authors believe long-term bracing to be a reasonable approach. One is the obese patient with weak abdominal muscles. A firm corset with flexible metal stays will reinforce the abdominal muscles. It has been demonstrated that if a lumbosacral corset is properly applied, the intradiscal pressure in the lumbar area will decrease by up to 30%.[38]

The aging patient with multilevel degenerative disease of the lumbar spine is the second type of patient for whom long-term bracing may be beneficial. As mentioned earlier, these older people sometimes do not tolerate exercise very well and in some cases exercise will aggravate their back condition. These patients can attain significant relief of pain with a well-fitted brace.

Physical Therapy

Some form of exercise is probably the most commonly prescribed therapy for patients recovering from low back problems. There are two regimens commonly advocated: isometric flexion exercises and hyperextension exercises. These programs are purported to reduce the frequency and intensity of low back pain episodes, although there is no scientific evidence to support this contention.

Isometric flexion exercises are the more popular regimen.[11, 26, 28] They are based on William's theory that by reducing the lumbar lordosis, back pain is decreased. This goal is achieved by strengthening both the abdominal and lumbar muscles, thereby creating a corset of muscles to support the lumbar spine.

Hyperextension exercises strengthen the paravertebral muscles. These exercises generally are used after a patient has satisfactorily performed a course of isometric flexion exercises. The goal is to have the paravertebral muscles act as an internal support for the lumbar spine. McKenzie believes that extending the spine will move the nucleus pulposus anteriorly.[32] Theoretically, these exercises can be used to keep the discs in their anatomic position. Unfortunately, again, there is no proof that this occurs. The McKenzie program also uses lateral bending and rotation with the regimen individualized to the patient's symptoms and ability to perform the exercises.

We believe that an exercise regimen is very important for the rehabilitation of most low back pain patients. An exercise regimen should not be instituted while the patient is experiencing acute pain but should be started after the symptoms have subsided to the point where no list or paravertebral muscle spasm is present. The exercises are increased gradually; if the patient has any recurrence of acute symptoms, the exercises are stopped. The patient is then closely monitored; when his symptoms again decrease, the exercises can be resumed. We prefer isometric flexion exercises. It should be stressed that there is no proof that exercises decrease recovery time or reduce the frequency of recurrences. Empirically, they appear to have a positive psychological effect and give the patient an active role in his treatment program. Patients with spinal stenosis sometimes have their symptoms exacerbated by exercises. When this occurs the exercises should either be decreased in number or stopped altogether. In other words, in this particular situation, if the symptoms are aggravated, exercises should not be used.

Back School

The concept of a back school originated in the 1970s with Zachrisson-Forsell in Sweden.[48] The theory is that if a patient understands the anatomic, epidemiologic, and biomechanical factors that give rise to low back pain, he or she can handle the problem in a better manner.

An audiovisual approach to teaching this material was developed. The patient is first introduced to the goal of the program. Then the basic anatomy and physiology of various back disorders are presented in a classroom setting, so each patient realizes his or her problem is not unique. Next, the patient is taught proper biomechanics of the spine and how to apply these principles to daily activities to reduce the forces applied to the spine. Finally, an exercise program is outlined. This multifaceted approach has been quite successful and has yielded more encouraging results than routine physiotherapeutic modalities.[17] There have been many varia-

tions on the program outlined above. Some of these back school programs are complex and costly, involving as much as 15 hours of classroom time. It is our opinion that the simpler the program, the better accepted it will be by the patient.

Few well-controlled studies exist validating the use of low back schools for patients with spinal stenosis.[29] Moffett et al. compared the results of a low back school with an exercise-only group of chronic low back pain patients.[33] Initially, both groups improved, but after 16 weeks the back school group tended to improve further, while the exercise-only group returned to their baseline activity level. At longer follow-up, however, the only significant difference between the groups was an increased knowledge of low back principles in the back school group. Use of the back school concept with acute low back pain has yielded more positive results. Unfortunately, no conclusions may be reached at this time concerning the effectiveness of low back school in spinal stenosis; further research must first examine patient compliance, test information retention, and assess subsequent behavioral modifications. It is believed that patients with spinal stenosis who get reasonable but not optimal results from medication will benefit from some form of education and understanding of their problem.

Modalities

There are many other treatment modalities used for spinal stenosis. These include hot packs, cold packs, light massage, ultrasound, transcutaneous electrical nerve stimulation, and diathermy.[13, 37] All of these are well tolerated and even pleasant. Most patients experience some immediate relief of symptoms but unfortunately there is no long-lasting impact on the disease process. There is no scientific evidence that any of these treatment modalities offers any long-term benefit or even adds to the efficacy of decreased physical activity alone.

CONCLUSION

The vast majority of patients with lumbar spinal stenosis can be managed by nonoperative means. Patients must be educated to understand the goals of therapy and must have realistic expectations for the level of recovery. The treating physician must be patient, and needs to be aware of the limitations of the various therapeutic options.

We believe that treatment should begin with the simplest modes of therapy and ultimately, only if necessary, progress to surgery. The patient is placed on limited physical activity and given a nonsteroidal anti-inflammatory agent for a period of 3 to 6 weeks. If no improvement in symptoms is noted during this time, a change of nonsteroidal drug may be warranted. If, at the end of this period, the patient continues to have debilitating symptoms, a trial of injection therapy (epidural steroids) may be considered. Some patients, especially if they have some response to the medications, may benefit from the addition of a corset or brace. Exercise is contemplated if the patient shows a decrease in his or her symptoms. Eighty percent to 85% of patients managed by this approach will go on to lead reasonably active lives.

REFERENCES

1. Alcoff J, Jones E, Rust P, et al: Controlled trial of imipramine for chronic low back pain. *J Fam Pract* 1982; 14:841–846.
2. Amlie E, Weber H, Home I: Treatment of acute low back pain with piroxicam: Results of a double-blind placebo-controlled trial. *Spine* 1987; 12:473–476.
3. Basmajian JV: Acute back pain and spasm. A controlled multicenter trial of combined analgesic and antispasm agents. *Spine* 1989; 14:438–439.
4. Benzon HT: Epidural steroid injections for low back pain and lumbosacral radiculopathy. *Pain* 1986; 24:277–295.
5. Bogduk N, Cherry D: Epidural corticosteroid agents for sciatica. *Med J Aust* 1985; 143:402–406.
6. Cuckler JM, Bernini PA, Wiesel SW, et al: The use of epidural steroids in the treatment of lumbar radicular pain: A prospective, randomized, double-blind study. *J Bone Joint Surg [Am]* 1985; 67:63–66.
7. Curtis P: Spinal manipulation: Does it work? *Occup Med: State of the Art Rev* 1988; 3(Jan-Mar):31–44.
8. Dahl SL: Nonsteroidal anti-inflammatory agents: Clinical pharmacology/adverse effects/usage guidelines, in Wilkens RF, Dahl SL (eds): *Therapeutic Controversies in the Rheumatic Diseases.* Orlando, Fla, Grune & Stratton, Inc, 1987, pp 27–68.
9. Dan NG, Saccasan PA: Serious complications of lumbar spinal manipulation. *Med J Aust* 1983; 2:672–673.
10. Dapas F, Hartman SF, Martinez L, et al: Baclofen for the treatment of acute low back syndrome: A double-blind comparison with placebo. *Spine* 1985; 10:345–349.
11. Davies JE, Gibson T, Tester L: The value of exercises in the treatment of low back pain. *Rheumatol Rehabil* 1979; 18:243–247.
12. Deyo RA, Diehl AK, Rosenthal M: How many days of bed rest for acute low back pain? *N Engl J Med* 1986; 315:1065–1070.
13. Dimaggio A, Mooney V: Conservative care for low back pain: What works? *J Musculoskeletal Med* 1987; 4:27–34.
14. Doran DM, Newell DJ: Manipulation in treatment of low back pain: A multi-center study. *Br Med J* 1975; 7:161–164.
15. Fast A, Alon M, Weiss S, Zer-Aviv FR: Avascular necrosis of bone following short-term dexamethasone therapy for brain edema. *J Neurosurg* 1984; 61:983–985.
16. Ferrante M: Epidural steroids in the management of spinal stenosis. *Semin Spine Surg* 1989; 1:177–181.
17. Frymoyer JW: Back pain and sciatica. *N Engl J Med* 1988; 318:291–300.
18. Gallinaro P, Cartesegna M: Three cases of lumbar disc rupture and one of cauda equina associated with spinal manipulation (chiroprosis). *Lancet* 1983; 1:411.
19. Garvey TA, Marks MR, Wiesel SW: A prospective randomized double-blind evaluation of trigger-point injection therapy in low back pain. *Spine* 1989; 14:962–964.
20. Glover JR, Morris JG, Khosla T: Back pain: A randomized clinical trial of rotational manipulation of the trunk. *Br J Ind Med* 1974; 31:59–64.
21. Hadler NM, Curtis P, Gillings DB, et al: A benefit of spinal manipulation as adjunctive therapy for acute low-back pain: A stratified controlled trial. *Spine* 1987; 12:703–706.
22. Hart FD: Naproxen and gastrointestinal hemorrhage. *Br Med J* 1974; 2:51–52.
23. Hoehler FK, Tobis JS, Buerger AA: Spinal manipulation for low back pain. *JAMA* 1981; 245:1835–1838.
24. Holdstock DF: Gastrointestinal bleeding: A possible association with ibuprofen. *Lancet* 1972; 1:541.
25. Jaffe G: A double blind multi-center comparison of naproxen and indomethacin in acute musculoskeletal disorders. *Curr Med Res Opin* 1976; 4:373–380.
26. Kendall PH, Jenkins JM: Exercises for backache: A double-blind controlled trial. *Physiotherapy* 1968; 54:154–157.
27. Lansa FL: Endoscopic studies of gastric and duodenal injury after the use of ibuprofen, aspirin, and other nonsteroidal anti-inflammatory agents. *Am J Med* 1984; 77:19–24.
28. Lidstrom A, Zachrisson M: Physical therapy on low back pain and sciatica: An attempt at evaluation. *Scand J Rehabil Med* 1970; 2:37–42.
29. Linton SJ, Kamwendo K: Low back schools: A critical review. *Phys Ther* 1987; 67:1375–1383.
30. Mathews JA, Mills SB, Jenkins VM, et al: Back pain and sciatica: Controlled trials of manipulation, traction, sclerosant and epidural injections. *Br J Rheumatol* 1987; 26:416–423.
31. McCarron RF, Wimpee MW, Hudkins PG, et al: The inflammatory effect of nucleus pulposus. A possible element in the pathogenesis of low back pain. *Spine* 1987; 12:750–753.
32. McKenzie RA: *The Lumbar Spine.* Waikanae, New Zealand, Spinal Publications, Ltd, 1981.
33. Moffett JA, Chase SM, Portek I, et al: A controlled, prospective study to evaluate the effectiveness of a back school in the relief of chronic low back pain. *Spine* 1986; 11:120–122.
34. Mooney V, Cairns D: Management of patients with chronic low back pain. *Orthop Clin North Am* 1978; 9:543–557.

35. Morris JM: Low back bracing. *Clin Orthop* 1974; 103:120–132.

36. Nachemson A: The load on lumbar disks in different positions of the body. *Acta Orthop Scand* 1965; 36:426–434.

37. Nachemson A: The lumbar spine—An orthopaedic challenge. *Spine* 1976; 1:59–71.

38. Nachemson A, Morris JM: In vivo measurements of intradiscal pressure: Discometry, a method for determination of pressure in the lower lumbar disc. *J Bone Joint Surg [Am]* 1964; 46a:1077–1092.

39. Pheasant H, Bursk A, Goldfarb J, et al: Amitryptyline and low back pain: A randomized double-blind cross-over study. *Spine* 1983; 8:552–557.

40. Rosen CD, Kahanovitz N, Bernstein R, et al: A retrospective analysis of the efficacy of epidural steroid injections. *Clin Orthop* 1988; 228:270–272.

41. *The Scientific Status of the Fundamentals of Chiropractic Analysis and Recommendations.* Bethesda, MD, National Institute of Neurological and Communicative Disorders and Stroke. April 8, 1975.

42. Swerdlow M, Sayle-Creer W: A study of extradural medication in the relief of the lumbosciatic syndrome. *Anaesthesia* 1970; 25:341–345.

43. Tsairis P: Corticosteroid therapy in the management of lumbar radiculopathy. *Contemp Orthop* 1988; 17:53–57.

44. Vignon G: Comparative study of intravenous ketoprofen versus aspirin. *Rheumatol Rehabil* 1976; 15:83–84.

45. Ward NG: Tricyclic antidepressants for chronic low back pain: Mechanisms of action and predictors of response. *Spine* 1986; 11:661–665.

46. Wiesel SW, Cuckler JM, DeLuca F, et al: Acute low back pain: An objective analysis of conservative therapy. *Spine* 1980; 5:324–330.

47. Willner S: Effect of a rigid brace on back pain. *Acta Orthop Scand* 1985; 56:40–42.

48. Zachrisson-Forsell M: The back pain school. *Spine* 1981; 6:104–106.

27

Decompressive Laminectomy

Thomas W. McNeill, M.D.

This chapter is an attempt to outline the techniques of surgical decompression for stenosis that I have found residents and fellows can learn easily and use safely. I attempt to explain in detail the various surgical tricks and methods for dealing with both routine and unexpected problems that arise in the course of performing spinal decompressing procedures. The following may seem to be excessively detailed and possibly even pedantic, but experienced surgeons appreciate that good surgery requires careful attention to detail. Lastly, these methods should never be considered the only method or the "best" method; however, my experience has been gratifying.

The application of these techniques is only one of the steps in the process of providing care for the patient with stenosis. Prior to the consideration of surgical decompression one must consider indications, alternatives, and efficacy of treatment with specific emphasis on quality and durability of results. Care following surgery has equal importance.

HISTORY

James W. Markham has provided a detailed history of laminectomy which can be found in A. Earl Walker's *A History of Neurological Surgery.*[9] In antiquity, Paulus Aegineta attempted removal of injured spinous processes and laminae. Ambroise Paré operated for depressed bone splinters of the spine in 1549. Through the next several centuries there are sporadic reports of spinal operations for various injuries, including the removal of sublaminar musket balls and laminectomy for treatment of paraplegia following a fall from a horse. In the 20th century, the modern concepts and techniques of "laminectomy" were described by Bailey, Elsberg, and Frazier.[1, 4–6] Verbiest[14] (see Chapter 1) should be given credit for recognizing "spinal stenosis" as a distinct group of related conditions and applying the principles of spinal decompression to their treatment. Almost all of the credit for the techniques that I shall describe are owed to these pioneers.[1, 4–6, 9]

INDICATION

In most instances of spinal stenosis (Paget's disease being the sole exception), nonsurgical "conservative" modalities cannot permanently alter the pathologic anatomy of spinal stenosis but may alleviate the symptoms for a variable period of time. Therefore, few, if any, patients should be subjected to surgical treatment until a reasonable trial of alternative methods has been completed and has failed. We consider a patient to be a surgical candidate when he or she can no longer walk 200 m, has severe intractable radicular symptoms, or has developed chronic cauda equina syndrome with significant neurogenic bladder or rectal dysfunction.

PREOPERATIVE PLANNING

Once it has been determined that surgical treatment for symptomatic spinal stenosis is appropriate and acceptable to the patient, then the preoperative phase is begun. Most of the patients that require surgical decompression for spinal stenosis are elderly and often have significant intercurrent disease. An individualized, comprehensive plan of medical care and management is required for most elderly surgical patients. Stenosis surgery is no different in this regard.

A formal written preoperative check list has proved very helpful in our institution (Table 27–1). Patients should be asked to stop all nonsteroidal anti-inflammatory medications before surgery. The actual time is dependent on the individual drug being taken, as the half-life of the various drugs differ, but 1 week is a safe rule of thumb except for aspirin which requires 2 weeks (Table 27–2). Patients with peripheral vascular disease, peripheral neuropathy, or intractable back pain tend to do poorly with elective decompression for symptomatic stenosis. The symptoms of the stenosis, neuropathy, and peripheral vascular disease overlap and the surgery only addresses one cause of the discomfort and disability. Additionally, decompression does not address the symptom of lower back pain. If the patients are experiencing symptoms of incontinence, urgency, or hesitancy, then urodynamic and sphincter electromyography (EMG) should be considered since longstanding spinal stenosis may be the cause of a chronic variety of cauda equina syndrome.[10] If the

TABLE 27–1.

Preoperative Check List*

	Yes	No
1. Are all previous studies available?	___	___
2. Will additional studies need to be done?	___	___
A. Radiographs	___	___
B. CT	___	___
C. MR	___	___
D. EMG	___	___
E. NCV	___	___
F. Myelogram	___	___
G. Postmyelogram CT	___	___
H. Selective blocks	___	___
I. Others ___	___	___
3. Consultations?	___	___
A. Medical	___	___
B. Neurologic	___	___
C. Vascular	___	___
D. Urologic	___	___
4. Stop NSAID type ( ); days ( )	___	___
5. Autologous blood?; no. of units ( )	___	___
6. Fusion?	___	___
7. Preoperative teaching done?	___	___

*CT = computed tomography; MR = magnetic resonance; EMG = electromyography; NCV = noncontrast venography; NSAID = nonsteroidal anti-inflammatory drug.

TABLE 27–2.

The Half-Life of Selected Nonsteroidal Anti-Inflammatory Drugs (NSAID)*

Drug	Half-Life (hr)
Carboxylic acids	
Salicylates	
Acetylsalicylic acid	4–15
Salicylsalicylate	4–15
Indoleacetic acids	
Indomethacin	3–11
Sulindac	16
Phenylalkanoic acids	
Ibuprofen	2
Ketoprofen	2
Suprofen	2–4
Naproxen	13
Fenamic acids	
Meclofenamate	2–3
Pyrazoles	
Phenylbutazone	40–80
Oxicams	
Piroxicam	30–86

*Adapted from Andersson GBJ, McNeil TW: *Lumbar Spine Syndromes.* Vienna, Springer-Verlag, 1989, p 55.

planned surgery is of sufficient magnitude (i.e., multiple levels need to be done), then 1 or 2 units of autologous blood may be appropriate. Lastly, patients with unrealistic expectations do poorly. A detailed explanation of the surgery, its risks, and expectations should be presented to the patient and his or her family. It is most important to emphasize that most of these procedures are not intended as a cure for lower back pain, and that the quality of the results may deteriorate with time.

Decompressing surgical procedures for the treatment of lumbar spinal stenosis require a detailed preoperative surgical plan which addresses both the pathologic changes seen on the various imaging studies and the presenting clinical syndrome. There is no one surgical procedure which is appropriate for all patients with lumbar spinal stenosis. As discussed in Chapter 4, there are three zones of the spinal canal which may need to be decompressed to a varying extent at each involved level. Excision of the lamina, ligamentum flavum, and sometimes even part of the disc will often be necessary to decompress the central canal (Fig 27–1). Laminaplasty may be an alternative in some instances of central canal stenosis, and anterior central corpectomy may be required in posttraumatic central canal stenosis. The medial facet and flavum will need to be removed in order to decompress the lateral recess along with synovial cysts, osteophytes, and disc fragments when present (Fig 27–2). Decompression of the neurofora-

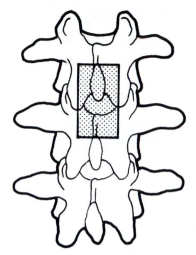

FIG 27–1.
Central decompression: the area of concern in central decompression.

men can be accomplished through distraction instrumentation or bony and ligamentous removal, or both. Wherever possible, disc, annulus, and facet should be preserved but not at the cost of failing to adequately decompress an involved nerve root. If it should be necessary to remove so much bony and ligamentous tissue that one motion segment is "destabilized," then fusion of that segment will be necessary. The probable need for fusion of a motion segment should be determined prior to surgery. Thus, patients should be advised of the possibilities, ask to give consent as necessary, and the appropriate equipment should be available.

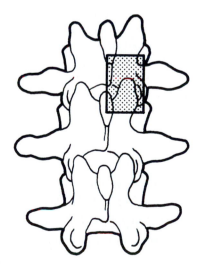

FIG 27–2.
Lateral decompression: the area of concern in lateral decompression. This much bone need not be removed in each case, however.

INSTRUMENTATION

Fancy equipment is not required to successfully complete most surgical decompressions for stenosis. Under ideal circumstances the equipment described in this section should be part of every spinal surgeon's kit and available in every operating room facility.

The operating table should permit the taking of intraoperative radiographs and fluoroscopy. The table should allow the patient to be placed in a kneeling position. Three types of spinal positioning devices are helpful as no one frame or positioner is ideal in every circumstance. A kneeling frame such as the Cloward saddle or Andrews frame or either a Wilson frame or a Relton-Hall frame should cover most patient positioning needs (Fig 27–3). The positioning frame selection should be able to accommodate a large protuberant abdomen and intraoperative radiographs or fluoroscopy when necessary. Great care must be taken to avoid abdominal pressure as this is an important method for the prevention of excessive intraoperative bleeding from dilated epidural veins. These frames need not be expensive. One of the best frames that I have seen was made from wood by the surgeon in his own home workshop.[3] Our Relton-Hall frame was made 20 years ago in the hospital shop and has served well since.

A headlight and surgical telescopes (loupes) make this surgery easier, safer, faster and far less fatiguing. The operating microscope has not been of much help to me in these operations, but may, of course, be used by those familiar with such equipment.

Table 27–3 contains a detailed list of the instruments that are mentioned in the description of the surgical technique to follow.

INTRAOPERATIVE MEDICATION

These procedures may require several hours of surgery and should not be considered minor. Therefore, we recommend prophylaxis with antibiotics, preoperatively, intraoperatively, and postoperatively. Further, we irrigate the wound with an antibiotic solution during the procedure unless the dura has been opened, in which case only saline is used.

Thrombin-soaked Gelfoam (absorbable gelatin sponge) and cottonoid sponges are useful to control

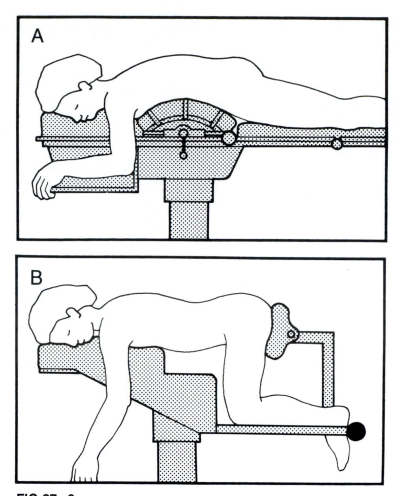

FIG 27–3.
Positioning frames: **A,** Wilson frame. **B,** kneeling frame.

minor bone bleeding or minor venous bleeding. Some surgeons prefer bone wax to control bone bleeding when electrocautery proves inefficient.

Epidural medication such as methylprednisolone acetate (Depo-Medrol) and morphine appear to be useful in some cases. A recent study[13] suggests that methylprednisolone acetate and epidural morphine both reduce the need for pain medications in the postoperative period. For small procedures, steroids alone are safe and effective. In major procedures and where fusion is also necessary, epidural morphine is also useful. Methylprednisolone acetate (80 mg) is placed directly in the epidural space on the nerve roots before closure. If morphine is to be used, special precautions are necessary. The dose is 3 to 5 mg diluted to 0.5 mg/mL which is placed in the epidural space by intraoperative catheter which is then removed. This gives 36 hours of significant analgesia. Care must be taken not to allow the drug to be injected intrathecally for the intrathecal dose is

one-tenth that of the epidural dose. When morphine is to be used, the patient will need an apnea monitor for 24 hours with a morphine antagonist at the bedside. In the instance of accidental intrathecal injection of a large dose of morphine, the patient may need a respirator for 36 hours and titration with a constant drip of an intravenous (IV) antagonist (*N*-allylnormorphine).

SURGICAL TECHNIQUE-LAMINECTOMY AND FORAMENOTOMY

The exposure is made through a midline posterior incision which is carried down to the spinous processes (Fig 27–4). The ligamentous and fascial at-

TABLE 27–3.

Instrumentation

A. Headlight
B. Wide-angle surgical telescopes, ×2.5
C. Cautery
    a. Monopolar, with coagulation and cutting current
    b. Bipolar for use within the spinal canal
D. Fluoroscopic and radiographic equipment
E. Elevators
    a. Cobb elevators, both wide and narrow
    b. Narrow Adson elevators, both curved and straight
F. Osteotomes—narrow Cloward type, both curved and straight
G. Disc rongeurs—narrow (3 mm) with long handles, both straight and angled
H. Kerrison rongeurs (40 degrees) three widths
I. Penfield dissectors, no. 2, 3 and 4
J. High-speed turbine burr
K. Dandy ligamentum flavum forceps
L. Bone impactors
M. Woodson dental elevator
N. Coronary artery dilators (2, 3, and 4 mm)
O. Dural hook
P. Fine-point curved needle holder and 6-0 eye silk
Q. Rongeurs
R. Curettes
S. Retractors

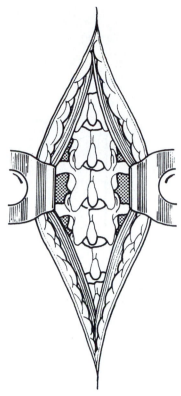

FIG 27–4.
Surgical exposure with self-retaining retractor.

tachments to the spinous processes are incised and the paraspinal musculature is elevated using elevators with a wide spatula. The elevator should be so wide as to have no risk of inadvertently falling between the laminae. Care must be taken to avoid entering a spina bifida occulta which may be present in as many as 5% of patients and every effort should be made to avoid unnecessary injury to facets. Exposure is maintained with a self-retaining retractor (see Fig 27–4). Hemostasis is achieved with electrocautery. The vessels which give the most trouble are the small arterioles between the facets at the level of the pars interarticularis and the sacral veins entering the sacral posterior root foramen. Electrocautery is adequate for the former, but packing with Gelfoam and thrombin or bone wax may be required for the sacral veins. The best policy, to reduce this problem, is to avoid wide exposure of the sacrum since decompression seldom needs to extend further than the S1 root in any case. Control of bleeding is important—do not proceed with the decompression until the field is dry. Controlled hypotensive anesthesia is not very helpful and should be avoided in patients with stenosis because of intercurrent cardiovascular or renal disease and because of the risk of additional vascular injury to the cauda equina.[7]

In decompressing bilateral stenosis there is seldom any advantage to retaining the spinous process,

intraspinous ligament, or supraspinous ligament since degeneration of the intraspinous ligament and shortening of the space between segments has rendered these structures incompetent. Removing these structures makes the surgery much simpler. In unilateral decompression, the spinous processes and ligaments should be retained to limit exposure and bleeding. At each level (Fig 27–5,A) in which the lamina must be removed to achieve an adequate decompression, it is practical to begin by removal of the spinous process and interspinous ligament, which is easily done with a rib cutter or rongeur. Bone bleeding is controlled with Gelfoam and thrombin or bone wax. The flavum is cleaned of muscle tissue at each level and then the superior attachment of the flavum is loosened with a 2- or 3-mm curette from facet to facet (Fig 27–5,B). Special care must be taken in the midline since the dura may be attached to the bone in this location. The flavum is then detached from the undersurface of the lamina using a narrow Cobb elevator, taking care to always control the depth of penetration and keeping contact with bone at all times (Fig 27–5,C). The elevator must be kept sharp on its edges and the flavum elevated with a side-to-side motion with a slight twist to cleanly pry the flavum loose. Af-

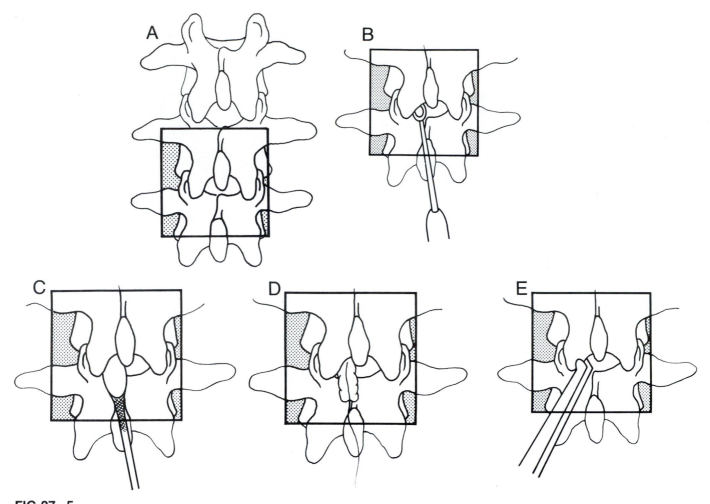

FIG 27–5.
Surgical technique: **A,** lamina, flavum, and facets of adjacent segments. **B,** curette for detaching the ligamentum flavum. **C,** narrow Cobb elevator for further detachment of the ligamentum flavum. **D,** cottonoid sponge to protect dura. **E,** Kerrison rongeur for removal of lamina.

ter the spinal canal has been entered, a cottonoid sponge is placed between the bone and the flavum and dura (Fig 27–5,D). The bone is then removed with appropriately sized rongeurs working from distal to proximal (Fig 27–5,E). The same procedure is done at each level. Removal of the lamina is easily and safely accomplished with successive middle, right, and left bites with a Kerrison rongeur. Avoid allowing the rongeur to become trapped in a narrow slot by changing the angle of the bite each time. Protect the dura with a moist cottonoid sponge which should always be between the dura and the lamina being removed. Suction should be directed to the surface of the cottonoid so as not to injure the dura or nerve roots. I prefer to leave the flavum until all of the laminae have been removed since, in longstanding stenosis, the dura may be firmly adherent to the degener-

ated flavum and necrotic epidural fat. Continuous removal of flavum and bone with a Kerrison rongeur may result in unnecessary durotomy where the two structures have become tightly adherent, thus prolonging the surgery and increasing the risk. Even in spite of this precaution, the dura is sometimes unavoidably opened in these cases (see Chapter 32).

Contrary to the procedure for removal of the lamina, the lateral recess and neuroforamina are decompressed from proximal to distal (Fig 27–6,A). This is done to prevent injury to the roots. A root may be amputated by inadvertently carrying the Kerrison rongeur up into the axilla of a root which is completely invisible from the distal to proximal view. Roots become invisible because of a severely medialized facet which surrounds it.

The lateral recesses are decompressed starting

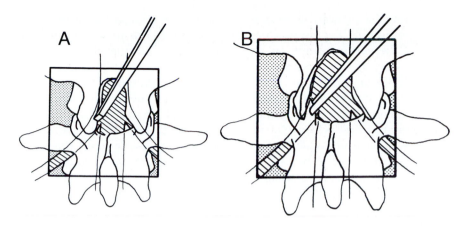

FIG 27–6.
A, nerve root decompression: This view is from proximal to distal as the nerve decompression should be done. **B,** view after osteotomy of the medial one third of the inferior facet and of the Kerrison rongeur removing the medial portion of the superior facet.

with exposed dura proximally and carefully detaching the flavum from the dura. Once the flavum has been removed laterally, it may become evident that the dura and nerve root origin is folded under the medial edge of the facet so tightly that even the smallest Kerrison or Sella punch will not fit safely between the facet and dura. In this instance, I find that the medial edge of the inferior facet can be safely removed with a narrow osteotome. This is done slightly obliquely, diverging from the midline structures. This can be done safely since the neural structures are protected by the underlying superior facet of the level below. Once the medial portion of the superior facet is exposed, it may still be impossible to safely slip the rongeur under it. Again, the osteotome can be used safely but only to crack the medial one third of the facet loose. Do not drive the osteotome through the bone. The bone of the superior facet is quite brittle and cracks easily since this portion of the facet is thin cortical bone. The medial portion of the superior facet may come loose after the crack has been made, or a Kerrison punch will now ride under without producing undue pressure on the nerve root origin. Once the level of the pedicle is achieved, the nerve root should be clearly visible. The pedicle is the key to the dissection of the nerve root. Always orientate yourself at each level to the center of the pedicle, which is marked by the inferior edge of the facet. Make allowances for the severely hypertrophic facet which may extend distally also. During the exposure of the lateral recess, one may encounter large synovial cysts and old encapsulated disc fragments. These must be removed, but a smooth degenerated hard annular bulge should not

be excised, as removal of the overlying bone will almost always free up the nerve and will result in less nerve root scar. These smooth annular bulges usually do not require surgical treatment. Try, also, to preserve at least 8 mm of the pars to prevent later stress fracture of the thinned bone.

In most instances, at least half of each facet joint can be preserved and an adequate decompression of the root at that level can be achieved. On rare occasions, an entire facet will need to be removed or breaks off in the course of decompression. In these instances, and in degenerative spondylolisthesis, fusion should be considered, especially when the involved segment remains mobile (see Chapter 11).

An individual neuroforamen is considered patent when the nerve root is seen to exit freely or a 2- or 3-mm coronary dilator or Penfield no. 3 dissector can be passed easily through the foramen along with the root.

Degenerative spondylolisthesis is a special case in surgical decompression for stenosis. Here, the abnormality is a combination of the central canal stenosis caused by the ring-on-ring "noose" effect of the slip and the distal lateral recess stenosis caused by the inevitable severe facet degeneration at the involved level. The whole cauda equina from the level of the slip down is affected by the noose effect, resulting in symptoms of pseudo-claudication. Radicular symptoms are also frequently present in patients with degenerative spondylolisthesis. These radicular symptoms are caused by entrapment of the root at the level below the slip level. For example, if the slip has occurred at the L4–5 level with the L4 level anterior to the L5 level, it will be the L5 root which will be trapped by the hypertrophic L4–5 facet. The superior facet of L5 will be the portion of the joint producing the more severe part of the nerve entrapment in the lateral recess. The surgery for decompression must address both of these pathologic elements.

In the decompression of degenerative spondylolisthesis, I begin with a complete bilateral laminectomy of the slipped segment followed by a nerve root decompression of the distal root which is always done from proximal to distal. Fusion is then attempted laterally, unless there has been nearly complete disc resorption producing an immobile segment. In younger patients and patients in whom previous fusion has failed, the addition of internal fixation appears to have some theoretical merit. However, the routine use of internal fixation in limited lumbar fusions remains at best controversial.[2]

Other special cases are stenosis caused by anterior bony fragments from healed burst fractures, the far-out syndrome, and degenerative scoliosis. The surgical treatment of these conditions is discussed in Chapters 12, 14, and 15.

RESULTS OF SURGICAL DECOMPRESSION FOR STENOSIS

In a recent report from Singapore by Wong and Bose,[17] three of five patients with degenerative spondylolisthesis had poor results due to persistent back pain. None of these patients were fused. Overall, Wong and Bose had approximately 9% failures and 28% fair results in the treatment of all groups of patients with spinal stenosis. These failures and marginal results were largely due to persistent disabling lower back pain. Wiltse et al.,[16] Paine,[11] Verbiest,[14] and Wong and Bose[17] all stated that the decompressive surgery for spinal stenosis was reliable for the relief of radicular symptoms and pseudoclaudication but not of back pain. Wong and Bose concluded that preoperative lower back pain was a negative predictor of outcome.[17]

If the patients had severe lower back pain preoperatively, they were more likely to have a poor outcome from surgery because of persistence of the lower back pain postoperatively. Therefore, more attention should be directed toward the back pain component of the disease. Weinstein et al.[15] used spinal stenosis patients to demonstrate the usefulness of a pre- and postoperative grading system to quantify the results of surgical treatment; they demonstrated, for the short term (1–4 years), that the patients consistently improve, but that the most severely affected are less likely to approach normal than the moderately affected. Patient satisfaction was high (85%) in Russin and Sheldon's series.[12] Herkowitz and Kurz.[8] concluded that decompression plus fusion gave the best results in patients with degenerative spondylolisthesis unless the spine was quite "stiff" preoperatively, in which instance the fusion should be avoided.

REFERENCES

1. Bailey P, Elsberg CA: Spinal decompression: Reports of seven cases and remarks on the diagnosis of and justification for exploratory operations. *JAMA* 1912; 58:675–679.
2. Bernhardt M, Swartz DE, Clothiaux PL, et al: Posterolateral lumbar and lumbosacral fusion with and without pedicle screw fixation, in *Proceedings of the International Society for the Study of the Lumbar Spine.* Boston, June 13–17, 1990, pp 7–8.
3. Brandon S: Kneeling frame. Personal communication, 1988.
4. Elsberg CA: Surgery of intramedullary affections of the spinal cord, anatomic basis and technique with report of cases. *JAMA* 1912; 59:1532–1536.
5. Elsberg CA: Experiences in spinal surgery. Observations upon 60 laminectomies for spinal disease. *Surg Gynecol Obstet* 1913; 16:117–132.
6. Frazier CH: Certain problems and procedures in the surgery of the spinal column. *Surg Gynecol Obstet* 1913; 6:552–560.
7. Garfin SR, Cohen MS, Massie JB, et al: Nerve-roots of the cauda equina: The effect of hypotension and acute graded compression on function. *J Bone Joint Surg [Am]* 1990; 72:1185–1192.
8. Herkowitz KN, Kurz LT: Degenerative spondylolisthesis: Prospective study comparing decompression vs decompression with fusion, in *Proceedings of the International Society for the Study of the Lumbar Spine.* Boston, June 13–17, 1990, p 39.
9. Markham JW: Surgery of the spinal cord and vertebral column, in Walker AE (ed): *A History of Neurological Surgery.* Baltimore, Williams & Wilkins Co, 1951, pp 364–393.
10. McNeill TW: Pelvic visceral dysfunction: Cauda equina syndrome, in Weinstein JN, Wiesel SW (eds): *The Lumbar Spine.* Philadelphia, WB Saunders Co, 1990, pp 449–455.
11. Paine KWE: Results of decompression for lumbar spinal stenosis. *Clin Orthop* 1976; 115:96–100.
12. Russin LA, Sheldon J: Spinal stenosis: Report of a series with long term follow-up. *Clin Orthop* 1976;115:101–104.
13. Schell BE, Andersson GBJ, Sinkora G, McNeill TW: A

comparison of epidural morphine and corticosteroids in controlling postoperative pain. International Society for the Study of the Lumbar Spine, Rome, June 1988.

14. Verbiest H: Results of treatment of idiopathic developmental stenosis of the lumbar vertebral canal—a review of twenty-seven years of experience. *J Bone Joint Surg [Br]* 1977; 59:181–188.

15. Weinstein JN, Scafuri RL, McNeill TW: The Rush-Presbyterian-St. Luke's lumbar spine analysis form: A prospective study of patients with "spinal stenosis." *Spine* 1983; 8:891–893.

16. Wiltse LL, Kirkaldy-Willis WH, McIvor GWD: The treatment of spinal stenosis. *Clin Orthop* 1976; 115:83–91.

17. Wong HK, Bose K: Results of surgical treatment of spinal stenosis, in *Proceedings of the International Society for the Study of the Lumbar Spine*, Boston, June 13–17, 1990, p 40.

28

Pedicle Screw Fixation: Indications, Techniques, and Systems

Mark B. Kabins, M.D.

James N. Weinstein, D.O.

Segmental pedicle screw fixation is rapidly becoming a popular method of surgical fixation of the spinal column. The strongest portion of the vertebra is the pedicle, which transmits all forces from the posterior elements to the vertebral body. The pedicle withstands all of the transmitted stresses of rotation, side bending, and extension of the spine. Thus, the pedicle has been labeled by Steffee et al.[99, 100] as the "force nucleus" of the vertebral body. It is an ideal structure to lock into and control with posterior instrumentation when spinal fixation is needed.

Pedicle screw fixation provides rigid immobilization of the spine while requiring only the presence of an intact pedicle. By comparison, Harrington and Luque instrumentation require an intact lamina for segmental fixation, and thus are frequently not applicable following extensive laminectomy. Fewer motion segments need be instrumented with pedicle screw fixation than are required by other forms of conventional instrumentation (i.e., Harrington, Luque). It is believed that this fixation not only provides stability for the unstable spine but can also aid in promotion of fusion between segments (i.e., L4–5 level; floating lumbar segments; multilevel fusions). Thus, the concept of "rodding long and fusing short" becomes somewhat obsolete.

There are now several pedicle screw systems available, and most are used in the treatment of various forms of spinal abnormalities. Although there are inherent advantages and disadvantages with each system, specific indications for the use of these systems have not been clearly established in the literature. Nevertheless, successful use of each system requires appropriate preoperative indications and correct application of the device.

The purpose of this chapter is to (1) examine the indications for pedicle screw fixation in spinal stenosis; (2) review the history along with the results and complications of vertebral screw and pedicle screw fixation; (3) survey a variety of pedicle screw systems presently available; (4) examine the anatomy of the pedicle and the surgical application of the pedicle screw; and (5) review basic biomechanical data assessing pedicle screw instrumentation.

INDICATIONS

The primary indications for pedicle screw fixation in spinal stenosis are in stabilizing "unstable" segments following decompression (laminectomy), and to augment the formation of a solid fusion between levels. Nevertheless, the extent of instability required to warrant such a procedure is not unanimously agreed upon.[7, 30, 42, 82, 85, 106, 114, 116]

Booth,[7] in addition to others, believes that stability can be maintained as long as a total of one facet joint at each level is retained. That is, a unilateral hemifacetectomy or even complete facetectomy can be performed without significant compromise to stability. A bilateral hemifacetectomy will likewise leave enough facet joint to prevent spondylolisthesis. Bilateral complete facetectomies, however, render the spine unstable. In contrast, Ray[85] stated that removal of one facet joint, even in the presence of an apparently normal disc space, may lead to torsional instability. Hopp and Tsou[42, 106] stated that bilateral hemifacetectomy (removal of the medial half of the facet) removes the anterior shear resistance of the facet. This, together with excision of the posterior ligaments, may eventually lead to further instability.

Booth[7] has stated that his relative indications for fusion following decompression for spinal stenosis also include patients under age 50 years, patients with low intercrestal lines, and patients with "dynamic spinal stenosis." These latter indications are more controversial and are topics of dispute.

Spinal stenosis with radiographic evidence of instability[22, 42, 106] (Macnab traction spur; centrum sclerosis adjacent to a degenerative disc; excessive motion between levels on dynamic flexion and extension films: translation that exceeds 3 mm at L3–4 or L4–5 at L5–S1 or angulation of one motion segment of more than 10 degrees) is believed by many to be a relative indication for fusion and instrumentation following decompression.

Wiltse stated that he always fuses for

> . . . (1) severe instability, (2) potential severe instability, (3) progressive deformity, (4) after reduction or repositioning of the vertebrae, (5) after internal fixation, (6) after decompression for degenerative spondylolisthesis, (7) after any operation for isthmic spondylolisthesis, (8) after a Gill operation, and (9) after decompression for the far out syndrome (an exception might be the case with very a narrow disc space with exuberant osteoarthritic spurs).[114]

Although the indications for instrumentation and fusion will vary with the operating surgeon, we believe that prior to the onset of significant kyphosis, posterior instrumentation alone with a pedicle screw system offers the best solution to pre- and postlaminectomy instability. In the presence of kyphotic deformity, an anterior stabilizing procedure would most likely also be needed.

Use of pedicle screw fixation should be considered in adults undergoing "floating" lumbar fusions, multilevel fusions, and in particular, fusions incorporating the L4–5 level.

This is supported by review of the literature indicating the difficulty in obtaining a solid fusion at the L4–5 level and between "floating" lumbar segments, regardless of the fusion type.[17, 83] The pseudarthrosis rate at the L4–5 level is reported to be the highest of any single level.[15, 19, 48, 105]

Using posterolateral fusions techniques without instrumentation, Kelly,[50] in 1963, reported a 44% fusion rate from L4–S1 and 100% from L5–S1. Later, Wiltse et al.,[115] in 1968, reported a 79%(11/14) fusion rate from L4–S1, compared with a 97%(33/34) rate from L5–S1. In 1979, Frymoyer et al.[29] reported a 26% pseudarthrosis rate in 96 patients (25/96) following discectomy and posterior fusion, with "almost all" occurring at L4–L5. Likewise, Lehmann et al.,[62] in 1987, reported a pseudarthrosis rate of 30% in 96 patients (29/96) undergoing lumbar arthrodesis at the L3 level and below.

In 1990, Kabins et al.[47] reviewed 41 patients treated with posterolateral floating fusions at the L4–5 level supplemented with VSP (variable screw placement, Steffee[99]) instrumentation (Fig 28–1, A,B). Patients were instrumented with either unilateral (18) or bilateral (23) plates. The authors found the use of unilateral instrumentation appealing in that it may decrease the potential morbidity seen with more rigid bilateral systems (i.e., osteoporosis secondary to stress shielding; segmental instability or degeneration above and below the fused level),[29, 61, 62, 75] in addition to decreasing the inherent risks of placing a greater number of pedicle screws.[108, 109, 111, 119] Average radiographic follow-up was 23 months. Overall, there were 35 of 41 patients (85%) with solidly healed fusions. In the patients fused with autograft, 97% (16/17 unilateral; 18/18 bilateral) were solidly healed. Two (4.9%) pseudarthroses occurred in 41 patients, yet optimal initial fixation was not achieved in either patient. Results with unilateral instrumentation were comparable to bilateral, and in both cases better than most historical controls for in situ, noninstrumented grafts. There was no correlation between the use of interbody grafting and the posterolateral fusion outcome, a technique suggested by some surgeons.[63, 99, 102] Posterolateral allogeneic grafts demonstrated significantly worse results. In contrast to the work of Brown et al.,[11] who reported a significant difference in fusion outcome ($\chi^2 = 14.035$, $P = .001$) for smokers (compared with nonsmokers) undergoing noninstrumented posterolateral fusions from L4–S1, smoking did not affect fusion outcome. Perhaps this difference reflected the contribution of the hardware. Unfortunately, subjective pain relief and functional outcome were less predictable, and not significantly related to fusion outcome.

These results were comparable to that of Schwaegler et al.[94] who reported no pseudarthroses among 39 patients treated with one-level fusions

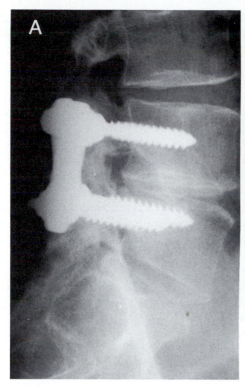
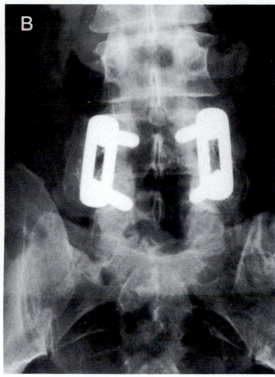

FIG 28–1.

Lateral **(A)** and AP **(B)** radiographs of a 50-year-old white man 2 years following an L4–5 decompression, posterolateral fusion, and bilateral VSP (variable screw placement, Steffee) fixation for degenerative disc disease. Radiographs demonstrate the presence of a solid fusion. His clinical outcome was rated "good." He had "mild intermittent pain" and returned to "normal daily activity."

supplemented with bilateral VSP instrumentation, and followed on average for over 2 years. In contrast, 21% of the noninstrumented group developed pseudarthroses. No hardware failures were reported. Dean et al.[18] reported similar findings. These optimistic results may, however, overstate the true percentage of solid fusions. The ability of plain films to assess fusion outcome has been shown to have limited value.[10, 54] The presence of a fixation device likely reduces accuracy further. Also, the criteria for determining fusion status differ in most studies.

Nevertheless, not all retrospective studies assessing the efficacy of pedicular fixation have yielded such favorable results. For example, Kabins et al.[48] reported a 65% fusion rate (26/40 patients) in patients with previously failed lumbar surgery whose subsequent treatment included posterolateral grafting with pedicular (VSP) instrumentation. Fusion rates for these patients were maximized when posterior interbody grafts (PLIFs) were used in combination with autogenous posterolateral grafts (8/8, 100%). Complications were greater than in their previously reported group of patients treated in a similar manner. Patients with postoperative pseudarthrosis (15%) demonstrated significantly poorer clinical outcomes ($P < .03$). Overall, 68% were clinically improved, yet only 38% returned to work.

It should be emphasized that spinal stenosis alone is seldom an indication for use of pedicular instrumentation. Most decompressions can be adequately accomplished without destabilizing the spine. However, spinal stenosis associated with degenerative spondylolisthesis may require postoperative fusion and stabilization. Upon retrospective review, Johnsson et al.[46] demonstrated a significantly ($P < .01$) greater incidence of further slippage in patients decompressed for degenerative spondylolisthesis, compared to spinal stenosis alone. They reported a 65% incidence of further slippage following decompression for degenerative spondylolisthesis. An abundance of literature[14, 27, 28, 46, 53, 71, 86, 116] now supports fusing the decompressed level in degenerative spondylolisthesis. Nevertheless, placement of an in situ, noninstrumented graft will not eliminate motion, and progression of the deformity (slip) can occur. In this setting, the pseudarthrosis rate is likely to be higher.

In 1990, Herkowitz and Kurz[41] reported results of a prospective study comparing decompression alone with decompression and fusion for 57 patients with one-level degenerative spondylolisthesis. Patients undergoing fusions reported less postoperative back and leg pain. Postoperative horizontal translation (slip) occurred in 22% of patients undergoing decompression and fusion, compared to 62% in the decompression group alone. In contrast, Kabins et al.[47] reported no further postoperative slippage and a 100% fusion rate in 15 patients receiving VSP instrumentation and posterolateral grafts for L4–5 degenerative spondylolisthesis (Fig 28–2,A,B). Interestingly, patients undergoing unilateral instrumentation for degenerative spondylolisthesis reported significantly better clinical results than all other patients with other diagnoses, instrumented unilaterally or bilaterally.

To study the effects of instrumentation upon the formation of the fusion mass, McAfee et al.,[75] in 1989, examined adult beagles destabilized at L5–6, and reconstructed with posterolateral grafts supplemented with hardware (Harrington distraction, Luque rectangular, or Cotrel-Dubousset transpedicular instrumentation). Control groups consisted of noninstrumented and noninstrumented, nongrafted specimens. Through quantitative histomorphometric studies, the volumetric density of bone was found at 6 months to be significantly lower for fused vs. unfused spines. In addition, those instrumented with the transpedicular system demonstrated the lowest volumetric density. However, there was a greater probability of achieving a solid fusion if instrumentation had been used. In addition, as the rigidity of the instrumentation increased, the probability of achieving a successful fusion also was greater. Nonetheless, nondestructive mechanical testing following instrumentation removal demonstrated a significant increase in the rigidity of the fusion mass when the original graft was supplemented with instrumentation. This seemingly paradoxical finding probably occurred as a result of the greater total area of graft incorporation in the more rigidly instrumented specimens. Apparently, this more than compensated for loss of rigidity due to device-related osteopenia. Thus, these results support the notion that rigid instrumentation may augment, and in fact enhance the formation of a fusion mass.

HISTORY OF VERTEBRAL SCREW AND PEDICLE SCREW FIXATION

The history of vertebral screw fixation dates back to 1944 when King[51, 52] first described the placement

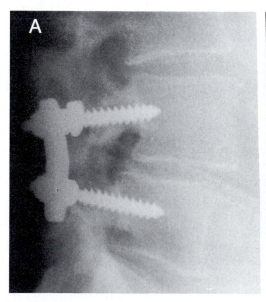
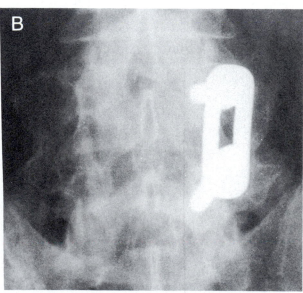

FIG 28–2.
Lateral **(A)** and AP **(B)** radiographs of a 64-year-old man 2 years following an L4–5 decompression, posterolateral fusion, and unilateral VSP (Steffee) fixation for degenerative spondylolisthesis. Radiographs demonstrate the presence of a solid fusion. His clinical outcome was rated "excellent." He had "no pain" and returned to "normal daily activity."

of screws (¾ in. for women, 1 in. for men) parallel to the inferior border of the lamina and across (perpendicular to) the facet joints of lumbar vertebrae in an attempt to avoid postoperative external immobilization and prolonged bed rest. Patients were, however, encouraged to stay in bed for 3 weeks following surgery, a practice not uncommon in those days. A pseudarthrosis rate of approximately 10% was reported in patients fixed with screws and grafted from L5–S1. One (2.3%) patient experienced "nerve-root irritation" as a result of a poorly positioned screw which was subsequently removed.

In 1949, Thompson and Ralston[105] reported a pseudarthrosis rate of 55.1% (27/49) using a similar technique in 49 patients undergoing L4–S1 instrumentation and grafting. Results were better (5/41, 12.2% pseudarthrosis rate) in 41 additional patients instrumented and grafted from L5–S1. Patients were allowed out of bed 2 to 3 weeks following surgery, and no external support was used. Bosworth,[8] in 1957, also reported poor results and stated that screw fixation did not prove to be of value compared to the difficulties encountered in screw placement.

Boucher,[9] in 1959, and Pennel et al.,[81] in 1964, described a method of internal fixation using longer (1½–2 in.), machined, stainless steel screws placed through the facet joints. Screws at L5–S1 were placed along the longitudinal axis of the body, nearly transversing the full anteroposterior (AP) diameter of the sacrum. Screws were typically placed through the inferior facet and into the pedicle and vertebral body below. Boucher[9] recognized that screws placed through the pedicle provided improved fixation. There were no hardware failures in 160 patients undergoing single-level fusions. There were, however, two broken screws in 14 patients undergoing multilevel fusions. Root irritation from poorly positioned screws occurred in two (1.1%) patients. Four of 49 (8.2%) patients with spondylolisthesis developed a pseudarthrosis.

In 1970, Buck[12] first described the use of screw fixation in the direct repair of isthmic-lytic defects in 16 patients with spondylolisthesis. Fully threaded screws were placed at the inferior edge of the lamina, through the pars interarticularis, and into the pedicle and vertebral body. Screws were partially withdrawn for autogenous grafting, and then driven home. One patient's fusion failed as both screws loosened and the lamina became unstable. Gaps measuring over 4 mm were felt to be "beyond the practical limit of repair."

In 1977, Evans et al.[26] reviewed 190 patients treated in a similar manner as those treated by Boucher[9] and Pennel et al.[81] As in previous reports, failure most often occurred at the L4–5 level (33% for single-level L4–L5 fusions). They reported a 15% failure rate at the L5–S1 level.

In contrast, Andrew et al.,[3] in 1985, found no difference in outcome between single-level L4–5, L5–S1, or two-level fusions. In their study, 59 patients were followed on average for 9 years. Screws 1¼ in. long were used along with posterior, corticocancellous grafts (avoiding the increased time requirement and potential morbidity of a posterolateral fusion). They reported no broken or loose screws, and with the exception of one patient, all attempted fusions "appeared" solid. Four screws were "malpositioned," giving rise to sciatica. Fifty-seven patients (97%) returned to their previous occupation within 6 months.

Jacobs et al.,[44] in 1989, likewise reported good results using translaminar facet joint screws. Using the technique previously described by Magerl,[73, 74] they reported 93% (82 patients) clinical improvement and 91% (80) solid fusion in 88 consecutive patients followed prospectively on average for 16 months. AO 4.5-mm cortical screws approximately 50 mm long were placed at the base of the spinous process, through the lamina, across the facet, ending at the attachment of the transverse process to the pedicle.

Clearly, these more recent results are better than those of most previous studies. This difference may reflect better surgical technique, improved instrumentation, or indications, or a combination of these. Nevertheless, the overall results of vertebral screw placement are mixed. The high fusion rates reported at the L5–S1 level are not unlike those seen for noninstrumented patients. Generally, complications, including infection, nerve damage, facet fracture, screw loosening, and breakage were rare.

In 1970, Roy-Camille and Demeulenaere[87] first described the use of posterior plates with screws positioned sagittally through the pedicles and articular processes. The use of this pedicle screw-plate system began in 1963. The plates were designed following anatomic studies that demonstrated the average interpedicular distance in the lumbar spine to be approximately 2.6 cm. Collar-reinforced holes were spaced every 1.3 cm to allow placement of 4.5 -cm screws within the pedicles, and adjacent, smaller screws (when needed) into the facet joints. Special plates were also designed for short fusions and lumbosacral fusions. Two screws could be placed through one central hole within the plate and into the pedicle for improved purchase. The plating system of Roy-Camille and colleagues was applied in the treatment of a number of spinal problems and the results were encouraging—a nearly 100% success rate in lumbosacral fusions. The instrumentation was also capable of partially reducing slips in high-grade spondylolisthesis.

The work of Roy-Camille et al[88–91] set the foundation for pedicle screw instrumentation. Cabot[13] described a midline lumbosacral plate that was hooked onto the spinous processes and also fixed transpedicularly with screws. Louis and Maresca[66, 67] subsequently modified Roy-Camille's technique and instrumentation. Louis[64, 65] later reviewed 455 cases of his modified screw-plate fixation system followed on average for 31.6 months. Solid fusions occurred in 97.4% of his single-staged posterior approaches, and in 100% of combined approaches. However, the criteria used to establish this high fusion rate is questionable. Louis stated "since dynamic roentgenograms failed to demonstrate instability . . ., the diagnosis of nonunion was considered probable in those patients whose persistent lumbar pain subsided immediately after they began wearing plaster corset braces."[65]

Transpedicular screws were quickly modified to be used in other situations. Harrington and Dickson,[38] in addition to Sijbrandij[95] and others,[23, 24, 110] have inserted screws into pedicles and vertebral bodies along with modified Harrington instrumentation for the reduction and fixation of spondylolisthesis.

Harrington and Tullos[39] are credited with being among the first authors in the United States to describe transpedicular screw fixation. In 1967, two children with progressive and symptomatic spondylolisthesis were reduced and instrumented with a Harrington A frame supplemented with L5 pedicle screws. "Lag screws" were placed through the pedicles of L5 and wired to Harrington distraction rods to aid in the reduction of the slip.

External transpedicular fixation of the lower thoracic and lumbar spine was originally developed by Magerl[73, 113] in 1977. His system ("fixateur externe") consists of two pairs of long Schanz screws and an adjustable external fixation device. Screws are placed by either open or closed technique. The fixation device, consisting of two transverse bars, three rods, and triangular locking plates, provides rigid stability, allowing for early mobilization without external support. The system can be applied in distraction, compression, or in a neutral mode. Magerl found the stability of the system to be enhanced by preloading the Schanz screws in distraction, and by adding translaminar screws through the facet joints. In 1984, Magerl[74] reviewed 52 patients (42 with acute

spinal trauma, 8 with osteomyelitis) followed for a minimum of 1 year. There were no deep infections, and all superficial screw tract "irritation" resolved with the screws in place, or upon removal. Loosening of the screws occurred in 1 patient, requiring subsequent removal of the device. Optimal results, without loss of reduction, were obtained when the device was kept in place on average for 18 to 19 weeks. In most cases the damaged intervertebral discs collapsed following removal of the fixator, despite facet screw fixation and fusion. Although results with this system were encouraging, Magerl specifically did not recommend its use for common degenerative spinal lesions.

Following Magerl's initial description of external four-point fixation with Schanz screws, Dick et al.[21] developed a similar internal device, which they called the "fixateur interne." This system also utilized 5-mm Schanz screws to create long lever arms to facilitate manual reduction. The screws are connected to the 7-mm threaded longitudinal rods by clamps which are mobile in all directions, allowing for compression, distraction, kyphosis, lordosis, and rotation. Biomechanical testing with anterior bending moments demonstrated its increased rigidity in comparison to Magerl's external fixator. Preliminary reviews by Dick[20] in 1987, and Aebi et al.[1, 2] in 1987 and 1988 revealed the diversity of the system. Dick reinstrumented 3 of 183 patients because of construct failure. Neurologic deficits occurred only in those reduced because of severe slips. Aebi et al. reported two construct failures with resultant kyphotic deformity in 30 patients followed for a minimum of 6 months.

In 1986 Olerud and Sjöström[78] reported results in 18 patients with severe low back pain who were stabilized externally. Transpedicular Schanz screws attached to a modified Hoffmann fixator were used. Sixteen (89%) patients were reported to have experienced dramatic improvement. The authors suggested that this device could be used as definitive treatment for spinal instability or as a clinical trial to determine levels to be fused at a later date. It could also be used to determine the stability of previous fusion sites. Eight patients who initially presented with painful fusions responded with marked relief when stabilized. Three were not considered radiographically healed. This indicated to Olerud and Sjöström that either the fusion was not healed despite the radiographic appearance, or that the stability of the fusion was not enough to prevent painful movements between vertebrae. Roentgenstereophotogrammetric techniques[80] have demonstrated that despite a solid, bilateral, posterolateral fusion, significant movement can occur between grafted vertebrae.

Following the original work of Roy-Camille and co-workers, and the modifications of Louis, several other designs of transpedicular screw-plate fixation systems were developed.

The use of an AO tibial dynamic compression plate within the spine was initially described by Müller et al.[77] in 1979, and later reviewed by Thalgot et al.[104] in 1989. Like previously designed systems, the screw-plate interface is not rigid and micromotion occurs. The AO DCP plate has long, oval-shaped holes which provides greater angular freedom for the 6.5-mm, fully threaded cancellous screws to be placed. Forty-six patients followed between 1.0 and 2.5 years were studied. Asymptomatic screw loosening occurred in five patients (11%), and three patients (6.5%) had broken screws. Nerve root irritation requiring screw removal also occurred in three patients. In all, 72% of patients (33/46) were reported to have solidly healed fusions. The use of a different AO plate, called the "notched plate," was introduced following the DCP plate, but this has not been widely used.

In 1982, Steffee and co-workers[99-103] developed a new segmental, spinal plate and pedicle screw system that could be used from the lower thoracic spine to the sacrum. After originally using standard AO neutralization plates with fixed holes, they developed a slotted plate with "nests" to permit easier insertion and positioning of the modified, cancellous screws. Steffee et al., like surgeons before them, recognized the importance of contouring the plates to conform to the physiologic curves of the spine. They also stressed the importance of using the largest single screw suitable for each pedicle.

Steffee et al.[100] stated, in their initial publication, that their mean follow-up was too short to provide a meaningful retrospective review. They reported 90% excellent to good functional and clinical ratings. Their reported complications in a preliminary follow-up of 120 patients included 7 deep wound infections, 2 radiculopathies secondary to the graft placement, 8 hardware failures, and 5 patients who developed a pseudarthrosis requiring subsequent hardware removal. They also reported that the incidence of hardware failure decreased substantially following modifications in the instrumentation.

Subsequently, West et al.,[108, 109] Whitecloud et al.,[111] and Zucherman et al.[119] have retrospectively examined their results and complications in patients instrumented with the VSP (Steffee) system. Since

each applied the instrumentation in treatment of a number of different problems, clinical results were mixed and are difficult to assess. The presence of postoperative pseudarthrosis ranged from 11% to 18%. West et al.[108] reported that their rate was highest in patients who had a previous pseudarthrosis (38%). They went on to state that all patients who developed a pseudarthrosis were clinical failures, either by self-assessment, or because of the need for further surgery. Within each diagnostic group, the failure rate was 21% for the spondylolisthesis group, 20% for the degenerative group, and 48% for the pseudarthrosis repair group. Deep and superficial wound infections within the three studies rarely occurred (range: 0%–5%) and were statistically no different from reports of noninstrumented fusions.

In 1986, Eduardo Luque[68] introduced another method of interpedicular segmental fixation using pedicle screws wired to Luque rods. A preliminary review of 20 cases, followed on average for 14 months, demonstrated continued anatomic "correction of pathology" in 16 (80%) patients. In 1988, Luque and Rapp[70] introduced a new, "semirigid," cannulated screw and slotted plate system. They stressed the system's function as a posterior tension band, and that load sharing by the anterior column was necessary for maintenance of stability. Thus, all patients with fractures were externally immobilized in plaster jackets for 3 months or until the fracture and fusion were solid. Eighty cases were followed on average for 18 months. Loss of anatomic correction occurred in approximately 20% of cases. No conclusions addressing pseudarthrosis formation were made in either study. Luque's most recent review, in 1990,[69] evaluated 57 patients with spinal "instability" instrumented with the semirigid screw and plate system. With an average follow-up of 2.6 years, he reported one loose screw, one broken screw, and two (3.5%) cases of pseudarthrosis. The majority of patients experienced improvement in pain.

Following extensive biomechanical testing, Krag et al.[56-58] designed a pedicular screw-rod system called the Vermont spinal fixator (VSF). Like those before them, the authors argued that the interpedicular screw fixation was superior to standard Harrington or Luque fixation for the following reasons: (1) They were designed for "short segment" spinal defects, spanning only two to three vertebrae, not the five to seven typically needed by Harrington rods to achieve adequate stabilization. (2) True rigid, three-dimensional, three-column fixation was achieved, providing immobilization by suppressing flexion, extension, and rotational movements. Thus, the screw-plate (or rod) system functions as a fixator, not as a distractor or compressor. It is our opinion, as well as that of others, that rigid fixation can only be achieved in the presence of a stable anterior column. Pedicle screw fixation alone cannot always be relied upon for three-column stability, especially if there is anterior column instability. (3) It readily reduces fractures and spondylolistheses without violation of the spinal canal with hooks or wires.

The VSF system, which consists of screws, articulating clamps, bolts, and connecting rods, provides rigid fixation, while allowing for three-dimensional adjustability. To prevent loosening, the threads which the clamp bolt engage inside the rod clamp are made of a special pattern known as Spiralock. Additional advantages of this design include its ability to be repeatedly tightened, loosened, and retightened without degradation; its improved load distribution; and its lack of need for a separate locking nut. A preliminary review of the first 46 consecutive patients treated with this instrumentation revealed three broken screws and one loose screw. Follow-up was too short to adequately assess fusion outcome.

The Wiltse pedicle screw system was yet another popular system introduced in the 1980s.[36, 37, 43] This system consists of pedicle screws connected to stainless steel rods by saddle clamps. The use of rods (instead of plates) increased the adaptability of the system, allowing for placement on irregularly contoured spines. This is a potential advantage over other systems less tolerant of changes in pedicle direction. Steffee[99] has argued that the VSP system can be applied to deformed spines through the use of "working plates," where meticulous adjustments are made at each level to properly align the spine. The Wiltse pedicle system, the AO fixateur interne, and the VSF offer greater degrees for freedom of screw direction.

Since the saddle clamps of the Wiltse system are small, they can usually be placed with minimal disturbance of the facet joint. One or two rods can be used on each side. The one-rod system offers the advantage of saving time and the possibility of not further damaging the facet at the upper end of the fusion. Nevertheless, Guyer et al.[36] do not recommend unilateral rod placement.

In 1989, Horowitch et al.[43] reviewed 99 patients instrumented with the Wiltse system. Follow-up averaged 20 months. Hardware failure was seen in 7 (7%) patients. Screw breakage was seen in 5 (5%) patients, rod breakage in 2 (2%), clamp loosening in 1 (1%), and screw loosening in 3 (3%). Radiographs

demonstrated the presence of union in 68 (68%) patients, and nonunion in 32 (32%). Overall, 70 patients (70%) stated that they received some benefit from surgery.

Other forms of posterior instrumentation that utilize pedicular screws include the Cotrel-Dubousset system,[16, 33] the ISOLA spinal system, the Jacobs pelvic fixator,[45] the Texas Scottish Rite system, and Zielke instrumentation.[84, 96]

New pedicle screw systems are continuously becoming available,[49] and old systems are being modified and updated. Long-term follow-up studies, in addition to randomized, prospective studies, are needed to evaluate the efficacy of pedicular fixation. Surgical experience in pedicle screw fixation along with familiarity of the instrumentation and knowledge of its limitations is critical to obtaining good results.

ANATOMY OF THE PEDICLE AND PLACEMENT OF THE PEDICLE SCREW

Knowledge of the morphometry of the thoracic and lumbar spine as it applies to transpedicular screw placement has increased immensely following the work of Saillant[93] in 1976. Further morphometric studies have since been performed by Krag et al.[56, 60] in 1986 and 1988, Zindrick et al.[117] in 1987, Berry et al.[6] in 1987, and Olsewski et al.[79] in 1990. Without question, growing interest in pedicle screw fixation has been the basis for the growth in knowledge. The goals of this section are to touch upon the salient features of pedicular morphology as it relates to pedicle screw size and placement, in addition to reviewing biomechanical testing of screw placement.

Pedicle size and angulation in both the transverse and sagittal planes have been studied in detail by computed tomography (CT) analysis, in addition to plain roentgenograms and direct specimen evaluation. Zindrick et al.[117] found no significant difference between measurements made by CT scans and radiographs. Krag et al.[60] likewise found no significant difference between CT scans and direct physical measurements. Olsewski et al.,[79] on the other hand, stated that measurements on radiographs and CT scans of the transverse angles of the pedicles, and the distances from the posterior aspect of the laminar cortex to the anterior aspect of the cortex of the vertebral body from the L2 to L5 vertebrae were greater than the actual dimensions obtained from direct measurements. Direct measurements of the transverse and sagittal diameters of the pedicle of the L5 vertebra, however, were greater than radiographic measurements.

It is critical for the operating surgeon to recognize and understand measurements of pedicular

anatomy. This helps prevent errors in screw placement and allows the largest screw size to be placed correctly within the pedicle and vertebral body for improved purchase.

With the exception of L5, the pedicle is oval in shape and is narrowest in the transverse plane. It is this plane that determines maximum allowable pedi-

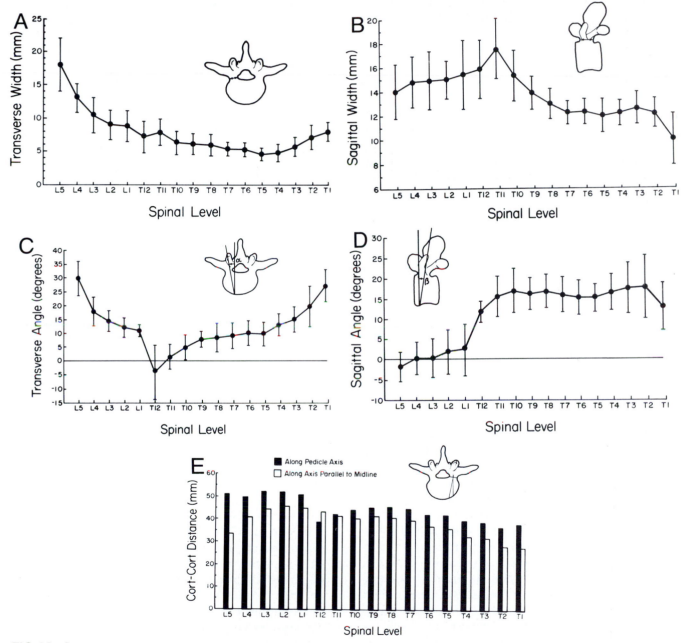

FIG 28–3.
A, transverse pedicle isthmus widths. **B,** sagittal pedicle isthmus widths. **C,** transverse pedicle angles. **D,** sagittal pedicle angles. **E,** distance to the anterior cortex through the pedicle angle axis vs. through the line parallel to the

midline axis of the vertebra. (From Zindrick MR, Wiltse LL, Doornik A, et al: *Spine* 1987; 12:160–166. Used by permission.)

cle screw diameter. Since the pedicle is much wider in the sagittal plane, screw migration and settling can occur without pedicle fracture or disruption.

In the transverse axis (Fig 28–3,A), Zindrick et al.[117] reported the widest pedicular isthmic diameter to be at L5 (mean: 18 mm; range: 9.1–29mm). This width decreased as the lumbar and thoracic spine was ascended (L1 was found to have a measured mean value of 8.7 mm, with a range of 4.5–13 mm). Sagittal pedicular isthmus width (Fig 28–3,B) within the lumbar spine was found to be least at L5 (mean: 14 mm; range: 9.5–19 mm), and to increase and peak at T11 (mean: 17.4 mm; range: 12.5–24.1 mm). This width subsequently declined when traveling cephalad in the thoracic spine.

Transverse angles of the pedicle (Fig 28–3,C) were found to angle medially in the lumbar spine (L5 mean: 29.8 degrees; range: 19–44 degrees). This decreased to neutral at L1 and angled laterally at T12 (mean: −4.2 degrees). This angle then increased medially as the thoracic spine was ascended. In the sagittal plane (Fig 28–3,D), L5 was found to angle caudally, with L4 and L3 at approximately neutral. As the lumbar spine was further ascended, this angle slowly increased cephalad. Once at T12, this angle sharply increased (mean: 11.6 degrees) cephalad. As one traveled further up the thoracic spine, this angle once more increased slowly.

The results of Krag et al.[60] closely paralleled those of Saillant[93] and Zindrick[117, 118]. They reported pedicle diameters (when measured perpendicular to the axis of the pedicle) to be fairly constant between T9 and L1, with a value of approximately 7 mm. A gradual increase then occurred from L1 to L5 (L5 mean: 13 mm).

Olsewski et al.[79] studied sex differences in pedicular anatomy. They determined that the average transverse and sagittal diameters of the pedicles and the distance from the posterior aspect of the cortex of the vertebral body along the central axis of the pedicles were 5% to 25% greater in men than women. However, the transverse and sagittal angles of the pedicle did not differ significantly.

Knowledge of the distance to the anterior cortex is also important in preventing anterior cortical perforation and possible injury to vital structures. Pedicle root length was found to be nearly constant from T9 to T12 (mean: 19 mm), and then to gradually decrease caudad (L5 mean: 15 mm). Krag et al.[60] noted that this finding was consistent with the decreasing volume of the cauda equina in the caudal direction. Vertebral body length was found to be almost constant from T9 to L5 (overall mean value: 32 mm).

The distance to the anterior cortex (Fig 28–3,E) has been found to vary depending upon the site of entry and the orientation of the screw. Three basic approaches have been described (Fig 28–4). Roy-Camille et al.[91] initially described the "straight ahead" approach in which screws are placed parallel to the sagittal plane and parallel to the vertebral end plates. The entrance point, following a posterior approach, was described to be situated at the crossing of two lines: a horizontal line passing through the middle of the transverse process, and a vertical line given by the articular processes 1 mm under the facet joint.

Later, Magerl,[74] Weinstein et al.,[107] and others[1, 2, 20, 21, 56] described the "anteromedial approach" in which the entrance point is situated at the lateral and inferior corner of the superior articular facet (the "nape of the neck"). This approach dictates a longitudinal guideline just lateral to the facet joint, intersecting with a horizontal line identical to that described by Roy-Camille et al. Screw orientation is parallel to the axis of the pedicle and end plate, but converges in the transverse plane.

Krag et al.[57] subsequently modified the anteromedial approach by placing the entry point further lateral and caudal, while angling the screws medially and cephalad. Thus, screws were no longer placed parallel to the vertebral end plate. Yet, it was emphasized that screws were not to violate the superior end plate. This "up and in" approach, like the anteromedial approach, offers several advantages: (1) The screw heads are placed further from the facet joint and are thus less likely to cause facet irritation and degenerative changes. (2) In comparison to the straight ahead approach described by Roy-Camille et al., the distance to the anterior cortex is increased at all levels (except at T11 and T12) with angulation of the screws in the anteromedial direction (parallel to the axis of the pedicle). In fact, they have stated that a 15-degree change in the anteromedial direction can result in an 8- to 10-mm increase in length of vertebral bone prior to anterior cortical perforation. In addition, the pedicular diameter tends to be larger for screws placed along the axis of the pedicle than along the midline axis in lumbar vertebrae. (3) The up and in orientation interlocks the instrumented vertebrae, preventing lateral translation of the superior vertebra upon the inferior one, even without a transverse rod or plate connector.

The appropriate depth for pedicle screw placement within the vertebral body continues to be debated. Krag et al.[55, 56, 59] have stated that the pedicle itself seems to be a stronger site for screw placement

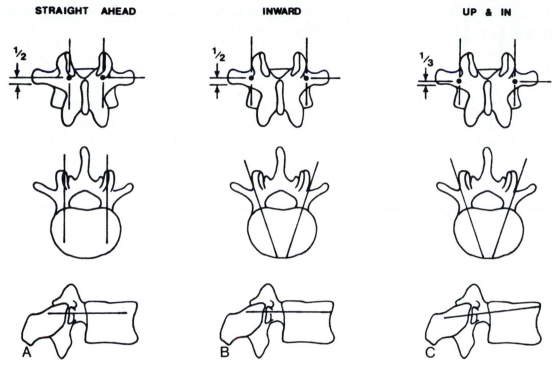

STRAIGHT AHEAD　　　　　**INWARD**　　　　　**UP & IN**

FIG 28–4.
Entry point and orientation alternatives for transpedicular screws. The "straight ahead" approach, initially described by Roy-Camille et al.,[91] places the screws parallel to the transverse and sagittal planes. The "inward" approach, initially described by Magerl,[74] places the screws in the anteromedial direction, along the axis of the pedicle. The "up and in" approach, initially described by Krag et al.,[57] places the entrance site farthest away from the facet joint (caudad and lateral). Screws are orientated anteromedial and anterocephalad. (From Krag MH, Fredrickson BE, Yuan HA: Spinal instrumentation, in Weinstein JN, Wiesel SW (eds): *The Lumbar Spine.* Philadelphia, WB Saunders Co, 1990; pp 916–940. Used by permission.)

than the vertebral body. Although both contain cancellous bone, the trabeculae in the pedicle appear to be stronger and thicker. Also, the pedicle has a thick cortex that can provide firm screw engagement. Thus, fully threaded pedicle screws should always be seated into the vertebral body in order for the threads to grip the entire length of the pedicle. Zindrick et al.[118] confirmed these findings by testing the pullout strength of partially threaded 6.5-mm cancellous (Steffee) screws with the threaded portion placed within the pedicle, in comparison with the vertebral body. They found the mean pullout strength to be 77% greater when the threaded portion was engaged within the pedicle. Likewise, the mean pullout force was 109% greater for 6.5-mm fully threaded cancellous screws compared with 6.5-mm partially threaded screws, when both were inserted to the anterior cortex.

The cadaver testing of Krag et al.[55, 56] of pedicle screws placed at varying depths within the vertebral body (50% vs. 80% penetration) suggests that deeper-seated screws tolerate higher forces prior to failure (Fig 28–5). Screws 6 mm wide placed at 80% depth demonstrated a 32.5% improvement in strength prior to failure for twisting loads, and a 29.3% improvement for extension loads.

On the other hand, Zindrick et al.[118] found no significant difference between screws seated at 50% depth and those seated adjacent to the anterior cortex. Screws placed through the anterior cortex, however, were significantly stronger than those seated adjacent to the cortex. The distal tip of the more deeply seated screws had a larger arc of motion and required more bony material to be displaced as the screw was cycled. The authors stated that the pedicle was large enough cephalad and caudad to accommodate this "windshield wiper" motion. Although increased screw purchase during axial pullout testing and cyclic loading was demonstrated by screws placed through the anterior cortex, clinical data have demonstrated that this is not necessary in the lumbar spine. In fact, it may pose an increased risk to the patient by causing damage to anterior vital structures.

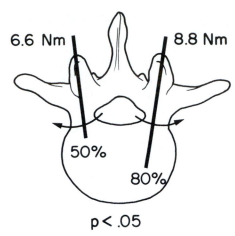

FIG 28–5.
Screw penetration of 80% tolerated 32.5% higher loads prior to cutout than did 50% penetration. (From Krag MH, Beynnon BD, Pope MH, et al: *Clin Orthop* 1986; 203:75–98. Used by permission.)

Sacral fixation differs in that many surgeons recommend screw placement through the anterior cortex (when placed through the S1 pedicle) for improved purchase. Bifurcation of the great vessels typically occurs at L4, leaving no major vascular structure immediately anterior to the promontory of the sacrum. In addition, there are no reports of increased morbidity following this approach at this level.

The award-winning work of Mirkovic et al.[76] examined sacral screw placement in 22 human cadaveric specimens to assess the risk of injury to anterior neurovascular and visceral structures. Screws (6.5-mm cancellous) were placed medially along the S1 and S2 pedicular trajectories, as well as laterally (25 degrees inferior, 30 and 45 degrees lateral) into the ala. All screws were placed through the anterior cortices. Anterior examination demonstrated remarkable consistency in the position of the anterior structures. The internal iliac vein and artery and the L4 and L5 nerve roots were most commonly at risk for injury from a protruding screw tip. The sigmoid colon was generally protected by its long mesentery. Screws placed medially through the S1 pedicle were least likely to injure the neurovascular bundle. Screws placed through the S2 pedicle tended to aim directly at the neurovascular structures. Thirty percent of laterally positioned (30 degrees) screws placed the internal iliac vein at risk, while 55% of those aimed 45 degrees laterally placed the lumbosacral trunk at risk. A lateral safe zone existed just superior to the arcuate line. Radiographically, a modified pelvic inlet view provided the most accurate assessment of screw penetration and transverse angulation.

The screw position in the sacrum may affect the pullout strength of the screw. Zindrick et al.[118] found the weakest pullout strength (mean: 185 newtons) to be at the S2 level with screws placed through the pedicle (Fig 28–6). Somewhat higher values were found with screws placed straight (anterior) into the sacral ala (mean: 668 newtons). The S1 pedicle site failed at an average of 870 newtons. Forty-five-degree lateral angulation of the screw into the ala provided the strongest fixation (mean: 1,007 newtons).

The significance of these findings is questionable. Krag et al.[57] have pointed out several potential shortcomings of the study. First, there was high interspecimen variation for the strength required for screw pullout. Second, pullout testing was performed along the axis of the screw, yet this does not appear to be a clinically important mode of failure. They have further suggested studying screw failure under bending loads to more closely re-create potential clinical failure.

Asher and Strippgen[4] have measured the path lengths of screws placed through the S1 pedicle and into the promontory of the sacrum and compared these values to other paths to identify optimal transsacral fixation. Eighteen cadaveric specimens of

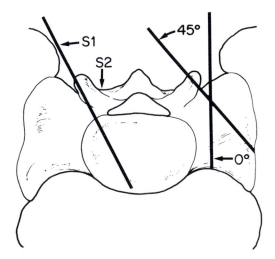

FIG 28–6.
Sacral screw placement and pullout strengths. *Left to right:* screw placed anteromedially into the S1 pedicle (mean: 870 newtons); screw placed straight anteriorly into the S2 pedicle (mean: 185 newtons); screw angled 45 degrees laterally into the sacral ala (mean: 1,007 newtons); screw placed straight anteriorly into the sacral ala (mean: 668 newtons). (From Zindrick MR, Wiltse LL, Widell EH, et al: *Clin Orthop* 1986; 203:99–112. Used by permission.)

known sex were studied. Paths through the S1 pedicle into the sacral promontory averaged 49.7 mm in men and 46.9 mm in women. This compared to 38.8 mm and 37.2 mm for paths from the S1 transverse tubercle angled laterally into the ala for men and women, respectively. Using hand-held spring scales to test the relative strength of fixation, the authors found "the longest, and apparently most secure fixation" in screws passed from the S1 pedicle into the promontory.[4]

It is apparent that the ideal screw entry site, orientation, and placement within the sacrum are unsettled. This explains the wide variety of techniques currently described for sacral screw placement.[24, 36, 65, 73, 100] We have found screw fixation through the S1 pedicle and anterior cortical wall of the promontory of the sacrum to provide optimal purchase without apparent increase in morbidity. Our technique for screw placement is similar to that in the lumbar spine where screws are placed into the nape of the neck, caudad and lateral to the facet joint. Screws are placed cephalad and lateral to the S1 foramen, angling anteromedially into the vertebral body. Fluoroscopy is used with adjustment for the lordotic sacrum.

There is seldom an indication for fixation below S1. Pedicle screws placed through the S1 pedicle and into the anterior cortex usually provide sufficient fixation. Relative indications for fixation below S1 include reduction of a high-grade slip, a long lumbar fusion, or poor S1 fixation.[101] Screws should not be placed into the S2 pedicle because there is insufficient bone for adequate purchase. Screws angled into the ala of the sacrum or the posterior ilium are occasionally indicated to augment S1 pedicle screws. Steffee has devised buttress clamps which fit onto the slotted plate. Undershooting clamps are used for screws placed in the sacral ala, and overshooting clamps are used for screws placed into the ilium. For instrumentation below S1, Steffee has described the following landmark: the point of entry for screws placed into the sacral ala is on a line drawn between the posterior foramina, directed between the first and second foramen. As long as the screw is directed laterally, the nerve root is not in jeopardy.

Proper placement and positioning of the screw within the spine can be difficult, even for the experienced surgeon. Establishing the correct starting point for screw placement can be accomplished through direct visualization of the pedicle following complete laminectomy, through examination of external landmarks, through radiographic analysis, or by a combination of the above.

In 1988, Weinstein et al.[107] examined eight cadaveric spines in which pedicle screws were placed bilaterally from T11 to S1 using fluoroscopic control and the placement techniques of Roy-Camille and Weinstein (Fig 28–7). A relatively experienced and an inexperienced surgeon placed the screws. Independent radiographic analysis of screw placement using AP and lateral films was performed, followed by sectioning of the spines to determine true screw location. Failure was considered to be cortical perforation at any location.

The overall failure rate was 21% with most (92%) representing cortical perforations within the spinal canal. Radiographs were unreliable for determining the angle of screw entry and in evaluation of screw placement. A high rate of false-positive (range: 6.5%–8.1%) and false-negative (range: 12.9%–14.5%) results occurred following radiographic analysis of screw placement. Success was not significantly related to approach, surgeon's experience, screw size, or spine level. There was, however, an appreciable practice effect following cadaveric sectioning and examination. Study of relative success rates indicated a trend toward greater success with Weinstein's approach in the lower lumbar spine: L3–S1 (Fig 28–8).

Initially, 5.5-mm screws were used from T11 to

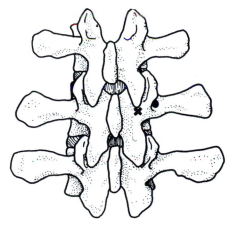

FIG 28–7.
AP view. Entrance points for pedicle screw placement in the lumbar spine as described by Roy-Camille *(X)* and Weinstein *(dot)*. The Roy-Camille entrance point is at the intersection of two lines: a horizontal line passing through the middle of the insertion of the transverse process, and a vertical line given by the articular processes 1 mm under the facet joint. The entrance point for the Weinstein (anteromedial) approach is at the lateral and inferior corner of the superior articular facet. (From Weinstein JN, Spratt KF, Spengler D, et al: *Spine* 1988; 13:1012–1018. Used by permission.)

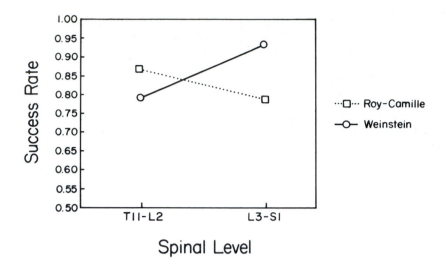

FIG 28–8.

Graphic representation of the differences in pedicle fixation success rate depending on approach (Roy-Camille vs. Weinstein) and spine level (T11–L2 vs. L3–S1). (From Weinstein JN, Spratt KF, Spengler D, et al: *Spine* 1988; 13:1012–1018. Used by permission.)

L1, and 7-mm screws were used distally. Interestingly, 40% of the failures were at the L2 and L3 level. Since data indicated that transverse pedicular diameter at L2 and L3 was 8.9 mm (range: 4–13 mm) and 10.3 mm (range: 5.3–16 mm) respectively, screw size was changed midway through the study to 5.5 mm. Nevertheless, 33% of the remaining failures were still at this level.

Gertzbein and Robbins[32] subsequently studied the accuracy of pedicular screws placed in vivo. Forty consecutive patients instrumented with the fixateur interne were evaluated using postoperative CT scans. Four percent of screws were inserted lateral to the pedicle, and 6% demonstrated 4 to 8 mm of canal encroachment medially. Five percent of patients developed minor neurologic complications that spontaneously resolved. A learning effect was also demonstrated by an improved accuracy in the last 25% of screws placed.

Finally, it should be stressed that true lateral radiographs can also be poor at determining screw depth and anterior cortical penetration. Whitecloud et al.[112] studied five cadaveric specimens, instrumented from T12 to S1, radiographically to determine the accuracy of a true lateral radiograph. Not only did they poorly predict screw depth but the actual discrepancy increased as they proceeded down the lumbar spine. This occurred because anterior screw penetration moved further lateral from the midline in the more caudal vertebrae. Thus, the greatest discrepancy was found at the L4–5 level. At this level, with 100% apparent radiographic penetration, the average actual screw penetration was 13

mm beyond the anterior cortex. The authors went on to state that the optimal radiographic axis-angle to study screw penetration was 5 degrees above the true lateral axis for T12–L3, and 10 degrees above the axis for L4–S1. Krag et al.[59] have stated that an "off-lateral" view of 20 to 30 degrees provides a more accurate analysis of screw depth than does a true lateral view.

SURGICAL APPROACH AND TECHNIQUES

A number of approaches to the pedicle and techniques for placement of pedicle screws have been described.* The following represents our approach.

The patient is placed under general anesthesia and is positioned prone on a frame designed to reduce intraabdominal pressure. This reduces venous pressure and hence epidural venous bleeding. Hypotensive anesthesia is often used concomitantly. The use of an autotransfusion unit is also recommended. Prophylactic antibiotics are given preoperatively.

A standard midline incision is made and the paraspinal musculature is meticulously reflected to prevent further blood loss. Exposure is carried to the outer margins of the transverse processes at the levels to be instrumented and fused. Extreme care is

References 20, 25, 36, 40, 57, 65, 70, 73, 78, 91, 100.

taken during the entire procedure not to violate or injure facet joints which are not to be included within the fusion. A laminectomy or decompression, or both, are then carried out, as indicated. Excision of the hypertrophied ligamentum flavum with a limited laminectomy, combined with decompression of the intervertebral foramina, is usually sufficient.[86] Partial facetectomies are often performed to further decompress the canal or foramina.

The napes of the neck of the pedicles to be instrumented are then located using external landmarks as described in the previous section. Care is taken to stay lateral and caudal to the facet joint. The posterior cortical wall at the entrance site is gently removed with a high-speed burr. A Penfield dissector no. 4 is then used to identify the entrance hole through the pedicle. Fluoroscopy in the axial plane of the pedicle is used simultaneously to help document this position. A "bull's-eye" or "coaxial view" using fluoroscopy positioned obliquely is desired (Fig 28–9). Additional views (i.e., lateral view) may also be helpful in determining position and orientation. A gearshift probe is then inserted. This is slowly advanced, following the path of least resistance (anteromedially) into the vertebral body. An appropriately sized tap (5.5 mm) is then used to

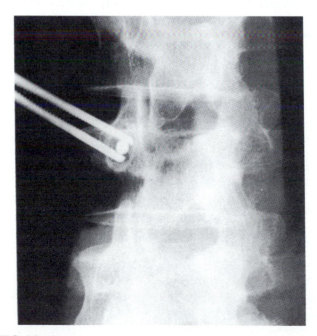

FIG 28–9.
A "bull's-eye" or "coaxial" view of the pedicle and drill bit through an oblique projection. (From Krag MH, Frederickson BE, Yuan HA: Spinal instrumentation, in Weinstein JN, Wiesel SW (eds): *The Lumbar Spine.* Philadelphia, WB Saunders Co, 1990, pp 916–940. Used by permission.)

widen the pathway and prevent splintering of the pedicle. A pedicle "feeler" is used circumferentially to confirm the absence of a breach in the wall of the pedicle. The screw is then placed. A basic guideline for screw sizes is as follows: 7.0 mm, S1, L5, L4; 6.25 mm, L3, L2; 5.5 mm, L1 T12.

Posterolateral intertransverse grafting is then performed in the usual fashion,[17, 50, 72, 98, 115] decorticating with a burr and using strips of corticocancellous graft from the iliac crest.

When using the VSP system, the plate is contoured to approximate the patient's "physiologic lordosis." The plate is then locked onto the screws in the appropriate position within the slot using "nesting nuts" and locknuts. The nesting nuts are made with Spiralock (as used in the VSF) to help prevent loosening. Spreaders can be placed between screws (prior to tightening of the nuts) to distract and open the intervertebral foramina. A "working" plate can be placed prior to the decompression to aid exposure and reduction. Appropriate use of oblique and transverse washers between the screwhead and plate helps provide for a flush fit at the screw-plate interface. This decreases motion at the interface, which increases the rigidity of the construct, and decreases the risk of screw breakage and plate loosening. Washers can also be used to uplift the plate if facet joint impingement is present. The foramina may be rechecked for patency prior to closure. Cross-bracing between plates is occasionally performed to increase the rigidity of the system, as well as the purchase of the device. The machined portion of the screw is cut close to the locknuts. A standard wound closure is performed over suction drainage.

Postoperative external immobilization in a soft brace is optional. Soft braces provide comfort and remind the patient of his recent procedure.

BIOMECHANICS

Pedicle screw design is evolving. Screws with wider proximal cores are generally stronger and less likely to break. The stresses placed upon the screws are greatest proximally, at or near the screw-plate (or rod) interface. It is at this location that the construct most often fails. This occurs through loosening of the screw-plate (or rod) interface, or through proximal screw breakage. Thus, as screws have evolved, the proximal core and platform (base-nut) diameters have increased to compensate for these

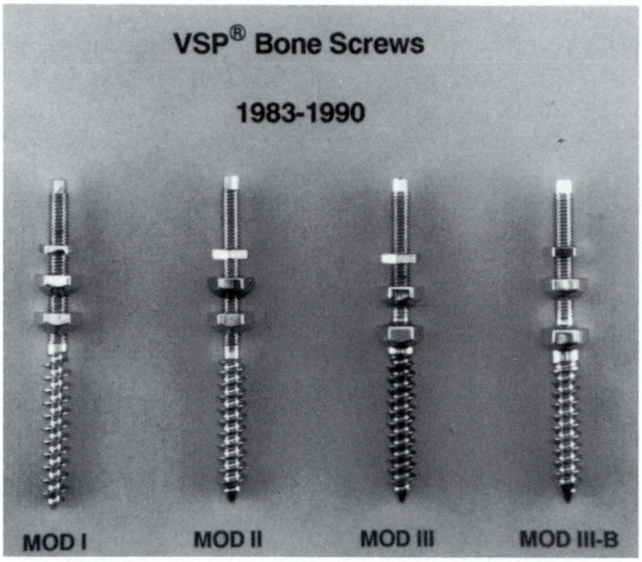

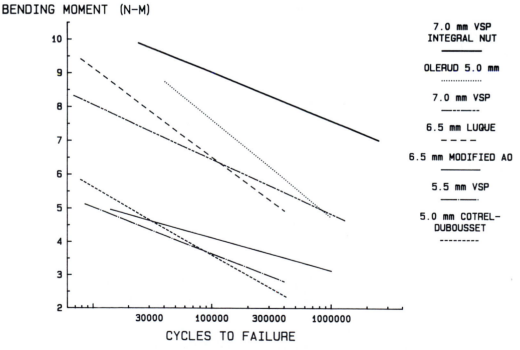

FIG 28–10.
Evolutionary design changes in VSP (Steffee) screw. (Courtesy of AcroMed, Inc., Cleveland.)

higher stresses (Fig 28–10). The most recent design modification of the VSP (Steffee) system features an integral fixed lower nut that is machined from the same bar stock and is thus stronger and more resistant to breakage. Also, various washers and articu-

lating clamps are now available which allow for a concentric (flush) fit between the screw and plate. This allows loads to be more evenly transmitted between the screws and the linking device. Screw pull-out resulting in construct failure is relatively uncommon, except in the osteoporotic spine, and following multiple level fusions in which large lever arm forces arise. Generally, pedicle screws are designed to have larger thread diameters distally, with smaller core diameters, and a greater pitch for improved purchase.

Geiger et al.[31] studied the fatigue lives of various transpedicular screws using cantilever bending tests in an effort to mimic physiologic loads (Fig 28–11). Logarithmic regression analysis demonstrated that the 7-mm VSP (Steffee) integral nut screw withstood the greatest number of cycles at the largest bending moments. The 5-mm Olerud, 7-mm VSP (Steffee), and 6.5-mm Luque screws demonstrated similar fatigue lives, but less than that of the integral nut screw. The 6.5-mm modified AO, 5.5-mm VSP (Steffee), and the 5-mm Cotrel-Dubousset screws exhibited the poorest response to recurrent bending loads. Retrospective clinical studies concur with these findings. For example, Gurr and McAfee[33] reported that hardware failure using Cotrel-Dubousset instrumentation most typically, and specifically oc-

FIG 28–11.
Fatigue life vs. bending moment. The VSP (Steffee) integral nut screw withstood the largest number of cycles at the highest loads. The 5.0-mm Cotrel-Dubousset, 6.5-mm mod- ified AO, and 5.5-mm VSP screws could not endure a significant number of cycles at a moderate load. (Courtesy of J.M. Geiger, N.A. Udovic, and J.L. Berry.)

curred due to bending of the 5-mm screws at the upper thread-shank junction. Geiger et al.[31] stated that the outer diameter of the screw did not play a significant role in fatigue life, yet geometric factors were highly instrumental in causing failure. Most screws had significant stress risers inherent in their own design which reduced fatigue life. Geiger et al. stressed the importance of "load sharing" and the presence of an intact "anterior column" for maximization of screw longevity.

Krag et al.[56] systematically studied design features of pedicle screws in an evaluation of pullout strengths. Results were as follows: (1) Smaller core diameters (3.8 vs. 5.0 mm) provided significantly greater resistance (19%–26%) to pullout only when coupled with 6-mm thread diameters (6 mm vs. 7 mm). However, smaller core diameters (3.8 mm vs. 5.0 mm) reduced flexural rigidity by 56%. (2) V and B (buttress) tooth patterns provided similar resistance to pullout. (3) A shorter pitch (2 mm vs. 3 mm) provided 21% greater resistance to pullout only for 6-mm B threads. Although this study provided valuable information, no definitive conclusions were made.

Experimental pullout testing comparing various commercially available pedicle screw designs was performed by Skinner et al.[97] in 1990. Steffee screws (6.5 mm) provided the greatest resistance to pullout, followed by the 5-mm AO Schanz screw, the 6-mm Howemedica screw (initially used by Olerud), and the 3.5-mm Roy-Camille screw. Enlargement of the major diameter of the screw increased pullout strengths. In addition, a longer pitch allowed greater displacement of the screw prior to failure. A smaller core size also improved results.

As one would expect, Zindrick et al.[118] found pedicle screws to have poor fixation in osteoporotic cadaveric spines. However, methyl methacrylate augmentation restored the pullout strength of these screws to near normal values. Pressurized methacrylate increased pullout strength further, nearly doubling that obtained when using nonpressurized methacrylate.

This procedure requires methacrylate to be injected down the pedicle and into the vertebral body. Screws are then placed while the acrylic is soft. Careful and meticulous technique is warranted. Extruding methacrylate through breaches in the pedicle must be avoided at all costs. Nerve root and thecal sac damage can occur during polymerization of the methacrylate. One of our patients developed a radiculopathy following pedicle screw fixation augmented with methacrylate. A subsequent explor-

atory procedure revealed excess methacrylate within the foramen compressing the nerve root. The patient improved following its removal.

In an attempt to improve pullout strength further, Ruland et al.[92] examined load-to-failure pullout strengths on 54 cadaveric spinal segments using a "triangulated" system. Specifically, Steffee and Cotrel-Dubousset screws were linked transversely with plates in an attempt to increase fixation within the same vertebra prior to placement of the longitudinal plate or rod. Triangulated pedicle screws demonstrated significantly greater fixation than conventionally placed screws. In fact, the limiting factor in the strength of the construct (unlike that of conventionally placed screws) was the intrinsic strength of the vertebral body bone. Failure typically occurred away from the metal-bone interface ($P = .0004$). The authors stated that the strength of the fixation in a triangulated system was superior to that of a single screw because failure was dependent upon the mass of bone between the screws, rather than on the amount of bone between the screw threads. Thus, ideal application of a triangulated system may be in the elderly and osteoporotic population.

Geiger et al.[31] also studied the biomechanical properties of various linking devices (Fig 28–12, A–C). They found superior bending strengths, rigidities, and fatigue lives with the ¼-in. Luque rod, Harrington distraction rod, VSP plate, ¼-in. ISOLA rod, and ISOLA plate/rod. These devices demonstrated sufficient mechanical properties to endure the bending loads experienced by the spine over multiple levels. The VSP plate was the most rigid (stiffest) (11.6 kN/mm) interconnecting device tested. VSP instrumentation is rigid enough to be used unilaterally or bilaterally for short segments. This potential advantage, however, should not be extrapolated to other, less rigid systems. The Luque plate, Olerud rod, and Cotrel-Dubousset rod had moderate bending strengths, rigidities, and fatigue lives. These devices have sufficient mechanical properties to transport forces for only a few levels in the lumbar spine. The ³⁄₁₆-in. Luque rod, ³⁄₁₆-in. ISOLA rod, and the Harrington rack were unable to withstand significant bending loads. Thus, their use requires the presence of an intact anterior column. The ⅛-in. and ³⁄₁₆-in. threaded Harrington rods endured even less prior to failure, leading the authors to discourage the use of this instrumentation at locations where significant bending loads can occur.

There have been many biomechanical studies performed to evaluate the entire internal fixation

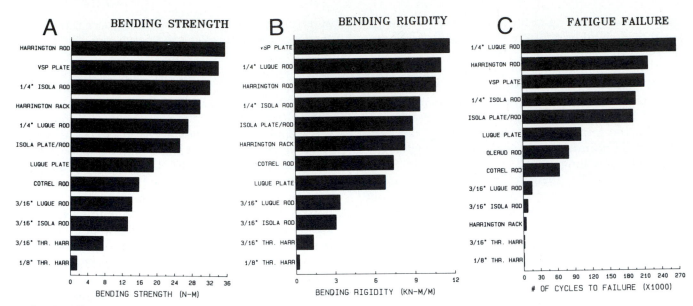

FIG 28-12.
Superior bending strength **(A),** rigidities **(B),** and fatigue lives **(C)** were exhibited by the ¼-in. Luque rod, Harrington distraction rod, VSP (Steffee) plate, ¼-in. ISOLA rod, and the ISOLA plate/rod. These devices demonstrated sufficient mechanical properties to endure the bending loads experienced in the lumbar spine. The ³⁄₁₆-in. Luque rod, ³⁄₁₆-in.

ISOLA rods, and Harrington rack had insufficient properties to withstand a significant amount of loading. Therefore, anterior column support is an essential prerequisite with use of this fixation. (Courtesy of J.M. Geiger, N.A. Udovic, and J.L. Berry.)

system (rather than individual components) in both animals and humans.

Gurr et al.[34] performed an in vitro study using a calf spine model to evaluate the response of various forms of instrumentation to cyclic loads including rotation, axial compression, and flexion (Fig 28–13 and Table 28–1). Spines were destabilized following bilateral laminectomies and facetectomies at L4 and L5, in addition to discectomy (L4–L5) and resection of the L4 pars interarticularis. They were then instrumented with a variety of systems including Har-

TABLE 28-1.
Flexion Rigidity in the Destabilized Calf Spine Model Following Laminectomy, Facetectomy, Pars Resection, and Discectomy at L4–5*

Subset†	Groups
1	Destabilized spine, intact spine, Harrington
2	Harrington, Luque, 3-level modified Steffee‡
3	Luque, 3-level modified Steffee, 3-level Cotrel-Dubousset
4	Three-level Cotrel-Dubousset, 5-level modified Steffee
5	Five-level modified Steffee

*From Gurr KR, McAfee PC, Shih C-M: *J Bone Joint Surg [Am]* 1988; 70:680–691. Used by permission
†Subsets are listed in order of rigidity, with *l* having the least and *5* the greatest flexural rigidity.
‡Plates were changed to notched rods.

rington, Luque, Cotrel-Dubousset, and modified (plates were changed to notched rods to better accommodate the spine) Steffee systems. Their findings were as follows: (1) instrumented spines were most unstable in rotation and flexion, not in axial compression; (2) five-level transpedicular Cotrel-Dubousset rods provided the greatest rigidity; (3) three-level modified Steffee and Cotrel-Dubousset instrumentation restored torsional, compressive, and flexural rigidity. This fixation was far superior to the standard five-level Harrington and Luque instrumentation.

A similar study was later performed by Gurr et al.[35] evaluating the response of instrumented calf spines following anterior L3 corpectomy and placement of an iliac crest graft. The most rigid posterior constructs were once more the Cotrel-Dubousset and standard Steffee plate systems (Fig 28–14).

In 1989, Ashman et al.[5] studied the biomechanical properties of five different types of pedicular instrumentation (DKS/Zielke, VSP, AO fixateur interne; Luque semirigid instrumentation; AO notched plates) using a corpectomy model.

Thirty fresh human cadaveric specimens harvested from T11 to L3 and vertebrectomized at L1 were instrumented from T12 to L2 with one of the above-mentioned systems. Relative axial and torsional stiffness was similar for all implants. There-

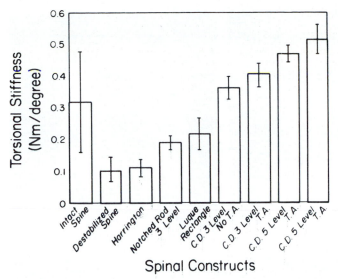

FIG 28–13.

A, mean torsional stiffness of each construct with standard deviations. Fresh spinal segments from calves were destabilized with bilateral laminectomy, facetectomy, resection of the pars interarticularis, and resection of the disc at L4–5, and then instrumented and tested for torsional stability. Five-level Cotrel-Dubousset *(C.D.)* pedicular fixation with transverse approximating *(T.A.)* rods provided the greatest stability. See also Table 28–1. (From Gurr KR, McAfee PC, Shih C-M: *J Bone Joint Surg [Am]* 1988; 70:680–691.

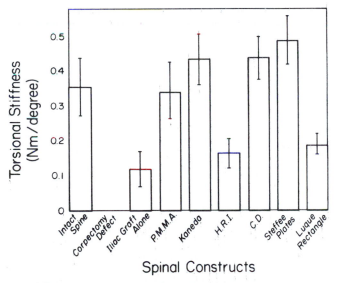

FIG 28–14.

Torsional stiffness using an instrumented calf spine model destabilized by anterior corpectomy at L3 and discectomies at L2–3 and L3–4. The stiffest posterior fixation included the Steffee screw-plate system and the Cotrel-Dubousset *(C.D.)* device applied from L1 to L5. *P.M.M.A.* = polymethyl methacrylate; *H.R.I.* = Harrington rod instrumentation. (From Gurr KR, McAfee PC, Shih C-M: *J Bone Joint Surg [Am]* 1988; 70:1182–1191. Used by permission.)

fore, the authors concluded that each device imparted approximately the same stability to the spine in this highly unstable model. Implants with more rigid screw-plate (rod) interfaces (VSP, fixateur interne) developed greater measured stresses at the base of the screws. At relatively low loads (175–270 newtons), the shanks of these screws were found to be subjected to stresses which exceeded the endurance level for 316L stainless steel. Steffee instrumentation using 6.5-mm cancellous screws tolerated the least number of cycles at 450 newtons prior to failure. Likewise, other rigid systems (DKS/Zielke; AO fixateur interne) failed early. The screws can pivot freely in the Luque and AO notched plate systems eliminating the high bending stresses on the proximal portion of the screw. These systems, however, require the presence of an intact lamina for four-point fixation in reduction of the spine. The less rigid systems resisted flexion moments by the plate resting upon the lamina with the screws experiencing primarily tension loads. This contrasts to the more rigid systems where the screws experienced cantilever bending stresses. The results of this vertebrectomy model cannot necessarily be extrapolated to other models (diagnoses) where anterior column stability exists (i.e., in most patients with spinal stenosis).

CONCLUSION

The field of pedicle screw instrumentation has grown enormously following Boucher's initial description in 1959[9] of screws placed posteriorly through the facet joint and into the pedicle. Roy-Camille has been appropriately credited as being the father of segmental transpedicular screw fixation. Biomechanical studies have confirmed initial theories stating that pedicular screw systems provide better overall positional control and stability than conventional forms of instrumentation (i.e., Harrington, Luque), while immobilizing fewer motion segments, and generally not requiring the presence of an intact lamina, facet joint, or spinous process. Preliminary clinical results have been encouraging, yet long-term results are not available.

Optimal rigidity for the pedicle screw system is unknown. Excessively rigid systems may stress-shield the fusion mass, while possibly increasing the stresses at adjacent intervertebral levels leading to accelerated instability and degenerative changes. It

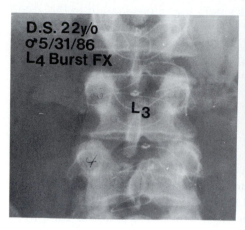
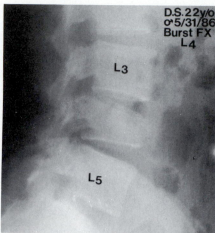
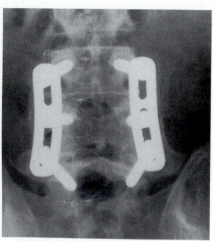
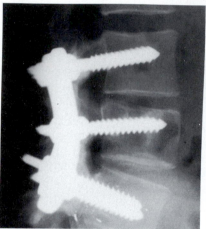
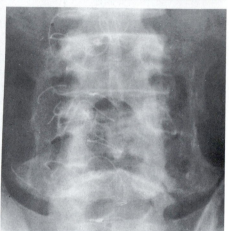

FIG 28–15.
(A) AP and **(B)** lateral radiographs of a 22-year-old man with an L4 burst fracture. **(C)** AP and **(D)** lateral radiographs 40 months following a posterior decompression, pedicle screw instrumentation (VSP), reduction of the fracture, and autogenous posterolateral grafting. **E,** AP radiograph following hardware removal. The extent to which the instrumentation may have augmented and enhanced the formation of this abundant, well-incorporated fusion mass is not known.

is not known how the findings of McAfee et al.[75] assessing device-related osteoporosis in beagles apply to humans (Fig 28–15,A–E).

Recently, a rash of new systems have flooded the market, each with different design modifications and emphasis. As our knowledge and experience grow, we will be better able to determine the limitations, indications, and usefulness of each system.

REFERENCES

1. Aebi M, Etter C, Kehl T, et al: Stabilization of the lower thoracic and lumbar spine with the internal spinal skeletal fixation system: Indications, techniques, and first results of treatment. *Spine* 1987; 12:544–551.
2. Aebi M, Etter C, Kehl T, et al: The internal skeletal fixation system: A new treatment of thoracolumbar fractures and other spinal disorders. *Clin Orthop* 1988; 227:30–43.
3. Andrew TA, Brooks S, Piggott H: Long-term follow-up evaluation of screw-and-graft fusion of the lumbar spine. *Clin Orthop* 1986; 203:113–119.
4. Asher MA, Strippgen WE: Anthropometric studies of the human sacrum relating to dorsal transsacral implant designs. *Clin Orthop* 1986; 203:58–62.
5. Ashman RB, Galpin RD, Corin JD, et al: Biomechanical analysis of pedicle screw instrumentation systems in a corpectomy model. *Spine* 1989; 14:1398–1405.
6. Berry JL, Moran JM, Berg WS, et al: A morphometric study of human lumbar and selected thoracic vertebrae. *Spine* 1987; 12:362–367.
7. Booth RE: Spinal stenosis. *Instruct Course Lect* 1986; 35:420–435.
8. Bosworth DM: Surgery of the spine. *Instruct Course Lect* 1957; 14:39–47.
9. Boucher HH: A method of spinal fusion. *J Bone Joint Surg [Br]* 1959; 41:248–259.

10. Brack S, Zucherman J, Hsu K, et al: The myth of the solid posterior lateral fusion, in *Proceedings of the North American Spine Society*, 1990.
11. Brown CW, Orme TJ, Richardson HD: The rate of pseudarthrosis (surgical nonunion) in patients who are smokers and patients who are nonsmokers: A comparison study. *Spine* 1986; 11:942–943.
12. Buck JE: Direct repair of the defect in spondylolisthesis: Preliminary report. *J Bone Joint Surg [Br]* 1970; 52:432–437.
13. Cabot JR: *Cirugia del dolor lumbosacro*, vol 1. Madrid, Industrias Graficas España SL 1971, p 129.
14. Chang KW, McAfee PC: Degenerative spondylolisthesis and degenerative scoliosis treated with a combination segmental rod-plate and transpedicular screw instrumentation system: A preliminary report. *J Spinal Dis* 1989; 1:247–256.
15. Cleveland M, Bosworth DM, Thompson FR: Pseudarthrosis in the lumbar spine. *J Bone Joint Surg [Am]* 1948; 30:302–312.
16. Cotrel Y, Dubousset J, Guillaumat M: New universal instrumentation in spinal surgery. *Clin Orthop* 1988; 227:10–23.
17. Dawson EG, Lotysch M, Urist MR: Intertransverse process lumbar arthrodesis with autogenous bone graft. *Clin Orthop* 1981; 154:90–96.
18. Dean SM, Hall BB, Johnson RG: Analysis of posterolateral lumbar fusion and VSP pedicle screw and plate fixation, in *Proceedings of the 57th Annual Meeting of the Academy of Orthopaedic Surgeons,* 1990.
19. Depalma AF, Rothman RH: The nature of pseudarthrosis. *Clin Orthop* 1968; 59:113–118.
20. Dick W: The "fixateur interne" as a versatile implant for spine surgery. *Spine* 1987; 12:882–900.
21. Dick W, Kluger P, Magerl F, et al: A new device for internal fixation of thoracolumbar and lumbar spine fractures: The "fixateur interne." *Paraplegia* 1985; 23:225–232.
22. Dupuis PR, Yong-Hing K, Cassidy JD, et al: Radiologic diagnosis of degenerative lumbar spinal instability. *Spine* 1985; 10:262–276.
23. Edwards CE: Spinal screw fixation of the lumbar and sacral spine: Early results treating the first 50 cases, in *Proceedings of the Scoliosis Research Society Annual Meeting*, 1986.
24. Edwards CC, Levine AM: Early rod-sleeve stabilization of the injured thoracic and lumbar spine. *Orthop Clin North Am* 1986; 17:121–145.
25. Esses SI, Beddar DA: The spinal pedicle screw: Techniques and systems. *Orthop Rev* 1989; 18:676–682.
26. Evans MJ, Sullivan MF, Kirwan EOG: Screw arthrodesis of the lumbar spine. *J Bone Joint Surg [Br]* 1977; 59:498.
27. Feffer HL, Wiesel SW, Cuckler JM, et al: Degenerative spondylolisthesis, To fuse or not to fuse. *Spine* 1985; 10:287–289.
28. Fitzgerald JAW: Degenerative spondylolisthesis. *J Bone Joint Surg [Br]* 1976; 58:184–192.
29. Frymoyer JW, Hanley EN, Howe J, et al: A comparison of radiographic findings in fusion and nonfusion patients ten or more years following lumbar disc surgery. *Spine* 1979; 4:435–440.
30. Frymoyer JW, Selby DK: Segmental instability—Rationale for treatment. *Spine* 1985; 10:280–286.
31. Geiger JM, Udovic NA, Berry JL: Bending and fatigue of spine plates and rods and fatigue of pedicle screws, in *Proceedings of the 56th Annual Meeting of the American Academy of Orthopaedic Surgeons*, Las Vegas, 1989.
32. Gertzbein SD, Robbins SE: Accuracy of pedicular screw placement in vivo. *Spine* 1990; 15:11–14.
33. Gurr KR, McAfee PC: Cotrel-Dubousset instrumentation in adults: A preliminary report. *Spine* 1988; 13:510–520.
34. Gurr KR, McAfee PC, Shih CM: Biomechanical analysis of posterior instrumentation systems after decompressive laminectomy. *J Bone Joint Surg [Am]* 1988; 70:680–691.
35. Gurr KR, McAfee PC, Shih CM: Biomechanical analysis of anterior and posterior instrumentation systems after corpectomy. *J Bone Joint Surg [Am]* 1988; 70:1182.
36. Guyer DW, Wiltse LL, Peek RD: The Wiltse pedicle screw fixation system. *Orthopedics* 1988; 11:1455–1460.
37. Guyer DW, Wiltse LL: Pedicle screw fixation of the lumbar spine. *Surg Rev Orthop* 1989; 2:17–21.
38. Harrington PR, Dickson JH: Spinal instrumentation in the treatment of severe progressive spondylolisthesis. *Clin Orthop* 1976; 117:157–163.
39. Harrington PR, Tullos HS: Reduction of severe spondylolisthesis in children. *South Med J* 1969; 62:1–7.
40. Henstorf JE, Gaines RW, Steffee AD: Transpedicular fixation of spinal disorders with Steffee plates. *Surg R Orthop* 1987; 3:35–43.
41. Herkowitz HN, Kurz LT: Degenerative spondylolisthesis—Prospective study comparing decompression versus decompression with fusion, in *Proceedings of the International Society for the Study of the Lumbar Spine*, Boston, June 13–17, 1990.
42. Hopp E, Tsou PM: Postdecompression lumbar instability. *Clin Orthop* 1988; 227:143–151.
43. Horowitch A, Peek RD, Thomas JC Jr, et al: The Wiltse pedicle screw fixation system—Early clinical results. *Spine* 1989; 14:461–467.
44. Jacobs RR, Montesano PX, Jackson RP: Enhancement of lumbar spine fusion by use of translaminar facet joint screws. *Spine* 1989; 14:12–15.
45. Jacobs RR, Schlaepfer F, Mathys R, Jr, et al: A locking hook spinal rod system for stabilization of fracture-dislocations and correction of deformities of the dorsolumbar spine: A biomechanic evaluation. *Clin Orthop* 1984; 189:168–177.
46. Johnsson K-E, Willner S, Johnsson K: Postoperative instability after decompression for lumbar spinal stenosis. *Spine* 1986; 11:107–110.
47. Kabins MB, Weinstein JN, Found EM, et al: Isolated L4-L5 floating fusions using the variable spinal plating system: Unilateral vs. bilateral, in *Proceedings of the North American Spine Society*, 1990.
48. Kabins MB, Weinstein JN, Spratt KF, et al: Clinical efficacy and outcome of pedicle screw instrumentation in patients with previously failed lumbar surgery, in *Proceedings of the North American Spine Society*, 1991.

49. Karlström G, Olerud S, Sjöström L: Transpedicular segmental fixation: Description of a new procedure. *Orthopedics* 1988; 11:689–700.

50. Kelly RP: Intertransverse fusion of the low back. *Trans South Surg Assoc* 1963; 74:193.

51. King D: Internal fixation for lumbosacral fusion. *Am J Surg* 1944; 66:357–361.

52. King D: Internal fixation for lumbosacral fusion. *J Bone Joint Surg [Am]* 1948; 30:560–565.

53. Knox BD, Harvell JC, Nelson PB, et al: Decompression and Luque rectangle fusion for degenerative spondylolisthesis. *J Spinal Dis* 1989; 2:223–228.

54. Kolvalsky ES, Brodsky AE, Khalil MA: Correlation of radiologic assessment of lumbar spine fusions with surgical exploration, in *Proceedings of the North American Spine Society*, 1990.

55. Krag MH, Beynnon BD, DeCoster TA, et al: Depth of insertion of transpedicular vertebral screws into human vertebrae: Effect upon screw-vertebra interface strength. *J Spinal Dis* 1988; 1:287–294.

56. Krag MH, Beynnon BD, Pope MH, et al: An internal fixator for posterior application to short segments of the thoracic lumbar or lumbosacral spine: Design and testing. *Clin Orthop* 1986; 203:75–98.

57. Krag MH, Fredrickson BE, Yuan HA: Spinal instrumentation, in Weinstein JN, Wiesel SW (eds): *The Lumbar Spine*. Philadelphia, WB Saunders Co, 1990, pp 916–955.

58. Krag MH, Van Hal ME, Beynnon BD: Clinical experience with Vermont spinal fixator (VSF): Initial 46 cases, in *Proceedings of the North American Spine Society*, 1989.

59. Krag MH, Van Hal ME, Beynnon BD: Placement of transpedicular vertebral screws close to anterior vertebral cortex: Description of methods *Spine*, in press, 1990.

60. Krag MH, Weaver DL, Beynnon BD, et al: Morphometry of the thoracic and lumbar spine related to transpedicular screw placement for surgical spinal fixation. *Spine* 1988; 13:27–32.

61. Lee CK: Accelerated degeneration of the segment adjacent to lumbar fusion. *Spine* 1988; 13:375–377.

62. Lehmann TR, Spratt KF, Tozzi JE, et al: Long-term follow-up of lower lumbar fusion patients. *Spine* 1987; 12:97–104.

63. Lin PM: Posterior lumbar interbody fusion technique: Complications and pitfalls. *Clin Orthop* 1985; 193:90–102.

64. Louis R: Single staged posterior lumbo-sacral fusion by internal fixation with screw plates, in *Proceeding of the International Society for Study of the Lumbar Spine*, 1985.

65. Louis R: Fusion of the lumbar and sacral spine by internal fixation with screw plates. *Clin Orthop* 1986; 203:18–33.

66. Louis R, Maresca C: Les arthrodéses stables de la charnière lombo-sacrée (70 cas). *Rev Chir Orthop* 1976; 62(suppl 2):70–79.

67. Louis R, Maresca C: Stabilisation chirurgicale avec réduction des spondylolyses et des spondylolisthesis. *Int Orthop (SICOT)* 1977; 1:215.

68. Luque ER: Interpeduncular segmental fixation. *Clin Orthop* 1986; 203:54–57.

69. Luque ER: Semirigid interpeduncular fixation in correction of instability of the low back, in *Proceedings of the North American Spine Society*, 1990.

70. Luque ER, Rapp GF: A new semirigid method for interpedicular fixation of the spine. *Orthopedics* 1988; 11:1445–1450.

71. Macnab I: Spondylolisthesis with a intact neural arch—the so-called pseudo-spondylolisthesis. *J Bone Joint Surg [Br]*, 1950; 32:325–333.

72. Macnab I, Dall D: The blood supply of the lumbar spine and its application to the technique of intertransverse lumbar fusion. *J Bone Joint Surg [Br]* 1971; 53:628–638.

73. Magerl F: External spinal skeletal fixation, in Weber BG, Magerl F (eds): *The External Fixator*. New York, Springer-Verlag, 1985, pp 290–365.

74. Magerl FP: Stabilization of the lower thoracic and lumbar spine with external skeletal fixation. *Clin Orthop* 1984; 189:125–141.

75. McAfee PC, Farey ID, Sutterlin CE, et al: Device-related osteoporosis with spinal instrumentation. *Spine* 1989; 14:919–926.

76. Mirkovic S, Abitbol JJ, Steinmann J, et al: Anatomic considerations for sacral screw placement, in *Proceedings of the North American Spine Society*, 1990.

77. Müller ME, Allgöwer M, Schnieder R, et al: Techniques recommended by the AO Group, in *1979 Manual of Internal Fixation*, ed 2. Berlin, Springer-Verlag, 1979.

78. Olerud S, Sjöström L, Karlström G, et al.: Spontaneous effect of increased stability of the lower lumbar spine in cases of severe chronic back pain. *Clin Orthop* 1986; 203:67–74.

79. Olsewski JM, Simmons EH, Kallen FC, et al: Morphometry of the lumbar spine: Anatomical perspectives related to transpedicular fixation. *J Bone Joint Surg [Am]* 1990; 72:541–549.

80. Olsson TH, Selvick G, Willner S: Mobility in the lumbosacral spine after fusion studied with the aid of roentgenstereophotogrammetry. *Clin Orthop* 1977; 129:181–190.

81. Pennel GF, McDonald GA, Dale GG: A method of spinal fusion using internal fixation. *Clin Orthop* 1964; 35:86–94.

82. Posner I, White AA III, Edwards WT, et al: A biomechanical analysis of the clinical stability of the lumbar and lumbosacral spine. *Spine* 1982; 7:374–389.

83. Prothero R, Parkes JC, Stinchfield FE: Complications after low-back fusion in 1000 patients. *J Bone Joint Surg [Am]* 1966; 48:57–65.

84. Puschel J, Zielke K: Transpedicular vertebral instrumentation using VDS instruments in ankylosing spondylitis, in *Proceedings of the Scoliosis Research Society 19th Annual Meeting*, 1984.

85. Ray CD: Extensive lumbar decompression: Patient selection and results, in White AH, Rothman RH, Ray CD (eds): *Lumbar Spine Surgery, Techniques and Complications*. St Louis, Mosby-Year Book, Inc, 1987, pp 164–174.

86. Reynolds JB, Wiltse LL: Surgical treatment of degenerative spondylolisthesis. *Spine* 1979; 4:148–149.

87. Roy-Camille R, Demeulenaere C: Ostéosynthèse du

rachis dorsale, lombaire et lombosacrée par plaque métalliques vissées dans les pédicules vertébraux et les apophyses articulaires. *Presse Med* 1970; 78:1447–1448.

88. Roy-Camille R, Saillant G, Berteaux D, et al: Osteosynthesis of thoracolumbar spine fractures with metal plates screwed through the vertebral pedicles. *Reconstr Surg Traumatol* 1976; 15:2.

89. Roy-Camille R, Saillant G, Bisserie M, et al: Surgical treatment of spinal metastatic tumors by posterior plating and laminectomy, in *Proceedings of the 51st Annual Meeting of the American Academy of Orthopaedic Surgeons,* 1984.

90. Roy-Camille R, Saillant G, Lapresle P, et al: A secret in spine surgery: The pedicle, in *Proceedings of the 51st Annual Meeting of the American Academy of Orthopaedic Surgeons,* 1984.

91. Roy-Camille R, Saillant G, Mazel C: Internal fixation of the lumbar spine with pedicle screw plating. *Clin Orthop* 1986; 203:7–17.

92. Ruland CM, McAfee PC, Cunningham BW, et al: Triangulation of pedicular instrumentation. A biomechanical analysis, in *Proceedings of the North American Spine Society,* 1990.

93. Saillant G.: Étude anatomique des pédicules vertébraux: Application chirurgicale. *Rev Chir Orthop* 1976; 62:151–160.

94. Schwaegler P, Cram R, Lorenz M, et al: A comparison of single level fusions with and without hardware, in *Proceedings of the North American Spine Society,* 1990.

95. Sijbrandij S: A new technique for the reduction and stabilization of severe spondylolisthesis. *J Bone Joint Surg [Br]* 1981; 63:266–271.

96. Simmons EH, Capicotto WN: Posterior Zielke instrumentation of the lumbar spine with transpedicular fixation, in *Proceedings of the Scoliosis Research Society Annual Meeting,* 1986.

97. Skinner R, Maybee J, Transfeldt E, et al: Experimental pullout testing and comparison of variables in transpedicular screw fixation. A biomechanical study. *Spine* 1990; 15:195–201.

98. Stauffer RN, Coventry MB: Posterolateral lumbar fusion. *J Bone Joint Surg [Am]* 1972; 54: 1195–1204.

99. Steffee AD: The variable screw placement system with posterior lumbar interbody fusion, in Lin PM, Gill K (eds): *Principles and Techniques in Spine Surgery.* Rockville, MD, Aspen Publishers, 1989, pp 81–93.

100. Steffee AD, Biscup RS, Sitowski DJ: Segmental spine plates with pedicle screw fixation—A new internal fixation device for disorders of the lumbar and thoracolumbar spine. *Clin Orthop* 1986; 203:45–53.

101. Steffee AD, Sitkowski DJ: Reduction and stabilization of grade IV spondylolisthesis. *Clin Orthop* 1988; 227:82–89.

102. Steffee AD, Sitkowski DJ: Posterior lumbar interbody fusion and plates. *Clin Orthop* 1988; 227:99–102.

103. Steffee AD, Sitkowski PAC, Topham LS: Total vertebral body and pedicle arthroplasty. *Clin Orthop* 1986; 203:203–208.

104. Thalgott JS, LaRocca H, Aebi M, et al: Reconstruction of the lumbar spine using AO DCP plate internal fixation. *Spine* 1989; 14:91–95.

105. Thompson WAL, Ralston EL: Pseudarthrosis following spine fusion. *J Bone Joint Surg [Am]* 1949; 31:400–405.

106. Tsou PM, Hopp E: Postsurgical instability in spinal stenosis, in Hopp E(ed): *Spine—Spinal Stenosis, State of the Art Reviews,* vol 1. Philadelphia, Hanley & Belfus, Inc, 1987, pp 533–550.

107. Weinstein JN, Spratt KF, Spengler D, et al: Spinal pedicle fixation: Reliability and validity of roentgenogram-based assessment and surgical factors on successful screw placement. *Spine* 1988; 13:1012–1018.

108. West JL, Bradford DS, Ogilvie JW: Steffee instrumentation: Two-year results, in *Proceedings of the 23rd Annual Meeting of the Scoliosis Research Society,* 1988.

109. West JL, Bradford DS, Ogilvie JW: Complications in Steffee plate pedicle screw fixation, in *Proceedings of the North American Spine Society,* 1989.

110. White AH, Zucherman JF, Hsu K: Lumbosacral fusions with Harrington rods and intersegmental wiring. *Clin Orthop* 1986; 203:185–190.

111. Whitecloud TS III, Butler JC, Cohen JL et al: Complications with the variable spinal plating system. *Spine* 1988; 14:472–476.

112. Whitecloud TS III, Skalley TC, Morgan, EL, et al: Radiographic measurement of pedicle screw penetration, in *Proceedings of the North American Spine Society,* 1989.

113. Wiltse LL: A review of "stabilization of the lower thoracic and lumbar spine with external skeletal fixation" by Friedrich P. Magerl, M.D. *Clin Orthop* 1986; 203:63–66.

114. Wiltse LL: Salvage of failed lumbar spinal stenosis surgery, in Hopp E (ed): *Spinal Stenosis,* in *State of the Art Reviews,* vol 1. Philadelphia, Hanley & Belfus, Inc, 1987, pp 421–456.

115. Wiltse LL, Bateman JG, Hutchinson RH, et al: The paraspinal sacrospinalis-splitting approach to the lumbar spine. *J Bone Joint Surg [Am]* 1968; 50:919–926.

116. Wiltse LL, Kirkaldy-Willis WH, McIvor GWD: The treatment of spinal stenosis. *Clin Orthop* 1976; 115:83–91.

117. Zindrick MR, Wiltse LL, Doornik AB, et al: Analysis of the morphometric characteristics of the thoracic and lumbar pedicles. *Spine* 1987; 12:160–166.

118. Zindrick MR, Wiltse LL, Widell EH, et al: A biomechanical study of interpeduncular screw fixation in the lumbosacral spine. *Clin Orthop* 1986; 203:99–111.

119. Zucherman J, Hsu K, White A, et al: Early results of spinal fusion using variable spine plating system. *Spine* 1988; 5:570–579.

29

The Surgical Reconstruction of Degenerative Lumbar Stenosis and Olisthesis

Charles C. Edwards, M.D.

Jeffrey R. McConnell, M.D.

When operative treatment is indicated for degenerative lumbar stenosis, the surgical goals are to (1) adequately decompress neural tissues by direct or indirect means, or both; (2) restore and maintain anatomic spinal alignment, (3) fuse unstable or painful motion segments, and (4) do so with the least amount of surgery and morbidity. To accomplish these four goals, the surgeon must first identify the anatomic origins of major signs and symptoms and correlate them with disease pathomechanics in order to formulate the most efficient surgical plan for each patient.

PATHOMECHANICS

Spondylosis

Lumbar spondylosis results from progressive degenerative changes in the spinal motion segment. The facet joints and intervertebral disc of each motion segment are physiologically linked as a "three joint complex."[11, 25] When a degenerative lesion affects the facet joints, it will also eventually affect the intervertebral discs and vice versa. This occurs because degenerative tissues are less effective in distributing loads through the spinal column. When one portion of the motion segment fails, increased stresses are passed to the other portions, leading to chronic overload and degenerative changes.

Both mechanical and inflammatory mechanisms can initiate the degenerative process. For example, a lumbar fusion concentrates the stresses that are normally dissipated over several motion segments to the motion segment above and below the fusion mass. The resulting mechanical overload leads to facet and disc degeneration. Likewise, lumbar or thoracolumbar kyphosis necessitates adjacent compensatory hyperlordosis to restore spinal alignment. Hyperlordosis can overload the facet joints and accelerate degenerative change. The repetitive overloading, abnormal motions, and vibrations associated with some sports and occupations can also initiate mechanical failure of the disc or facets with degenerative change and lumbar spondylosis.

Degeneration of lumbar motion segments may also follow primary facet arthritis or disc degeneration because of the biochemical changes associated with aging. Loss of facet integrity from erosive synovitis, like surgical resection, leads to translational instability with increased shear stresses across the intervertebral disc. Conversely, spondylosis may originate with failure of the disc. This can occur primarily from proteoglycan loss and disc dehydration, herniation of the nucleus pulposus, or trauma. It can occur secondarily from surgical resection or chemonucleolysis. Either cause renders the disc unable to effectively transmit compressive loads through the motion segment, thereby increasing the load shared by the facet joints.

The pain associated with lumbar spondylosis originates from root compression and from the surrounding soft tissues. Local nerve root compression can result from bulging discs, facet joint osteophytes, or synovial cysts. Loss of facet and disc integrity can lead to instability of the motion segment. Excessive motion causes abnormal stretching of facet capsules, ligaments, and other soft tissues. It further inflames already compressed nerve roots. Instability may, in turn, lead to translational or angular deformity of the spine. Deformity magnifies the loads crossing the motion segment with added tissue stretch, fatigue of muscles attempting to maintain spinal alignment, and compression and tension on the nerve roots. Finally, abnormal local stress, nerve impingement, and inflammation may stimulate a secondary regional neurovascular response characterized by hypersensitivity of the surrounding soft tissues, including dorsal nerve roots, fascia, and skin.

Stenosis

Stenosis of the spinal canal or neural foramen is one manifestation of degenerative spondylosis. Degeneration of the disc and facets leads to motion segment instability. In an effort to stabilize the motion segment, facet capsules thicken and facet osteophytes grow through enchondral ossification. In this process they decrease the space available for exiting nerve roots. If degenerative olisthesis occurs, translation of one vertebra relative to another will act as a guillotine to further decrease the volume of the spinal canal.

Stenosis can occur in the central canal, lateral nerve recess, or neural foramina. *Central stenosis* is caused by hypertrophy of the inferior facets, redundant ligamentum flavum, bulging discs, and posterior rim traction osteophytes.[24] Degenerative spondylolisthesis accentuates central stenosis from translation of the posterior elements into the canal.[12] *Lateral recess* stenosis is typically caused by osteophytes on the anteromedial edge of the superior facets or by hypertrophic fibrocartilage from a spondylolytic defect.[27] *Foraminal stenosis* usually follows disc degeneration and facet erosion with axial collapse such that the superior facet of one vertebra approaches the pedicle of the vertebra above. Superior facet osteophytes and lateral disc bulge can accentuate the foraminal stenosis.[31]

Olisthesis

The normal facet joint serves as a buttress to block vertebral translation in both the coronal and sagittal planes. Facet integrity may be compromised by surgical resection or erosion from mechanical overload or synovitis. Degenerative olisthesis in the lumbar spine occurs when the facet joints and intervertebral discs are unable to resist shear stresses acting across the motion segment.

The direction or pattern of a degenerative lumbar olisthesis is largely predictable. The direction of slip is determined by the predominant force acting on that vertebra relative to its position in the coronal and sagittal planes. *Degenerative spondylolisthesis* (anterior slippage) occurs in the lordotic lower lumbar spine where shear stresses through the disc are directed anteriorly and caudally. *Retrolisthesis* is often associated with compensatory hyperlordosis in the midlumbar spine where shear stress is directed posteriorly. It is likely to occur above a fused lumbosacral flat back or above a spondylolisthesis with lumbosacral kyphosis. *Lateral olisthesis* occurs when the distal vertebra is oriented obliquely in the frontal plane as in a lumbosacral scoliosis. When reconstructing any degenerative olisthesis, corrective forces must be applied to the spine to directly counteract the predominant deforming force.

Degenerative Spondylolisthesis.—This most commonly occurs at the L4–5 level where lumbar lordosis is greatest. Since the body's center of gravity is anterior to the lumbar spine, the lumbar spine is inclined to slide forward on the lordotic (anteriorly flexed) L5 vertebral body.[30] Anterior shear stresses are concentrated in the L4–5 disc which is often the first disc to degenerate. Anterior shear forces lead to softening of the disc and facet synovitis with erosion. Anterior translation of the proximal spine follows. With relative loss of anterior column support from progressive disc degeneration and vertebral body erosion, the L4–5 segment also rotates into relative kyphosis.

Neural compromise in degenerative spondylolisthesis is often secondary to the combined effects of central, lateral, and foraminal stenosis (Fig 29–1). Central stenosis results from the dural sac being "pinched" between the lamina of L4 and the posterosuperior edge of the L5 vertebral body. The hypertrophied or redundant L4–5 ligamentum flavum usually accentuates the central stenosis at the step-off. Lateral recess stenosis is due to the anteromedial overgrowth of the L5 superior facet osteophytes. As the slip progresses, there is great stress concentra-

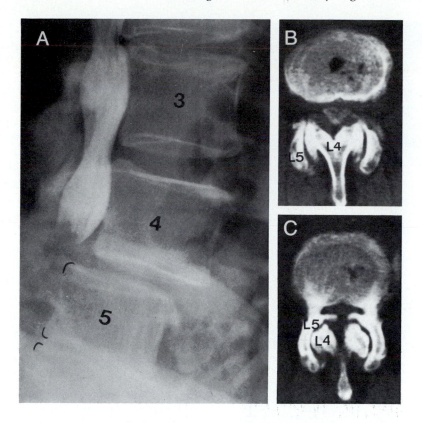

FIG 29–1.

Degenerative L4–5 spondylolisthesis. **A,** 22% anterior slip of L4 on L5 with reduced disc space and complete myelographic block at the level of the slip. **B,** CT-myelogram demonstrates severe erosive facet joint arthritis with anterior subluxation of the inferior facet of L4 on the superior facet of L5 and hypertrophy of the ligamentum flavum. **C,** CT-myelogram at the level of the L5 pedicle demonstrates large osteophytes which arise from the anteromedial aspect of the L5 superior facets and cause significant lateral stenosis.

tion on the anterior lip of the L5 superior facet with resulting erosion. In an effort to restore stability, osteophytes grow about the anterior and medial edge of the L5 facet. In time, they nearly fill the lateral recess to impinge on the L5 root. Anterior projection of the L5 facet osteophytes combined with posterior bulging of the collapsed L5 disc annulus with or without inferior L4 osteophytes produces foraminal stenosis and compression of the exiting L4 roots. Therefore, to surgically reconstruct an unstable degenerative spondylolisthesis, it is necessary to resect any offending L5 superior facet osteophytes, restore axial height, translate the L4 vertebra posteriorly, maintain lumbar lordosis, and resist anterior shear and flexion forces until successful fusion.

Retrolisthesis.—Retrolisthesis may follow degenerative spondylosis and is characterized by posterior translation of the proximal spine accompanied by asymmetric posterior disc collapse and facet subluxation.[15] Lateral and foraminal stenosis occurs when the superior vertebral body and its bulging an-

nulus shift posteriorly toward the superior facet of the vertebra below (Fig 29–2). Correction of retrolisthesis involves restoration of disc height and forward translation of the proximal vertebra.

Lateral Olisthesis.—This results from the coupling of lateral and rotational shear forces through the intervertebral disc. (Fig 29–3). It most commonly follows a degenerative scoliosis or pelvic obliquity (Fig 29–3,A and B). The spinal canal area is diminished as the pedicle shifts medially into the dural sac. The nerve root exiting *away* from the direction of slip is pulled medially by the pedicle of the slipping vertebra and stretched over the lateral body of the distal vertebra. Additional lateral recess stenosis may occur from the anteriorly subluxated and osteoarthritic inferior facet (Fig 29–3,C). The facet joint on the concave (lower) side of the slip is overloaded and hypertrophic (Fig 29–3,D). It often causes recess and foraminal stenosis compounded by an asymmetrically collapsed disc. Reconstruction of lateral olisthesis requires establishing a relatively level base for the lis-

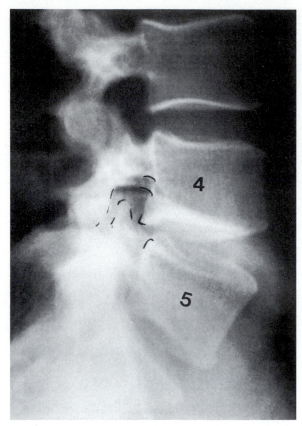

FIG 29–2.
Degenerative L4–5 retrolisthesis. Facet erosion and loss of disc space height have resulted in posterior translation of the superior vertebra with migration of the superior facet into the L4–5 neural foramina to cause foraminal stenosis.

thetic vertebra followed by the application of distraction and translational and derotational forces to reduce the slip and indirectly decompress the roots.

TREATMENT PRINCIPLES

The primary goal in the treatment of degenerative lumbar stenosis with or without olisthesis is to provide adequate decompression of neural tissues. Direct surgical decompression is needed to remove facet osteophytes, hypertrophic facet capsules, synovial cysts, or redundant ligamentum flavum causing symptomatic radiculopathy and neurogenic claudication. Reduction of significant translational deformity will facilitate indirect decompression of neural tissues by restoring normal spinal alignment. The need for spinal fusion is based upon the presence or likelihood of segmental instability.

Stenosis

A *stable pattern* of degenerative stenosis is characterized by patients who are at minimal risk for developing postdecompression instability. These patients tend to be older persons in whom limited spinal loading is anticipated. Symptoms are predominantly related to compromise of neural tissue with little or no complaints of low back pain. Preoperative radiographs demonstrate advanced degenerative disc disease with anterior osteophyte formation and the absence of significant angular or translational deformity[16][20] (Fig 29–4). Flexion-extension films demonstrate little or no motion in the degenerated segments. Direct decompression alone is usually adequate in patients with a stable pattern of degenerative stenosis. Only those structures causing symptomatic radiculopathy or claudication should be resected while preserving the integrity of the facet joints and pars interarticularis.

As patient selection criteria are relaxed or the surgical decompression becomes more extensive, the incidence of postdecompression instability with pain and further neural compromise increases.[20, 22] Likewise, the incidence of postoperative spondylolisthesis after decompression alone for lumbar stenosis may approach 20% as series include more patients with unstable patterns or extensive decompressions.[9–13]

A number of predisposing factors for postdecompression *instability* have been identified.[23] These include younger and more physically active patients, female sex, and the demonstration of instability on preoperative flexion-extension radiographs[19, 22, 38] (Fig 29–5). Lumbar instability is suggested by sagittal plane rotation (flexion-extension) greater than 22 degrees and translation greater than 4.5 mm or 15%.[37] Other factors include near-normal disc space height,[38] prior decompression at the same level, and the presence of nonunions.[17] The risk of postoperative instability is also directly related to the extent of decompression at the time of surgery. Total facetectomy, even created unilaterally, significantly decreases segmental stability.[1] Multiple-level decompressions and penetration of the disc space also reduce stability.[21, 26, 32, 36]

In those patients at risk for developing postdecompression instability, instrumented fusion is probably indicated. The role of instrumentation in this setting is to prevent postoperative vertebral subluxation after decompression, decrease postoperative pain, and enhance the rate of successful fusion, particularly if there is a preexisting nonunion.[17]

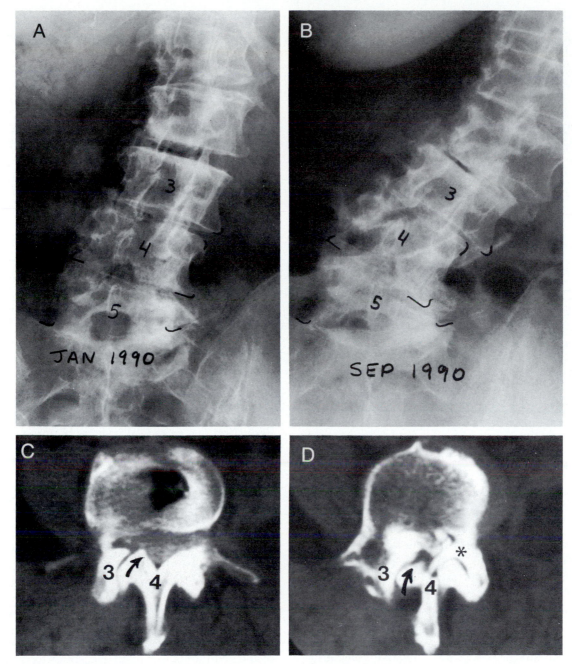

FIG 29–3.
Degenerative lateral olisthesis. **A** and **B,** AP radiographs at 9-month intervals demonstrate progressive L3–4 lateral olisthesis secondary to increasing obliquity between L4 and L5. **C** and **D,** CT-myelogram of the same patient shows that L3 has rotated about the eroded hypertrophic L4 superior facet (*). The combination of lateral and rotatory subluxation and hypertrophic L5 facet osteophytes produce both central and lateral recess stenosis.

Degenerative Olisthesis

The treatment of degenerative olisthesis depends upon the degree of instability and nerve compression. The presence of several millimeters of degenerative olisthesis does not necessarily indicate segmental instability. As with stenosis, loss of disc space height, formation of large anterior osteophytes, and little motion on flexion-extension radiographs suggest a *stable* pattern. Very focal direct decompression alone may suffice. Partial facetectomy and tapered removal of superior facet osteophytes

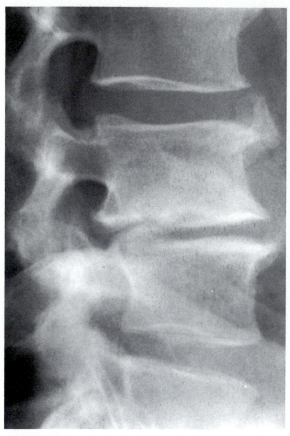

FIG 29–4.
Stable lumbar spondylosis. Minimal olisthesis, marked loss of disc space height, and prominent anterior osteophytes suggest "stable pattern" spondylosis in a patient with degenerative stenosis.

will adequately decompress the lateral recess without sacrificing facet joint integrity. Undercutting the lamina (laminaplasty) instead of total laminectomy may successfully relieve central stenosis.

An *unstable degenerative olisthesis* is present when associated with the other predisposing factors for degenerative instability outlined above. Major decompressive surgery for an unstable olisthesis greatly increases the chance of postoperative instability and further slippage, even with attempted fusion in situ. Indeed, adequate canal decompression for major olisthesis often requires resection of the entire lamina or even pedicle (in the case of lateral olisthesis) which serves to further destabilize the motion segment. The incidence of increased slippage after decompression alone has been reported to be as high as 88%.[2–5, 13–19, 23, 28, 34, 38] Many of these patients required reoperation and fusion for back pain or recurrent neurologic symptoms. The severity

of symptoms in degenerative spondylolisthesis has no correlation with the magnitude of the slip,[4, 23, 33] but a significant correlation exists between symptoms and the degree of translatory instability demonstrated by traction-compression radiographs.[14]

If unstable or major degenerative olisthesis or angular deformity exists, then instrumented reduction and fusion is especially recommended. It offers four advantages over noninstrumented in situ fusion. Specifically, instrumented reduction and fixation will (1) indirectly decompress neural tissues by reducing the deformity; (2) decrease postoperative pain; (3) restore normal spine alignment and compensation in both the sagittal and coronal planes; and (4) enhance the rate of fusion. When neural compression is caused by vertebral translation, bulging discs, or subluxated facets, *in*direct decompression can reduce the amount of vertebral resection needed. Distraction while maintaining lumbar lordosis will flatten bulging discs and restore foraminal size; thus, disc resection is unnecessary and the extent of foraminotomy is decreased. When a major olisthesis is present, direct decompression would require complete laminectomy and perhaps resection of pedicles or posterior vertebral bodies which would increase surgical morbidity and blood loss. Reduction makes radical resections unnecessary.

PREOPERATIVE EVALUATION

The first step in preoperative evaluation is to establish the cause of the patient's back pain and neurologic symptoms, if present. The more precise the location and understanding of the origin of pain, the better and more predictable the end result. Patient evaluation begins with a detailed medical history including prior spine surgery and clinical results. Each of the symptoms is ranked according to its degree of severity or concern to the patient. Questions are directed to determine if back pain is secondary to instability, facet arthrosis, disc disease, deformity, or nonunion. Does the leg pain follow specific dermatomes or represent neurogenic claudication?

Physical findings should objectively confirm the patient's subjective complaints by eliciting spinous process tenderness to strong palpation at specific and reproducible motion segments. Careful neurologic examination should elicit subtle root dysfunction compatible with the patient's radicular symp-

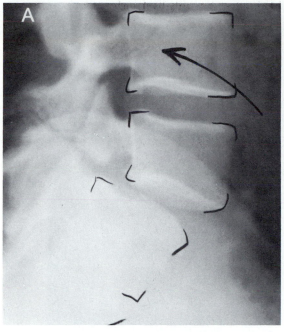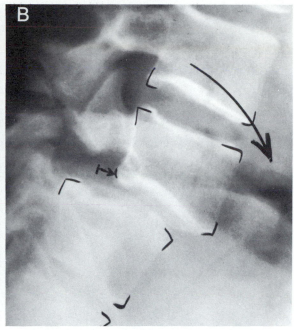

FIG 29–5.
Unstable lumbar spondylosis. **A** and **B,** flexion and extension radiographs demonstrate a degenerative spondylolisthesis pattern with moderate disc space, nominal anterior osteophytes, and significant translation and angulation on bending films.

toms. Standing, coronal, and sagittal decompensation secondary to significant deformities may explain back muscle fatigue or spinal pain from compensatory lordosis and scoliosis.

Radiographic studies should include anteroposterior (AP) and lateral views in the standing and supine positions to determine coronal and sagittal plane deformities. Flexion-extension views will elicit pathologic instability with forward displacement greater than 2 mm when standing up from a supine position.[29] Traction-compression radiographs may reveal translational instability not readily demonstrated by routine flexion-extension or supine-standing radiographs.[14] Quantitative measurement of flexion-extension films will determine nonunion. Computed tomography (CT) with myelography is indicated in those patients with radicular or neurogenic claudication syndromes and allows excellent visualization of the structural defects causing central or lateral canal stenosis. It is important to identify and mark on the CT films the precise location of each root impingement causing radiculopathy or claudication.

In order to assess whether or not a borderline instability is symptomatic, it is often helpful to immobilize the patient in a body cast with a unilateral thigh spica for a period of 3 weeks. If the patient shows significant improvement in the cast, this may help establish that fusion is warranted. Although spinal deformity is obvious on the radiograph, it is important to determine precisely which segments in or around the deformity are symptomatic and limit surgery to only the symptomatic levels when treating older patients with degenerative olisthesis.

Once the surgeon understands the pathomechanics of a particular patient's case, it is time to proceed with preoperative planning for the surgical procedure. However, before embarking on the reconstruction of a lumbar spine with unstable degenerative olisthesis, kyphosis, or scoliosis, we recommend the following *planning sequence:*

1. Analyze standing and bending films to determine the direction of forces causing the present or potential spinal deformity.
2. Select opposing corrective forces you would like to apply in order to directly counteract the forces of deformation and the planes of instability. Mark vectors to be applied on the preoperative AP and lateral films with a wax pencil (Fig 29–6,A).
3. Determine the levels of fixed nerve root impingement due to structures such as facet osteo-

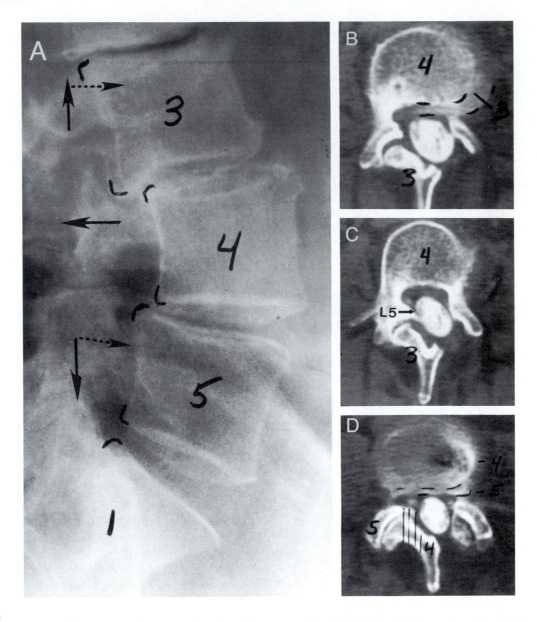

FIG 29–6.
Preoperative planning. **A,** degenerative spondylosis with L3–4 retrolisthesis and L4–5 spondylolisthesis, causing L5 radicular pain. *Arrows* indicate the corrective forces needed for reduction of deformity and indirect decompression. **B,** CT-myelogram demonstrates L3–4 retrolisthesis with an open L3–4 facet which must be cleared of soft tissue to permit reduction. **C,** osteophytes protruding from the medial aspect of the L4 superior facet irritate the L5 root *(arrow).* This root and dural sac lie posterior in the canal owing to the L3–4 retrolisthesis. Correction of retrolisthesis will move the root anteriorly to provide indirect decompression, making direct resection unnecessary. **D,** L4–5 facet erosion allows slight anterior subluxation (spondylolisthesis). Medial osteophytes on the superior facet of L5 cause lateral stenosis. Reduction of the spondylolisthesis will *not* relieve lateral recess stenosis. *Hatch marks* indicate the required direct resection of the osteophytes.

phytes or synovial cysts that will *not* be relieved by reduction of the deformity alone. Plan direct surgical decompression on the basis of preoperative radicular symptoms, neurologic findings, and the CT-myelogram. For example, before reduction of a degenerative spondylolisthesis, anteromedial osteophytes on the superior facet must be resected. Mark the structures to be resected on the preoperative CT scan (Fig 29–6,D).

4. Select or design the instrumentation construct to most effectively apply the corrective forces needed for reduction and stable fixation.

5. Determine the presence of anterior bony bridges or posterior blocks to reduction which must be resected before spinal instrumentation and mark them on the plain and CT films.

6. Decide the most proximal and distal vertebra which must be instrumented to maintain stable fixation without excessive length of instrumentation.

7. Select the optimum sites of spinal attachment. In general, hooks are safer and more efficient in the thoracic spine while screws are safer and more effective in the low lumbar and sacral spine.

8. Determine the order of reduction. For most translational deformities, first distract, then translate, and finally, compress. For angular deformities, apply three-point loading, then compress the convexity and distract the concavity.

9. Mark the location of any rod cross-links to enhance the stability of long constructs or those to be left in net distraction.

INSTRUMENTATION SELECTION

To achieve indirect decompression and either neutralize instability or correct listhesis, we require instrumentation that is able to attach to any deformity and then gradually apply corrective forces to individual vertebrae in all directions.

To fulfill these requirements, one of us (C.C.E.) combined the advantages of a ratcheted rod system derived from Harrington with pedicle screw fixation as popularized by Roy-Camille and added transverse adjustability. The resulting modular system was designed to fulfill four biomechanical principles:

1. *Versatility of attachment:* Linkages (i.e., hooks or adjustable connectors) between the screws and rods permit placement of screws in the most advantageous position and orientation for each vertebra.

2. *Three-dimensional control:* Axial control (segmental compression with or without distraction) is provided by ratcheted spinal rods. Independent control of vertebral translation in the coronal, sagittal, and rotational planes is achieved with adjustable rod-screw connectors and rod cross-links.

3. *Stress relaxation:* Independent axial and transverse adjustability makes it possible to slowly move individual vertebrae in any direction. The ability to apply corrective forces in small gradations over time allows the surgeon to slowly stretch out contracted tissues even after many years of deformity. The spi-

nal rods are then loaded within their elastic range to maintain corrective forces, and hence reduction, until fusion.

4. *Load sharing:* The various instrumentation constructs are designed to apply only the forces needed to correct the deformity or instability without unnecessary residual restraints which could stress-shield bone and interfere with healing. The resulting semirigid fixation appears to promote fusion and lessen subsequent breakdown of the adjacent motion segments. Hence, the instrumentation is biocompatible and late removal is usually unnecessary.

Four components of the modular system are used in the treatment of stenosis with instability or degenerative olisthesis (Fig 29–7):

1. *Spinal screws:* The ball-tip self-tapping screws and the sequential insertion technique lessen the risk of injury. Various lengths provide unicortical pedicle or bicortical sacral alar fixation. Large threads help prevent loosening while the tapered minor diameter lessens breakage. Screwhead geometry helps preserve normal spinal alignment during either compression or distraction.

2. *Universal rods:* Fully ratcheted and bidirectional spinal rods allow segmental compression, distraction, or neutralization.

3. *Anatomic hooks:* The hooks serve as linkages between the screws and rods to facilitate assembly, permit variable screw orientation, and absorb impact loads.

4. *Adjustable connectors:* Connectors between the rods and screws control the position of individual vertebrae in the transverse plane. The connectors make it possible to gradually reduce kyphosis, lateral listhesis, retrolisthesis, or spondylolisthesis, and actively derotate scoliotic vertebrae.

The components of the Edwards modular system are assembled to form various constructs depending on the biomechanical needs of the case at hand. The *compression construct* is used for patients with intact facets or interbody grafts in whom the goal of fixation is to promote fusion. When disrupted facets preclude compression, the simple screw-rod-screw *neutralization construct* is substituted. The *distraction-lordosis (D-L) construct* uses pedicle screw fixation to effect short segment distraction and lordosis for reduction of degenerative olisthesis. The *lateral olisthesis* and various *scoliosis constructs* are employed for the more complex multi-

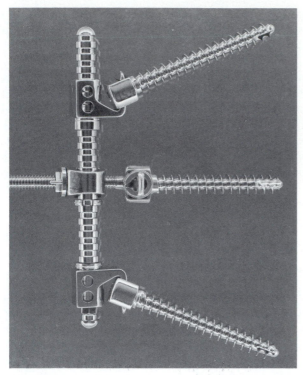

FIG 29–7.
Modular system components including spinal screws, Universal rods, anatomic hooks, and adjustable connector. Components are arranged to form a distraction-lordosis construct.

plane deformities. When treating major olisthesis or other deformities, all of the constructs apply corrective forces very gradually to facilitate stress relaxation and reduce the need for anterior or transcanal release procedures.

THE OPERATION

Patient Preparation and Positioning

Predonated autogolous blood and cell-saver apparatus are requisites for major spine reconstructive surgery. Blood loss is further reduced by proper patient positioning on an appropriate frame to decompress the abdomen. The arms should be padded well to prevent nerve compression with less than 90 degrees of shoulder abduction to prevent traction injury.

Exposure

A midline posterior approach to the lumbar spine is utilized. Care is taken to preserve the inter-

spinous ligaments and facet joint capsules of the levels proximal and distal to those being fused to prevent junctional instability. The entire supraspinous ligament is left attached to the spinous processes, when possible, to facilitate subsequent reattachment of the paraspinous muscle fascia and help reduce dead space in the wound. To maximize the fusion area, lateral gutters are cleared out to the tip of the transverse processes and particular attention is paid to removing soft tissues on the lateral wall of the superior facets of the proximal vertebra to be fused. The transverse processes are decorticated and facet joint cartilage is removed prior to instrumentation for best access.

Decompression

Direct decompression within the vertebral canal is limited to those structures that will still cause impingement *after* reduction of any olisthesis. This will minimize epidural bleeding and neural tissue manipulation. The anteromedial and sometimes superior osteophytes of the superior facets are beveled with a Kerrison punch to relieve lateral recess stenosis. Each nerve root to be decompressed is traced out laterally through its respective foramen. We recommend angled punches with flat shoes that project as little as possible into the canal. Care is taken to preserve the integrity of the pars interarticularis when decompressing neural foramina. The underside of laminae and facets are beveled so exiting nerves encounter no sharp ridges. Routine discectomies are not performed unless there is disc herniation or extreme posterior rim osteophytes. If the disc space is entered, then consideration should be given to placement of an interbody graft to serve as a spacer to support the anterior column.

Spinal Attachment

After necessary root decompressions and resection of any blocks to reduction, laminar hooks and spinal screws are placed in accordance with the preoperative plan. When instrumenting the patient with central stenosis, screws are preferred since they provide secure fixation without entering the already narrowed canal. To maximize the safety and strength of screw fixation, one of us (C.C.E.) has since 1984 recommended the following screw insertion techniques with a screw complication rate of less than 1%. For *sacral* fixation, bicortical screws are placed across the lateral sacral ala, a location that usually provides greater ease of insertion and strength of fixation than the alternatives.[6, 39] First, a 2-mm drill bit enters the sacrum in the dimple found at the base of the L5–S1 facet and is directed approximately 35 degrees lateral and 25 degrees caudad to parallel the superior end plate of S1. The bit is manually pushed to contact the anterior cortex of the sacrum where an AP radiographic image should show the tip of the bit 1 to 2 cm from the anterior sacroiliac joint. The hole is expanded with a 3.5-mm bit. The drill should just penetrate the anterior alar cortex but remain within the anterior reflection of the sacroiliac ligament. A depth gauge is used to carefully feel around the medial edge of the anterior alar hole in order to select the correct screw length.

When medial sacral screw orientation is preferred, the sacral screw is inserted just lateral to the L5–S1 facet directed 25 degrees medially through the S1 pedicle toward the junction of the anterior cortex and the S1 end plate in the midline. Medial screws are considered for lumbarized S1 vertebrae when the S1 alae are poorly developed. They are also used to facilitate assembly for one-level L5–S1 instrumentation and in the correction of lateral olisthesis.

For lumbar *pedicle* fixation, the posterior cortex over the pedicle is removed with a burr. A 3-0 curette probe is used to locate the center of the pedicle and 2-mm drill bits are inserted. After correct orientation is confirmed radiographically, the hole is expanded with a 3.5-mm probe or drill in 1-cm increments. All four quadrants of the hole are palpated with a depth gauge to ensure that there is no pedicular penetration after each increment and prior to screw insertion.[9] In most cases, a screw length is selected that will approach but not penetrate the anterior vertebral body cortex. A seating reamer is used to prepare a bed for lateral screwhead support prior to inserting screws with a standard hex screwdriver. Once good position of all screws is radiographically confirmed, it is time to assemble the appropriate instrumentation construct.

INSTRUMENTATION CONSTRUCTS

The instrumentation construct required for each patient will vary with the abnormality and is determined during the preoperative evaluation.

Compression Construct for In Situ Fixation With Intact Facets or Interbody Graft

The compression construct is indicated for primary fusions and nonunions. It facilitates physiologic axial loading and blocks tension and shear to promote union.[10] (Fig 29–8). However, the compression construct requires intact facets, residual fusion mass, or anterior interbody graft to maintain foraminal height and provide rotational stability. Hence, foraminotomies and interbody grafts should be performed prior to compression construct fixation in most cases with instability and stenosis. When treating central stenosis, it is best to avoid hooks in the canal. Therefore, proximal and distal attachment is accomplished with spinal screws. For single-level L5–S1 fusions, both pairs of screws are orientated medially to simplify assembly.

The compression construct is assembled as follows: Insert the proximal and distal screws as described above. Place cancellous bone plugs into the debrided facet joints. To assemble the construct, pass a cephalad-facing low anatomic hook through the slot of the distal screw. Pass the octagon end of the Universal rod distally through the hook linkage and apply a narrow washer in the groove at the end of the rod to fix the rod to the hook and distal screw. Another low anatomic hook is placed facing caudad over the proximal end of the rod and inserted into the slot of the proximal screw. The spreader is then positioned adjacent to the proximal hook to apply compression.

Screw fixation on both sides of each nonunion is recommended for optimal results when treating multiple nonunions. Midposition vertebrae are attached to the rods with pedicle connectors. During the application of compression, the midposition connectors are shortened to prevent excess lordosis and enhance rotational stability.[8]

Neutralization Construct for In Situ Fixation Without Compressible Facets

The posterior neutralization construct combines proximal angled hole screws, distal straight hole screws, and Universal rods for short segment fixation of primary fusions when bilateral compression cannot be applied (Fig 29–9). The technique for assembly of the neutralization construct is as follows: Proximal attachment is accomplished with angled hole screws. The screws are angled 15 to 20 degrees cephalad and medially to keep the instrumentation from impinging on the adjacent unfused facet joints. For distal attachment, angled hole screws should be

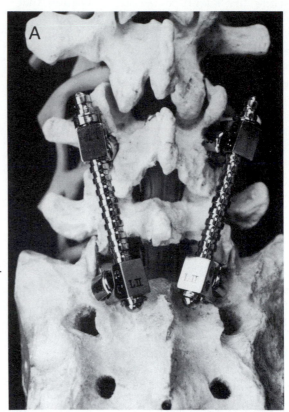

FIG 29–8.
Compression construct. **A,** screw-to-screw L4–S1 compression construct demonstrating appropriate L4 screw placement to avoid L3–4 facet joint impingement. **B** and **C,** AP and lateral radiographs demonstrating a screw-to-screw L4–S1 compression construct in a patient with intact facet joints status post-decompression *(arrows).* Sacral screws enter the sacrum at the base of the L5–S1 facet and just cross the anterior cortex of the lateral ala.

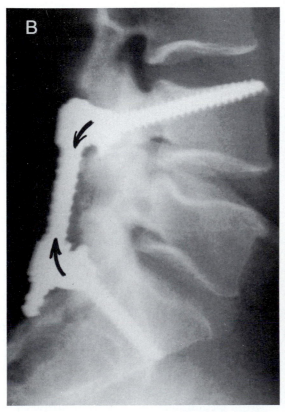

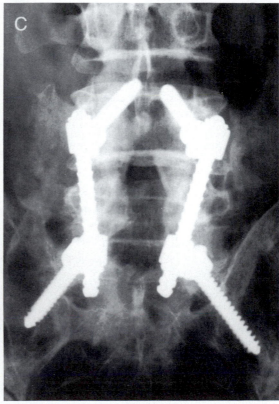

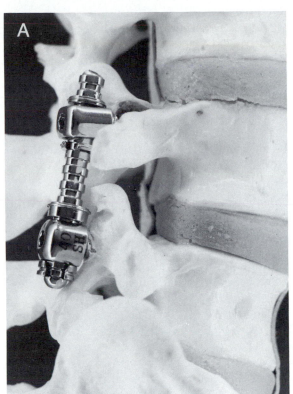

FIG 29–9.
Neutralization construct. **A,** L4–5 neutralization construct model with a proximal angle-hole screw and distal straight-hole screw for low profile. **B,** preoperative AP radiograph of a patient with a prior extensive L4–5 decompression. There is surgical absence of the pars interarticularis and inferior facet on the right *(arrows)* which precludes use of a compression construct without an interbody graft. **C,** postoperative AP radiograph showing a neutralization construct. Washers are placed above and below the screws to allow autocompression across intact facets on the left *(arrows)*. However, washers are placed between the screws to prevent autocompression and maintain foraminal height on the right *(arrows)*.

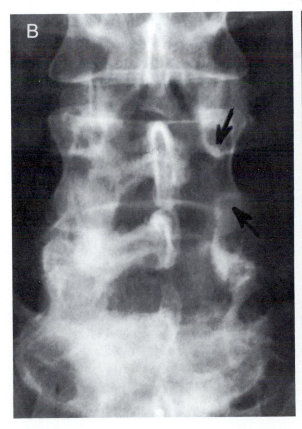

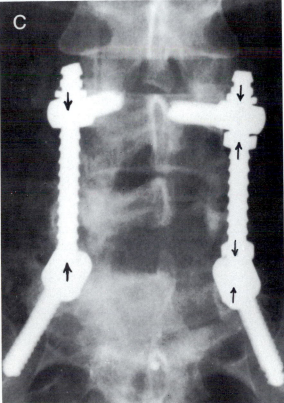

used for S1 and straight hole screws for lumbar vertebrae. The distal screws are inserted parallel to the vertebral end plates. Flex or extend the operating table or slightly contour and then rotate the rod as needed to align with the distal screw hole. Slide the rod through the distal screw holes and apply washers adjacent to each screw to fix the position of the spine until union.

Distraction-Lordosis Construct for Stenosis and Degenerative Spondylolisthesis

The D-L construct is indicated when central stenosis or instability is due in part to loss of intervertebral height, lordosis, or sagittal alignment.[7] For instability with central stenosis, the D-L construct will restore normal lordosis, flatten bulging discs, and enlarge foramina to reduce the amount of direct decompression required.[18] After decompression of stenosis, fixed-angle distraction screws are placed proximally and distally in the presence of stenosis and instability to maintain lumbar lordosis during distraction.

For *degenerative spondylolisthesis* between L3–4 or L4–5, distraction restores normal height to flatten bulging discs, and enlarge foramina, while lengthening the midposition connectors causes the lower two vertebrae (i.e., L5 and the sacrum) to rotate into flexion underneath the slipped proximal vertebra (L4). This reduces the olisthesis and counteracts translational instability (Fig 29–10).

Assembly of the D-L construct follows removal of anteromedial osteophytes from the superior facets. Proximal distraction screws are angled 15 degrees cephalad to avoid the adjacent unfused facets, and distal screws parallel the vertebral end plate. For reduction of spondylolisthesis a standard screw is always used distally to allow L5–S1 to rotate into flexion about the screwhead for correction of the L4–5 slippage. For midpoint fixation, a standard screw is seated more deeply than usual to accommodate a connector between the screw and the rod. A straight Universal rod is attached to the proximal and distal screws with low hooks facing away from the rod. The primary distraction washer is placed and gentle distraction is applied to disengage the olisthetic vertebrae. Midpoint connectors are then added to the rod and held perpendicular to the rod as they are extended. The connectors are lengthened until reduction of all olisthesis and the desired lordosis is confirmed radiographically. Gentle distraction is then sequentially applied until normal disc height is restored.

Retrolisthesis Construct

Correction of retrolisthesis involves the restoration of disc space height and forward translation of the proximal vertebra. This construct is assembled in the same manner as described for the D-L construct for degenerative spondylolisthesis. However, instead of lengthening the midpoint connectors, they are gradually shortened. The posterior pull of connectors combined with the anterior push of the rod reaction force on the adjacent proximal vertebra will reduce retrolisthesis and stabilize the spine in translation. After reduction of the deformity, the surgeon releases all but minimal distraction to permit physiologic loading (Fig 29–11).

Lateral Olisthesis Construct

Lateral olisthesis usually follows degenerative scoliosis or pelvic obliquity. However, the proximal scoliosis is usually asymptomatic. If the curvature proximal to the listhesis is reasonably compensated and can be accepted, lateral slippage can be reduced with a short construct (Fig 29–12). Nerve root decompression is achieved directly by removing osteophytes and indirectly by restoring alignment. Coronal compensation is improved by establishing a level base below the lateral olisthesis. Prior to the reduction of a lateral olisthesis, all blocks to reduction must be removed. This includes resection of the facet osteophytes and a partial facetectomy on the convex side to allow unimpeded compression with unilateral shortening of the posterior column.

The lateral olisthesis construct requires fixation at one level above and two levels below the slip. For example, when treating L4–5 lateral listhesis, standard screws are inserted at L4, L5, and S1 (Fig 29–12,A). The S1 screws are inserted in the medial direction so that the hook and screw linkage is lateral. This increases the effective moment arm for the compression-distraction rods in correcting the L5 obliquity. The distal low hook linkages at L5–S1 are applied in distraction on the concave side and compression on the convex side. The first step in reduction is sequential L5–S1 concave distraction and convex compression to establish a level base for L4 and vertical orientation for the spinal rods.

The second step of reduction is connection of the olisthesis. Connectors are placed between the screws in the slipped vertebrae and proximal end of the rods. Connector stems are positioned opposite the direction of the slip. First, the slipped vertebra is gently distracted to disimpact the L4–5 vertebrae.

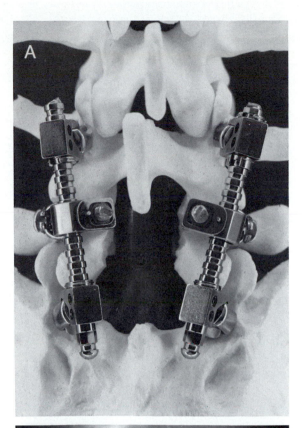

FIG 29–10.
Distraction-lordosis construct. **A,**
model of an L4–S1 distraction-
lordosis construct. Universal rods are
attached to screws with low hooks at
L4 and S1 and with adjustable
connectors at L5. **B,** preoperative
radiograph of a unstable degenerative
L4–5 spondylolisthesis with L5–S1
spondylosis. **C,** postoperative
radiograph of the same patient treated
with a distraction-lordosis construct
demonstrating full reduction of the
olisthesis and maintenance of lumbar
lordosis. The first step in reduction is
gentle distraction to disengage the
vertebrae and open the foramen. The
L5 connectors are then lengthened to
rotate (flex) L5 about the S1 screws
under the L4 vertebra until full
correction of the olisthesis is
documented radiographically. *Arrows*
indicate direction of reduction forces
at L4 and L5.

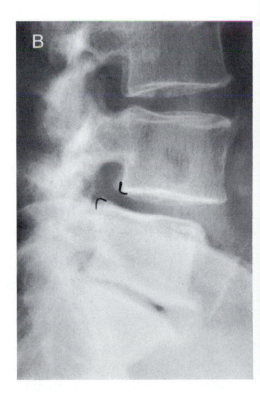

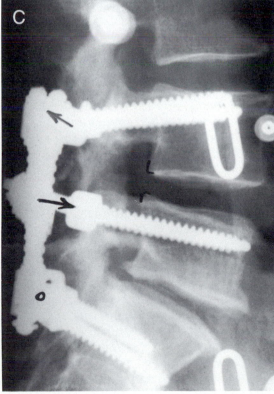

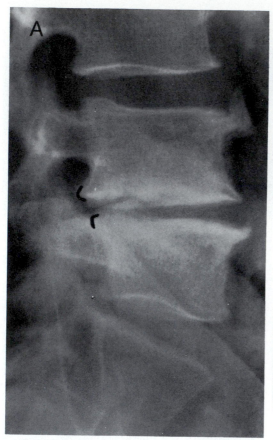

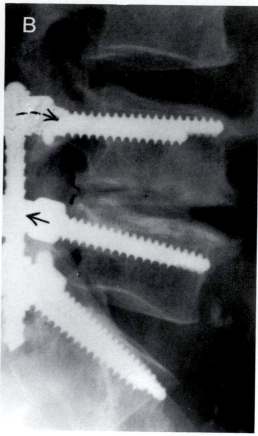

FIG 29–11.
Retrolisthesis construct. **A,** preoperative radiograph demonstrating degenerative retrolisthesis of L4 on L5. **B,** correction of the olisthesis with a retrolisthesis construct. After initial gentle L4–5 distraction, the connectors at L5 are shortened *(solid arrow),* thereby generating an anterior translational force (rod reaction) at the L4 vertebral body to reduce the olisthesis *(dashed arrow).* Compression is then applied to preserve or enhance lordosis.

The connectors are then shortened to reduce the lateral olisthesis. Thereafter, gentle compression is applied on the convexity. Rod washers, connector lock washers, and at least one cross-link are applied to maintain correction.

Scoliosis Construct for Symptomatic Scoliosis With Olisthesis

If the scoliosis associated with olisthesis is symptomatic or requires instrumentation, then the lateral olisthesis is reduced within a longer construct. Screws are placed in the stable vertebrae above and below the scoliosis. Screws with connectors are assembled on either side of the olisthetic vertebrae. Distraction is applied across the concavity. The pedicle connectors are then shortened or lengthened to reduce the olisthesis. Finally, compression across the apex of the convexity is applied and the rods are approximated with an adjustable cross-link.

Custom Constructs for Multiple-Level Spondylolisthesis of Retrolisthesis

These deformities are also called "stairstep" spines. The first step in reconstruction is to establish a stable base with two points of screw fixation (i.e., S1 and S2) below the most distal slip. Reduction then proceeds proximally in ascending order (Fig 29–13). Connectors attached to the olisthetic vertebrae are slightly distracted, then lengthened or shortened to correct sagittal olisthesis, and finally mildly compressed to allow axial loading. The more distal slip is always reduced first, thereby extending the stable base onto which the next more proximal listhesis is reduced.

Custom Constructs for Combined Deformities

Various combinations of lateral, retro-, and spondylolisthesis, combined with rotational and ky-

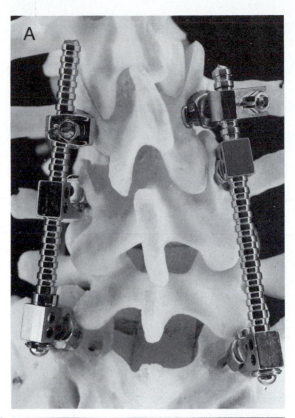

FIG 29–12.
Lateral olisthesis construct. **A,** model demonstrating an L4–S1 lateral olisthesis construct. **B,** preoperative radiograph demonstrating an L3–4 lateral olisthesis with associated obliquity between L4 and L5. **C,** postoperative radiograph of the same patient treated with an L3–5 lateral olisthesis construct. A stable base for the reduction of the lateral olisthesis is created by first correcting the L4–5 obliquity. Segmental distraction is applied on the concavity and compression on the convexity at the L4–5 level. Distraction is then applied at the L3–4 level to restore disc space height. Connector stems are orientated on the side of the rod opposite the direction of lateral olisthesis. The adjustable connectors at L3 are then shortened to correct lateral translation. Finally, compression is applied at L3–4 on the convex side. *Arrows* indicate direction of applied forces.

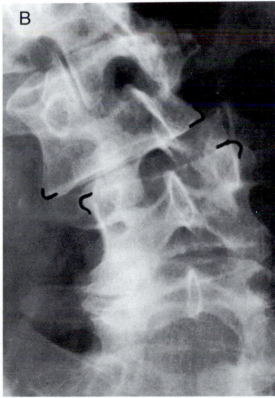

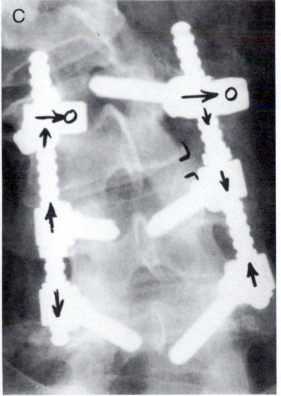

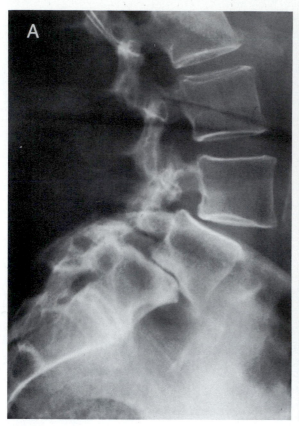
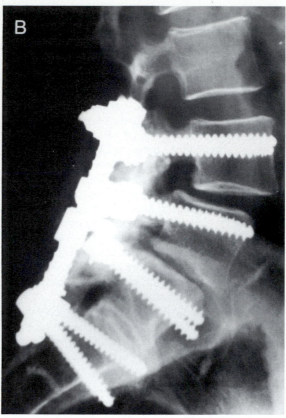

FIG 29-13.
Stairstep spinal deformity. **A,** preoperative lateral radiograph demonstrating degenerative spondylolisthesis at both L4-5 and L5-S1. **B,** postoperative radiograph 1 year after treatment with a spondylolisthesis construct. The stable base caudal to the most distal slip is first established with two points of fixation in the sacrum. The L5-S1 olisthesis is corrected with gentle distraction and shortening the connec- tors attached to spinal screws at L5. This effectively extends the stable base proximally to L4. The next olisthesis can then be corrected by distracting and shortening the adjustable connectors at L4. After reduction, distraction is released to permit axial loading. (Case courtesy of Michael McCutcheon, M.D.)

photic deformities, often characterize degenerative lumbar scoliosis. Reconstructing these multiplanar deformities for optimum indirect decompression, restoration of coronal and sagittal compensation, and stable fixation is both an intellectual and surgical challenge. Fortunately, some of these combined deformities occur in recognizable patterns. A detailed description of their treatment is beyond the scope of this chapter. However, through careful preoperative planning utilizing the principles outlined in this chapter, the surgeon can design the optimum modular instrumentation construct required for each case.

FUSION AND POSTOPERATIVE CARE

Resection of all scar tissue from prior operations is necessary to restore a soft tissue envelope condu- cive to bony union with adequate vascularity for the graft bed and with a source of osteoprogenitor cells from surrounding muscle for bone production. Care is taken to decorticate the lateral superior facet walls and transverse processes for maximum graft contact surface. Denuded facet joints and the lateral graft bed are packed with fresh cancellous bone prior to inserting the rods. Wound retractors are rotated during surgery to avoid ischemic myonecrosis.

Fusion is also facilitated by optimizing local biomechanics. (1) Compression should be applied across motion segments whenever possible. If the disc is violated, then an interbody graft should be applied to serve as an axial spacer. (2) Distraction needed to facilitate decompression should be restrained and combined with lordosis to direct axial loads across the facets and fusion mass. (3) When instrumentation extends across three or more lumbar motion segments or when two or more segments are left in distraction, the number of fixation points should be increased and rod cross-links are added to increase construct stability.

Following multiple-level lumbar reconstruction, we advise postoperative brace protection. When in situ fixation is planned, a polypropylene Total Contact Orthosis (TCO) with Velcro straps is fabricated prior to surgery. However, when major reductions are anticipated, a plaster TCO mold is fabricated 3 to 4 days postoperatively on a Risser frame. For most reconstructions extending to the sacrum, we add a unilateral thigh cuff to stabilize the lumbosacral junction (Fig 29–14). In a study of over 800 cases using modular instrumentation and TCO bracing with or without a thigh cuff, the fusion rate was enhanced by 5% when the thigh cuff was added.

Patients are ambulant in physical therapy immediately after receiving their brace except in cases with marked osteoporosis or extreme reductions. Stair climbing is discouraged for 4 to 6 weeks. At 6 to 8 weeks, the patient is encouraged in progressive walking exercises in the brace. At 2 months, the brace is removed for showers. At 10 to 14 weeks, the

thigh cuff is removed if radiographs show maintenance of alignment and there is no unusual spine tenderness. The TCO brace is then used for an additional 4 to 6 weeks. If at 7 to 9 months, quantitative flexion-extension films reveal evidence of early union, then the patient is instructed in partial sit-ups, deep knee bends, and general stretching exercises. Low-impact aerobic exercises are also encouraged.

RESULTS

The Spinal Fixation Study Group was formed in 1986 to transfer new concepts and techniques for reconstructive spinal surgery to other surgeons and generate a clinical data base for the continued evolution of these new procedures and the modular spinal system. The group's prospective series included over 3,000 cases by the end of 1990. Of these, 164 cases with degenerative spondylolisthesis were treated with the D-L construct. Results using the techniques outlined in this chapter have been favorable to date with consistent reduction of listhesis, indirect nerve root decompression, and a primary union rate of 88%. Another 223 patients were treated for stenosis without listhesis using either the D-L, compression, or neutralization constructs. The primary fusion rate for these constructs also averaged 88%.

Overall complications using the modular system have been acceptably low. In the group's series, the infection rate was 2%. Transient radiculopathy occurred in 3.1% of patients and was often associated with direct decompression. With current implant design, the screw breakage rate has been held to 0.5%. Only one sacral and one pedicle screw pullout have been recorded.

Using the surgical and biomechanical principles outlined in this chapter, it has been possible to treat successfully a wide variety of degenerative conditions in the lumbar spine. By first identifying the forces of deformation and resulting planes of instability, the appropriate modular system construct can be designed to apply corrective forces, restore normal spinal alignment, and indirectly decompress neural tissues.

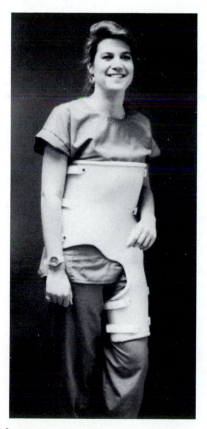

FIG 29–14.
Postoperative bracing. Polypropylene total contact orthosis with thigh cuff extension for initial postoperative protection. The front and back halves of the clamshell can be removed separately for daily skin care.

REFERENCES

1. Abumi K, Panjabi MM, Kramer KM: Biomechanical evaluation of lumbar spinal stability after graded facetectomies. *Spine* 1990; 15:1142–1147.

2. Bolesta MJ, Bohlman HH: Degenerative spondylolisthesis. *Instr Course Lect* 1989; 38:157–168.

3. Brown MD, Lockwood JM: Degenerative spondylolisthesis. *Instr Course Lect* 1983; 32:162–169.

4. Cauchoix J, Benoist M, Chassaing V: Degenerative spondylolisthesis. *Clin Orthop* 1976; 115:122–129.

5. Dall BE, Rowe DE: Degenerative spondylolisthesis: Its surgical management. *Spine* 1985; 10:668–672.

6. Edwards CC: The sacral fixation device: Design and preliminary results in *Proceedings of the Scoliosis Research Society*, 1984, p 135.

7. Edwards CC: Early results correcting spondylolisthesis. *Orthop Trans* 1989; 13:72.

8. Edwards CC: *Spinal Reconstruction Using a Modular System: Surgical Manual*. Baltimore, Spinal Research Foundation, 1990.

9. Edwards CC, Levine AM, Weigel MC: A modular system for 3-dimensional correction of lumbosacral deformities. *Orthop Trans* 1987; 11:19.

10. Edwards CC, Weigel MC: A prospective study of 51 low lumbar nonunions. *Orthop Trans* 1988; 12:608.

11. Farfan HF: Effects of torsion on the intervertebral joints. *Can J Surg* 1969; 12:336–341.

12. Farfan HF: The pathological anatomy of degenerative spondylolisthesis: A cadaver study. *Spine* 1980; 5:412–418.

13. Feffer HL, Wiesel SW, Cuckler JM: Degenerative spondylolisthesis: To fuse or not to fuse. *Spine* 1985; 10:287–289.

14. Friberg O: Lumbar instability: A dynamic approach by traction-compression radiography. *Spine* 1987; 12:119–129.

15. Frymoyer JW, Selby DK: Segmental instability: Rationale for treatment. *Spine* 1985; 10:280–286.

16. Grabias S: The treatment of spinal stenosis: Current concepts review. *J Bone Joint Surg [Am]* 1980; 62:308–313.

17. Herkowitz HN: The role of fusion in decompression surgery of the lumbar spine. Presented at the Spine Study Group 7th Symposium, Orlando, Fla, April 27, 1990.

18. Herkowitz HN, El-Kommos H: Instrumentation of the lumbar spine for degenerative disorders. *Op Tech Orthop* 1991; 1:91–96.

19. Herron LD, Trippi AC: L4–5 degenerative spondylolisthesis: The results of treatment by decompressive laminectomy without fusion. *Spine* 1989; 14:534–538.

20. Hopp E, Tsou PM: Postdecompression lumbar instability. *Clin Orthop* 1988; 227:143–151.

21. Iida Y, Kataoka O, Sho T, et al: Postoperative lumbar spinal instability occurring or progressing secondary to laminectomy. *Spine* 1990; 15:1186–1189.

22. Johnsson KE, Redlund-Johnell I, Uden A: Preoperative and postoperative instability in lumbar spinal stenosis. *Spine* 1989; 14:591–593.

23. Johnsson KE, Willner S, Johnsson K: Postoperative instability after decompression for lumbar spinal stenosis. *Spine* 1986; 11:107–110.

24. Kirkaldy-Willis WH: The relationship of structured pathology to the nerve root. *Spine* 1984; 9:49–52.

25. Kirkaldy-Willis WH, Wedge JH, Yong-Hing K: Pathology and pathogenesis of lumbar spondylosis and stenosis. *Spine* 1978; 3:319–328.

26. Lee CK: Lumbar spinal instability (olisthesis) after extensive posterior spinal decompression. *Spine* 1983; 8:429–433.

27. Lee CK, Rauschning W, Glenn W: Lateral lumbar spinal canal stenosis: Classification pathologic anatomy and surgical decompression. *Spine* 1988; 13:313–320.

28. Lombardi JS, Wiltse LL, Reynolds J: Treatment of degenerative spondylolisthesis. *Spine* 1985; 10:821–827.

29. Lowe RW, Hayes TD, Kaye J: Standing roentgenograms in spondylolisthesis. *Clin Orthop* 1976; 117:80–84.

30. Macnab I: Spondylolisthesis with an intact neural arch—the so-called pseudospondylolisthesis. *J Bone Joint Surg [Br]* 1950, 32:325–333.

31. Macnab I: The pathogenesis of spinal stenosis, in Hopp E (ed): *Spine: State of the Art Reviews*, vol 1. Philadelphia, Hanley & Belfus, Inc, 1987, pp 369–381.

32. Posner I, White AA, Edwards WT: A biomechanical analysis of the clinical stability of the lumbar and lumbosacral spine. *Spine* 1982; 7:374–388.

33. Rosenberg NJ: Degenerative spondylolisthesis: Predisposing factors. *J Bone Joint Surg [Am]* 1975; 57:467–474.

34. Rosenberg NJ: Degenerative spondylolisthesis: Surgical treatment. *Clin Orthop* 1976; 117:112–120.

35. Rosomoff HL: Neural arch resection for lumbar spinal stenosis. *Clin Orthop* 1981; 154:83–89.

36. Shenkin HA, Hash CJ: Spondylolisthesis after multiple bilateral laminectomies and facetectomies for lumbar spondylosis. *J Neurosurg* 1979; 50:45–47.

37. White AA, Panjabi MM: *Clinical Biomechanics of the Spine*, ed 2. Philadelphia, JB Lippincott Co, 1990.

38. White AH, Wiltse LL: Spondylolisthesis after extensive lumbar laminectomy, *J Bone Joint Surg [Am]* 1976; 58:727–728.

39. Zindrick MR, Wiltse LL, Widell EH, et al: A biomechanical study of intrapedicular screw fixation in the lumbosacral spine. *Clin Orthop* 1986; 203:99–111.

30

Bone Transplantation

Michael Bonfiglio, M.D.

Transplantation of organs, limbs, and bone is a very old concept. The subject has captured the imagination of man through artists of medieval times. Works of the great painters often adorned hospitals, especially paintings recording the miracles of the medical saints such as SS. Cosmas and Damian who grafted a white leg onto the body of a black who had an amputation for a cancer of the leg,[23] a scene portrayed in an altarpiece by the 15th century Spanish painter Jaime Huguet. Such a composite allograft obviously ignored the immunologic aspects of transplantation.

It was not until the experimental and clinical work of Ollier in the 19th century and of Barth,[6] Axhausen,[5] and Macewen[30] at the turn of the century that a clearer picture of bone graft repair developed. The term used by Barth, *schleichender Ersatz,* to describe the process of bone graft repair, was translated (probably by Phemister[38]) as "creeping substitution," to describe the slow vascular invasion of dead bone, bone resorption by osteoclasts, and bone deposition by osteoblasts. There was considerable discussion by early writers on the subject as to the contribution of components of bone, particularly periosteum, to the repair and to the viability of the cells after transplantation. Most agreed that periosteum did contribute to the take of the graft, but Phemister[38] noted that even without the periosteum the graft did incorporate, albeit at a slower rate. It was not until modern methods were used that the contribution of the graft cells to osteogenesis and to the take of the graft could be demonstrated.[2, 3, 16]

A number of excellent reviews on bone transplantation are worthy of the reader's time.[11, 13, 15, 34, 37, 39, 40, 45]

The usual bone transplants used in orthopaedic surgery are fresh autografts, free or vascularized; allografts, fresh, frozen, or freeze-dried; and xenografts. Even though xenografts are processed to reduce immunogenicity, they do not qualify as graft material.

There is little doubt that fresh *autogenous bone graft* is the superior bone transplant in situations when graft union to a properly prepared host bone bed is critical. As noted, surface cells of fresh autogenous bone, cancellous or cortical, *do survive* and participate in the early stages of the repair process to unite the graft to the host bone. Proper attention to preparation of the recipient site and removal of the graft from the donor site is essential to protect the viability of the cells of the graft. Thereafter, the repair of the graft substance follows the well-known process of resorption by vascular invasion and replacement (creeping substitution) by living bone within the form of appositional new bone along cancellous trabeculae and by formation of new haversian systems within cortical bone before remodeling to a functional state.

Allografts from living donors are for obvious reasons rarely used, but allografts of bone stored in a bone bank by cryopreservation techniques are commonly employed. The primary source of skeletal tissue is from fresh cadaver donors of organs such as kidney, heart, lung, pancreas, and liver. An additional source is bone recovered from surgical procedures (femoral head and rib). Fresh osteochondral allografts procured at the time of retrieval of these other organs have been used when cartilage survival is needed to repair articular defects and to preserve joint function.[18] Bone processed by freeze-drying and stored at room temperature accounts for a smaller portion of bone used in clinical practice.[31]

Many nonhuman bone substitutes have been devised: beef bone; cow horn; deantigenized, deproteinized, and decalcified bones; calcium hydroxyapatite; ceramic; calcium carbonate; plaster of Paris pellets; polymethyl methacrylate; and bone morphogenetic protein, to name a few. All suffer from a lack of predictable results in use compared with corticocancellous autogenous bone. These nonhuman implants are not discussed here.

The repair and remodeling of autografts and allografts must be understood if maximal benefit for the patient is to be achieved. There is no doubt that allografts evoke an immune response in the experimental animal as well as in the human.[10, 13, 14, 25, 35] These responses are primarily cellular (hypersensitivity type) and mild humoral antigen-antibody reactions.[10] Although the immune reaction is more intense, as in the use of a fresh allograft from a living donor, bone graft rejection is usually a minor problem compared to a slough of allograft skin or rejection of a kidney or other organ. Even when the immune response is modified experimentally or clinically to improve the take of the graft,[14, 35] the volume of bone to be replaced or incorporated into a functional state still constitutes the major aspect of the reconstitution of a bone graft.[9] As autogenous bone is repaired it is gradually remodeled into a biomechanically functional entity.[22, 38] Allograft bone is repaired much more slowly and less predictably because as long as any allograft remains it is subject to resorption, immune response, and weakening.[8] Grafts used to repair segmental defects after resection for tumors,[32] disease, or injury are subject to greater stress and therefore fracture during the repair process. Fractures in allografts usually show a poor healing response (15% at best) unless supplemented by autogenous bone.[7] Autogenous cortical bone repair is accompanied by a comparable incidence of stress fractures, but a higher proportion of the latter heal without the need for further surgery.[22]

An example of each type of graft used in lumbar spine fusion will be presented to illustrate the differences in response to autogenous and allograft bone. First, however, the repair of experimental and human clinical autogenous and allograft bone transplants is reviewed. Suggestions on retrieval of autogenous bone and the complications at donor sites will also be discussed. The use of allografts from bone banks should follow the principles described by Friedlaender and others.[21, 24]

AUTOGENOUS BONE

The usual sources of autogenous bone grafts are local bone (e.g., the corticocancellous pieces of spinous processes and laminae), the ilium,[1] the tibia (corticocancellous), and rib. There has been increasing effort directed toward the use of vascularized autografts of fibula, and rib and iliac crest in the repair of large bone defects.[45] However, in spine surgery their use has been limited to very special circumstances such as an anterior spine fusion with the combination of a vascularized autogenous rib pedicle graft and a femoral neck allograft, in patients with posttraumatic kyphosis with a neurologic deficit.[33] In general, such a time-consuming and specialized procedure is not needed for patients with spinal stenosis, degenerative lumbosacral spine disease, or spondylolisthesis.

Autogenous bone transplants have been shown to produce new bone from the surviving periosteal and endosteal surface cells.[2, 3, 10, 16, 38] Before the host response has developed, this proliferation of new bone gives the fresh autogenous graft a clear advantage over any other form of transplant.[27]

Rapid repair of a corticocancellous graft 7 weeks after insertion in a staged spinal fusion for scoliosis is shown in Figure 30–1,A. There is new bone forming along the cortex of the corticocancellous iliac crest graft and in the adjacent bed. The cortex is undergoing vascular invasion and creeping substitution with new bone forming around the new vascular channels (Fig 30–1,B).

Another patient had had a spinal fusion for degenerative disc disease 1 year previously. Because of persistent back pain and a suspected failed fusion, the fusion site was explored and a portion of the graft retrieved. At one end of the graft there was evidence of the fibrous nonunion site, but the graft itself had undergone a considerable amount of remodeling (Fig 30–2,A). Appositional new bone formed along the trabeculae of cancellous bone and vascular invasion of the cortical bone results in the formation of new haversian systems as part of the internal reconstruction of the bone (Fig 30–2,B). Cortical bone of the iliac graft usually undergoes repair in a somewhat slower but no less effective manner. Cortical bone repair progresses from approximately 50% replacement after 1 year up to 90% replacement after 10 years (author's observation).

Repair of cancellous bone takes considerably less time (on the order of 6 months to 2 years). Based on

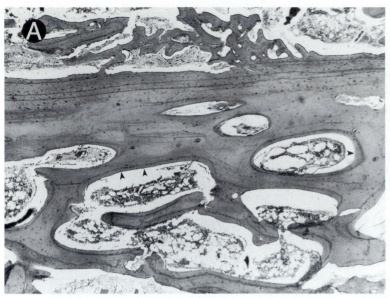

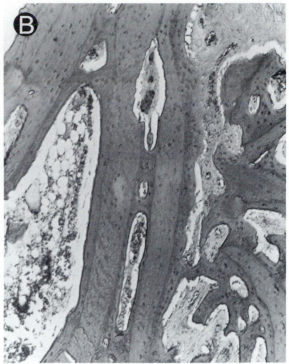

FIG 30–1.

A, repair of a corticocancellous iliac autogenous bone graft 7 weeks after insertion into a prepared bed of a Hibbs spinal fusion for scoliosis. Note new bone seams along endosteal spaces *(arrowheads)* and host new bone along the cortex (×42). **B,** vascular invasion within the cortex with new bone formation within the vascular channels (×84).

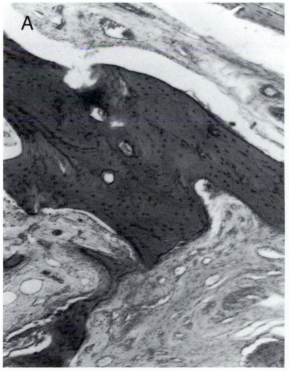

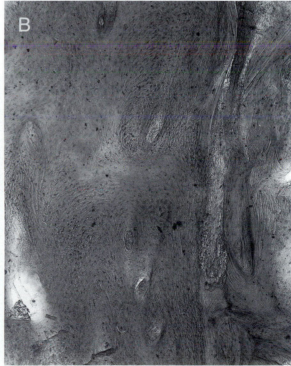

FIG 30–2.

A, autogenous bone graft repair at 1 year. Retrieval was from a failed spinal fusion as seen by fibrous nonunion at one end of the graft (×75). **B,** extensive remodeling into new haversian systems and lamellar bone has occurred. A small area of necrotic bone is being resorbed by osteoclasts at the end of a vascular bud "cutting cylinder" (×72).

observations of repair of the necrotic femoral head in children (Legg-Calvé-Perthes disease) and adults (posttraumatic and nontraumatic aseptic necrosis), the calculated rate of creeping substitution was estimated at 0.5 mm/month.[17] Cancellous bone graft repair is subject to stresses during creeping substitution and may fracture and fragment during the repair. Protection of the repair site is essential for the expected period of healing of the graft at the fusion site.

The repaired graft functions long before complete replacement of necrotic bone occurs. In some instances islands of necrotic bone of cortical grafts may persist adjacent to lamellar bone of new haversian systems for many years without turnover.

Had internal fixation with pedicular screws or plates been used with the bone graft the nonunion of the graft with the bed may have been avoided (See case 1).[4, 28, 29] (Fig 30–3,A–C).

In order for the autograft to have the best chance

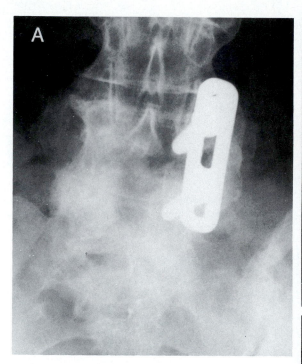

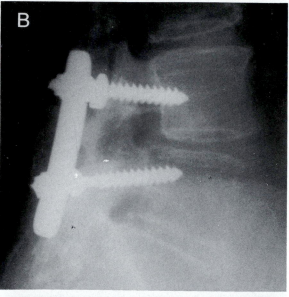

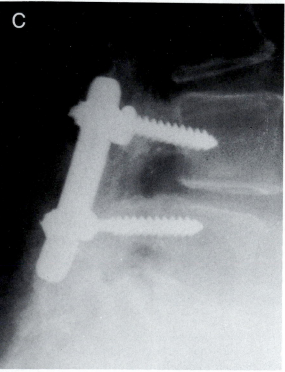

FIG 30–3.
A, AP radiograph at 24 months shows solid fusion of L4–S1 with autograft. Lateral flexion **(B)** and lateral extension radiographs **(C)** show no motion.

for union with the recipient bed, care must be taken to prepare the bed properly and to harvest the graft with care to protect the exposed surface cells of both the bed and the graft. The preparation of the recipient site should include decortication of the spinous process, laminae, and transverse processes. The decorticated fragments of bone are in fact local bone graft and should be treated as gently as harvested graft from the selected donor site. Subperiosteal stripping of those structures alone is performed to receive the graft when a non-Hibbs-type fusion and a corticocancellous graft is to be put in place (with or without sublaminal wires). Excessive cautery should be avoided. The wound should be packed with sponges soaked in warm (37°C) lactated Ringer's solution. All fixation should be done (wires or pedicular screws put in place) preferably before the autogenous bone is harvested to minimize the transfer time from donor site to recipient bed. If the surgeon prefers to harvest the graft first, then the graft pieces should be kept covered in a tray between the folds of a towel soaked in warm (37°C) lactated Ringer's solution. During the removal of the graft from the ilium or tibia or rib, warm lactated Ringer's solution is preferable to saline solution for wound lavage. In either case the autogenous graft whether one or two larger pieces for wiring technique or many 3- to 5-mm- × 4- 6-cm pieces for posterolateral fusion slabs, should be protected from contamination by room air or drying of the graft cells. Only when the surgical decompression of the spinal stenosis is complete and the fixation (if any) is in place should the graft be transferred to the prepared bed, the fixation wires, if any, tied, and the muscle brought over the graft for closure of the wound.

The improved results of spinal fusion in recent years are due in part to the stabilizing effect of better fixation techniques on the repair of the bone graft–recipient bed fusion mass, as the following case demonstrates.

> **Case 1.**— A 76-year-old man presented with the symptoms and signs of spinal stenosis of over 54 years' duration characterized by chronic low back pain and radiculopathy. The most recent episode of 3 months' duration included a shuffling gait and numbness in his legs. On examination, hypesthesia and dysesthesia of the L4–5 dermatomes were present. Weakness of dorsiflexion of the ankle and great toe was noted. Radiographs, computed tomography (CT) scans with contrast myelogram confirmed the diagnosis of degenerative lumbar spine disease and acquired spondylolisthesis at L4–5. Decompression of L4–S1 was performed bilaterally with bilateral posterolateral fusion with corticocancellous autogenous bone re-

trieved from the posterior superior spine of the ilium and iliac crest through a separate incision. On the left side, a bed for placement of the graft strips was prepared and the screws with a washer-spacer for the Steffee plate were put into the pedicles of L4 and L5 before the bone graft was placed across the decorticated transverse processes and the facet joints and lateral gutter. A 1 ½-in. slotted plate was attached to the two screws and screwed with the nuts and locking bolts. At 24 months an anteroposterior (AP) radiograph shows solid fusion of L4–S1 (see Fig 30–3,A). Lateral radiographs in flexion (see Fig 30–3,B) and extension show no motion at the fusion site. The autografts have consolidated and remodeled into a stress-bearing longitudinal mass.

It is evident that when the fixation device loosens, pseudarthroses of the fusion mass are more likely to occur.[4, 28]

Before proceeding to the discussion of allografts it is important to review complications at autogenous bone donor sites.

Donor Site Complications

In harvesting any graft from a donor site the surgeon should be cognizant of the potential complications so that these can be minimized. The final surgical result may relieve the original problem only to have a donor site complication supplant it.

The posterior iliac spine is most frequently used as donor bone if spinal fusion is needed after treatment of the spinal stenosis, degenerative disc disease, or spondylolisthesis. If the same midline incision is extended to reach the site, care should be taken to protect the sacroiliac ligament and adjacent muscles by staying subperiosteally on the lateral aspect of the process. Strips of corticocancellous bone are taken with either a gouge, thin osteotome, or chisel down to the endosteal aspect of the medial cortex, but preferably not through it so as to prevent sacroiliac joint instability or fracture of the posterior third of the ilium. Fracture of the anterior spine or wing of the ilium may occur with graft removal from the anterior part of the ilium. Hernia and meralgia paresthetica (see below) have also been reported, as well as chronic pain after iliac graft removal, particularly from the anterior two thirds of the ilium.[42] Any skin incision can lead to a painful scar or neuroma with hypoesthesia or anesthesia affecting the donor site area. At the anterior and lateral iliac crest, cutting the ilioinguinal nerve or its branches results in a residual meralgia paresthetica, a painful neuroma, sensory skin loss syndrome of the anterolateral aspect of the hip and thigh.

Although rib grafts are not suitable for fusion in spinal stenosis, such graft retrieval may be complicated by pneumothorax or chest wall hypoesthesia or anesthesia or neuroma from injury to the intercostal nerve, and by a painful scar.

Grafts removed from the tibia put that site at risk for fracture (up to 3%) usually at the ends of the graft excision site where a stress riser is created by cross-cutting the bone with a saw, osteotome, or chisel. Care should be taken to drill corner holes before using the chisel or osteotome to lift the graft from the bone.

Retrieval of the proximal third of the fibula has been complicated by ligamentous instability of the lateral collateral ligament. Peroneal nerve paralysis (temporary, partial, or complete) may result from injury during the surgery. The distal third of the fibula should be avoided as a donor site lest laxity of the tibiofibular ligament and the interosseous membrane lead to ankle instability.

It is obvious that each donor site is also subject to the commonly recognized complications of any surgery, e.g., infection, hemorrhage, and hematoma, skin and subcutaneous tissue injury, and cutaneous nerve damage.

ALLOGRAFTS

Because of the extra time need to operate on a donor site and the morbidity associated with the procedure, the clinical use of allograft bone has increased and bone banks developed. The use of allograft bone should follow the guidelines developed for bone banking by Friedlaender[24] and Doppelt et al.[21] Standards for tissue banking have been developed by the American Association of Tissue Banks, McLean, Virginia.

As noted earlier, the primary source of most bone for cryopreservation is from fresh cadavers within 12 hours of death. All donors should be disease-free, especially from hepatitis or human immunodeficiency virus (HIV). Currently, bone is deep-frozen at −70 to −90°C. Storage at −20°C is acceptable for a short time (less than 1 year). Cadaveric bone also serves as the source for freeze-dried bone. The details of retrieval, testing for sterility, and packaging are available in the literature[21, 24] and from the bone bank source. The surgeon should be aware of what his supplier does to ensure a safe allograft. The risk of allograft use is infectious hepatitis and, more recently, HIV infection. The risk of HIV transmission is estimated at 1 in 1.5 million donors.[12, 40] Ten percent to 15% of donor bone is discarded because of bacterial contamination, hepatitis, or a history of malignancy, either ante mortem or post mortem.[40]

Allograft repair follows the same pathways as noted for autografts except for the immune reaction and the rate of repair. The immune reaction has been shown experimentally to follow the same laws as for other tissues.[10, 35] It is known to be greatest in fresh bone allograft tissue and markedly reduced by freezing or freeze-drying. This has been noted in the experimental animal and in humans. This observation has led to the increased use of cryopreserved bone in clinical situations, including spinal fusions.[4, 20, 31, 34, 36, 37, 41, 44]

The repair by creeping substitution is at a slower rate than that observed in an autograft.[10] Resorption areas with a small inflammatory cellular infiltrate in fibrovascular connective tissue suggest a mild immune response. Histologic section from an allograft recovered from the ulna 3 months after a failed application of an onlay corticocancellous graft used to fix a bone fracture of the forearm shows appositional new bone on dead bone with empty osteocyte lacunae and a few new vessels in haversian canals (Fig 30–4,A). One area of the graft shows osteoclastic resorption and granulation tissue with a few chronic inflammatory cells. Resorption areas of the graft are present in an allograft removed 2 years after a failed spinal fusion (Fig 30–4,B). There has been considerable repair and remodeling.

In some experimental animals and uncommonly in clinical situations in humans, resorption is extensive with the graft replaced by fibrous tissue rather than bone.[10, 13, 26] Presumably the tissue is rejected by the host tissue. There is some evidence that the use of immunosuppressive drugs ameliorates the immune response and improves the take of the allograft.[14, 35] From a practical point of view, this is not necessary and the slower repair is accepted. Clinical use of allografts[20, 31, 34, 41] in spinal fusion is almost, but not quite, comparable to the use of autografts[19] when internal fixation with rod systems or plate and screws are used.[4, 28] In fact, Knapp and Jones[29] found a high fusion rate with local bone only and internal fixation.

An example of the use of corticocancellous allografts with plate and pedicle screw fixation is shown in Figure 30–5. The graft showed resorption and slower incorporation when compared with that observed with autogenous bone in case 1.

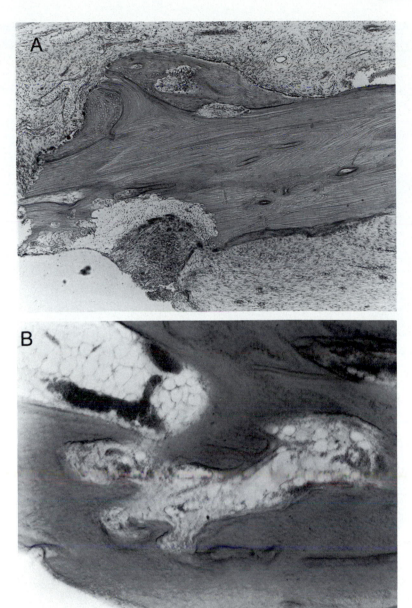

FIG 30–4.
A, corticocancellous allograft removed at 3 months shows appositional new bone along the surface but minimal vascular invasion of the cortex. Fibrous tissue with scattered inflammatory cells surrounded the graft. In one area active re-sorption by inflammatory granulation tissue is occurring (×56). **B,** large resorption areas are present in an allograft removed 2 years after a failed spinal fusion. There has been considerable remodeling of the graft (×76).

Case 2.—A 62-year-old woman had a long history of low back pain and bilateral leg pain, worse with extension and better with flexion. The patient had disc surgery at L4–5 previously with temporary relief of symptoms. Instability at L4–5 and severe narrowing of the neuroforamina with extension was shown with flexion-extension radiographs. Myelogram and CT scan revealed multiple levels of spinal stenosis and a left L4–5 herniated disc. Decompression of the L4–5 right and left neural foramina was performed and a herniated disc fragment ventral to the left L5 nerve

root was removed. The right L4 nerve root was decompressed. A bilateral intertransverse process and facet and spinous process L4–5 fusion with allografts and local autogenous bone was performed. Steffee fixation was applied on the right side. At 2 months, the mass of allograft bone is clearly shown on both the AP and lateral views (Fig 30–5A,B). There is considerable resorption of the allograft fragments on both AP and lateral radiographs at 18 months (Fig 30–5,C,D). The same amount of resorption was present at 6 months. At the time of the last follow-up 2 years and

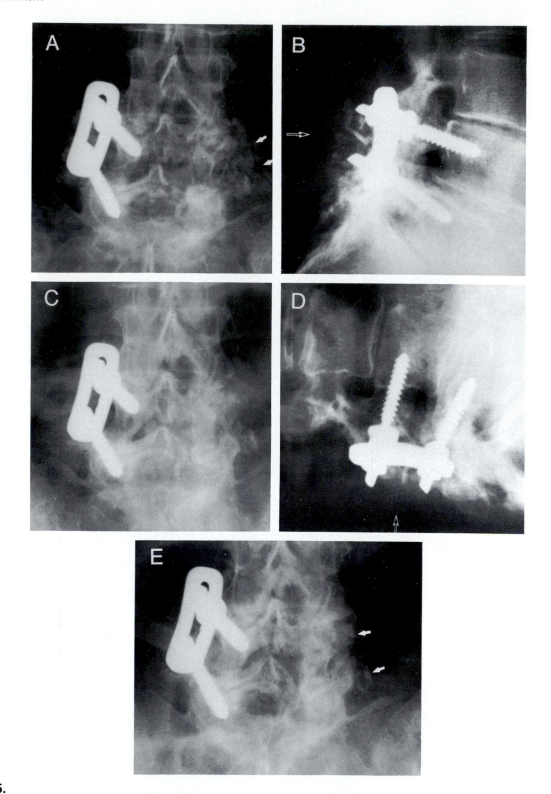

FIG 30–5.
AP **(A)** and lateral **(B)** radiographs show the screw and plate fixation and fragments of allograft bone *(arrows)*. At 18 months, AP **(C)** and lateral **(D)** radiographs show partial resorption of allografts *(arrow)*. **E,** AP radiograph shows per-sistent partial resorption of the fusion mass *(arrows)* but there was no evidence of motion at the site in flexion-exten-sion lateral radiographs (not shown).

10 months after surgery, the patient had tolerable low back and radicular pain. The radiographs were read as solid fusion despite what appears to be persistent partial resorption of the allograft (Fig 30–5,E). The lack of motion on flexion and extension lateral films probably supports that conclusion, but, as noted, one cannot be certain without exploration of the fusion site and histologic confirmation. This approach is not practical, nor is it accepted practice.

In general, repair with autografts is faster and more certain when the fusion site is examined by a surgical second look to assess the presence of a pseudarthrosis in cases of scoliosis fusion.[20] Some studies suggest that in the lumbosacral spine the final result may depend on factors other than fusions.[28, 43] Some patients with solid fusion still have pain and functional impairment, while others with pseudarthrosis do not.

REFERENCES

1. Abbott LC: The use of iliac bone in the treatment of ununited fractures. *Instr Courses Lect* 1944; 2:13–18.
2. Albrektsson T: Repair of bone grafts. *Scand J Plast Reconstr Surg* 1980; 14:1–12.
3. Albrektsson T: The healing of autologous bone grafts after varying degrees of surgical trauma. *J Bone Joint Surg [Br]* 1980; 62:403–410.
4. Aurori BF, et al: Pseudoarthrosis after spinal fusion for scoliosis. *Clin Orthop* 1985; 199:153–158.
5. Axhausen G: Die pathologisch-anatomischen Grundlagen der Lehre von der freien Knochentransplantationen beim Menschen und beim Tier. *Med Klin* (suppl) 1908; 23–58.
6. Barth A: Histologische Untersuchen über Knochenimplantationen. *Beitr Pathol Anat Allg Pathol* 1985; 17:65–142.
7. Berrey BH, et al.: Fractures of allografts. *J Bone Joint Surg [Am]* 1990; 72:825–833.
8. Bonfiglio M: Repair of bone transplant fractures. Repair bone transplant fractures. *J Bone Joint Surg [Am]* 1958; 40:446–456.
9. Bonfiglio M: Transplantation of massive bone allografts (editorial). *N Engl J Med* 1976; 294:1258.
10. Bonfiglio M, Wayburn SJ: Immunological responses to bone. *Clin Orthop* 1972; 87:19–27.
11. Brown KLB, Cruess RL: Bone and cartilage transplantation in orthopaedic surgery. *J Bone Joint Surg [Am]* 1982; 64:270–279.
12. Buck BE, Malinin TI, Brown MD: Bone transplantation and human immunodeficiency virus. *Clin Orthop* 1989; 240:129–136.
13. Burchardt H: The biology of bone graft repair. *Clin Orthop* 1983; 174:28–42.
14. Burchardt H, Glowczewskie FP, Enneking WF, et al.: Short-term immunosuppression with fresh segmental fibular allografts in dogs. *J Bone Joint Surg [Am]* 1981; 63:411–415.
15. Chase SW, Herndon CH: The fate of autogenous and homogenous bone grafts: A historical review. *J Bone Joint Surg [Am]* 1955; 37:809–841.
16. Craig Gray J, Elves MW: Osteogenesis in bone grafts after short term storage and topical antibiotic treatment. *J Bone Joint Surg [Br]* 1981; 63:441–445.
17. Cohen J, Bonfiglio M, Campbell CJ: *Orthopaedic Pathophysiology.* New York, Churchill-Livingston, Inc, 1990, p 276.
18. Czitrom AA, Keating S, Gross AE: The viability of articular cartilage in fresh osteochondral allografts after clinical transplantation. *J Bone Joint Surg [Am]* 1990; 72:574–581.
19. Dawson EG, Lotysch M III, Urist MR: Intertransverse process lumbar arthrodesis with autogenous bone graft. *Clin Orthop* 1981; 154:90–96.
20. Dodd CAF, Ferguson CM, Freedman L, et al.: Allograft versus autograft bone in scoliosis surgery. *J Bone Joint Surg [Br]* 1988; 70:431–434.
21. Doppelt SM, Tomford WW, Lucas AB, et al: Operational and financial aspects of the hospital bone bank. *J Bone Joint Surg [Am]* 1981; 63:1472–1481.
22. Enneking WF, Morris JL: Human autologous cortical bone transplants. *Clin Orthop* 1972; 87:28–35.
23. Farmer DH: *The Oxford Dictionary of the Saints.* Oxford, Clarendon Press, 1978, p 92.
24. Friedlaender GE: Bone banking: Current concepts review. *J Bone Joint Surg [Am]* 1983; 64:307–311.
25. Friedlaender GE: Current concepts review: Bone grafts. *J Bone Joint Surg* 69A(5):786–790, June 1987.
26. Goldberg VM, Stevenson S: Natural history of autografts and allografts. *Clin Orthop* 1987; 225:7–16.
27. Harris IE, Weinstein SL: Long-term follow-up of patients with Grade III and IV spondylolisthesis. *J Bone Joint Surg [Am]* 1987; 69:960–969.
28. Kabins MB, Weinstein JN, Found EM, et al.: Isolated L4–L5 floating fusions using the variable screw placement system: Unilateral versus bilateral. Submitted to *Spine,* 1990. Presented to North American Spine Society, Monterey, Calif, August 1990.
29. Knapp DR Jr, Jones ET: Use of cortical cancellous allograft for posterior spinal fusion. *Clin Orthop* 1988; 229:99–106.
30. Macewen W: Intrahuman bone grafting and reimplantation of bone. *Ann Surg* 1909; 50:959–968.
31. Malinin TI, Brown MD: Bone allografts in spinal surgery. *Clin Orthop* 1981; 154:68–73.
32. Mankin HJ, Fogalson FS, et al: Massive resection and allograft transplantation in the treatment of malignant bone tumors. *N Engl J Med* 1976; 294:1247–1257.
33. McBride GG, Bradford DS: Vertebral body replacement with femoral neck allograft and vascularized rib strut graft. *Spine* 1983; 8:406–415.
34. McCarthy RE, Peck RD, Morrissy RJ, et al.: Allograft bone in spine fusion for paralytic scolioses. *J Bone Joint Surg [Am]* 1986; 68:370–375.
35. Musculo DL, Caletti E, Schajowicz F, et al.: Tissue-typing and human massive allografts of frozen bone. *J Bone Joint Surg [Am]* 1987; 69:583–595.
36. Nasca RJ: The use of cryopreserved bone in spinal surgery. *Spine* 1987; 12:222–227.
37. Ollier L: Recherches expérimentalies sur les greffes osseuses. *J Physiol Homme Anim* 1860; 3:88–108.

38. Phemister DB: The fate of transplanted bone and regenerative powers of its various constituents. *Surg Gynecol Obstet* 1914; 19:303–333.

39. Prado DJ, Rodrigo: Contemporary bone graft physiology and surgery. *Clin Orthop* 1985; 200:322–342.

40. Skinner HB: Alternatives in the selection of allograft bone. *Orthopaedics* 1990; 13:843–846.

41. Stabler CL, Eismont FJ, Brown MD, et al.: Failure of posterior cervical spine fusions using cadaveric bone graft in children. *J Bone Joint Surg* 1985; 67:371.

42. Summers RN, Eisenstein SM: Donor site pain from the ilium. *J Bone Joint Surg [Br]* 1989; 71:677–680.

43. Tenturi T, Niemelä P, Laurinkari J, et al.: Posterior fusion of the lumbosacral spine. *Acta Orthop Scand* 1979; 50:415–422.

44. Urist MR, Dawson E: Intertransverse process fusion with the aid of chemo-sterilized autolyzed antigen extracted allogeneic bone. *Clin Orthop* 1981; 154:97–118.

45. Weiland AJ: Current concepts review: Vascularized free bone transplants. *J Bone Joint Surg [Am]* 1981; 63:166–169.

31

Biomechanics of Fusion

Vijay K. Goel, Ph.D.

Tae-hong Lim, Ph.D.

J. Gwon, M.D.

Jen-Yuh Chen, M.D.

J. Han, M.S.

The spatial relationship between the spinal structures, including the nerve roots, in a normal spine is important to enable a person to perform daily living activities without experiencing pain. Following trauma or degenerative changes these relationships may change to the extent that a surgical intervention may be indicated. The term *spinal stenosis* characterizes one such spatial change. It is a descriptive and nondiagnostic term, indicative of a narrowing of the spinal canal or the intervertebral foramen to the extent that pressure exerted on the nerve root entrapped within these structures may lead to "chronic" pain.[31] Surgical treatment is aimed at decompressing the neural structures. From a purely mechanical point of view, the surgery involves removal of spinal structures such as the laminae, facets, disc, etc. These dissections may be indicated for one side (unilateral) or both sides (bilateral) and may span one or several motion segments. Depending upon the amount and location of bony and soft tissue decompression, these procedures may lead to spinal instability because support structures are removed. It is often necessary, therefore, to surgically fuse lumbar segments to provide long-term stability. Internal fixation with instrumentation may be indicated to provide stability immediately following surgery and keep the motion segment(s) aligned until the fusion process is complete (healed). Despite an abundance of literature comparing the results of discectomy alone to the results of discectomy with lumbar fusion, for example, the long-term effects of lumbar arthrodesis are still not clear.[12, 37] Lumbar and lumbosacral spinal fusion for low back pain remains a somewhat disputed and controversial subject.[10, 27, 35]

The rationale for spinal fusion procedures as treatment for low back pain originates from the idea that painful symptoms due to a degenerated or unstable spinal motion segment can be relieved.[3, 5, 7, 9, 19, 25, 26, 29, 30, 32, 36] On the other hand, some authors feel that spinal fusion procedures should not be encouraged, as adverse iatrogenic effects outweigh the positive results. For example, a number of studies report an increase in spinal stenosis or spondylolisthesis both above and below the fusion level, which they believe was caused by excessive stress on the adjacent intervertebral motion segment.[18, 23, 32, 33, 38] A rather high complication rate was observed by Lehmann et al.[27] in a 30-year follow-up of patients with fusions performed prior to 1964. These included an increase in the prevalence of both spinal stenosis and instability which was present as high as two levels above the fusion. For these reasons, biomechanical evaluations of different surgical procedures and various fixation systems are needed to afford a basic understanding of the issues associated with the use of internal fixation devices. This chapter reviews experimental and theoretical biomechanical investigations undertaken at the authors' laboratory, as well as data obtained by other researchers.

EXPERIMENTAL INVESTIGATIONS

The in vitro experimental investigations reported in the literature so far may best be described under three categories. The studies in the first category deal with the component design of the system itself.[2, 6, 24, 34] For example, what should be the shape and size of the screws and the dimensions of the plate constituting a pedicle screw fixation system?

In the second category are investigations dealing with the overall strength afforded by the use of a particular instrumentation.[4, 17, 20, 39] The results of such studies have shown that most of the devices currently in use are effective in restoring stability to the injured specimens in flexion and extension, although the degree of effectiveness varies among different devices. These studies, however, do not provide insights into the load-displacement behavior of the injured and stabilized levels and adjacent levels. Experiments addressing these aspects constitute the third category. The experiments require the testing of multilevel spine segments. The methodology used for preparing and testing such specimens and the results obtained by us are briefly described in the following paragraphs.[8, 14, 15, 16, 28]

Fresh cadaveric ligamentous spines (T12–sacrum) were potted at the sacrum for housing in a testing fixture. A loading frame was secured rigidly to the topmost vertebra of a specimen for the application of clinically relevant loads (Fig 31–1). A set of three infrared light–emitting diodes (LEDs) were rigidly secured to each of the five vertebral bodies (L1–L5). The spatial locations of these LEDs, in response to the applied load, were recorded using the Selspot II motion measuring system. The resulting spatial data were then transformed into three displacements (anteroposterior [AP], lateral, and axial) of a point on the vertebra (e.g., the geometric center H) and three rotations (flexion or extension rotation, $\pm R_x$; axial rotation, $\pm R_y$; and lateral bending, $\pm R_z$) of the vertebra with respect to the global axes system fixed to the

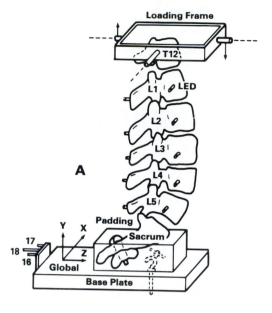

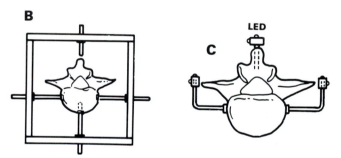

FIG 31–1.
The steps involved in preparing a specimen for testing are shown. **A,** the relative position of the loading frame, infrared red light–emitting diodes *(LED)*, Plastic Padding base, base plate, and the directions of the global axes fixed to the base are shown. The *arrows* at the loading rods indicate arrangement of load lines to apply flexion moment to the specimen. **B,** details of the loading frame and rods. **C,** method for attaching three LEDs to a vertebra.

base of the specimen (Fig 31–1). Thus, the three-dimensional, load-displacement behaviors of intact specimens in flexion (FLX), extension (EXT), right and left lateral bending (RLB, LLB), and left and right axial rotation (LAR, RAR) were recorded sequentially. The specimens were then divided into five groups of ten specimens each for further testing.

Group I. The specimens were destabilized at the L4–5 level to create a bilateral nerve root decompression. The supraspinous and interspinous ligaments were also transected at the L3–4 and L5–S1 levels, and two 19-gauge stainless steel wires were placed on both sides of the midline from the L3–4 to

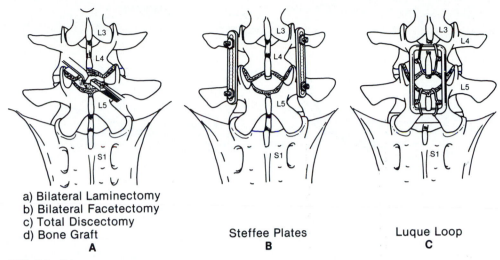

a) Bilateral Laminectomy
b) Bilateral Facetectomy
c) Total Discectomy
d) Bone Graft
      A

Steffee Plates
B

Luque Loop
C

FIG 31–2.
A, the extensive injury model to achieve spinal decompression is shown (*a, b,* and *c*). A bone graft (*d*) is inserted in the disc space. The injured specimen is stabilized sequentially using **(B)** Steffee plates and **(C)** Luque loop.

the L4–5 interspace and, similarly, from the L4–5 to the L5–S1 interspace. A small amount of the ligamentum flavum was also removed at the median raphe to allow passage of the wires. The specimens were stabilized with Luque loops of appropriate sizes, shown schematically in Fig 31–2,C.

Group II. The specimens in this group were injured by creating a bilateral laminectomy, bilateral facetectomy, and total discectomy across the L4–5 motion segment (Fig 31–2,A). The injury model is an extension of the group I model with the addition of a total discectomy. A bone graft was inserted into the disc space and then the segment was further stabilized sequentially using Steffee plates and then the Luque loop (Figs 31–2,B,C). This group provided a comparison between two fixation systems (Steffee and Luque) used to stabilize the same injury.

Group III. The specimens in this group were used to assess the efficacy of the Luque loop and Steffee plates in stabilizing the L5–S1 level instead of the L4–5 level. The injury model was similar to that of group II.

Group IV. In this group, the injuries and stabilizations of groups II and III were combined to determine the stabilization characteristics for the Steffee plates and the Luque loop used to stabilize the L4–L5 and L5–S1 segments instead of one segment only.

Group V. In this group, the injury was a bilateral partial laminectomy, facetectomy, and transection of the ligamentum flavum, the interspinous and supraspinous ligaments of the L4–5 motion segment, followed by stabilization using a number of devices shown in Fig 31–3. The effect of using one Steffee

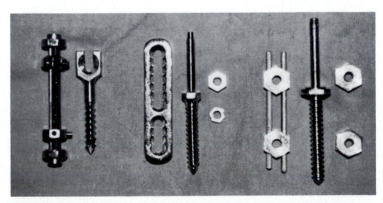

FIG 31–3.
A few of the devices tested by the authors. The conventional Steffee system is shown in the middle.

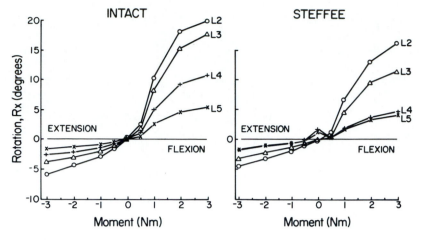

FIG 31–4.
The primary flexion-rotation component (R_x) of an L1–S1 specimen as a function of the applied flexion and extension moment. The intact specimen, and the same but "injured" specimen stabilized across the L4–5 segment using bilateral Steffee plates are shown.

plate (unilateral) as opposed to two Steffee plates (bilateral) in stabilizing the injured specimen was also investigated in this group.

The specimens were tested after each injury and after each stabilization procedure using a protocol adopted for testing of the intact specimens: the positional information of all of the LEDs were stored. The LED spatial location data of the intact, injured, and stabilized specimens were further reduced to calculate the six displacement parameters described above. The flexion and extension rotation angles, R_x, as a function of the applied moment for the intact and stabilized tests of a typical specimen are shown, respectively, in Fig 31–4. In the graphed experiment, the L4–5 motion segment was stabilized using the Steffee plate system. The flexion-rotation following stabilization was very small compared with the corresponding intact specimen. Thus, the Steffee device was effective in providing rigidity across the "injured segment." Comparisons of this type were made, as functions of device, level of fixation, load magnitude, and load type, and included all vertebral levels, i.e., both the stabilized and adjacent segments.

Results and Discussion

In the flexion mode, the Luque loop reduces the motion across the injured level, in comparison with intact specimen behavior, by about 60%. The loop, however, is not effective in providing stability in other loading directions. The closed-loop Luque system seems to provide stability on the following principles. In flexion-extension, the tension induced in

the wire during twisting helps to transmit loads from L4 to the closed loop, and then to the L5 vertebra. The stability provided against axial rotation and lateral bending loads is primarily due to frictional force between the loop and the laminae of the L4 and L5 vertebrae. This frictional force is a function of the normal force component due to the tension in the wires. In vivo, the wires become loose with time and, therefore, the stabilizing effect diminishes. The fact that the frictional force is small helps explain the lack of stability in axial rotation and lateral bending modes.

The inability of the closed loop to provide significant fixation in the group I model in axial rotation and lateral bending raises questions about its ability to impart a definite stability in cases of spinal decompression, when rigidity in response to lateral bending loads may also be desirable. The situation may be further compromised if more than one motion segment needs to be stabilized, because obtaining a solid fusion may be even more difficult to achieve in such cases. The studies carried out on groups II, III, and IV were designed with these questions in mind. The percentage of reduction in major rotation components in various loading modes, in comparison with the intact case, is shown in Table 31–1. The effectiveness of the Luque loop in stabilizing the injured motion segments in all groups seems to be similar. It reduces motion by about 50% in flexion and extension compared to the intact data, but is not very effective in other load types. Furthermore, its ability to provide rigidity in the flexion mode is better when used to stabilize more than one motion segment. The Steffee system,

TABLE 31–1.

Change in Motion Following Stabilization With Respect to the Intact Specimen for Various Groups*

Load Type	Injury Group	Injured and Stabilized Level	Primary Rotation	Average Change in Motion Across the Stabilized Segment (%)†	
				Steffee System	Luque Loop
FLX	II	L4–5	R_x	−74.1	−65.4
	III	L5–S1	R_x	−42.7	−38.7
	IV	L4–S1	R_x	−67.9	−68.7
EXT	II	L4–5	R_x	−51.8	−50.5
	III	L5–S1	R_x	−14.4	−21.5
	IV	L4–S1	R_x	−41.9	−9.6
LB	II	L4–5	R_z	−75.6	+24.7
	III	L5–S1	R_z	−58.0	+36.7
	IV	L4–S1	R_z	−70.4	+3.7
AR	II	L4–5	R_y	−63.9	+15.0
	III	L5–S1	R_y	−52.0	+58.7
	IV	L4–S1	R_y	−41.3	+21.8

*FLX = flexion; EXT = extension; LB = lateral bending; AR = axial rotation; R_x = flexion or extension rotation; R_z = lateral bending; R_y = axial rotation.

†Changes are decreases (−) or increases (+) with respect to intact spine (its motion was taken as zero).

a rigid screw-plate system, on the other hand, is very effective in stabilizing the injured segment (reduces the motion by about 70% compared to the intact case), and restores stability to the injured level(s) in all loading directions. Results similar to those obtained for the Steffee system were also obtained for the other plate-screw fixation systems tested by us. In the flexion-extension mode, the use of one Steffee plate leads to a less rigid system than using two plates (40% vs. 70% reduction). The stability with one plate is also less than with two in the lateral bending (13% vs. 65% reduction in motion with respect to the intact specimen behavior) and in axial loading (9% vs. 50% reduction in motion with respect to the intact specimen behavior). A recent study has found that the Steffee system appears to possess appropriate strength to maintain lumbosacral alignment needed for the reduction and stabilization of spondylolisthesis.[1] The Luque loop, on the other hand, is not effective in reducing spondylolisthesis.

It must be mentioned, however, that the role of rigid stabilization in healing of disrupted motion segments of the spine is uncertain.[11] Excess motion in any plane may lead to progressive instrument loosening and increase the chances of development of a pseudarthrosis in the fused segments, with resultant loss of fixation and eventual loss of reduction of spinal alignment. How much stiffness is optimal is not known, however. It may be that all instrumentation systems achieve adequate stiffness to permit load-bearing during heal-

ing, or conversely, none do, and the patient requires protection in all cases. Thus, it is not possible at this stage to single out a system that is the best or optimal, based on the biomechanical performance alone.

ANALYTIC STUDIES

The experimental approach suffers from certain drawbacks. It is difficult to simulate the effect of lordosis and the stabilizing effects of the muscles in an experiment. It is also neither practical to test a specimen subjected to the complex loads seen in vivo nor possible to estimate experimentally the stresses and strains within the spinal structures as a function of injury or stabilization. It is also not realistic to quantify the loads being imposed on spinal elements. Besides this, the experimental approach alone provides limited data, not sufficient to resolve all of the issues associated with the use of a fixation device.

Experimental investigations such as the ones summarized above have enabled investigators to understand the effects of instrumentation on the levels adjacent to the stabilized levels during the physiologic range of motion of the spine in terms of the load-displacement behavior. This is an important clinical contribution. A number of other clinical issues such as the loosening or breakage of screws, re-

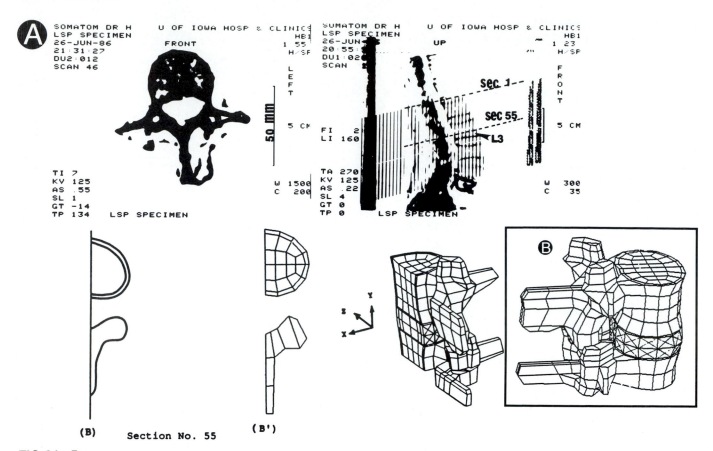

FIG 31–5.
A, the serial cross sections from the CT film were enlarged, digitized, and stacked sequentially on top of each other to generate a number of finite element models of the spine. **B** *(inset),* the complete three-dimensional finite element model of an intact L3–4 motion segment. The ligaments are not shown for lack of clarity.

distribution of loads, etc., still need to be understood. Furthermore, in an experimental protocol, it is almost impossible to address all the parameters which can be varied within a given system, not to mention the large number of fixation systems available. The experimental studies also cannot explain satisfactorily the basis for changes (e.g., spinal stenosis, disc degeneration, stress-induced osteopenia, etc.) seen clinically at the injured and stabilized and adjacent levels. Since it is known that the living tissue responds to changes in the stresses and strains, the quantification of parameters like the stresses and strains in the spinal elements, the nucleus pressure, and forces within spinal structures, including the fixation device itself, may provide a better understanding of the relationship between the clinical observations following surgery and mechanical factors. Such an investigation may also afford us an opportunity to improve the designs. This mandates development of highly detailed analytic models as a complement to the experimental studies.

Finite Element Models of an Intact Motion Segment

The finite element technique has been widely used to analyze the mechanical behavior of complex structures like the spine.[15] The following is a very brief description of the steps involved in preparing a three-dimensional finite element model of an intact lumbar spine segment and modifications thereof to simulate a few of the clinically relevant injuries and stabilization procedures.[13, 15, 22, 28]

Geometric Data

The geometric data of the L3–4 motion segment were acquired from 1-mm-thick computed tomography (CT) scans (transverse slices) of a cadaveric ligamentous spine specimen (Fig 31–5,A). The three-dimensional mesh for an intact one–motion segment finite element model is shown in Figure 31–5,B.

Material Properties and Element Types Used

The elements chosen for the formulation of the models are as follows. The material properties as-

TABLE 31–2.

Properties of Materials Used for Intact and Stabilized Finite Element Models*

Material†	Young's Modulus (MPa)	Shear Modulus (MPa)	Poisson's Ratio	Cross-Sectional Area (mm²)‡
Cortical bone	12,000	4,615	0.30	
Cancellous bone	100	41.7	0.20	
Bony posterior elements	3,500	1,400	0.25	
Annulus				
Ground substance	4.2	1.6	0.45	
Fiber	175			
Nucleus pulposus	1,667.7§			
Ligaments				
AL	7.8 (<12.0%) 20.0 (>12.0%)			63.7
PL	10.0 (<11.0%) 20.0 (>11.0%)			20.0
LF	15.0 (< 6.2%) 19.5 (> 6.2%)			40.0
TL	10.0 (<18.0%) 58.7 (>18.0%)			1.8
CL	7.5 (<25.0%) 32.9 (>25.0%)			30.0
IS	10.0 (<14.0%) 11.6 (>14.0%)			40.0
SS	8.0 (<20.0%) 15.0 (>20.0%)			30.0
Steffee plate	180,000		0.30	
Screw	180,000		0.30	
Bone graft	3,500		0.25	

*Data from Goel VK, Weinstein JN: *Biomechanics of the Spine—Clinical and Surgical Perspective.* Boca Raton, Fla, CRC Press, 1990.

†AL = anterior longitudinal; PL = posterior longitudinal; LF = ligamentum flavum; TL = transverse; CL = capsular; IS = intraspinous; SS = supraspinous.

‡Corresponding to a full model.

§Bulk modulus.

signed were obtained from the literature (including our own data) and are listed in Table 31–2.[15]

The cortical shell and the cancellous bone core of the vertebral body, and the posterior bony elements, were modeled as three-dimensional isoparametric eight-nodal (brick) elements. The material properties were assumed to be homogeneous and isotropic. The annulus fibrosus was modeled as a composite material comprised of a series of fiber bands (lamellae) embedded in the ground substance around the nucleus. The fibers were modeled as "tension-only" three-dimensional linear spar elements (cable elements). The fact that these elements are active in tension and not in compression allowed an appropriate simulation of the role of fibers in the disc. The ground substance of the annulus was modeled as three-dimensional isotropic eight-nodal elements. The hydrostatic characteristics of the nucleus pulposus were simulated with a three-dimensional incompressible fluid element, represented by its bulk modulus. The ligaments, being active in tension only, were also modeled as bilinear cable elements similar to the fibers in the annulus. These elements were oriented along the respective ligament fiber directions.

A three-dimensional interface element (gap element), capable only of supporting a compressive load normal to its surface, was used to simulate the gap across the facets. A total of six gap elements were assigned to each facet articulation. The average initial gap between the articulating surface, based on the CT film, was taken as 0.45 mm.

Boundary and Loading Conditions

The inferior surface of the most inferior vertebral body and its inferior facets were not allowed to move in any direction (Fig 31–6,A). All nodes located on the midsagittal plane were restricted in the X direction because of the assumed sagittal symmetry in half-models. The axial compressive loads (maximum of 1,905 newtons for the intact model and 413 newtons for the stabilized models) were simulated by applying uniform pressures on the surface of the most superior vertebral body and facets. The finite element models described above were executed using the nonlinear finite element program ANSYS, and solutions were obtained in an iterative manner. The output was processed further to yield load-displacement curves, and data on changes in the nucleus pressure, on disc bulge, on forces in various spinal structures (including the forces across the facets), on strains in the ligaments and the annulus fibers, and on stress fields within the bony elements and ground substance of the annulus.

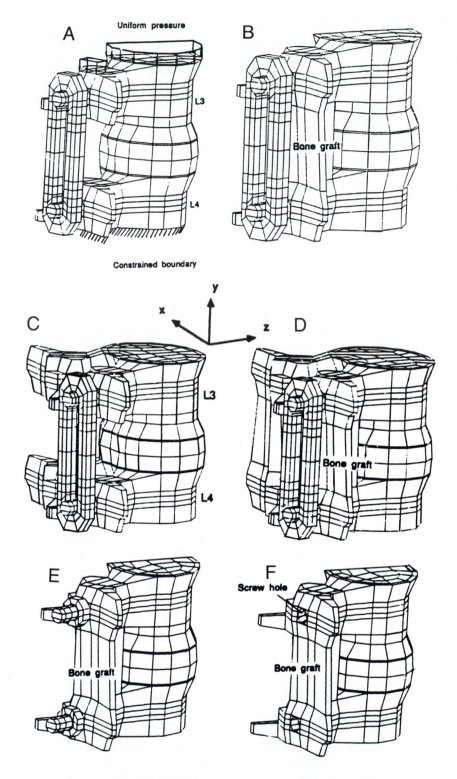

FIG 31–6.

Finite element models of a stabilized one motion segment simulating bilateral fusion. The degenerated disc was left intact. **A,** the model with bilateral plates and before healing of the fusion mass (P2BFBH). **B,** the model with bilateral plates and after healing of the fusion mass (P2BFAH). **C,** the model with unilateral plates and before healing of the fusion mass (P1BFBH). **D,** the model with unilateral plates and after healing of the fusion mass (P1BFBH). **E** and **F,** models after healing in which plate(s) and screws are removed. Similar models for the bilateral plating with interbody bone graft were also developed. The nucleus was discectomized and an interbody bone graft was inserted in these models.

Finite Element Models of a Stabilized Motion Segment

The intact finite element model described above was appropriately modified to simulate the use of a screw-plate system, as exemplified by the Steffee system, and various fusion techniques that are currently in use for stabilizing a decompressed segment. For example, the plates may be used with a bilateral fusion (BF) mass or with an interbody bone graft (BG). In the former case the degenerated disc is left intact. Likewise, surgeons at the University of Iowa have used only one plate in conjunction with bilateral fusion technique with the assumption that the decrease in rigidity may reduce the adverse effects attributable to the use of two plates without compromising the healing process.[21] Consequently, three models were developed: bilateral plates and bilateral fusion before healing of the fusion mass (P2BFBH; see Fig 31–6,A); unilateral plate and bilateral fusion before healing of the fusion mass (P1BFBH, Fig 31–6,C); and bilateral plates with an interbody bone graft before healing of the graft (P2BGBH, not shown). These models simulate the segment behavior immediately following surgery. The appropriate elements of the intact model were modified to simulate the variations. The degenerated disc in the P2BFGH and P1BFBH models was modeled by replacing the nucleus with a material twice as stiff as that of the ground substance. The bilateral fusion mass was not simulated owing to its inability to transmit any load prior to fusion. On the other hand, the interbody bone graft is capable of transmitting compressive loads prior to healing. This was simulated within the model P2BGBH. However, the bone graft was not allowed to transmit any tensile load. The healing process enables the bone mass or the interbody bone graft to transmit tensile loads as well. The extreme situation when the bone mass–interbody bone graft is fully healed was simulated by including additional elements to simulate bone mass and permitting bone graft–bone mass to resist tensile loads (P2BFAH, P1BFAH, Fig 31–6,B,D, and P2BGAH, not shown). The elements corresponding to the metal plates and screws were also deleted to study the effects of removing the device following healing (Fig 31–6,E,F).

Results

Intact Model Results

The intact models were used to study the response of an intact spine subjected to axial compressive loads. Comparison of the predicted gross re-

sponse characteristics of the intact one–motion segment model (such as load-displacement behavior, intradiscal pressure, strains in ligaments) with available experimental measurements indicated satisfactory agreements.[13] The responses of the stabilized models are next compared with the intact model predictions.

Stabilized Motion Segment Results

Stiffness Response.—The main motion components were the axial compression (D_y) and the coupled flexion rotation (R_x) (Table 31–3). The predicted displacement data for all of the stabilized models decreased as compared with the intact case. The maximum stiffness was found in the models that simulated the interbody bone graft (P2BGBH, P2BGAH, etc.). The least increase in rigidity was predicted for the unilateral plate models (P1BFBH, P1BFAH, etc.). The "after-healing" model predictions were stiffer than the corresponding predictions for the "before-healing" models. The stiffness decreased following removal of the devices, the magnitudes being in between the before- and after-healing model predictions. The application of only one plate for stabilizing the motion segment led to coupled rotations because of the asymmetry induced in this model.

Stress Response.—The maximum and average von Mises stress values in various structures in response to 413 newtons of compression force are given in Table 31–4 for all of the models, including the intact model predictions. In the cortical region of the models simulating stabilized specimen behavior before healing (BH models), the procedures resulted in a localized increase in stress, although the average von Mises stresses were smaller compared with those of the intact case. Localized increases in stresses were found at the posterior region in the case of bilateral fixation with bilateral fusion (P2BFBH, average 1.51 MPa, maximum 2.04 MPa), at the anterolateral region in the case of unilateral fixation with bilateral fusion (P1BFBH, average 1.51 MPa, maximum 2.03 MPa), and at both of the anterior and posterior regions for the case of bilateral fixation with interbody bone graft (P2BGBH, average 1.78 MPa, maximum 2.53 MPa).

After healing, no local increase in stresses was found for the bilateral and unilateral fixation with bilateral fusion models, and average stresses decreased further compared with the respective before-healing situation. These decreases resulted from the solid bilateral fusion. As expected, the posterior interbody bone graft model did not show any change in stress distribution following healing.

TABLE 31–3.

Axial Displacement and Rotations of the L3 Vertebra of the Intact and Stabilized Models in Response to 413 Newtons of Axial Compression Load

	Model*	D_y (mm)	R_x (°)	R_y (°)	R_z (°)
	INTACT	−0.34	0.35		
Before healing (BH)	P2BFBH	−0.23	0.35		
	P1BFBH	−0.27	0.36	0.01	−0.28
	P2BGBH	−0.02	0.00		
After healing (AH)	P2BFAH	−0.10	0.23		
	P1BFAH	−0.13	0.28	−0.02	−0.02
	P2BGAH	−0.02	0.00		
Device removed	BFNP	−0.15	0.35		
	BFNPS	−0.16	0.37		
After healing	PFNP	−0.02	0.01		
	PFNPS	−0.03	0.01		

*D_y = axial displacement; R_x = flexion or extension rotation; R_y = axial rotation; R_z = lateral bending; INTACT = half-intact model; P2 = bilateral plates; P1 = unilateral plate; BG = interbody bone graft; NP = no plates; NPS = no plates and screws; BF = bilateral fusion; PF = posterior fusion.

The stress patterns in the cancellous bone region following stabilization were similar to those for the cortical bone region except that there were no local increases in the stress values. In the before-healing models, the decrease in stresses was the greatest in the P2BFBH model and least for the P1BFBH model. Following healing, the stresses in the bilateral fusion models decreased further indicating that the healed bone mass on either side had assumed a load-sharing role. As expected, the decrease in stress magnitudes for the interbody bone graft is capable of transmitting compressive loads before its healing as well. Removal of the devices following healing of the bilateral fusion mass helped lessen the decrease

TABLE 31–4.

Von Mises Stresses (MPa) in Various Structures of the Models in Response to 413 Newtons of Axial Compression Load*

Models†		Cortical Bone	Cancellous Bone	Disc	Bone Graft	Plate	Superior Screw	Inferior Screw
INTACT	Max	1.98	0.19	0.29				
	Av	1.83	0.11	0.21				
P2BFBH	Max	2.04	0.15	0.18		29.23	39.62	42.20
	Av	1.51	0.07	0.12		16.75	6.47	7.24
P1BFBH	Max	2.03	0.18	0.25		33.59	43.02	44.49
	Av	1.50	0.08	0.15		18.53	5.76	6.70
P2BGBH	Max	2.53	0.10		1.96	4.10	9.80	3.85
	Av	1.78	0.05		0.85	1.78	2.46	1.26
P2BFAH	Max	1.30	0.08	0.09	2.64	6.92	39.25	42.98
	Av	1.03	0.04	0.06	1.06	2.43	10.85	9.16
P1BFAH	Max	1.38	0.12	0.11	3.10	8.97	45.90	52.10
	Av	1.05	0.06	0.07	1.27	2.98	10.93	7.71
P2BGAH	Max	2.49	0.10		1.92	3.83	9.64	3.63
	Av	1.80	0.05		0.77	1.82	2.64	1.15
BFNP	Max	1.28	0.11	0.13	3.53		14.64	5.57
	Av	0.90	0.05	0.05	1.56		4.34	1.75
BFNPS	Max	1.54	0.16	0.14	3.30			
	Av	1.02	0.07	0.09	1.44			
PFNP	Max	3.19	0.08		2.39			
	Av	1.80	0.04		0.91			
PFNPS	Max	2.38	0.13		2.38			
	Av	1.80	0.07		0.90			

*Stress distributions in the cortical and cancellous bones at the level immediately inferior to the superior screw are presented.
†For abbreviations, see footnote to Table 31–3.

in stresses as compared with the after-healing cases with plates still included in the models. The stresses, however, were still less than the before-healing model and the intact model predictions.

Discussion

Rigidity of the stabilized motion segment was investigated in terms of the decrease in the axial displacement and the flexion-rotation angle as compared to the intact model predictions. The stabilized models were stiffer than the intact model. This implies that the three fixation techniques analyzed by us all provide stability. Comparing the three techniques of spinal instrumentation and fusion investigated, displacements predicted for the unilateral fixation with bilateral fusion model were the closest to the displacements for the intact case. Unilateral fixation with bilateral fusion, however, was found to result in axial rotation and lateral bending rotations (coupled motions) compared with the case in which two plates were used to stabilize the same injury. This may influence the healing process before the fusion mass consolidates and provides stability. The rigidity provided by the unilateral fixation with bilateral fusion, however, seems adequate to obtain solid fusion and early mobilization of patients since clinical follow-up of patients undergoing this procedure has revealed solid fusion and no apparent complications.[21]

The predicted stress results suggest the presence of stress-shielding effects of the device as well as the healed fusion mass–bone graft in the stabilized motion segment. The plates may transmit 9% to 38% of the applied compression load depending on the stabilization technique used. The stresses in the cortical and cancellous bone regions immediately inferior to the superior screws were less in the stabilized motion segment than those in the intact motion segment. The results suggest that unilateral fixation with bilateral fusion mass is likely to induce the least amount of stress-shielding effects. The removal of devices after solid fusion leads to a marginal increase of stresses in the cancellous bone regions compared with the after-healing cases, but the stresses are still smaller than those in the intact motion segment. This shows that stress-shielding effects are likely to occur with a noninstrumented fusion as well.

A comparison of stresses in the bone mass–bone graft of the stabilized models with the stresses in the lamina of the intact model may help explain the clinical finding of spinal stenosis observed in some cases following stabilization. The stresses in the bilateral bone grafts (see Table 31–4) were higher than the stresses in the lamina of the intact motion segment (average 0.282 MPa in the intact one motion segment). The stresses in the posterior interbody fusion grafts were also greater than 0.77 MPa. The stress values showed a further increase following the removal of fixation devices in the stabilized models. These higher stresses may induce the abnormal growth of the graft following the solid fusion, and thus central stenosis could ensue at the stabilized segment.

The presence of higher stresses in the inferior screws as compared to the superior screws indicates that the inferior screws are more prone to failure for the procedures that use bilateral fusion mass.

Based upon the predicted results, a unilateral fixation with bilateral fusion with the degenerated disc intact may be preferable to the other two stabilization techniques, provided the surgeon has a choice. This procedure is less rigid and the degree of stress-shielding is also less compared to the other two techniques. The decrease in rigidity does not seem to effect the solid fusion process or the early mobilization of patients as evidenced by clinical data.

Acknowledgment

This work was supported in part by a grant from the National Institutes of Health (AR-32549) and a grant from AcroMed Inc., Cleveland.

REFERENCES

1. Ashman RB, Birch JG, Bone LB, et al: Mechanical testing of spinal instrumentation. *Clin Orthop* 1988; 227:113–125.
2. Brunski JB, Hill DC, Moskowitz A: Stresses in a Harrington distraction rod: Their origin and relationship to fatigue fractures in vivo. *J Biomech En* 1983; 105:101.
3. Callahan RA, Johnson RM, Margolis RN, et al: Cervical facet fusion for control of instability following laminectomy. *J Bone Joint Surg [Am]* 1997; 59:991.
4. Casey MP, Jacobs RR: Internal fixation of the lumbosacral spine: A biomechanical evaluation, in *XI Proceedings of International Society for the Study of the Lumbar Spine,* Montreal, June 3–7, 1984.
5. Cloward RB: Posterior lumbar interbody fusion updated. *Clin Orthop* 1985; 193:16.
6. Cook SD, Barrack RL, Georgettee FS, et al: An analysis of failed Harrington rods. *Spine* 1985; 10:313.
7. Deorio JK, Bianco AJ: Lumbar disc excision in children and adolescents. *J Bone Joint Surg [Am]* 1982; 64:991.
8. Du W: *Biomechanics of Steffee and Luque*

Instrumentation—An Experimental Investigation (thesis). University of Iowa, Iowa City, 1988.

9. Eie N, Solgaard T, Kepple H: The knee-elbow position in lumbar disc surgery: A review of complications. *Spine* 1983; 8:897.

10. Feffer HL, Wiesel SW, Auckler JM, et al: Degenerative spondylolisthesis: To fuse or not to fuse. *Spine* 1985; 10:287.

11. Ferguson RL, Tencer AF, Woodard P, et al: Biomechanical comparison of spinal fracture models and the stabilizing effects of posterior instrumentation. *Spine* 1988; 13:453.

12. Frymoyer JW: The role of spine fusion. *Spine* 1981; 6:289.

13. Goel VK, Kim YE, Lim T-H, et al: An analytical investigation of spinal instrumentation. *Spine* 1988; 13:1003–1011.

14. Goel VK, Nye TA, Clark CR, et al: A technique to evaluate an internal spinal device by use of the Selspot system—An application to the Luque closed loop. *Spine* 1987; 12:150.

15. Goel VK, Weinstein JN: *Biomechanics of the Spine—Clinical and Surgical Perspective.* Boca Raton, Fla, CRC Press, 1990.

16. Goel VK, Weinstein J, Liu YK, et al: Comparative biomechanical evaluation of the Steffee and Luque loop systems, in *XIV Proceedings of the International Society for the Study of the Lumbar Spine,* Rome, May 24–28, 1987, p 51.

17. Guyer DW, Yuan HA, Werner F, et al: Biomechanical comparison of seven internal fixation devices for the lumbosacral junction. *Spine* 1987; 12:569.

18. Hutter CG: Spinal stenosis and posterior lumbar interbody fusion. *Clin Orthop* 1985; 193:103.

19. Inoue S, Watanabe T, Hirose A, et al: Anterior discectomy and interbody fusion for lumbar disc herniation. *Clin Orthop* 1984; 183:22.

20. Jacobs RR, Nordwall A, Nachemson A: Reduction, stability and strength provided by internal fixation systems for thoraco-lumbar spinal injuries. *Clin Orthop* 1982; 171:300.

21. Kabins MB, Found EM, Weinstein JN: Isolated L4–L5 floating fusions using the variable spinal plating system: Unilateral vs. bilateral. Presented at Annual Meeting of North American Spine Society, Monterey, Calif, Aug 8–11, 1990.

22. Kim YE: *An Analytical Investigation of Ligamentous Lumbar Spine Mechanics* (dissertation). University of Iowa, Iowa City, 1988.

23. Kornblatt MD, Jacobs RR: The effect of bracing and internal fixation on lumbar spine fusion in 100 consecutive cases: A preliminary report. Presented at the *12th International Society for the Study of the Lumbar Spine.* Sydney, Australia, April 14–19, 1985.

24. Krag MH, Beynnon BD, Pope MH, et al: An internal fixator for posterior application to short segments of thoracic, lumbar, or lumbosacral spine: Design and testing. *Clin Orthop* 1986; 203:75.

25. Lee CK: Lumbar spinal instability (olisthesis) after extensive posterior spinal decompression. *Spine* 1983; 8:429.

26. Lee CK, Langrana NA, Yang SW: Lumbosacral spinal fusion: A biomechanical study. *Spine* 1984; 6:574.

27. Lehmann TR, Tozzi JE, Weinstein JN, et al: Long term follow-up of lower lumbar fusion patients. *Spine* 1987: 12:97.

28. Lim, Tae-hong: *Design of a Spinal Fixation Device and Its Evaluation: An Analytical and Experimental Approach* (dissertation). University of Iowa, Iowa City, 1990.

29. Mooney V: The role of spinal fusion. *Spine* 1981; 6:304.

30. Nachemson A: The role of spinal fusion. *Spine* 1981; 6:306.

31. Nasca RL: Surgical management of lumbar spinal stenosis. *Spine* 1987; 12:809–816.

32. Rothman SLG, Glen WV: CT evaluation of interbody fusion. *Clin Orthop* 1985; 193:47. [*See also other articles of the symposium Posterior Lumbar Interbody Fusion in this issue.*]

33. Schneck CD: The anatomy of lumbar spondylosis. *Clin Orthop* 1985; 193:20.

34. Skinner R, Maybee J, Venter R, et al: Experimental testing and comparison of variables in transpedicular screw fixation: A biomechanical study. Personal communications, 1986.

35. Stokes IAF, Wilder DG, Frymoyer JW, et al: Assessment of patients with low-back pain by biplanar radiographic measurement of intervertebral motion. *Spine* 1981; 6:233.

36. Sypert GW: Low back pain disorders—lumbar fusion. *Clin Neurosurg* 1986; 33:457.

37. Tibrewal SB, Pearcy MJ, Portek I, et al: A prospective study of lumbar spinal movements before and after discectomy using biplanar radiography: Correlation of clinical and radiographic findings. *Spine* 1985; 12:455.

38. Tile M: The role of surgery in nerve root decompression. *Spine* 1984; 9:57.

39. Zindrick MR, Wiltse LL, Holland RR, et al: A biomechanical study of intrapedicular screw fixation in the lumbosacral spine, in *XII Proceedings of International Society for the Study of the Lumbar Spine.* Sydney, Australia, April 14–19, 1985, p 50.

32

Dural Tears in Lumbar Spine Surgery

Edward J. Goldberg, M.D.

Gunnar B.J. Andersson, M.D., Ph.D.

Surgical decompression is an established and accepted treatment modality for lumbar spinal stenosis when symptoms are not alleviated by conservative measures* (See Chapter 26). Cerebrospinal fluid (CSF) leaks can, however, occur during the operation when there is violation of the pia-arachnoid that permits escape of the fluid into the extraarachnoid space.[84] The purpose of this chapter is to discuss the anatomy of the meninges, the epidemiology of dural tears, and the diagnosis and treatment of CSF leaks relevant to lumbar spine surgery.

EMBRYOLOGY AND ANATOMY

The dura mater or *pachymeninx* arises from mesenchymal cells at 40 days of gestation and initially appears ventral to the neural tube. The dura completely encloses the tube by day 52 and extends to the S4 vertebral body in the fetus.[12, 20] The pia mater, the innermost meningeal layer, commences formation on day 37 of gestation. It forms from mesenchyme and may receive a contribution from neural crest cells.[3 20]

The adult spinal dura, composed primarily of collagen and lesser amounts of elastic fibers, extends from the foramen magnum to the level of the S2 vertebra where it invests the filum terminale to form the coccygeal ligament. This ligament fuses with the periosteum of the coccyx. The roots of the lumbar

*References 13, 23, 24, 33, 38, 39, 62, 68, 83, 87, 88, 93.

spinal nerves and the dorsal root ganglia are covered by the dura (see Chapter 7). When the spinal nerves form within the intervertebral foramina, the dura becomes continuous with the epineurium.[12] In the lumbar spine the dura of the thecal sac and extrathecal intraspinal nerves is attached to the posterior longitudinal ligament and vertebral periosteum by the *Hofmann* ligaments. These ligaments prevent dorsal displacement of the dura.[82]

The pia mater consists of two layers. The inner *intima pia* follows the contours of the nervous tissue closely and is composed of reticular and elastic fibers. The *outer epipial* layer, of which collagen is the major constituent, contains the blood vessels that supply the spinal cord.[3 12] From this epipial layer arise the *denticulate* ligaments, which are bands of tissue that attach to the inner surface of the dura. These ligaments extend from the foramen magnum to the T12 vertebral level and maintain the position of the spinal cord relative to the vertebral column. In accord with dura, these ligaments also dissipate stress on the neural elements during spinal motion.[3]

The dural blood supply is provided by segmental arteries which enter the intervertebral foramina to form a capillary system within the dura. Neural innervation of the dura is from the meningeal rami of spinal nerves which accompany these arteries. Free nerve endings within the dura have been demonstrated and are responsible for the transmission of pain impulses. The pia-arachnoid membranes obtain their blood supply from anastomoses between the radicular arteries that pass to the spinal cord.[3]

The arachnoid, lying between the pia and dura mater, extends from its intracranial location along the roots of the cranial and spinal nerves. The space between the pia mater and arachnoid is the subarachnoid space and contains CSF.

When injury occurs to the dura mater alone, healing without the formation of adhesions to the subjacent pia and arachnoid ensues. Fibroblasts of the organizing blood clot which effect healing are limited by the intact arachnoid. Injury to the pia-arachnoid, however, results in adhesions of all three meninges. The fibroblastic ingrowth does not meet a barrier with an injured arachnoid and the overlying dura is involved in the inflammatory reaction. This may explain the scarring found at previous sites of CSF leaks.[46]

The CSF is produced primarily in the choroid plexuses in the ventricles of the brain with lesser amounts manufactured by the ependyma, glial cells, and capillary beds that supply the pia-arachnoid.[3] The CSF contains trace amounts of glucose, protein, Na^+, Cl^- and K^+, but no significant cell component (one to five cells/per cubic millimeter is considered to be within normal limits).[12] Approximately 600 to 700 mL/day of CSF are produced with 140 mL circulating in the subarachnoid space and ventricles at any one time.[12] The CSF made in the lateral and third ventricles passes into the fourth ventricle where it enters the cerebellomedullary cistern via the foramen of Magendie and the foramina of Luschka. From this site the CSF flows in the subarachnoid spaces surrounding the brain and intraspinal nerves. Most of the CSF is passively returned to the venous system via the arachnoid villi and a lesser amount by the ependyma, arachnoid capillaries, and lymphatics of the meninges. The CSF functions to protect the nervous system from trauma, as well as provide nutrition to and remove waste products from the neural cells.[12]

EPIDEMIOLOGY

The incidence of CSF leaks in the lumbar spinal surgery ranges from 0.3% to 13%.[15, 16, 28, 34, 60, 66, 87] The risk of dural injury is higher in spines previously operated on and in cases of very tight stenosis.[15, 58, 92]

Complications of a dural tear include a CSF fistula with an increased risk of meningitis, and pseudomeningocoele formation.* While the incidence of dural-cutaneous fistulas is unknown, the

*References 6, 16, 17, 26, 31, 34, 41, 58, 61, 63, 68, 69, 72, 74, 77, 79, 85, 94.

incidence of pseudocyst formation varies from 0.68% to 2.0%. Predisposing factors include epidural bleeding, traumatic myelograms, postoperative wound infections with sinus tracts, and unrecognized or poorly repaired dural defects.[61, 85, 92] The dural tear, which acts as a flap valve, allows the escape of CSF into the surrounding soft tissue which becomes walled off in a reactive fibrous sac.[63] Unlike a true meningocoele, however, the pseudocyst wall lacks an epithelial lining.[61]

DIAGNOSIS

When a CSF leak occurs intraoperatively, visual identification of the dural defect is usually possible, and allows an immediate repair to be performed.[16, 34, 45, 51, 74] The principles of repair are discussed below under Treatment. Performing a Valsalva maneuver may aid in localization of the dural violation.

To diagnose a CSF leak postoperatively, the physician must maintain a high index of suspicion. Clinical symptoms of nausea, vomiting, and headache exacerbated with the upright position and relieved during recumbency are characteristic.[22, 35, 58, 61] The etiology of postural headaches is believed to be secondary to a reduction in CSF volume due to leakage through the dural defect. The brain, without a full fluid cushion to support it, sags when the patient stands and the resultant traction on the pain-sensitive dura and blood vessels produces the headache.[35, 44] In cases of pseudocysts, back pain from a locally enlarging fluid accumulation and radicular symptoms from the herniation of nerve roots into the dural defect may occur.[6, 17, 26, 58, 61] Pseudocysts may also present with a large local fluctuant mass beneath the skin at the previous lumbar surgical site.[58, 61]

Several diagnostic methods can be utilized to confirm a CSF leak. Chemical tests, such as the determination of glucose and protein (normal values are 45–70 mg/dL and 15–45 mg/dL, respectively), have been unreliable.[16, 37, 56] Protein electrophoresis of a sample of CSF with demonstration of a unique band of transferrin located in the β_2-fraction has been successfully employed in the diagnosis of intracranial CSF leaks. This β_2-transferrin is pathognomonic for CSF and allows differentiation from serum, saliva, lymphatics, and nasal secretions.[32, 56] Its use in spinal CSF leaks, however, has not been reported. Intrathecal injection of fluorescein has been advocated to identify the site of a dural tear, but neurologic complications, including status epilepticus, have been reported.[37, 48, 90] The injection of methylene blue into the lumbar subarachnoid space has also been condemned because paraparesis, quadriplegia, hydrocephalus, and dementia have resulted.[18]

Contrast myelography may be helpful in the detection of an early or late CSF leak as the dye moves from a subarachnoid location into the epidural space. Myelography may be particularly beneficial in diagnosing a pseudocyst as filling of the pseudomeningocoele by contrast may be seen.[58, 61] Shahinfar and Schecter recommended a standing full column or supine technique to allow the contrast entrance into the dorsally located pseudocyst from the dural defect.[79] Delayed radiographs, performed as late as 24 hours after injection, should be obtained to permit adequate time for the filling of the

pseudocyst.[61, 79] (Fig 32–1,A and B). Not all CSF leaks or pseudomeningocoeles, however, are demonstrable with contrast myelography.[86]

Radionuclide myelography, performed by injection of technetium Tc 99m human serum albumin and iodine 131 serum albumin into the cisterna magna, has been reported to allow identification of the site of a lumbar dural defect. Scintigrams performed of the lumbar spine at various hours after administration showed the isotope move from the subarachnoid to the epidural space.[22, 35]

Plain computed tomography (CT) scans of the lumbar spine have been reported to yield diagnostic images of pseudomeningocoeles.[78, 86] The efficacy of CT in acute leaks, however, has not been documented. The pseudocyst appears as a rounded area of low density posterior to the thecal sac. The pseudocyst is of lower density than the thecal sac contents and its capsule exhibits a higher density

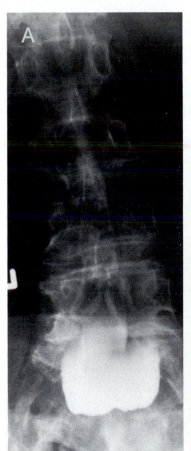
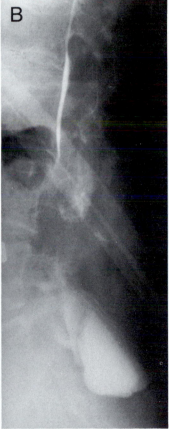
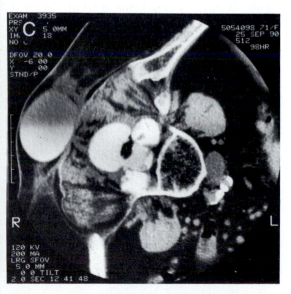

FIG 32–1.

AP **(A)** and lateral **(B)** views of a lumbar myelogram performed on a patient who had decompressive laminectomies of L4 and L5 for spinal stenosis 8 weeks earlier. Note the extravasation of dye from the subarachnoid location into the extradural space with filling of a large pseudomeningocele.

C, the postmyelogram CT scan demonstrates the posteriorly located pseudomeningocele filled with the myelographic dye. The stalk connecting the subarachnoid space with the pseudocyst can be seen adjacent to the left L5–S1 facet joint.

than the surrounding tissues.[86] A delayed postmyelographic CT scan may identify the site of the dural defect as well as the epidural collection of contrast after leaving the subarachnoid injection site (see Fig 32–1).

CSF leaks can also be evaluated by magnetic resonance imaging (MRI).[5, 76] Ross et al. reported that in the early postoperative period MRI is capable of demonstrating fluid collections but not of differentiating between seromas, wound abscesses, and pseudocysts. Postoperative hematomas, however, can be distinguished from CSF accumulation.[76] Pseudomeningoceles, seromas, and abscesses demonstrate low signal on T1- and high signal on T2-weighted images, whereas hematomas possess high signal characteristics on both T1- and T2-weighted images[5, 76] (Fig 32–2).

It is our opinion that no one radiographic examination consistently demonstrates a postoperative CSF leak and that a strong clinical suspicion is mandatory for the diagnosis. Refer to the section Authors' Preferred Management for suggestions regarding diagnostic imaging of CSF leaks.

TREATMENT

When a CSF leak is identified intraoperatively, immediate repair of the dural tears is recommended in order to prevent the previously discussed potential complications.[16, 34, 45, 51, 58, 61, 72, 75] Placing muscle or Gelfoam (absorbable gelatin sponge) alone on a dural defect is ineffective for repair.[16, 25, 58, 61] Gurdjian et al. reported that these substances do not close dural defects adequately when used alone and advised meticulous surgical closure.[25] Eismont et al. outlined the principles to obtain a watertight closure for dural repair[16]

1. The operative field should be dry and unobscured by bleeding. Suction maintains a bloodless field and cotton pledgets protect the neural elements. Adequate lighting and magnification loupes are recommended.

2. Dural silk sutures 4-0 to 7-0 gauge on a one-half circle reverse cutting or tapered needle are used. A running locked suture technique may be employed (Fig 32–3). An alternative method is to utilize simple sutures incorporating a fat or muscle graft. In this technique simple dural stitches are placed through the tear with their ends left long. A second needle is attached to the free suture end and both ends of the suture are passed through a piece of muscle or fat, which is tied down over the repaired tear (Fig 32–4). We have successfully utilized Gelfoam in this capacity. When the dural defect is too large to repair by the above methods, a graft which is sutured to the margins of the dural tear by simple sutures may be used (Fig 32–5). Human dural allograft; autogenous dermis, fat, and split-thickness skin grafts; porcine

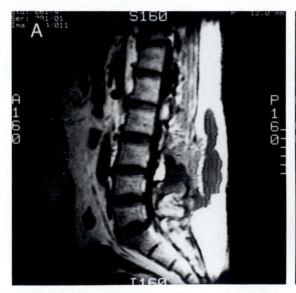
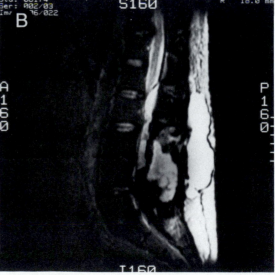

FIG 32–2.
A and **B**, T1- and T2-weighted images of MRI of the lumbar spine in a patient who presented with a CSF leak 6 weeks after laminectomies at L4 and L5. Note the low signal on T1- and high signal in T2-weighted images of the CSF located on the epidural space and subcutaneous tissues. The CSF in the epidural space extends as far cephalad as L1.

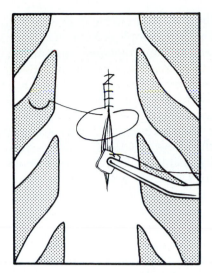

FIG 32–3.
A dural repair using a running locked dural suture on a ta-pered or reverse-cutting, one-half circle needle. Cotton pledgets protect the intradural elements while suction main-tains a bloodless field. (Redrawn from Eismont FV, Wiesel SW, Rothman RH: *J Bone Joint Surg [Am]* 1981; 63:1132–1136.)

dermis and peritoneum; calf pericardium; polyester fiber mesh (Mersilene); polyglactin 910, (Vicryl); pro-plast (Teflon polymer and carbon); and silicone-coated Dacron (Dura Film) have been utilized clini-cally or experimentally as dural patches.* We concur with Eismont et al. that lumbar fascia should be used for small defects and fascia lata for large tears.[16] We prefer autologous tissue to allograft, xenograft, or

References 10, 11, 14, 36, 40, 42, 49, 50, 54, 55, 57, 64, 71, 95.

nonbiologic materials. Adverse complications such as subarachnoid bleeding and increased neurologic deficit due to the infolding of the substitute causing neural compression have been documented with sil-icone-coated products.[2, 19 59, 65, 80] For dural tears in inaccessible locations, such as those in the anterior or lateral walls, a transdural approach may be per-formed.[16, 51] A small plug of fat or muscle anchored to a suture is passed to the dural defect via a central dorsal durotomy. In tears less than 2 to 3 mm, the plug of tissue is secured by the pulsatile flow of the spinal fluid and no anchoring sutures are required. With dural defects exceeding this size, two anchor-ing sutures are recommended (Fig 32–6). The dorsal durotomy is closed with a standard suture tech-nique.[51]

3. The repair is tested by performing the Val-salva maneuver in a reverse Trendelenburg position in order to increase intrathecal pressure. Reinforce-ment of the repair should be performed if egress of CSF is encountered.

4. The paraspinous muscles and overlying lum-bar fascia are closed individually using 0-gauge monofilament nonabsorbable sutures. The skin is closed with interrupted vertical mattress sutures placed 3 to 4 mm apart. No drains are used in order to minimize fistula formation should the CSF con-tinue to leak.

5. Four to 7 days of bed rest in the supine posi-tion is recommended after repair of lumbar dural tears. This permits early healing of the suture lines which have been found to fail at pressurization lev-els within the physiologic range when tested in vitro.[8]

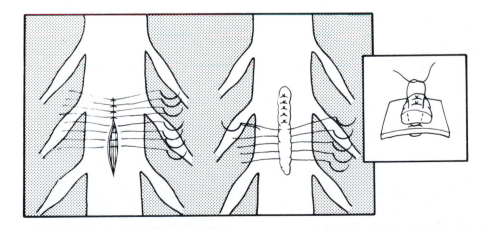

FIG 32–4.
An alternative method for repair of a dural tear in which sim-ple sutures incorporate a fat or muscle graft. Simple sutures are placed through the tears with their ends left long. A sec-ond needle is attached to the free suture end and both ends of the stitch are passed through a piece of fat or muscle, which is tied down over the repaired tear. (Redrawn from Eismont FJ, Wiesel SW, Rothman RH: *J Bone Joint Surg [Am]* 1981; 63:1132–1136.)

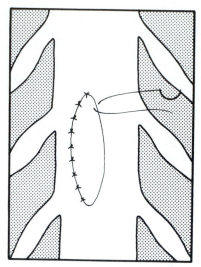

FIG 32–5.
Repair of a large dural tear by suturing a free lumbar fascia or fascia lata graft to the margins of the rent. Simple silk sutures are used. (Redrawn from Eismont FJ, Wiesel SW, Rothman RH: *J Bone Joint Surg [Am]* 1981; 63:1132–1136.)

When a CSF leak is first diagnosed postoperatively, two modalities of treatment are available: (1) subarachnoid drainage using a closed catheter system and (2) direct operative repair of the dural defect. Bed rest alone has not proved to be consistently efficacious, but is advised after surgical repair has been performed.[16, 41]

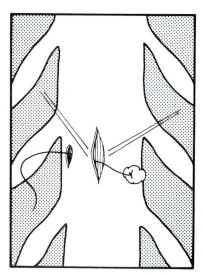

FIG 32–6.
A transdural approach for inaccessibly located dural tears. A dorsal central durotomy allows an anchored small plug of fat or muscle to be passed to the dural defect. The durotomy is closed in a routine manner. (Redrawn from Eismont FJ, Wiesel SW, Rothman RH: *J Bone Joint Surg [Am]* 63:1132–1136.)

Continuous subarachnoid external drainage of CSF was initially employed for dural-cutaneous fistulas secondary to intracranial procedures. Vourc'h[83] and Aitken and Drake[1] independently reported the success of lumbar spinal fluid drainage systems in the treatment of postoperative cranial CSF leaks. McCallum et al. utilized this technique in three patients for the treatment of dural leaks after operations of the spine.[52] Kitchel et al. described successful results using a closed subarachnoid drainage system in 14 patients with a postoperative CSF leak after spinal procedures and considered it as a nonoperative alternative to direct surgical repair of the dura.[41]

The mechanism by which a dural tear heals with the subarachnoid drainage system has been hypothesized to be due to the preferential flow of fluid through the catheter which results in less fluid passing by the dural defect and a decreased spinal fluid pressure. With a decreased pressure the dura is less distended and contracts to a size more amenable to healing.[41] McCoy demonstrated experimentally that granulation tissue forms at the site of CSF fistulas when fluid diversion is accomplished.[53]

The closed subarachnoid drainage procedure is done at bedside in the lateral decubitus position with the patient's knees, hips, and neck flexed to decrease the lumbar lordosis. A continuous epidural anesthesia tray and a sterile blood collection bag are utilized. After sterile preparation of the lumbar spine and infiltration with local anesthetic, a thin-walled continuous epidural needle is inserted between the second and third spinous processes into the subarachnoid space. Five milliliters of CSF are collected and sent for culture, cell count, and differential, as well as for determination of protein and glucose. These tests serve as baseline values to monitor for infection. The bevel of the needle is rotated cephalad and an epidural catheter is passed through the needle into the subarachnoid space for a distance of 5 to 10 cm. The catheter is kept in place as the needle is withdrawn. An intravenous line adapter is then connected to the subarachnoid catheter and the intravenous line is attached to the sterile collection bag. A sterile dressing is applied to the catheter site.

The collection bag is initially placed at the same level as the long axis of the spine and is subsequently adjusted to either above or below the level of the spine to obtain a flow of 200 to 300 mL/24 hr of CSF. A new sterile collection bag is used daily and a sample of spinal fluid is sent daily for culture, cell count and differential, and protein and glucose measurements to monitor for infection. The catheter is left in place for 4 days unless infection occurs. During that period the patient is kept supine and may logroll from side to side. Upon removal of the catheter, the patient is maintained at bed rest for an additional 24 hours to permit the shunt puncture site to heal. Ambulation is then permitted. Kitchel et al.[41] do not routinely use antibiotics whereas we prophylactically use a broad-spectrum antibiotic while the catheter is in place.

Operative repair of a CSF leak first diagnosed postoperatively follows the principles and techniques outlined above.[16] Surgery can be performed as the initial intervention or in cases where the subarachnoid drainage technique fails to yield a successful result.[16, 41] The outcome of direct operative repair of the dura is not compromised by the previous use of the closed catheter system.[41]

When a pseudocyst occurs in conjunction with a CSF leak, operative repair is recommended.[6, 16, 17, 31, 58, 61, 63, 72, 85, 94] The successful treatment of these lesions consists of closure of the dural defect by sutures, grafts, or flaps fashioned from the pseudocyst wall, and excision of the cyst.[58, 61] The pseudomeningocele is incised and its communication with the subarachnoid space is identified.[16, 58, 61] Repair of the dural defect is performed with care taken to avoid injury to the nerve roots which may herniate through the dural tear into the pseudocyst. Single ligature closures, Gelfoam, or muscle used alone, and incomplete resection of the pseudocyst, have led to recurrence and are not recommended.[61]

Epidural injections of autologous blood for the treatment of CSF leaks incurred after myelography, spinal anesthesia, and inadvertent dural penetration during epidural blocks have been utilized with variable success.[21, 67, 70, 73] Fifteen to 20 mL injected at the same level or one space below the dural defect appears most efficacious.[21, 73] It is recommended that this procedure be performed approximately 24 hours after puncture.[47] We consider employing this technique as the initial modality for persistent symptoms after myelography and believe that it should not be used in the treatment of surgical durotomies which are discovered intraoperatively or after surgery.

Fibrin adhesive sealant (FAS) has recently been investigated as a means to repair dural defects.[8, 9, 27] FAS consists of freeze-dried protein concentrate of human fibrinogen and freeze-dried bovine thrombin which form a firm fibrin clot after contact. The sealant bonds with collagen and is reabsorbed during the healing process.[4, 8, 29, 91] It has been used successfully in cardiovascular operations to seal bleeding anastomotic suture lines, control oozing from injured solid organs, and obtain hemostasis in oral surgery and in the resection of intracranial aneurysms.[4, 7, 8, 9, 91] Cain et al. performed in vitro studies on human cadaveric dura with durotomies and demonstrated that FAS alone or when supplementing sutures created a seal able to withstand bursting pressures approximately eight times greater than sutures alone.[8] Furthermore, minimal inflammatory reaction was observed histologically.[8, 9, 27] FAS provided strength in dural repairs comparable to cyanoacrylate polymer, another tissue sealant, without causing dural thinning, gliosis, cortical necrosis, or hemorrhage, as has been documented with the latter.[30, 43, 96] Cain et al. concluded that further investigation with FAS is warranted and its greatest use may be for dural defects that are surgically inaccessible to direct suture repair.[8]

RESULTS

The long-term results of properly performed dural repairs are favorable. In a large series of lumbar spine operations, Oppel et al. reported that dural leaks did not adversely affect the clinical outcome.[66] Jones et al.[34] examined 16 patients who had incidental intraoperative durotomies repaired primarily at the time of surgery at a mean follow-up of 25.1 months. This group was compared with a matched control group which did not incur a CSF leak. No significant difference was found between the two groups in regard to resolution of back and radicular pain, ultimate neurologic status, and overall success of the operation. The authors concluded that there appeared to be no significant sequelae of durotomies repaired primarily.[34]

AUTHORS' PREFERRED MANAGEMENT

Our recommendation for the treatment of a CSF leak noted intraoperatively is immediate repair. Either a running locked suture or simple suture incorporating a tissue plug technique can be utilized. For dural defects not amenable to suture methods, autologous fascial grafts should be used. Lumbar fascia is recommended for small defects and tensor fascia lata for larger rents.

When a CSF leak is initially suspected in the postoperative period, a contrast myelogram of the lumbar spine in the supine or standing position is obtained. A delayed CT scan is performed 4 hours after the myelogram in an effort to delineate the site of the dural defect. We do not routinely use an MRI postoperatively but believe it may differentiate an epidural hematoma from other fluid accumulations.

If the radiographic studies demonstrate a CSF leak without an associated pseudocyst, or fail to reveal a clinically suspected dural tear, we utilize a closed subarachnoid drainage system as described by Kitchel et al.[41] Should this fail to alleviate the patient's symptoms, then direct operative repair of the dural defect is performed. We do not feel that pseudocysts are amenable to the subarachnoid drainage technique because excision of the wall is important in preventing its recurrence. Hence, we proceed directly to surgical repair of the dural defect and pseudomeningocele.

SUMMARY

Dural tears are an unfortunate but potential complication of lumbar spine surgery with an incidence of 0.3% to 13%. Immediate meticulous repair of CSF leaks recognized intraoperatively should be performed in order to prevent fistula formation, meningitis, and pseudomeningocele formation. CSF leaks discovered postoperatively may be treated initially with a closed subarachnoid drainage system. If unsuccessful, direct operative repair should be undertaken. If a pseudocyst is present, surgical repair of the defect and excision of the walls are recommended. If meticulous closure of the dural rent is achieved, long-term sequelae can be minimized.

REFERENCES

1. Aitken RR, Drake CG: Continuous spinal drainage in the treatment of postoperative cerebrospinal-fluid fistulae. *J Neurosurg* 1964; 21:275–277.
2. Banerjee T, Meagher JN, Hunt WE: Unusual complications with use of Silastic dural substitute. *Am Surg* 1974; 40:434–437.
3. Bargmann W, Oksche A, Fix JD, et al: Meninges, choroid plexuses, ependyma, and their reactions, in Haymaker W, Adams RD (eds): *Histology and Histopathology of the Nervous System*. Springfield, Ill, Charles C Thomas, Publisher 1982, pp 560–596.
4. Barton BE, Moore EE, Pearce WH: Fibrin gene as a biologic vascular patch. A comparative study. *J Surg Res* 1986; 40:510–513.
5. Berns DH, Blaser SI, Modic MT: Magnetic resonance imaging of the spine. *Clin Orthop* 1989; 244:78–100.
6. Borgesen SE, Vang PS: Extradural pseudocysts. A cause of pain after lumbar-disc operation. *Acta Orthop Scand* 1973; 44:12–20.
7. Borst HG, Haverich A, Walterbusch G, et al: Fibrin adhesive. An important hemostatic adjunct in cardiovascular operations. *J Thorac Cardiovasc Surg* 1982; 84:548–553.
8. Cain JE Jr, Dryer RF, Barton BR: Evaluation of dural closure techniques. Suture methods, fibrin adhesive sealant, and cyanoacrylate polymer. *Spine* 1988; 13:720–725.
9. Cain JE Jr, Rosenthal HG, Bloom MJ, et al: Quantification of leakage pressures after durotomy repairs in the canine. *Spine* 1990; 51:969–970.
10. Campbell JB, Bassett CAL, Robertson JW: Clinical use of freeze-dried human dura mater. *J Neurosurg* 1958; 15:207–214.
11. Cantore G, Guidetti B, Delfini R: Neurosurgical use of human dura mater sterilized by gamma rays and stored in alcohol: Long-term results. *J Neurosurg* 1987; 66:93–95.
12. Carpenter MB: *Human Neuroanatomy*, ed 7. Baltimore, Williams & Wilkins Co, 1976, pp 1–20.
13. Ciric I, Mikhael MA, Tarkington JA, et al: The lateral recess syndrome. A variant of spinal stenosis. *J Neurosurg* 1980; 53:433–443.
14. Clark RP, Robertson JH, Shea JJ, et al: Closure of dural defects with Proplast. *Am J Otol* 1984; 5:179–182.
15. DeBurge A, Lasalle B, Benoist M, et al: Le traitement chirurgical des sténoses lombaires et ses résultats à propos d'une série de 163 cas opérés. *Rev Rhum Mal Osteoartic* 1983; 50:47–54.
16. Eismont FJ, Wiesel SW, Rothman RH: Treatment of dural tears associated with spinal surgery. *J Bone Joint Surg [Am]* 1981; 63:1132–1136.
17. Elsberg CA, Dyke CG, Brewer ED: Symptoms and diagnosis of extradural cysts. *Bull Neurol Inst NY* 1934; 3:395–417.
18. Evans JP, Keegan HR: Danger in the use of intrathecal methylene blue. *JAMA* 1960; 174:856–859.
19. Fisher WS, Six EG: Cervical myelopathy from dural substitute. *Neurosurgery* 1983; 13:715–717.
20. French BN: Midline fusion defects and defects of formation, in Yeomans, JR (ed): *Neurosurgery*, vol 3. Philadelphia, WB Saunders Co, 1982, pp 11–14.
21. Fry RA, Perera A: Failure of repeated blood patch in the treatment of spinal headache. The Association of Anaesthetists of Great Britain and Ireland, 1989, p 492.
22. Gass H, Goldstein AS, Ruskin R, et al: Chronic postmyelogram headache. Isoptic demonstration of dural leak and surgical care. *Arch Neurol* 1971; 25:168–170.
23. Getty CJM: Lumbar spinal stenosis. The clinical spectrum and the results of operation. *J Bone Joint Surg [Br]* 1980; 62:481–485.
24. Grabias S: The treatment of spinal stenosis. *J Bone Joint Surg [Am]* 1980; 62:308–313.

25. Gurdjian ES, Webster JE, Ostrowski AZ, et al: Herniated lumbar intervertebral discs—An analysis of 176 operated cases. *J Trauma* 1961; 1:158–176.

26. Hadani M, Findler G, Knoler N, et al: Entrapped lumbar nerve root in pseudomeningocele after laminectomy: Report of three cases. *Neurosurgery* 1986; 19:405–407.

27. Hadley MN, Martin NA, Spetzler RF, et al: Comparative Transoral dural closure techniques: A canine model. *Neurosurgery* 1988; 22:392–397.

28. Hagen R, Engesaeter LB: Unilateral and bilateral partial laminectomy in lumbar disc prolapse. A follow-up study of 156 patients. *Acta Orthop Scand* 1977; 48:41–46.

29. Haverich A, Walterbusch G, Borst HG: The use of fibrin glue for sealing vascular prosthesis of high porosity. *Thorac Cardiovasc Surg* 1981; 29:252–254.

30. Hood TW, Mastri AR, Chou SW: Neural and vascular tissue reaction to cyanoacrylate adhesives: A further report. *Neurosurgery* 1982; 11:363–364.

31. Hyndman OR, Gerger WF: Spinal extradural cysts, congenital and acquired. Report of cases. *J Neurosurg* 1946; 3:474–486.

32. Irjala K, Suonpaa J, Laurent B: Identification of CSF leakage by immunofixation. *Arch Otolaryngol* 1979; 105:447–448.

33. Johnsson KE, Willner S, Petersson H: Analysis of operated cases with lumbar spinal stenosis. *Acta Orthop Scand* 1981; 52:427–433.

34. Jones AAM, Stambough JL, Balderston RA, et al: Long-term results of lumbar spine surgery complicated by unintended incidental durotomy. *Spine* 1989; 14:443–446.

35. Kadrie H, Driedger AA, McInnis W: Persistent dural cerebrospinal fluid leak shown by retrograde radionuclide myelography: A case report. *J Nucl Med* 1976; 17:797–799.

36. Keller JT, Ongkiko CM Jr, Saunders MC, et al: Repair of spinal dural defects: An experimental study. *J Neurosurg* 1984; 60:1022–1028.

37. Kirchner FR, Proud GO: Method for the identification and localization of cerebrospinal fluid, rhinorrhea, and otorrhea. *Laryngoscope* 1960; 70:921–931.

38. Kirkaldy-Willis WH, Paine KWE, Cauchoix J, et al: Lumbar spinal stenosis. *Clin Orthop* 1974; 99:30–50.

39. Kirkaldy-Willis WH, Wedge JH, Yong-Hing K, et al: Lumbar spinal nerve lateral entrapment. *Clin Orthop* 1982; 169:171–178.

40. Kisner WH, Flynn TB: Dermal graft for dural defect. *Ann Plast Surg* 1981; 6:315–321.

41. Kitchell SH, Eismont FJ, Green BA: Closed subarachnoid drainage for management of cerebrospinal fluid leakage after an operation on the spine. *J Bone Joint Surg [Am]* 1989; 71:984–987.

42. Klen R, Metelka M, Parizek J: Freeze-dried-homogenous grafts of fascia lata in neurosurgery. *J Neurosurg Sci* 1977; 21:247–250.

43. Kline DG, Hayes GJ: An experimental evaluation of the effect of a plastic adhesive, methyl-2-cyanoacrylate, on neural tissue. *J Neurosurg* 1963; 20:647–654.

44. Kunkle CE, Ray BS, Wolfe HG: Experimental studies in headache: Analysis of the headache associated with changes in intracranial pressure. *Arch Neurol Psychiatry* 1943; 49:323–358.

45. Kurokowa K, Dunsker S, Mayfield FH: Spinal dural patch grafts in experimental animals. *J Neurol Neurosurg Psychiatry* 1975; 38:412.

46. Lear M, Harvey SC: The regeneration of the meninges. *Ann Surg* 1924; 80:536–544.

47. Loeser EA, Hill GE, Bennett GM, et al.: Time vs. success rate for epidural blood patch. *Anesthesiology* 1978; 49:147–148.

48. Mahaley MS, Jr, Odom GL: Complication following intrathecal injection of fluorescein. Case report. *J Neurosurg* 1966; 25:248–249.

49. Maurer PK, McDonald JV: Vicryl (polyglactin 910) mesh as a dural substitute. *J Neurosurg* 1985; 63:448–452.

50. Mayfield FH: Autologous fat transplants for the protection and repair of the spinal dura. *Clin Neurosurg* 1980; 27:349–361.

51. Mayfield FH, Kurokawa K: Watertight closure of spinal dura mater. Technical note. *J Neurosurg* 1975; 43:639–640.

52. McCallum J, Maroon JC, Jannetta PJ: Treatment of postoperative cerebrospinal fluid fistulas by subarachnoid drainage. *J Neurosurg* 1975; 42:434–437.

53. McCoy G: Cerebrospinal rhinorrhea. A comprehensive review and a definition of the responsibility of the rhinologist in diagnosis and treatment. *Laryngoscope* 1963; 73:1125–1157.

54. Meskhia NS, Beybzon ND, Imamaliev AS, et al: Biological material for bridging dura mater defects. Experimental and clinical study. *Acta Chir Plast* 1973; 15:33–38.

55. Messer HD, Strenger L, McVeety HJ: Use of plastic adhesive for reinforcement of a ruptured intracranial aneurysm. *J Neurosurg* 1963; 20:360–362.

56. Meurman OH, Irjala K, Suonpaa J, et al: A new method for the identification of cerebrospinal fluid leakage. *Acta Otolaryngol* 1979; 87:366–369.

57. Miglets AW, Saunders WH: Experimental dural replacement with split-thickness skin. *Laryngoscope* 1964; 77:1028–1039.

58. Miller PR, Elder FW, Jr: Meningeal pseudocysts (meningocele spurious) following laminectomy. Report of ten cases. *J Bone Joint Surg [Am]* 1968; 50:268–276.

59. Misra BK, Shaw JF: Extracerebral hematoma in association with dural substitute. *Neurosurgery* 1987; 21:399–400.

60. Moyes PD: Protruded lumbar intervertebral discs with special reference to surgical technique and preoperative and postoperative management: A clinical essay. *Can J Surg* 1970; 13:382–386.

61. Nash CL, Jr, Kaufman B, Frankel VH: Postsurgical meningeal pseudocysts of the lumbar spine. *Clin Orthop* 1971; 75:167–178.

62. Nelson MA: Lumbar spinal stenosis. *J Bone Joint Surg [Br]* 1973; 55:506–512.

63. O'Connell JEA: The cerebral spinal fluid pressure as an etiological factor in the development of lesions affecting the CNS. *Brain* 1953; 76:279–298.

64. O'Neill P, Booth AE: Use of porcine dermis as a dural substitute in 72 patients. *J Neurosurg* 1984; 61:351–354.

65. Ongkiko CM, Keller JT, Mayfield FH, et al: An unusual complication of Dura Film as a dural substitute. Report of two cases. *J Neurosurg* 1984; 60:1076–1079.

66. Oppel F, Schirmer M: Results and complicated course after surgery for lumbar disc herniation. *Adv Neurosurg* 1977; 4:36–51.

67. Ozdil T, Forrest Powell W: Post lumbar puncture headache: An effective method of prevention. *Anesth Analg* 1965; 44:542–545.

68. Pagni CA, Cassanari V, Bennasconi V: Meningocele spurious following hemilaminectomy in a case of lumbar discal hernia. *J Neurosurg* 1961; 18:709–710.

69. Paine KWE: Results of decompression for spinal stenosis. *Clin Orthop* 1976; 115:96–100.

70. Palahniuk RJ, Cumming M: Prophylactic blood patch does not prevent post lumbar puncture headache. *Can J Annesth* 1979; 26:132–133.

71. Parizek J, Mericka P, Spacek J, et al: Xenogeneic pericardium as a dural substitute in reconstruction of suboccipital dura mater in children. *J Neurosurg Sci* 1989; 70:905–909.

72. Pau A: Postoperative "meningocele spurious." Report of two cases. *J Neurosurg Sci* 1974; 18:150–152.

73. Quaynor H, Corbey M: Extradural blood patch—why delay? *Br J Anaesth* 1985; 57:538–540.

74. Rosenblum DJ, DeRow JR: Spinal extradural cysts with report of an ossified spinal extradural cyst. *AJR Am J Roentgenol* 1963; 90:1227–1230.

75. Rosenthal JD, Hahn JF, Martinez GJ: A technique for closure of leak of spinal fluid. *Surg Gynecol Obstet* 1975; 140:948–950.

76. Ross JS, Masryk TJ, Modic MT, et al: Lumbar spine: Postoperative assessment with surface-coil MR imaging. *Radiology* 1987; 164:851–860.

77. Schreiber F, Haddad B: Lumbar and sacral cysts causing pain. *J Neurosurg* 1951; 8:504–509.

78. Schumacher HW, Wassmann H, Podlinski C: Pseudomeningocele of the lumbar spine. *Surg Neurol* 1988; 29:77–78.

79. Shahinfar AH, Schechter MM: Traumatic extradural cysts of the spine. *AJR J Roengtenol* 1966; 98:713–719.

80. Simpson D, Robson A: Recurrent subarachnoid bleeding in association with dural substitute. Report of three cases. *J Neurosurg* 1984; 60:408–409.

81. Spangfort EV: The lumbar disc herniation. A computer-aided analysis of 2,504 operations. *Acta Orthop Scand Suppl* 1972; 142:1–95.

82. Spencer DL: Mechanisms of nerve root compression due to a herniated disc, in Weinstein JN, Wiesel SW (eds): *The Lumbar Spine.* Philadelphia, WB Saunders Co, 1990, pp 141–145.

83. Spengler DM: Degenerative stenosis of the lumbar spine. *J Bone Joint Surg [Am]* 1987; 69:305–308.

84. Spetzler RF, Wilson CB: Dural fistulae and their repair, in Yeomans JR (ed): *Neurosurgery,* vol 4. Philadelphia, WB Saunders Co, 1982. pp 2209–2227.

85. Swanson HS, Fincher EF: Extradural arachnoidal cysts of traumatic origin. *J Neurosurg* 1947; 4:530–538.

86. Teplick JG, Peyster RG, Teplick SK, et al: CT identification of postlaminectomy pseudomeningocele. *AJR Am J Roentgenol* 1983; 140:1203–1206.

87. Tile M, McNeil SR, Zarins RK, et al: Spinal stenosis. Results of treatment. *Clin Orthop* 1976; 115:104–108.

88. Verbiest H: Results of surgical treatment of idiopathic developmental stenosis of the lumbar vertebral canal. *J Bone Joint Surg [Br]* 1977; 59:181–188.

89. Vourc'h G: Continuous cerebrospinal fluid drainage by indwelling spinal catheter. *Br J Anaesth* 1963; 35:118–120.

90. Wallace JD, Weintraub MI, Mattson RH, et al: Status epilepticus as a complication of intrathecal fluorescein. *J Neurosurg* 1972; 35:659–660.

91. Wepner F: The use of fibrin adhesion system for local hemostasis in oral surgery. *J Oral Maxillofac Surg* 1982; 40:555–558.

92. Wiesel SW: The multiply-operated lumbar spine. *Instr Course Lect* 1985; 34:68–77.

93. Wiltse LL, Kirkaldy-Willis WH, McIvor GWD: The treatment of spinal stenosis. *Clin Orthop* 1976; 115:83–91.

94. Winkler H, Powers JA: Meningocele following hemilaminectomy: A report of two cases. *NC Med J* 1950; 11:292–294.

95. Xu BZ, Pan HX, Li KM, et al: Study and clinical application of a porcine biomembrane for the repair of dural defects. *J Neurosurg* 1988; 69:707–711.

96. Zumpano BJ, Jacobs LR, Hall JB: Bioadhesive and histotoxic properties of ethyl-2-cyanoacrylate. *Surg Neurol* 1982; 18:452–457.

33

The Surgical Treatment of Failures of Laminectomy and Spinal Fusion

John P. Kostuik M.D., F.R.C.S.C.

The two major areas of surgery of the spine are decompressive procedures and fusion procedures. This chapter deals with failures of these procedures. The chapter is divided into two parts: (1) failures of laminectomy or decompressive procedures and (2) failures of fusion.

Failure to alleviate signs and symptoms and subsequent deterioration following a fusion or decompression procedure presents a difficult problem for both surgeon and patient. Failures following decompressive surgery vary from 5% to over 50% with a general average of about 15%.[122] This variation is due to the different forms of procedures, the pathologic conditions of the population analyzed, as well as the different criteria used to measure success.[48] It is well recognized that patients receiving third-party payment, i.e., workers' compensation, have a lesser success rate than patients whose economic outcome depends upon their own efforts.[89] Because of the development of the special physician-patient relationship, the surgeon performing the initial operative procedure often cannot objectively arrive at a decision with reference to further surgery in his own patient. The treating surgeon to some extent frequently buries his head in the sand and denies that a problem exists.

CAUSES OF FAILURE

The "three W's" have been described as encompassing the failures of spinal surgery. These are the *wrong* patient, the *wrong* diagnosis, and the *wrong* surgery. Included in the wrong preoperative diagnosis are improper indications.

It is simple to eliminate the wrong surgeon. In 1971 Jones[53] reviewed 180 residency training programs of which 88% believed spinal surgery was an important component of clinical practice. However, only 74% provided what was deemed to be adequate training. Today, spinal surgery is about to enter the 21st century. The current state of the art in this field is approximately comparable to joint replacement surgery 15 to 20 years ago. Because of the increasing complexity of spinal surgery, and the increasingly sophisticated techniques and instrumentation, the spinal surgeon of tomorrow will need to have completed a fellowship and be willing to devote the majority of his or her time to spinal problems in order for these complex techniques to be mastered.

The wrong patient is a more complex problem, and can be divided into two general categories: (1) the patient was chosen for treatment by fusion or decompression when the pathologic findings were such that the patient could not be expected to benefit from the operation, or (2) the patient's psychosocial circumstances and expectations simply precluded success. An example of the former is the utilization of spinal fusions for a patient with nonspecific, chronic, disabling low back pain, where the history, physical examination, and imaging studies indicate no definite abnormality. In these circumstances, failure rates as high as 80% are recorded, leading most authorities to conclude that spinal fusion has no role in the management of nonspecific spinal pain. Similarly, the psychosocial determinants of success and failure in spinal disease and surgery require emphasis as they relate to spinal surgery and its indications. The wrong operation is an even more complex issue, and ranges from inadequate imaging studies which led to misdiagnosis, all the way to a poor choice of surgical technique from the large menu of alternatives which currently are available to the spinal surgeon.

An inadequate preoperative assessment combined with the failure to understand the objectives of the patient, together with failure to understand the impact of psychosocial problems on outcome, can result in a disaster.

An increasing emphasis today has been placed upon the use of sophisticated imaging techniques. It should be remembered that a careful analysis of subjective pain complaints, namely, history taking, forms more than 90% of the basis of the decision to proceed to surgery. Objective physical findings and confirmatory imaging studies help to localize the source of the patient's complaints.

Though some failures can be described as being a result of the three W's, some complications occur which are beyond the surgeon's control including such things as arachnoiditis or extradural scarring.

Surgery is but one aspect in the total care of the patient. Although surgery plays a major role it is not the only event leading to a successful outcome. The role of rehabilitation and postoperative care is almost equally as important. This is particularly true in surgery for a previous failed procedure. The ultimate goal is pain relief, restoration of function, and patient satisfaction. Surgery is one of the steps in the rehabilitative process.

This chapter not only deals with the causes of failure in patients who have had decompressive procedures or fusion of the lumbar spine and reviews solutions[107] but also offers an analysis of what should be done initially in order to avoid a second operative intervention. Finally, presentations of patients with surgical failures and the treatment alternatives are discussed.

Although the three W's account for many failures, this approach does not account for the problems which follow a properly performed procedure in the correct patient for the right diagnosis. Such failures are represented by unavoidable complications or can result from progressing degenerative disease.

TABLE 33–1.

Classification of Failures of Decompressive Surgery

I. No improvement immediately following surgery with outright failure to improve mono- or polyradiculopathy
   A. Wrong preoperative diagnosis
      1. Tumor
      2. Infection
      3. Metabolic disease
      4. Psychosocial causes
      5. Discogenic pain
      6. Decompression done too late for disc sequestration (>6 mo)
   B. Technical error
      1. Missed level(s)
      2. Failure to perform adequate decompression
         a. Missed fragment including foraminal disc
         b. Failure to recognize spinal stenosis as part of lumbar disc herniation
         c. Conjoined nerve root
II. Temporary relief but recurrence of pain
   A. Early recurrence of symptoms (within weeks)
      1. Infection
      2. Meningeal cyst
   B. Midterm (within weeks to months)
      1. Recurrent disc prolapse
      2. Battered root
      3. Arachnoiditis
      4. Patient expectation ill founded
   C. Longer-term failures (within months to years)
      1. Recurrent stenosis or development of lateral stenosis from disc space collapse
      2. Instability

CLASSIFICATION OF FAILURES OF DECOMPRESSIVE SURGERY

Failures of decompressive surgery can be divided into two main types: (1) those in which radiculopathic symptoms predominate, and (2) those in which low back pain is the major problem (Table 33–2). Both, of course, may coexist.

TABLE 33–2.

Causes of Failure of Decompressive Surgery

Radiculopathy Predominant	Low Back Pain Predominant
Neural tumors	Osseous tumors
Infections—epidural abscess	Infections
Inadequate decompression	Discitis
Missed fragment	Osteomyelitis
Foraminal disc	Discogenic pain
Conjoined nerve root	Segmental instability
Recurrent disc prolapse	
Peridural fibrosis	
Meningeal cyst	
Arachnoiditis	

Approaches to the Patient With a Failed Spinal Decompression

History and Physical Examination

The clinical history is the most significant diagnostic measure in assessing probable causation of continuing symptoms. Finnegan et al.[29] identified three typical pain syndromes:

1. The patient has no initial relief of symptoms or his or her symptoms are worse. It is likely that the wrong diagnosis was made or the wrong operation was performed.

2. The patient has initial relief, sometimes accompanied by increased numbness or even weakness, followed by the gradual onset of recurrent radiculopathy over weeks to months. It is likely that nerve root injury has occurred with subsequent scarring.

3. The patient has complete relief of symptoms, but later, over months to years, develops recurrent radiculopathy—often suddenly. It is likely that recurrent disc prolapse has occurred.

Frymoyer et al.[36] emphasized the importance of long-term failures which they felt were usually the manifestation of an evolving degenerative process. In patients who had undergone decompression for radiculopathy, low back pain as a continuing problem may be a major factor regardless of whether or not an arthrodesis has been performed. The patient may have expected complete relief of all back symptoms, an expectation which is probably, in most cases, ill founded. The ability to differentiate the usual expected continuum of back pain from severe back pain for which an anatomic cause can be established is difficult.

In addition to the factors outlined above, other important factors in the history are the presence or absence of systemic symptoms, the patient's occupation, the psychosocial history, and the status of compensation or legal proceedings. Efforts must be made to obtain records of previous interventions.

The physical examination, although not as important as the history, does have a role. This role may not be particularly rewarding if low back pain is the predominant complaint. If residual deficits from prior surgery or neurologic problems are present, interpretation of the neurologic examination may be difficult. It is recognized that 40% to 50% of patients who have had previous discotomy have residual alterations in reflexes and sensation corresponding to the level of previous root involvement.[36, 85] Nerve tension signs are useful indications of failure when positive, since these are usually alleviated by surgery. The physical findings may be confusing as a result of the pathologic findings. Patients with recurrent stenosis may have minimal or misleading physical findings.[114] The presence of nonorganic physical findings, as described by Waddell et al.,[115] may help to identify patients who have an inappropriate pain pattern.

Imaging Studies

Imaging studies are the confirmatory basis for diagnosis. The most likely cause for continuing symptoms should be established on the basis of history and physical examination. The various imaging techniques are emphasized in greater detail in the section on failed fusions. In my opinion the use of computed tomography (CT)–enhanced myelography has proved thus far to be more effective than enhanced magnetic resonance imaging (MRI). CT-myelography is capable of diagnosing arachnoiditis. Although MRI is more effective for soft tissue analysis, I feel that CT-myelography is of added value as it more clearly demonstrates bony problems. This is particularly true in cases of spinal stenosis.

CT discography may be of value in assessing far-out lateral syndromes as well as annular tears.

Facet blocks are of little value as a diagnostic tool in the case of failed surgery because of dorsal scarring.[28]

Selected nerve root blocks have proved to be extremely valuable in differentiating various aspects of root pain. They are by no means infallible. An injection of 1 to 2 cc at the base of a nerve root may anesthetize an adjacent root. Moreover, they do not differentiate extrinsic from intrinsic compression or scarring.[62, 76]

The failures of decompressive surgery can also be classified according to immediate or early recurrence of symptoms, midterm failures, and long-term failures (see Table 33–1).

Immediate Failure: Wrong Diagnosis

Radiculopathy has a variety of causes including lumbar disc herniation and spinal stenosis. Most other causes are rare and include such things as infections and tumors. Wiesel et al.[123] found that only 109 of 5,362 failed to improve. Of these, only 14 patients with low back pain were ultimately found to have an underlying cause. Schofferman et al.[102] emphasized occult infections as an important cause of symptoms in patients with low back pain and radiculopathy. The incidence of spinal infections, including epidural abscesses, is 0.037/1,000; of disc space infection, 0.037/1,000; and of multiple myeloma, 0.07/1,000.[21] Other causes include neural tumors[72]; retroperitoneal tumors, including endometriosis; viral plexopathies; and peripheral neuropathies of metabolic, viral, or traumatic etiology. Other causes to be ruled out are vascular disease, metastatic neoplasms, and arthritic conditions of the hip.[1, 42, 67]

Treatment.—Treatment, especially surgery, should be tailored to the specific pathologic finding.

Psychosocial Causes

Psychosocial causes have been found in many surveys to be a major factor in failure of decompressive surgery.[29, 70, 89, 105] Important factors in predicting failure are workers' compensation, job dissatisfaction, low education, low income, heavy job requirements, cigarette smoking, psychological disturbances, and litigation.[25, 44, 107, 122]

In assessing the patient with prior failure of decompressive surgery, these factors must be clearly understood and may require a multidisciplinary approach.[70] It is particularly important in the presence of psychosocial factors to identify a specific anatomic cause if surgery is contemplated, even in a primary case of exploratory surgery.

Surgical intervention is inappropriate unless a specific anatomic cause is clearly defined. Prolonged rest is inappropriate.[22] The use of aggressive rehabilitation programs,[79] pain clinics,[83] progressive exercise programs,[75] and work-hardening programs should be considered. They have proved to be successful in many patients with underlying psychosocial causes of their failure.

Discogenic Pain

Discogenic pain per se has been difficult to understand. Crock[16] has described internal disc disruption. This has been demonstrated by discography with reproduction of the patient's symptoms in the presence of varying degrees of morphologic degeneration. In my opinion, degenerative disease of the disc results in a cascade of problems including facet pain as well as pain of discogenic origin. Walsh et al.[116] have shown that discography has a high degree of sensitivity and specificity in patients without prior surgery. On the other hand, Nachemson[84] disputes this. Esses, Botsford, and Kostuik[27] have shown that rigid external skeletal fixation applied percutaneously is a better predictor of outcome for fusion than radiography, discography, or facet blocks. One problem which many surgeons have failed to comprehend is that lumbar spine discography has a relatively high incidence of false-nega-

tives, primarily in those cases which show extensive degeneration, but where pain is not reproduced. Owing to the significant annular tears it is impossible, in my opinion, to increase the intranuclear pressure sufficiently upon injection to reproduce the patient's symptoms.

In the patient who has undergone previous lumbar discotomy and has persistent symptoms, discography may be of little value at that level, unless there is a positive reproduction of pain on disc distention. Some authors have found discography and CT scanning of value in such cases.

Crock,[16] Norton,[89] and Pilgaard[95] have reported surgical success in 95% of primary cases of discogenic pain. O'Brien et al.[90] suggest that these primary results may be duplicated in patients with prior surgical failures.

Treatment.—If surgery is considered in cases of disc disruption, the alternatives include anterior interbody fusion,[17, 18] simultaneous combined posteroanterior fusion, or posterior surgery alone.[90] In my opinion posterior interbody fusion after prior decompression is exceedingly difficult because of preexisting postoperative scarring which may be enhanced by the surgery and place the patient at greater neurologic risk.

Missed Levels

Factors which may lead to surgery being done at the inappropriate level in cases of primary disc herniation include (1) abnormalities of segmentation; (2) mislabeling of imaging studies; (3) failure to verify the side of the patient's complaints; (4) obesity; and (5) microsurgical approaches. There has been an increase in missed levels with the development of microsurgical approaches. Intraoperative radiographs may be difficult to obtain, particularly in obese patients.

Treatment.—Since the patient's pathologic condition has not been alleviated, it is felt that surgical intervention is warranted. If the diagnosis is made early, i.e., within a day or two, the patient should be returned to the operating room at that time. More often persistence of symptoms beyond a few weeks is the usual scenario. The patient should be reevaluated, bearing in mind that the wrong level or side may have been operated on. The surgeon should be frank with the patient, admit that he has made an error, and deal with the patient as expeditiously as possible.

Delayed Decompression

Although Weber[121] has shown that the outcome of the patient with a disc herniation and sciatica is the same at 1 year whether he is operated on or not, frequently patients who are operated on 6 months or later from the onset of sciatica do not do as well as those patients who have had surgery performed prior to this time. This is especially the case in the presence of a sequestered disc. Sequestration results in root scarring. Many patients have undergone decompression where there has been a preexistent longstanding history of back pain with a more recent history of sciatica. Discotomy or decompression is undertaken with the idea that this will alleviate both the sciatica and the back pain. This is a major error and removal of a disc or decompression of the contents of the epidural canal will do little to relieve longstanding back pain, which in my opinion often occurs as a result of instability. Although the sciatica may be helped, the back pain may be aggravated or persist. In such conditions, fusion should be considered following appropriate assessment, including discography and facet blocks.

Inadequate Decompression

Negative exploration has a high correlation with failure.[106] Macnab emphasized the importance of other causes of sciatica than disc herniation and recommended a thorough examination in patients with continued nerve root compression.[77] He included such causes as facet impingement, pedicular kinking, foraminal migration of disc material, spinal stenosis, and extraforaminal disc herniation (Table 33–3). In 18 of 68 cases no cause could be found. O'Connell[91] as well as Macnab[77] described variations in neurologic presentation other than the classic presentation. They described L4–5 disc herniations producing generally L5 pain and similarly an L5–S1 disc herniation producing S1 pain. Such a far-lateral herniated nucleus pulposus or two-level disc herniations may occur in up to 10% of cases.[91] Further, a central disc herniation can compromise more than one root or even produce the cauda equina syndrome. Conjoined roots, which in some series occur in up to 11% of cases, may be another cause for the variability in signs and symptoms. The far-out or far-lateral syndrome of disc herniation can affect the more proximal root rather than the root at the level of the herniation. This explains how an L4–5 far-out disc herniation produces L4 symptoms.[117] Modern imaging techniques are more successful in identifying these variations. As a consequence, negative explorations should become rare occurrences.

TABLE 33–3.

Causes of Continued Radiculopathy*

Causes	No. of Cases (N = 68)
Facet impingement	19
Pedicular kinking	12
Foraminal migration	9
Spinal stenosis	8
Extraforaminal disc	2
No cause identified	18

*Data from Mcnab I: *J Bone Joint Surg [Am]* 1971; 53:891–903.

Operative failure occurs as a result of an inadequate decompression. The surgery must be tailored to the pathologic changes. Extraforaminal stenosis in association with disc herniation may also be a cause of continued radioculopathy if the stenosis is not recognized. This has been emphasized by Burton et al.[10] and Macnab.[77]

Macnab[77] has suggested that in the presence of multilevel stenoses it is important to identify the root or roots which require decompression. He believes that on the basis of nerve root injection studies the positive root or roots may be more readily identified, thus allowing for a less extensive decompression. The decision as to how many levels to decompress in the presence of multilevel stenoses is often an enigma. The use of nerve root injection studies and, more recently, somatosensory evoked potentials done pre- and intraoperatively may be of value.

Other causes of inadequate decompression are found in cases of degenerative spondylolisthesis and isthmic spondylolisthesis. In degenerative spondylolisthesis decompression is usually done for L5 radiculopathy. However, the L4 root may be entrapped in the lateral recess. In the case of an L5 isthmic spondylolisthesis, the L5 root is most commonly affected by bony cartilaginous material. The S1 roots may be affected as well although less commonly and in a case of spondylogenic spondylolisthesis of L5 and S1 the L4–5 disc proximal to the olisthesis may also be herniated.

Treatment.—Repeat decompression following accurate localization is recommended. Because of the previous surgery, scarring may be extensive. At the time of surgery it is recommended that the surgeon proceed from areas of normal tissue, i.e., bone, to the edges of scar overlying the previous decompression. Using fine dissection a plane can usually be developed between the edge of the bone and the soft tissue without exposing the underlying dura.

Bone is then removed proceeding to the more normal epidural contents of the canal. Following this, as much bone or soft tissue as necessary should be removed. A commonly used criterion for adequacy of decompression is the ability to immediately retract the root for a minimum of 5 mm, and when the root is free a probe can be easily passed into the foramina. The disc space need not be approached unless there is evidence of the presence of residual significant disc material based on preoperative radiologic images.

Motion segment stability may be affected if considerable bone has been sacrificed or the facet joint is destroyed. In these patients, fusion may be necessary in addition to the decompressive procedure.

Inadequate Nerve Root Decompression

This is most commonly seen as a result of midline decompression without adequate nerve root decompression. In patients with lateral or foraminal stenosis decompression should include foraminotomy or resection of part of the inferior facet, or undercutting of the facet.

Conjoined Nerve Root

Although various studies have indicated an incidence of conjoined nerve root of between 2% and 14%, it is more likely that the true incidence is closer to the latter figure. As a result of failure to recognize this possibility at the time of surgery, the nerve root may become excessively scarred as a result of surgical trauma, or the actual root may be cut or evulsed or overlooked. CT-myelography provides perhaps the most accurate diagnosis of a conjoined root (see Chapter 22). Frequently, the misinterpretation is with a disc herniation. The surgical approach is similar to that for lateral recess stenosis.

Temporary Relief Followed by Early Recurrence (Days to Weeks)

Infection

The incidence of wound infection following decompression varies from 0.5% to a high of 4%.[40, 47, 106] This higher figure is more commonly encountered today with the use of microdiscectomy. Infections vary from mild wound infection to discitis to frank osteomyelitis and epidural abscess.

Discitis

Discitis may present in its classic form with significant uncontrollable back pain and extreme discomfort. Not infrequently, however, cases of discitis are not recognized and are diagnosed only in retro-

spect when sclerosis of the end plates is seen with significant settling of the disc space following discotomy. The erythrocyte sedimentation rate remains elevated and bone scanning at 10 days and MRI may be positive. The most common organism is *Staphylococcus aureus*. Though spontaneous fusion may occur in as many as 50% of patients, this has not generally been my experience.

Cultures, including wound aspirates, often remain negative, particularly if an antibiotic has been used, even for a short period.[31] Blood cultures, urine cultures, wound cultures, and, if necessary, a culture biopsy from the disc space may be needed in order to isolate an organism. Although in the past, immobilization and a spica cast have been recommended, in our experience, bed rest with bathroom privileges and intravenous antibiotics for 10 days followed by oral antibiotics are usually sufficient.

Pilgaard[95] noted that nonoperative treatment was usually sufficient and most patients went on to spontaneous fusion in from 6 months to 1 year. Postinfection discitis, in contrast to osteomyelitis, rarely requires surgical intervention.

Postoperative Osteomyelitis

Although the initial presentation is similar to discitis, the latter becomes more chronic, as symptoms persist and indeed increase. Osteomyelitis may also be associated with systemic problems, including anorexia, failure to thrive, and in some cases cachexia. The sedimentation rate remains elevated. Not always, however, are systemic symptoms present. The pathologic picture is one of disease progression starting with disc space narrowing and subsequent plate erosion leading to vertebral body collapse. In contrast to discitis, cultures are more likely to be positive.

Treatment.—If diagnosed early enough, the response to antibiotics is satisfactory. In most cases 6 weeks of antibiotic treatment intravenously is recommended. Intravenous antibiotics for a period of 10 days to 2 weeks followed by oral antibiotics may suffice, provided that the sedimentation rate is closely monitored.

Surgery is indicated if there is progressive vertebral body collapse associated with instability or the development of neurologic signs and symptoms. Treatment usually consists of anterior debridement and bone grafting together with appropriate antibiotics. Infection is rarely posterior and is more likely to be associated with an epidural abscess. Epidural abscesses are often associated with vertebral body osteomyelitis.

Epidural Abscess

An epidural abscess is extremely rare following surgery. Neurologic symptoms and signs may be rapid and confused with those seen as a result of hematoma. Surgical treatment is indicated with appropriate decompression and antibiotics.

Meningeal Cyst

A meningeal cyst is usually the result of an unrecognized durotomy with the development of a ball-valve phenomenon.[54, 81] The nerve root or roots become part of the cyst. Radicular pain may be present. A diagnosis can be made with the use of myelography with or without CT scanning or MRI scanning. Meningeal cysts are uncommon and occur in less than 1% of patients. They are more common following decompression for spinal stenosis than for disc excision (see Chapter 27).

Treatment.—Not all cysts are symptomatic and in need of treatment. Treatment consists of surgical excision of the cyst and closure of the dural opening. Care must be taken to see that the cyst does not contain nerve roots. If it does, these should be dissected free of the cyst before closing the defect. If the defect is large, a graft may be necessary for closure.

Midterm Failures (Weeks to Months)

Recurrent Disc Prolapse

This is the most common cause of failure. In some series[33, 34, 38] the recurrent herniation may occur at the same level on the same side or on the opposite side or at a new level.[38]

Patients initially do well, but may present as early as a few days, but more typically a few weeks following surgery with recurrent symptoms. The history and physical examination are compatible with disc herniation but because of residual deficits from the initial herniation, the physical examination may be difficult.

The amount of disc removed does not influence the risk of recurrence. Spengler[107] found that excision of the herniation only resulted in no increased incidence of recurrence in comparison to the more radical evacuation of the disc space. The past practice of excising a second disc based on myelographic findings in order to prevent herniation at this level should not be done.[91]

Treatment.—The treatment approach should be similar to that of a primary disc herniation. Conservative measures are first attempted. These include a few days of bed rest, analgesics, nonsteroidal anti-inflammatory drugs, and graduated mobilization.

Because of the natural reluctance for repeat surgery on the part of the surgeon and perhaps the patient, many of these patients are treated nonoperatively whereas if their presentation had been de novo, surgery would have been undertaken. Studies[43, 121] have shown that most patients do well without surgery. This is based on the natural history of disc herniation in which it is recognized that most patients followed over the long term, whether treated surgically or nonoperatively, have approximately the same outcome.[121] Some surgeons believe that the outcome is poor with recurrent disc herniation because of increased scarring with or without intervention.

The alternative to nonoperative care is repeat surgery. It is recommended at this time that a conventional incision be used rather than microdiscotomy. Frymoyer et al.[38] believed that the outcome of repeat surgery is similar to that of a primary disc excision.

In a consecutive series of 500 discotomies for disc herniation, I have experienced two recurrences. These were both encountered early in my experience. In both cases the disc space was curetted rather than a simple removal of the loose fragment.

Differential diagnosis must include failure to identify sequestrated fragments at the original surgery. These patients do not do well in the immediate postoperative period. Failure to find sequestrated fragments is a result of a failure to recognize how far disc fragments may migrate from the site of the point of exit from the disc.

Perineural Scarring

The incidence of perineural scarring resulting in postoperative symptoms as a result of root trauma has been reported to range from a low of 1% to 2%[106] to a high of 12%.[36] Burton et al.[10] reported an 8% failure rate due to perineural scarring. Perineural scarring is frequently associated with the presence of conjoint roots and excessive bleeding. Hoyland et al.[49] have implicated the use of cottonoid pledgets as a possible source of fibrosis.

The patient usually does well in the immediate postoperative period but then develops a recurrence of sciatica, often with no increased neurologic deficit. The patient's symptoms may initially be helped by nonsteroidal anti-inflammatory drugs but symptoms may persist and increase for a number of months.

The differential diagnosis is obviously one of recurrent disc herniation. The most extreme form of the "battered root" is, of course, direct nerve injury to one or more roots, including the cauda equina syndrome. The incidence of the latter varies from 0.4% to 4.0%. Spangfort[106] has reported on caudal injury with disturbance of bowel and bladder function. He noted only 5 out of 2,504 cases following disc excision. More recently, the addition of oversized free fat grafts to prevent epidural scarring may produce cauda equina syndrome as well.

Prevention includes proper surgical technique and proper identification of the pathologic changes. Whether or not the use of fat grafts prevents epidural scarring is controversial. In my opinion, it probably does not. Vascularized fat grafts may be preferable but often are technically difficult to perform.

Many surgical treatments are controversial. These include the application of various materials, including silicone, to prevent scarring; dural sleeve splitting; the removal of scar; and spinal fusion. More recently, the use of an electrical stimulator has been advocated. No one of these modalities has been shown to be of any particular value over another.

Epidural Fibrosis

Epidural fibrosis is the normal outcome of any decompressive procedure. Epidural fibrosis without the presence of direct trauma to roots is, in my opinion, unlikely to be a cause of symptoms. The use of enhanced CT or MRI may differentiate fibrosis from other causes of extrinsic neural compression. Attempts at prevention with the use of fat grafts remain controversial. The use of laminaplasty (restoration of the posterior elements) has, in my opinion, been more valuable than fat grafts in the prevention of epidural fibrosis.

Arachnoiditis

The most common cause of arachnoiditis has been the use of oil-based radiopaque contrast media for myelography. Other causes are bleeding during myelography, intrathecal injection of corticosteroids, and surgical trauma. Arachnoiditis is a nontreatable condition. Fortunately, there does not seem to be continued deterioration.

Long-term follow-up by Guyer et al.[41] showed no increase in symptoms with the passage of time ranging from 10 to 21 years. The use of oil-based contrast media was the most common cause in their series. Pain was a major reason for dysfunction with no increasing neurologic deficits noted.

Long-Term Failures (Months to Years)

A definition of long-term failure is difficult. The causes include recurrent disc herniation, which I have seen as late as 10 years following previous discectomy. Other causes are recurrent stenosis, including the development of lateral stenosis and foraminal stenosis due to progressive degeneration and disc narrowing, and instability following either discectomy or decompression.

Failure to recognize associated disease processes that may go on to increased morbidity may be one cause. Prevention is difficult. It has been well shown that the addition of spinal fusion is not preventive in most cases of discectomy and the routine decompression at multiple levels as practiced in the two decades following World War II, based on the presence of myelographic bulges, is no longer recommended.[38]

Recurrent Stenosis (Including Lateral Stenosis Secondary to Disc Space Collapse)

The incidence of disc space collapse following disc excision varies from 16% to 100%.[36, 40, 44, 85, 86] As a result of disc space narrowing and the development of secondary changes in the facets, recess stenosis may develop. The incidence is similar with respect to sex and occupation.[35, 86] Some authors[114] have related recurrent stenosis to the original size of the canal or to other structural problems.[103] Some patients develop symptoms of spinal stenosis which may be related to one or more roots. This usually occurs after a long period of relief of symptoms following the initial surgery. Patients are more likely to develop a lateral recess stenosis rather than a central or mixed stenosis. Frequently the cause is the excision of disc material in the presence of lateral stenosis. The latter may be recognized or not recognized. If a disc herniation is removed in the presence of lateral recess stenosis, the patient should be forewarned that there is a possibility of recurrence of symptoms. If the majority of the patient's symptoms appear to be the result of a disc herniation rather than the presence of associated stenosis, then in my opinion only the herniation should be dealt with.

Treatment.—Treatment should as far as possible be nonoperative including the use of nonsteroidal anti-inflammatory drugs, epidural blocks, and modification of activities. With failure of nonoperative treatment decompression is advocated.

Instability After Disc Excision

Back pain symptoms resulting from postoperative instability is said to occur in up to 10% of patients following disc excision.[27, 93, 109] The patients usually develop gradual onset of back pain which may occur months to years later. In my opinion this tends to be more common in patients who have had some degree of back pain prior to disc excision which was not thought to be significant by the treating surgeon and therefore not dealt with during otherwise appropriate postoperative care. Malcolm et al. reported an increased problem of instability following disc excision at the L4–5 level.[78] In my opinion, these patients are best dealt with by a prolonged conservative care program. The indications for spinal fusion are those for spinal fusion in general, namely, localized documented instability as evidenced by discography, facet blocks, and external skeletal fixation.[27, 92, 93]

Instability After Lumbar Decompression

The controversy over whether or not to add a fusion to a decompression for spinal stenosis still exists. As discussed in Chapters 9 and 31, sacrifice of 50% of both facets or complete sacrifice of a single facet significantly alters the motion segment kinematics.[99] I believe that decompression involving partial destruction of the facets on both sides at a single-level decompression often should be accompanied by fusion. If facets on one side are affected at two or more levels, then a fusion should also be added.

There is no doubt that postmenopausal women with some degree of osteoporosis are at greater risk of developing late instability. The patient in whom the disc heights are reasonably maintained, i.e., the younger patient, is also at greater risk of developing later instability following extensive lumbar decompression.[52] Levels proximal to L5–S1 disc space are more susceptible to later instability. The narrower the disc spaces and the greater the degree of degenerative changes (e.g., osteophyte formation), the less is the chance of developing late instability. Patients who have a degenerative spondylolisthesis and are only decompressed are at greater risk of developing late instability.

Treatment.—If instability has been demonstrated and confirmed by studies such as facet blocks, discography, the use of external fixation, or dynamic motion radiographs, then spinal fusion may be indicated. The ability to perform a spinal fusion in the presence of a previous extensive decompression may be difficult. The advent of pedicle fixation has, in my hands, improved the incidence of successful arthrodesis. If there have been multiple previous procedures, then an anterior fusion is preferred.[98]

FAILURES AFTER SPINAL FUSION

The early enthusiasm for lumbar spinal fusion as a treatment for low back pain with or without sciatica has decreased considerably because of the poor results. In the past 5 years, enthusiasm has again increased for a variety of reasons: the causes of failure have become better understood; new operative techniques, such as rigid internal fixation, have allowed fusion to be performed more predictably, and more difficult adult deformities can now be corrected; and new diagnostic tests such as MRI and discography have led to a better understanding of the causes of lumbar pain, particularly those associated with degenerative conditions. Although some of the diagnoses are still debated, e.g., "disc disruption," surgeons are treating them aggressively, and are demonstrating a greater percentage of good results.

At the same time, surgeons now are dealing with the late consequences of prior fusion, the treatment of which may require further stabilization. With the new developments there is an even greater need to understand the sources of failure that accompany spinal fusion, and how these problems can be managed when they appear.

In this section, I discuss the causes of failure after lumbar fusion, and the general approach to the patient with respect to history, physical examination, and useful imaging information. I then detail the causes of failure, how often they occur, how they are recognized, and how they are treated. Finally, an overview is given as to the methods by which good results may be obtained. Although spinal fusion is employed for a variety of pathologic conditions, this discussion focuses on failures which follow fusion for degenerative conditions.

A classification of failures after spinal fusion is shown in Table 33–4, in which failures are classified by time of appearance, as well as by the predominant symptoms. The importance of time of failure was emphasized by Finnegan et al.[29] in an analysis of failures of both decompression and fusion. When the patient has no immediate relief, the wrong diagnosis or the wrong operation should be suspected.

TABLE 33–4.

Causes of Failure After Spinal Fusion

Time of Appearance	Predominant Symptoms	
	Back Pain	Leg Symptoms
Early (weeks)	Infection	Nerve impingement by fixation devices or cement
Midterm (months)	Wrong level fused	
	Insufficient levels fused	
	Psychosocial distress	
	Pseudarthrosis	Fixation loose
	Disc disruption	
	Early adjacent disc degeneration	Early adjacent disc degeneration
	Inadequate reconditioning	
	Graft donor site	Graft donor site
Long term (years)	Late pseudarthrosis	Disc with pseudarthrosis
	Adjacent-level instability	
	Acquired spondylolysis	Adjacent-level stenosis
	Abutment syndrome	Adjacent-level disc
	Compression fracture above fusion	Stenosis above fusion

When the patient has immediate relief and then has recurrent symptoms within weeks to months following the operation, a new pathologic condition or a complication of the operation should be suspected. When the patient has good relief, and months to years later has recurrent symptoms, a new abnormality or progressing degeneration should be suspected. Table 33–4 organizes the causes of failures as a function of time after surgery.

It should be emphasized that reference is not made here to leg symptoms which relate to an original decompression performed in conjunction with a fusion, since this topic has been covered earlier. Rather, reference is to leg symptoms independent of the original abnormality, which in the case of prior fusion is more likely to suggest spinal stenosis rather than a single-level radiculopathy.

In addition to these general sources of failure, there are also specific systemic and local complications which follow spinal fusion. In some instances these complications may cause symptoms which are at times more devastating to the patient than the condition for which treatment was initially sought. These complications are detailed later in this chapter.

Approach to the Patient With Failure Following Fusion

A complete history and physical examination is essential, and historical records, operative reports, and imaging studies need to be reviewed. A history of never having pain relief from a previous operation strongly suggests the wrong preoperative diagnosis, the wrong operation, or the wrong patient, whereas, a long interval of relief and return to function followed by insidious onset of symptoms suggests a late degenerative lesion. Obviously, it the patient did not have relief, never returned to function, and had a long preoperative interval of disability, the possibility of psychosocial dysfunction should be strongly entertained. The physical examination rarely gives a precise diagnosis, particularly if the original surgery included a decompression. Limitation of spinal motion is a nonspecific symptom of failure rather than an observation identifying its causes.[36] Similarly, limitation of motion is frequently associated with psychosocial dysfunction, particularly in the patient who appears to have had the right operation and to have achieved a solid fusion. Leg symptoms should be carefully analyzed. If the patient had no leg symptoms and a normal neurologic examination prior to the first operation, and the current examination shows deficits, this is of major importance and suggests a high probability that there is new abnormality or complication due to a fixation device. If the patient had preoperative leg symptoms before the first operation, the neurologic findings are most likely residual, unless an entirely new set of objective deficits is present. If the patient has diffuse leg symptoms as part of the overall pain complaint, it is common for these to be localized to the graft donor site. However, the usual graft donor complaints seem to be highly associated with overall failure of symptomatic relief rather than due to a specific complication at the donor site.[37]

Psychological Testing

The psychosocial issues are of major importance in evaluating a patient with failed fusion, particularly those patients who have not had a pain-free interval and return to normal function prior to the new onset of symptoms.[2, 108]

Plain Radiography

Plain radiographs must be interpreted with care. In postoperative patients it is common to identify disc space narrowing and even excessive motions at the adjacent functional spinal segment. For example, a positive Knuttsen's sign is identified in 20% of patients at the L3–4 level in a fusion of L4 to the sacrum, but few have symptoms.[36] However, a number of radiographic signs are particularly useful: (1) the unequivocal presence of a pseudarthrosis; (2) a pars defect above a midline fusion, most commonly at the L3 lamina; and (3) an obvious failure of instrumentation with cutting out of devices attached to the lamina, or breakage of screws (a more subtle sign may be a halo around a pedicle screw, indicating motion in an apparently solid fusion).

Motion radiography is an important test in the identification of pseudarthrosis, as was emphasized by Bosworth and Cleveland in 1948.[11] Because some motion is common, particularly in a solid midline fusion, it is important to identify at least four degrees of motion before a pseudarthrosis can be strongly suspected.[36] The major difficulty lies in accurate centering and positioning of the patient for the flexion and extension views. Translation of 3 to 4 mm is diagnostic of abnormal motion.

Bone scintigraphy is rarely indicated, but is helpful on occasion in a patient suspected of having an infection, or occasionally when a pseudarthrosis is suspected, but the diagnosis is confirmed by flexion-extension films and tomography. Most spinal fusions show increased uptake up to 2 years following fusion, and significant "hot spots" within the general area of increased uptake or a localized area 2 years or more following fusion may be indicative of a pseudarthrosis (see Chapter 24).

CT Scans

The CT scan is invaluable in assessing the bony canal (see Chapter 19) and in one series is reported to demonstrate the cause of failure in 13% of cases, most of which were secondary to improper diagnosis prior to the first operation.[94] The test is particularly enhanced by the addition of myelographic dye, which remains the most sensitive method to identify spinal stenosis (see Chapter 22). In patients with apparent instability and stenotic symptoms, it is often helpful to obtain a flexion and extension view with the dye in place before proceeding to the CT scan. CT scans, especially if enhanced by myelographic dye, are valuable postsurgically for the assessment of canal content, but may easily miss a transverse pseudarthrosis if the cut is not at the appropriate level. These deficits may be overcome by three-dimensional CT. For example, Laasonen and Soini[64] studied 48 patients with a painful lumbosacral fusion by careful CT scanning. Sixteen patients had unsuspected fragmented grafts, and 9 had hairline pseudarthroses which may have caused their symptoms. Similarly, hypocycloidal frontal plane tomography was investigated by Dawson et al.[19] and revealed unsuspected pseudarthrosis in patients who had previous fusions for scoliosis. The imaging evidence for pseudarthrosis was later confirmed by surgical exploration. Pseudarthroses occur in two modes: (1) transverse and (2) plate pseudarthroses. The former is the traditional well-known form of pseudarthrosis. The latter is a failure of the graft material to unite with the underlying laminae or transverse processes, or both, despite the fact that the fusion mass, derived from the graft material, is solid.

Myeloscopy

Myeloscopy was initially believed to provide the answer to many of the problems of continued radicular pain following surgery. It has, however, not met with universal enthusiasm. In the country of its origin, the originator remains the only person participating in clinical trials. Its value may lie in the assessment of arachnoiditis.

Facet Blocks

The problem with facet blocks in a failed surgical case[82] is that the presence of scarring frequently inhibits an accurate infiltration and hence in the failed case it may be of limited value. It is of value in assessing levels proximal to a previous fusion. The local infiltration of anesthesia into a pseudarthrosis may help determine whether or not the pseudarthrosis is the cause of the patient's pain. Infiltration may be done into both anterior or posterior pseudarthroses. The infiltration of local anesthesia around internal fixation devices may help determine whether these are the cause of postoperative pain. However, the sensitivity and specificity of these techniques are unknown.

Discography

Discography can be used in two fashions: (1) to assess disc degeneration and (2) as a pain provocative test (see Chapter 21). As a method of assessing disc degeneration, MRI is valuable and, of course, is noninvasive. MRI is less sensitive in detecting the earliest disc changes such as annular tears.

Discography may be used to diagnose painful levels within an area of obvious disc degeneration as noted on plain radiographs, but is perhaps more reliably used in the discs proximal to obvious degenerative levels both to determine minor degrees of degeneration and as part of a pain provocative study.

Macnab[77] has stated that discography is valuable in determining whether posterior pseudarthrosis is the source of pain. He believed that reproduction of pain on discography at the suspected level of pseudarthrosis proved that the pseudarthrosis was the source of pain. I am not fully convinced of this. Technically, discography in the presence of a previously performed posterolateral fusion with or without pseudarthrosis may be difficult. We prefer to do discography from a posterolateral rather than a transdural approach.

In patients with previous surgery the use of discography may be of great value in the differentiation of pain. The patient with a previous fusion who continues to have pain but otherwise shows no evidence of psychosocial problems may have two sources of pain which can be diagnosed with the aid of discography. Firstly, levels proximal to a fusion can be evaluated. When the patient has had a previous fusion of L4 to the sacrum and presents with pain some time postoperatively, or many years postoperatively, the use of discography at levels above the fusion may help determine whether these are a source of subsequent or continuing pain.

Secondly, discography may be of value below the level of a previous fusion. In a small number of patients with continuing pain without psychosocial problems who radiographically on plain films, dynamic radiographs, and tomography show no evidence of pseudarthroses, subsequent pain was reproduced on discography.[118] A subsequent anterior procedure with disc excision and fusion and the addition of a bone graft despite the solid posterior fusion has resulted in relief of pain. We believe that these cases are examples of what Crock described as "internal disc derangement" (Figs 33–1 and 33–2).

Nachemson[84] has recently criticized discography. The reason given is that the outer part of the annulus has a multilevel nerve supply as does the dorsal longitudinal ligament. This may result in dif-

ficult and false interpretations. The criticism that previously normal pain-free patients may have pain from a discogram is not valid, since the point is whether or not the discogram reproduced the patient's typical pain in the same area and whether the pain was of the same quality. In a significantly degenerative disc as well, the application of pressure at the time of discography may not elicit pain. Since there are so many annular tears it is impossible to raise the intradiscal pressure to a degree sufficient to reproduce pain. In these instances the fluid medium used to inject and raise the pressure escapes too rapidly. There is no doubt that the injection of irritants at different sites of the motion segments can elicit back pain and leg pain.

Discography has, in our hands, helped us to dif-

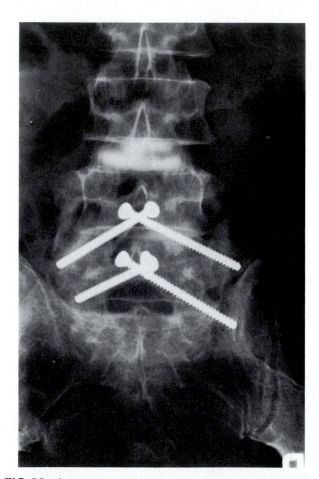

FIG 33–1.
A 53-year-old man, operated on for segmental instability of L4–S1. AO translaminar screws were used. Preoperative discography at L4–S1 and L5–S1 reproduced his pain. Postoperatively, pain persisted despite a solid fusion. Repeat discography at L4–5 reproduced his pain despite the solid fusion. An L3–4 discogram was normal. (Note: Same patient as in Fig 33–1.)

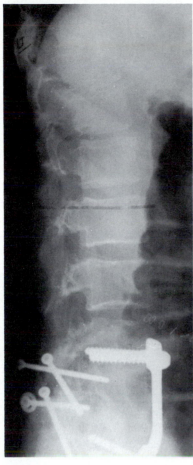

FIG 33–2.
Lateral view: Anterior L4–S1 interbody fusion (I-plate was added for fixation) relieved the pain. (Note: Same patient as in Fig 33–1.)

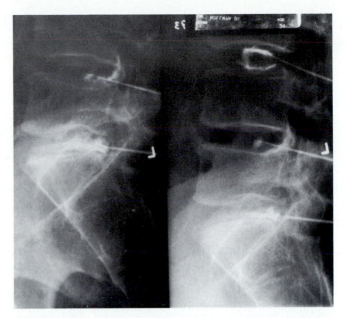

FIG 33–3.
This 39-year-old man presented with a 2-year history of disabling low-back pain. Plain films were unremarkable (except for a small traction spur). L4–5 was unstable on flexion-extension radiographs. Discograms were done. L3–4 was normal, L4–5 and L5–S1 were degenerate, and pain was reproduced on disc distention.

ferentiate the painful from the nonpainful levels and thereby has aided in the assessment of the number of levels requiring fusion. It has been of particular value in the failed back patient.

Use of External Fixation

Esses, Botsford, and Kostuik[27] recently compared preoperative testing with the AO external fixator (Figs 33–3 and 33–4), plain films, and discography in 30 patients with chronic low back pain. The clinical improvement with the use of rigid external fixation proved to be a good predictor of the results of posterior fusion in discography and pain reproduction by discography. However, this series was small and must be repeated with larger numbers. Although Esses et al.[27] have shown that external fixation may be a good predictor of outcome following spinal fusion, a similar study by Olerud[92, 93] did not come to the same conclusion. After initially report-

ing a success similar to that of Esses et al., further evaluation was less successful. This physical modality as a method of prediction of the outcome of a spinal fusion requires further evaluation.

Let us now look at the specific causes of failure which occur after lumbar spinal arthrodesis.

Causes of Early Failure

Infection

The rate of infection following lumbar surgery is variable. It depends on the era in which the operation was performed, the time of operation, history of prior surgery, the approach used, and the use of prophylactic antibiotics and instrumentation. Incidence rates ranging from less than 1% to greater than 10% have been reported. In general, the lower figures have been reported in the past decade. In 1966, Prothero et al.[96] reviewed 1,000 cases of midline and intertransverse process fusion and compared patient cohorts treated a decade apart. The operative indications were multiple; the overall infection rate of 3.4% was no different for the two time intervals. At about the same time, Freebody et al.[32] reported an incidence of wound infection of 3%. The highest rate of recently reported infection was 18% in patients treated with pedicle fixation, which was

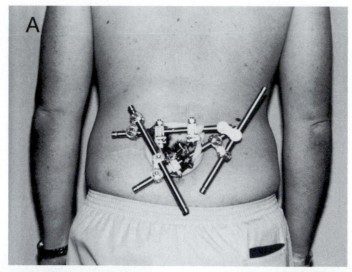

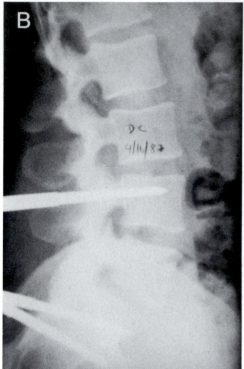
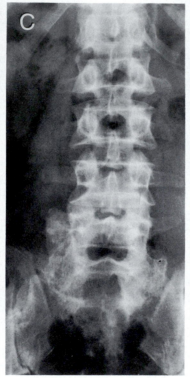
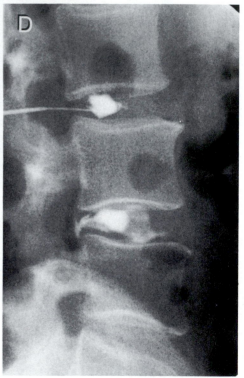

FIG 33–4.
A and **B,** a temporary external fixator was placed with relief of symptoms. **C,** the patient then underwent a two-level fusion of L4–S1. Despite a solid fusion, pain persisted. **D,** discograms done at L3–4 revealed a degenerative painful disc. L2–3 was normal. The fusion was extended one level and the pain was relieved. (Note: Same patient as in Fig 33–3.)

attributed to the long operative time which resulted from a steep learning curve, rather than to the use of instrumentation per se.[125] Others have noted a similar association and reached the same conclusion. Although there is no certain proof, Kostuik and Hall[61] believed that anterior fusion had a lower rate of infection than the posterior approach. In 100 anterior fusions performed for burst fractures, together with decompression and instrumentation, the authors noted one deep infection. In 67 cases of anterior fusion and instrumentation performed for degenerative disease or previous failed posterior surgery, no deep infections occurred.[58, 59] One deep infection occurred in 108 cases of anterior instrumentation and fusion for scoliosis. No infections occurred in 205 cases of kyphosis instrumented and fused anteriorly.

Whether this infection rate can be reduced by antibiotics is debatable. A generally accepted but not proven belief is that antibiotics are warranted with fusions, particularly if metallic devices are implanted. In an early retrospective and uncontrolled study, Fogelberg et al.[30] reported lower infection rates in both spine and hip surgery with the use of postoperative penicillin. In a similar uncontrolled study, Lonstein et al.[71] reported infection rates, respectively, of 2.8% with and 9.3% without antibiotics in patients treated for scoliosis with and without Harrington instrumentation. If antibiotics are employed for prophylaxis, a general body of basic and clinical research supports the drug being given preoperatively, intraoperatively, and for as little as 24 hours postoperatively. This teaching is opposed to the historical belief that antibiotics should be administered for longer postoperative intervals.

Presentation.—The classic time of presentation of deep wound infection is 5 to 7 days postoperatively. Rarely, infections are clinically observed in the first 24 hours. We have encountered one such patient with a streptococcal infection. The clue was a rapidly developing sore throat and a watery hematoma, suggesting bacteriologic fibrinolysis. Dependent on host immunologic competence and the virulence of the organism, the presentation ranges from high-grade fever and severe pain, to an indolent course, often accompanied by delay in diagnosis. Superficial signs may be notably absent in a large, muscular, or obese patient.

Treatment.—A superficial wound infection can be appropriately treated by antibiotics, and relief of any local wound tension, including drainage to the fascia. In deeper infections, the issue is whether or not to remove the instrumentation or graft, or both, and whether to debride and leave the wound open or debride and close the wound over suction drainage. This decision is dependent on the degree of sepsis, the condition for which the operation was performed, and the organism. In general, we have performed debridement, washed the bone graft, left the instrumentation in place, and closed the wound over suction drainage or a suction irrigation system. Exceptions to this general approach may be warranted when a gram-negative organism such as *Pseudomonas* is identified. Obviously, if the original indication was for severe spinal instability, particularly when associated with neurologic involvement, every effort should be made to retain the fixation device.

Wrong Level or Insufficient Number of Levels Fused

Patients with fusions at wrong or insufficient levels usually are only identified when a significant time interval has elapsed after the operation, although the failure of symptomatic relief is noticeable early. Often the postoperative symptoms are attributed to wound healing, and later, pseudarthrosis is often suspected. The most apparent source of failure of this type is when a surgeon fails to perform a fusion over the area of an obvious abnormality, which is equivalent to failure to decompress a known disc herniation. In the older literature, a common cause of failure was thought to occur when the surgeon overlooked two-level lumbar disc herniations when combined decompression and fusion was performed. It will be remembered that some clinical reviews indicate that two-level lesions occurred in up to 10% of patients.[86] For that reason, many reports stressed the importance of two-level decompressions, and fusion in all patients with suspected L5–S1 or L4–L5 disc herniations. Today's sophisticated imaging techniques make these earlier recommendations obsolete. However, this issue is more difficult when subtle pathologic conditions are being treated, such as disc disruption or degenerative scoliosis. Recommendation is made for performing discography at all lumbar levels, until a morphologically normal disc is identified and the patient has no pain reproduction. This is a controversial view. The use of MRI is also controversial in this regard; Zuckerman et al.[125] and Kornberg[57] each reported a small group of patients with normal MRIs that were later shown to have an unequivocally positive discogram.

In the older literature, the extent of the fusion was often based on the plain radiographic findings, such as disc space narrowing and osteophyte formation. When the primary indication was "lumbar disc disease," more than two-level degeneration was used as a contraindication to fusion of L4 to the sacrum. For this reason, many authorities believed a floating fusion at L4–5 should never be done. Fusion which involved L4–5 was thought to necessitate an L5–S1 fusion as well. However, Brodsky et al.[7] have shown that satisfactory results can be obtained with the floating fusion, provided the L5–S1 level is carefully analyzed. We have advocated that the extent of a fusion in complex degenerative conditions should be determined by preoperative facet blocks and discography, although the precise sensitivity and specificity of these tests have yet to be established. At this time there are no certain data which tell us how often missed levels cause failures of spinal fusion.

Presentation.—As previously noted, fusion at the wrong level is suspected only after a significant time delay in all but the most gross and obvious omissions. Back pain which fails to improve during the first 3 months would suggest this diagnosis, but frequently it is only when the fusion is solid that this type of failure is suspected. In these instances the differential diagnosis typically is pseudarthrosis, or the wrong patient was chosen. In the latter instance, the patient may be assumed falsely to have psychosocial or compensation issues which are the cause of symptoms.

Treatment.—Treatment is based on establishing that the fusion was inadequate in its extent, or that the wrong levels were fused. This decision necessitates the use of all of the preoperative analytic techniques outlined earlier in this chapter and in Section III.

Psychosocial Distress

The issues of psychosocial distress, compensation, and their effects on the incidence of later surgical failures need to be emphasized. The important time to identify these factors is before the operation, and not after it. Finnegan et al.[29] have stressed the importance of this. An analysis of entrants into rehabilitation programs also emphasizes the commonality of psychosocial distress and compensation in the etiology of fusion failures.[2] How commonly this failure occurs is uncertain. In one series where fusion was performed in conjunction with disc excision, 15% of patients had no obvious cause for their continued pain and disability.[36]

Early Failures: Nerve Root Impingement

Early failures due to preoperative misdiagnosis, intraoperative errors, or nerve root complications such as scarring which follow decompression are not included here. They were discussed earlier in this chapter. Today, the major cause of nerve root impingement which relates directly to fusion is usually the result of internal fixation devices, particularly those involving the pedicle. The most important insight into this problem is derived from the study of Weinstein's et al.[120] of screw misplacement. When experienced and inexperienced surgeons performed the operation in cadaver specimens (set up to simulate a real procedure including C-arm radiographic control), misplacement of the screws occurred in 21% of all pedicles, many of which were in close proximity to the nerve. The addition of methyl methacrylate to increase holding strength is an added risk factor for nerve damage, since thermal and mechanical damage can result.

This cause of failure also is observed in devices which depend on laminar fixation, and is usually due to a jumped hook. A particularly high rate of nerve root complications was noted with the Knodt rod. The problem usually occurs in the lumbosacral area, and necessitates rod removal in 20% to 50% of patients. In general, nerve root symptoms, when they occur with this device, are a late rather than early complication. Causes of nerve root impingement, specific to one or another fusion technique, include nerve root traction injury and graft extrusion. The incidence of graft extrusion with posterior lumbar interbody fusion varies. It was reported in 1 in 321 cases by Cloward,[12] in 4 in 500 cases by Lin,[68] and in 4 in 750 cases by Collis.[14] Lin[69] suggests an overall rate of 0.3% to 2.4%, but for inexperienced operators, the rate is a "disturbing" 9.0%. The rate of nerve root damage is less certain although Lin[69] noted a temporary dropped foot in 25 of 5,000 patients (0.005%), of whom all but 3 recovered in 6 months. With posterior fusion techniques, neurologic deficit or pain may occasionally result from graft material becoming dislodged, or from an unrecognized fracture of a facet, producing a fragment which causes nerve impingement. How often this occurs is unknown, but it is probably rare.

Presentation.—The diagnosis is most suspect in patients who have had no preoperative nerve root symptoms, but who early after their surgery have neurologic deficit or radicular pain. More difficult is a patient who had nerve involvement, a decompression in combination with the fusion, and in whom the postoperative picture is that of increased deficit or pain. In these instances, the differential diagnosis is difficult, as detailed earlier in this chapter. The diagnosis is also complicated because of the presence of metal which may make imaging techniques such as MRI impossible, or CT scans difficult to interpret because of image scatter. In these cases, it may be necessary to resort to polytomal tomography, with or without myelographic enhancement, although when the screw misplacement or fixation displacement is obvious, plain radiographs will suffice (see Fig 33–5).

These same diagnostic issues also come into play when later nerve root symptoms occur. Assuming the nerve root compression is within the area en-

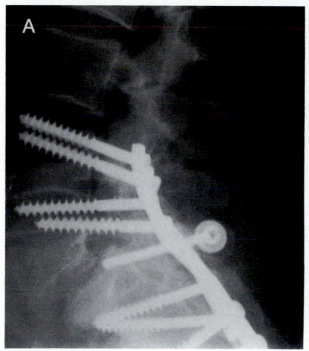
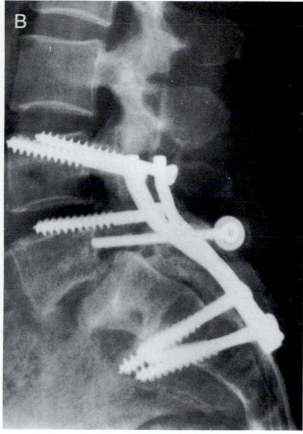

FIG 33–5.

A, a 42-year-old woman with grade II L5–S1 spondylolisthesis. Discography revealed a typically painful L4–5 disc. Facet blocks at L4–S1 relieved the pain. Arthrodesis was done using contoured AO-DCP plates and screws. One screw missed the L5 pedicle resulting in root pain, while two screws appear to be in the disc space of L4–5. The screw with the washer is a translaminar screw used to hold the lamina in place following laminaplasty. **B,** the screw was removed and symptoms abated. A solid fusion was obtained. The sacral screws are in the ala and thus appear too long in the lateral projection, while one L4–5 screw remains in the disc space.

compassed by the fusion, displacement of the fixation device should be considered. Usually, when this occurs, there may be obvious clues from plain radiography, i.e., a jumped hook, or the diagnosis may be suspected by the presence of a radiolucent "halo" around one or more portions of the device.

Treatment.—Dependent on the magnitude of symptoms and the neurologic deficits, the options range from doing nothing until the fusion is mature, to immediate removal in more severe cases, and replacement of the screw or placement of an alternative fixation device.

Midterm Failures: Back Pain Predominant

Pseudarthrosis

Pseudarthrosis is the most common cause of failure in spinal fusion. It is also the most difficult to es-

tablish as the source of failure, because many patients will have radiographic evidence of fusion failure with no symptoms.[20, 36] Conversely, repair of a pseudarthrosis often will not result in symptomatic relief. For example, one long-term follow-up study of patients that had undergone repeat fusion demonstrated satisfactory results in only 60% of the patients who had repair of a pseudarthrosis.[38] It is, however, anticipated that today, with better means of internal fixation, this will be improved upon. The calculation of the rate of pseudarthrosis is highly variable and dependent on the following factors: (1) the number of levels fused; (2) the fusion technique, including both the type (i.e., anterior interbody, midline posterior, etc.), as well as the presence or absence of internal fixation; (3) the source of bone graft; (4) the underlying pathologic condition for which the fusion was performed; (5) constitutional and other factors such as age and possibly sex of the patients, and smoking; (6) the type of external protection afforded the patient; and (7) the radiographic criteria utilized to assess for the presence or absence of pseudarthrosis. These issues are mentioned to emphasize that the rate of pseudarthrosis cannot be calculated unless full knowledge is present of the relevant variables which influence its occurrence. In posterior surgery a one-level fusion usually bears an incidence of pseudarthrosis of 5%. For two levels, this may increase to as high as 20%, and for three or more levels, to 40% or greater in fusions performed to the sacrum.[74]

In anterior surgery, the incidence of pseudarthrosis for one- or two-level anterior fusions is in the area of 20%. Given the current state of internal fixation devices, no clear statistics are available as to the incidence of pseudarthrosis. This is particularly true for failed back surgery. Jacobs et al.[51] have recently shown that with the use of AO translaminar screw fixation (see Figs 33–1 and 33–6) the incidence of pseudarthrosis is approximately 5%. These were in previously unfused patients. Kostuik and Enrico,[60] in a review of operations with internal fixation devices used to treat various causes of low back pain, showed that with the use of Luque sublaminar wires and ¼-in. Luque rods, the incidence of pseudarthrosis in lumbosacral fusion at three or more levels was about 15% (Fig 33–7). This study was done prospectively in a consecutive series. This was a significant decrease from 40% without internal fixation.

Kostuik et al.[58] reported an 18% incidence of pseudarthrosis in a series of 56 patients who had previously undergone unsuccessful posterior spinal fusion when anterior fusion was used with the aid of internal fixation devices. The fixation devices initially included the single-cable Dwyer or single-rod Zielke systems which were subsequently replaced by double-rod systems. When double-rod systems alone are analyzed, the incidence of pseudarthrosis decreased to 9%. Current improved methods of anterior fixation should lower this even more.

Clinical Presentation.—The clinical presentation of pseudarthrosis is highly variable, and ranges from no symptoms to significant persisting and disabling back pain.[20, 36] Rarely should pain be ascribed to a pseudarthrosis until a 6-month interval has elapsed, and even then, continued motion may not necessarily indicate that the fusion is a failure. For that reason, we usually do not consider a fusion to be a failure until 1 year has elapsed. Exceptions are when there are obvious reasons to make that conclusion, such as graft dislodgment, or an obvious failure of fixation. Frequently a pseudarthrosis will remain undetectable for years. In our opinion, no fusion is solid until 2 years have elapsed. Because pseudar-

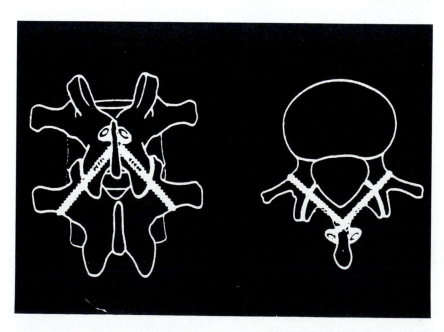

FIG 33–6.
AO translaminar screw technique: 4.5-mm cortical screws are used. Facets are denuded with a burr or curette of articular cartilage, and packed with cancellous bone graft. The laminae and transverse processes are decorticated with a burr. The screws aim for the base of the transverse process. (See also Fig 33–1.)

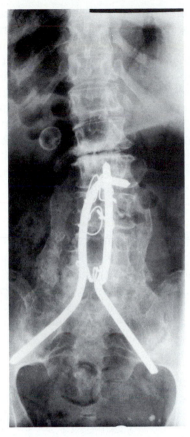

FIG 33–7.
This 48-year-old woman underwent an L3–S1 fusion using Luque rods and sublaminar wires. She did well for 10 years but developed mild back pain and degenerative changes above her fusion at L2–3.

throsis can be asymptomatic, it is important to evaluate patients for other sources of continued or recurrent symptoms. The strategies which have been used to determine a symptomatic pseudarthrosis were presented earlier in this chapter.

Treatment.—Because pseudarthrosis frequently accompanies other causes of failure, we consider treatment of this condition later in this chapter.

Disc Disruption

This issue has been discussed in general under the heading of wrong diagnosis. However, there is a small subset of patients who achieve a solid arthrodesis, yet have continuing symptoms. This usually occurs when the first operation has been a posterior fusion and the continuance or onset of new symptoms occurs in the face of a solid fusion. Biomechanical studies have suggested that an apparently continuous graft may nevertheless allow continued

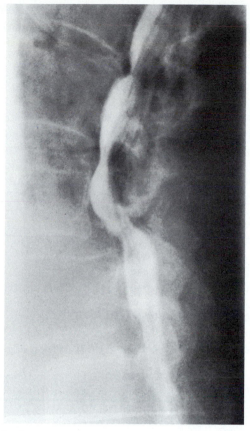

FIG 33–8.
An L5–S1 fusion performed 2 years previously. The patient developed a degenerative slip 18 months later. An acute disc sequestration was found in addition to the spondylolisthesis at L4–5. The fusion was extended to L4 with internal fixation following decompression.

deflections of a magnitude sufficient to cause symptoms.[65, 99, 124] In these instances, discography may be employed to determine the diagnosis, although this may be technically difficult because of obstructing bone between the transverse processes.

Treatment.—If a solid posterior fusion is present, the obvious solution is an anterior interbody technique. If "disc disruption" is part of the presentation of a pseudarthrosis, then anterior fusion or circumferential fusion, with or without instrumentation, may be considered (see Figs 33–1 and 33–2).

Early Adjacent Degeneration

Rarely does degeneration cause symptoms in the months which follow spinal fusion in a segment which was normal prior to operation. The exception may be in cases in which rigid internal fixation or possible circumferential fusion has been performed.

Hsu et al.[50] have reported accelerated degeneration with internal fixation, while Dewar[23] reported this complication occurring with circumferential fusion. This led him to abandon the technique.

Presentation.—The typical presentation of degeneration adjacent to a fusion is discussed later in this chapter, but it is important to stress here that the single unequivocal indication of accelerated degeneration is a new disk herniation at the level adjacent to the fusion (see Fig 33–8). More common is the development of disc degeneration without herniation, resulting in instability (Figs 33–8 and 33–9).

Treatment.—Treatment is identical to that for late degeneration and is presented therewith.

Graft Donor Site Problems

This issue is discussed later in this chapter.

Inadequate Reconditioning

There is very little data to establish how often patients are inadequately reconditioned. However, it must be a common problem, based on our clinical experience. Very often patients are referred either because they are thought to have an anatomic failure of fusion, or because they are thought to have psychosocial or compensation factors interfering with their recovery. Where those problems leave off and inadequate conditioning enters in less relevant than the knowledge that the two often go hand in hand. Frequently, the patients have had a long period of disability and deconditioning prior to the first operation, complicated by the fact that posterior fusion techniques denervate the paraspinal muscles.

Clinical Presentation.—Continued back pain, particularly pain which increases with physical activity (i.e., mechanical pain), must be suspected in all patients as a source of failure, unless the cause is obvious and anatomic. Thus, pseudarthrosis cannot be considered the source of symptoms until adequate physical rehabilitation has occurred without successful resolution of symptoms.

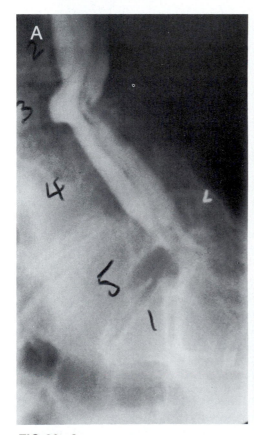
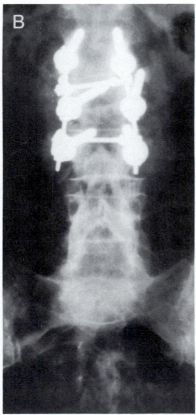
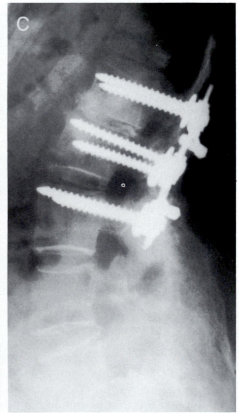

FIG 33–9.
A, this 58-year-old woman had spinal fusion 18 years previously. Myelogram demonstrates flow defects proximal to the fusion (L2–3) with retrolisthesis at L2–3 and L1–2. **B** and **C,** the fusion was extended to L1 with instrumentation (Zielke). Symptoms were relieved.

Treatment.—It can be argued that a chronically debilitated patient can be returned to function solely by outpatient physical therapy or by a work-hardening program. If these methods are chosen, the operating surgeon must take an active role in monitoring the program, and establishing a time-limited goal. Too often, a patient will continue month after month with a combination of inadequate reconditioning and emphasis on conservative modalities. General principles would suggest that a more intensive, multidisciplinary rehabilitation is appropriate in those patients who fail to respond to less structured programs. The surgeon constantly finds himself in the dilemma of when to repeat all studies and consider reoperation vs. continuing the rehabilitation program. There is no certain guideline other than the general principle that the more certain the anatomic cause of pain, the more reasonable is surgical intervention; the less certain, the greater the reason to continue a nonoperative approach.

Long-Term Failures

Late Pseudarthrosis

The general issues in pseudarthrosis have already been presented. It is uncommon for a patient who has previously had symptomatic relief to present after 1 year with pain due to a pseudarthrosis. There are two general exceptions: the first is a disc herniation under a fusion. In a follow-up study of minimum 10 years' duration and an average follow-up of 13.7 years, Frymoyer[35] found that no patient with a solid fusion had a disc herniation. Of 23 patients who required a second operation, 13 required fusion for back pain only, 4 for a recurrent disc herniation at the same level as their previous surgery, and 1 who had a new herniation at a new level, under the fusion. All patients with new or recurrent herniation had a pseudarthrosis. Thus, a patient presenting with a disc herniation under a fusion must be highly suspect of having an accompanying pseudarthrosis. A less certain source of failure is in a patient who had spinal fusion, and who later presents with symptoms and findings indicative of arachnoiditis. In this situation, it is less certain that the increasing symptoms can be alleviated by repair of the pseudarthrosis.

Treatment.—The principles are the same as for the previously detailed treatment of pseudarthrosis. Obviously, if a disc herniation accompanies the pseudarthrosis, the disc must be decompressed.

Adjacent Motion Segment Degeneration

Segments adjacent to a previously performed lumbar fusion are at risk for the development of a variety of later degenerative changes. These may either be asymptomatic or symptomatic, and may include the clinical and radiographic features of segmental instability, degenerative spinal stenosis, or lumbar disc herniation.[5, 66] These changes are four times more likely to occur at L4–5 (20%) when the original fusion was performed at L5–S1 for a degenerative condition than at L3–4 when the original fusion spanned L4 to the sacrum where the rate of failure is 4% to 5%.[36] Similarly, when the fusion was performed for thoracolumbar deformities, the magnitude of symptomatic degeneration increased the lower into the lumbar spine the original fusion was extended.[13, 46, 73, 80]

The dominant reasons for these degenerative changes are mechanical (see Chapters 6 and 9). Fusions cause increased stresses on adjacent segments, as measured experimentally and in humans with biplanar radiography.[65, 99, 110] Inadvertent damage to facets or denervation may be contributory.

Asymptomatic Degeneration

Asymptomatic degenerative changes may include osteophyte formation, disc space narrowing, hypermobility with or without translation (i.e., a positive Knuttson's sign), and spinal stenosis. A comparison of plain radiographic findings in patients treated with and without fusion 10 or more years after their operation is shown in Table 33–5. This table demonstrates the high rate of degenera-

TABLE 33–5.

Comparison of Plain Radiographic Findings in Fusion and Nonfusion Patients*

Variable	Fusion Patients (%)	Nonfusion Patients (%)	Significance
Traction spurs, L3–L4	14.3	34.3	$0.01 > P < .025$
Traction spurs, L4–L5	8.1	19.4	$0.01 > P < .025$
Traction spurs, L3–L4	50.0	22.5	$P = .005$
Facet subluxation, L1–L2	70.8	45.0	$0.01 > P < .025$
Facet subluxation, L3–L4	82.8	84.0	$P = .025$

*Adapted from Frymoyer JW, et al: *Spine* 1979; 4:435–440.

tive changes. These were usually unrelated to symptoms. Traction spurs above the fusion were more common in men with physically demanding jobs. Hypermobility was also more common in this group. A subsequent study by Lehman et al.[66] in 1987 analyzed patients 30 or more years after fusion, and included CT studies as part of the radiologic evaluation. Almost 50% of patients had radiographic evidence of segmental instability or spinal stenosis, or both. Again, these radiographic findings in general were unrelated to symptoms. The authors found that 85% of patients were satisfied with their outcome 30 or more years after their spinal fusion.

Because there is a high incidence of radiographic changes, the most difficult clinical task is to determine if the level above the fusion is causing symptoms in a patient who has back pain alone. In these instances, discography is the procedure of choice, in our opinion. If segmental instability is present, without an actual fixed deformity such as a new degen-erative spondylolisthesis, the problem is complex. In these instances discography, and possibly facet blocks, may again be useful to determine if the lesion is symptomatic.

Spinal Stenosis

The diagnostic problem becomes significantly easier if the patient has peripheral symptoms of claudication (Fig 33–10). Brodsky[5] in particular has stressed that this is the most common cause of recurrent symptoms after a fusion. Although he reported a large number of cases, it was impossible from his study to determine the actual incidence of this late cause of failure.

Disc Herniation

This is the easiest problem to diagnose with certainty, because the clinical symptoms, physical findings, and confirmatory images are typical. How often true disk herniation occurs varies widely. In the

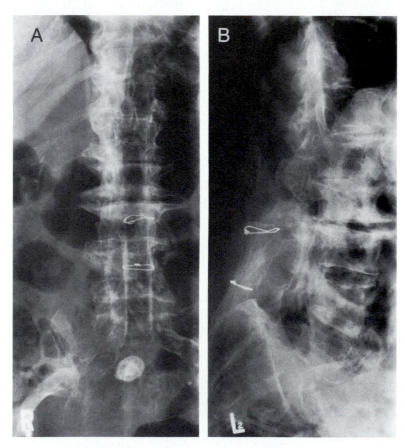

FIG 33–10.
A and **B,** this 76-year-old woman had a three-level midline tibial graft fusion 35 years previously with an excellent result. Subsequently the patient became paraparetic with grade I–II power and loss of bowel and bladder control. Preoperative myelogram (**C** and **D**) and CT (**E**) demonstrate a complete block with very severe spinal stenosis at the level immediately proximal to the fusion. One year following decompression, she walks with one cane and has complete bowel and bladder control.

(Continued.)

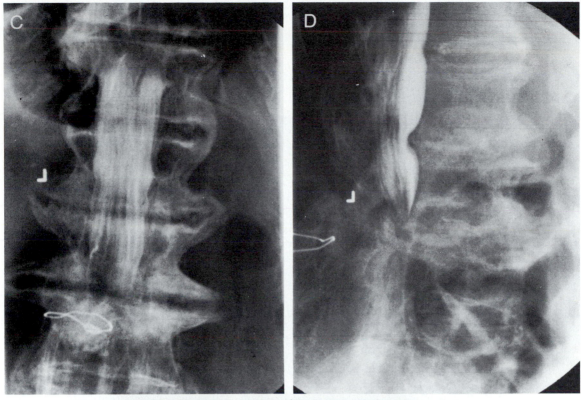

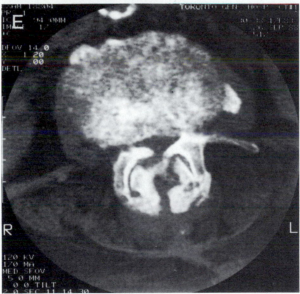

FIG 33-10 (cont.).

10-year study by Frymoyer et al.,[35] the rate of disc herniations at L3–4 in fusions from L4 to the sacrum was 4%, which is similar to that reported by De-Palma and Rothman.[20]

Treatment.—Treatment of failures above a fusion is largely based on the pathologic findings, but in our opinion should usually include an extension of the spinal fusion, combined with appropriate decompression based on the preoperative symptoms, physical findings, and radiologic images. In general, the accompanying fusion should include instrumentation, particularly when the segment is unstable. However, selected cases may be appropriately

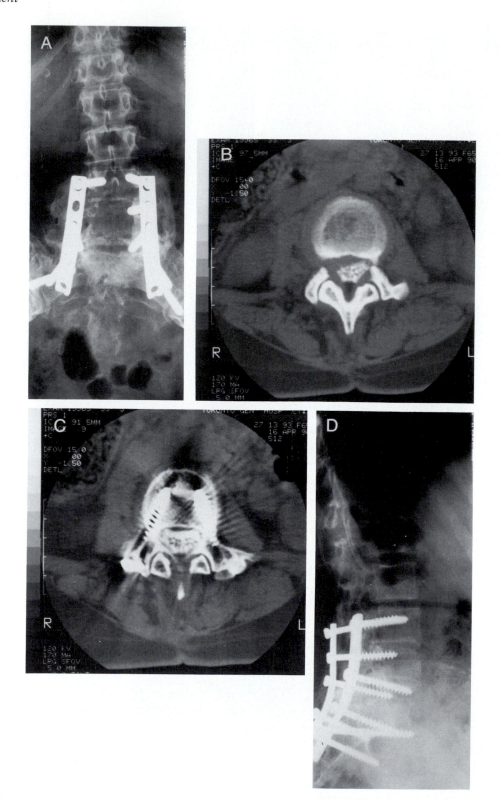

FIG 33–11.
A, this 67-year-old woman had prior decompression of L4–5 and L5–S1. She presented with a solid arthrodesis, but recurrent back and leg pain. Myelographically enhanced CT scans demonstrate a disc herniation at L3–4 **(B)**. The level below **(C)** demonstrates well-placed pedicle screws and a normal canal. **D,** decompression revealed a sequestrated disc. A fusion supplemented by plates was performed with symptom relief (lateral view).

treated by posterior fusion techniques, or anterior interbody fusions with instrumentation (Fig 33–11).

Spinal Stenosis Under A Fusion.

This problem is almost exclusively a problem with posterior midline fusions. Macnab[77] thought it occurred in 20% of all patients treated previously with that technique, but later Brodsky's[5] clinical experience suggested this was a significant overestimate of the problem. His opinion is supported by the finding of Lehman et al.,[66] that a stenotic appearance was common under a midline fusion many years after the operation, but rarely were symptoms of spinal stenosis present. The presumed cause is hypertrophy of the graft over time in response to Wolff's law. Stenosis has never been reported as occurring beneath a fusion performed in adolescence or adult life for scoliosis. The majority of cases reported by Macnab[77] had their fusions done prior to the common recognition of the spinal stenosis syndrome. Thus, it is quite possible that they had spinal stenosis prior to their fusion (Fig 33–12).

Clinical Presentation.—The condition is suspected in a patient with longstanding midline posterior fusion, insidious and progressive onset of symptoms of spinal stenosis, and imaging studies which demonstrate the absence of significant stenosis above the fusion, and a significant stenosis beneath it.

Treatment.—The treatment is decompression. This is made difficult by the massive amount of bone which overlies the lamina, the inability to identify the old lamina, and by frequently associated scar. In very difficult cases, it may be necessary to go to the next level to identify tissue planes, and move back from that level. In that event, the fusion should be

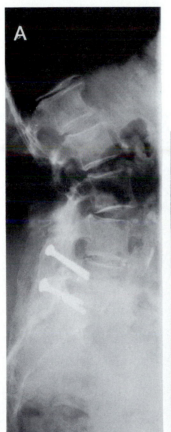
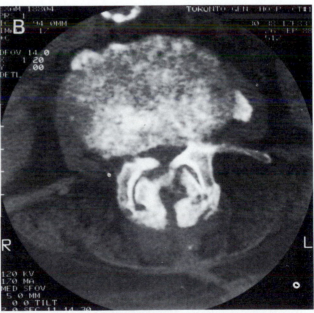

FIG 33–12.
A, this 51-year-old man underwent a two-level fusion 21 years previously. He later developed symptoms of spinal stenosis. A myelogram-CT from L2–L4 was done only and demonstrates stenosis. He underwent decompression of L3–4 with only partial relief of his symptoms. **B,** a repeat myelographically enhanced CT scan shows full decompres-sion at L2–4, but at L4–L5 spinal stenosis persists. A further decompression was done with improvement. It is anticipated that the instability at L2–3 and L3–4 may increase and require stabilization, which ideally should have been done at the time of the L2–4 decompression.

extended, unless the level is anatomically normal, and minimal bone sacrifice is necessary.

Late Causes of Failure

Acquired Spondylolysis

This is almost exclusively a late cause of failure of posterior midline fusions and is reported in 0% to 2.5% of patients treated by that technique[8, 36, 45, 97, 100, 113] (Fig 33–13). The cause is thought to be secondary to repetitive mechanical forces, and can be produced in the laboratory, after simulated posterior midline fusions.[99] Weakening of the neural arch by overzealous decortication, or possibly by interference with the blood supply, has also been suggested.[77] It has been rarely reported with transverse process fusion.[3]

Treatment.—The treatment is stabilization and fusion by anterior interbody or posterior intertransverse process fusion, with or without instrumentation.

Abutment Syndrome

This complication was noted in the early literature regarding posterior midline fusions[11] and has been reported in more recent literature to be an overlooked source of failure, particularly when the facets are involved.[17, 111] The cause is either overzealous initial graft placement, or later hypertrophy. The condition may be considered when motion pain occurs, particularly in extension, and radiographs show a large midline fusion mass, usually at L4, abutting on the spinous process of L3. Diagnostic anesthetic injections can be employed to confirm the diagnosis. Surgical management may include excision of the abutment, or extension of the fusion to the next adjacent level.

Graft Donor Site Problems

The graft donor site may be a source of problems in general, while specific donor sites are associated with unique complications, particularly nerve entrapments.

Pain

Graft donor site pain is a common complaint of all patients, particularly in the early postoperative phase. How long the pain persists is debatable. Kurz et al.[63] state it is common in up to 15% in the first 3 months. However, a long-term study[37] reported

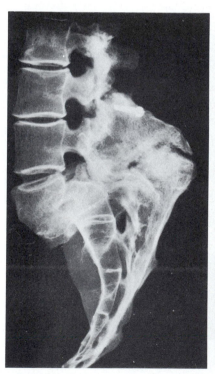
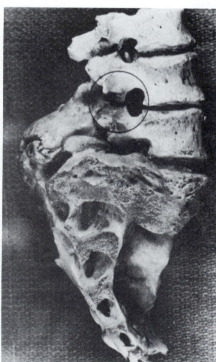
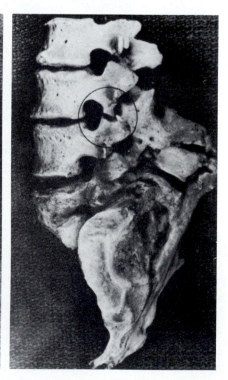

FIG 33–13.
Acquired spondylolysis above a fusion. This patient underwent an L4–S1 fusion for a severe spondylolisthesis when she was a young woman. She did well but later in life developed breast cancer and died. At autopsy the spine was harvested. A pseudoarthrosis at L4–5 was found plus an acquired spondylolysis at L3–4 which was not present initially. (Courtesy of the late Dr. R.I. Harris.)

that 37% of the patients had donor site pain 10 or more years after their operation. Statistical analysis made it uncertain if the pain was actually related to the donor site or was part of a general pain syndrome. When donor site pain was present, it was more common if the graft had been taken from the same side as the original sciatica, and there is a high association between persisting back pain, leg pain, and donor site pain. These complaints occurred independent of any radiographic changes, such as degeneration, that occurred at the donor site. A positive Trendelenburg's sign was seen in 18% of patients but appeared to be independent of the donor site.

Specific Complications

Specific complications can occur. Those which are painful and require later treatment include sacroiliac disruption, when the graft is from the posterior iliac crest, hernias in both anterior and posterior grafts, and fracture at the graft donor site, typically when the graft is taken from the anterior ilium. Heterotopic bone formation has also been thought to occasionally cause local pain, although in a long-term study, the presence of heterotopic bone bore little relationship to symptoms.[37] Sacroiliac instability occurs rarely, and is rarely included in large series as a significant complication. Fractures are usually an avulsion of the anterior wing of the ilium, and may necessitate internal fixation. Fractures extending into the acetabulum have been alluded to in the literature.[15]

Similarly, hernias are an infrequent complication and usually related to full-thickness grafts. Bosworth described this complication in posterior iliac graft donor sites, as well as a technique for its repair.[4]

Infection

The donor site as a local source of infection is reported by Kurz et al.[63] to be less than 1%.

Nerve Pain

Bone graft incisions may cause peripheral nerve injury, or later nerve symptoms may result from entrapments secondary to scar or occasionally heterotopic bone formation. The classic site is in the anterior iliac, where involvement of the lateral femorocutaneous nerve produces meralgia paresthetica. This complication is reported in 1% to 14% of patients.[119] Even more rarely, other cutaneous nerves such as the ilioinguinal, genitofemoral, or the femoral nerve may become involved.[15, 63, 105]

In posterior grafting, the cluneal nerves are most commonly involved (Fig 33–14). To avoid this problem, we advocate not using an incision over the crest which extends more than one handbreadth. A hockey stick incision, or tunneling procedure, or longitudinal incision is used as a method to avoid this problem. Drury[24] suggested that the diagnosis of cluneal nerve neuroma could be made by local anesthetic injections, and that resection of the neuroma could relieve that symptom.

In addition, a variety of more dramatic complications may include hemorrhage, particularly from gluteal arteries in posterior iliac grafts, and even visceral injuries.

General Complications

Table 33–6 lists the array of complications that have been associated with lumbar spinal fusions, some of which are specific to a particular technique, and others of which are generic.

Surgical Treatment

Because there are so many different causes for failure after spinal fusion, the operative choices are numerous and must be carefully selected. Again, the general principle applies: the more certain the history, physical examination, and imaging studies, the more likely is success. In general, the most predictable results will be achieved in patients with leg symptoms rather than with low back pain alone. Alternatively, uncertainty about diagnosis will predictably lead to less certain results, particularly in patients with longstanding disability and psychosocial dysfunction. In this regard, pseudarthrosis is one of the most difficult conditions to assess as a source of symptoms, and not surprisingly the outcome from repair of pseudarthrosis is the most difficult to predict.

It should also be evident that the second, third, or even fourth operation introduces additional risks, including higher rates of infection and lower rates of successful fusion, as well as specific problems related to scarring, and devascularization of bone and soft tissues.

A few general principles of surgical treatment are useful. They are categorized by the type of previous surgery performed.

Failed Previous Posterior Surgery

When adequate bone stock is present, the patient may again be approached posteriorly, particularly when a new level of abnormality is present which necessitates decompression and a new or repeat fusion. We believe that refusion in general should be accom-

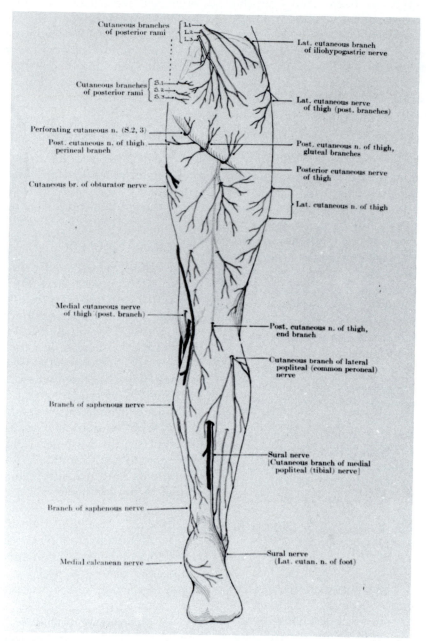

FIG 33–14.
The cluneal nerves pass over the iliac crest approximately 8 cm from the posterior iliac spine.

TABLE 33–6.

Complications Associated with Spinal Fusions

Local	General
Posterior	
Early	
Hemorrhage	Blood transfusion readings
Ecchymoses	Hemolysis
Wound dehiscence	Anemia
Neurologic	Urinary retention
Laminar fracture	Sepsis
Pedicle fracture	Metabolic
Sepsis	Psychosis
Vascular (anterior)	Drug overdose
Iliac crest fracture	Hypotension
Anterior	
Early	
Hemorrhage	Cholecystitis
Vascular (vessel)	Pancreatitis
Ureteric damage	
Renal damage	
Splenic damage	
Bowel damage	
Sympathetic disruption	
Iliac crest hemorrhage	
Iliac crest fracture	
Wound dehiscence	
Sepsis	
Graft extrusion	
Intermediate	
Wound sepsis	
Fracture at fixation points	
Instrumentation failure	
Vascular aneurysm	
Retroperitoneal fractures	
Ureteric obstruction	
Hydronephrosis	
Incisional hernia	
Iliac crest fracture	
Nerve irritation secondary to donor site	
Late	
Late sepsis	
Instrumentation failure	
Donor site problems	
Retroperitoneal fibrosis	
Ureteric obstruction	
Hydronephrosis	
Vascular aneurysm	
Incisional hernia	

panied by the use of internal fixation, of which pedicle screw devices seem to be the most useful (Fig 33–15). If the decompression required is wide, and involves additional facet sacrifice, serious consideration should be given to a second-stage anterior procedure. This need is particularly evident if there is inadequate bone stock for fusion, or rigid posterior fixation cannot be obtained (Fig 33–16).

Failed Previous Posterior Surgery with Wide Laminectomy

If decompression is not necessary, and stabilization is the major objective, this is best obtained with an anterior fusion. The presence of a wide laminectomy usually leaves inadequate bone stock for posterior repeat fusion, particularly when there is extensive scarring and a poor blood supply (Figs 33–17, 33–18, and 33–19).

Failure of Two or More Previous Posterior Fusions

Under these circumstances an anterior fusion is indicated to achieve stability. Whether this is accompanied by anterior instrumentation will depend on the number of levels, as well as the specific levels, and the assessment of whether stability might be achieved without instrumentation (Fig 33–20).

Failure of Previous Anterior Surgery

If there has been previous anterior surgery, and a resultant pseudarthrosis, a posterior approach with internal fixation is the method of choice. However, patients who have had both prior anterior and posterior surgery are again better approached anteriorly. In either event, it is advisable to insert stents up both ureters to prevent inadvertent cutting of these structures, which are at risk because of retroperitoneal scarring. Even though the ureters still may be cut, the complication is easier to recognize and repair with the stents in place.

It is also important to realize that the additional retroperitoneal scarring caused by the new procedures may result in urinary tract obstruction. Fortunately, this complication is rare. However, repeat anterior surgery in the lumbosacral area, in particular, has a definite risk of vascular complications, involving both venous and arterial structures. The surgeon must be prepared to deal with the consequences of the injuries. It is also prudent to consider postoperative anticoagulation therapy, because of an increased risk of thromboembolism.

Combined Procedures—Anterior and Posterior Surgery

The selection of patients for a combined procedure is of increasing interest. As already noted, this approach is indicated when a posterior approach is mandated for decompression, but where prior decompression and fusion have left inadequate bone stock either for a fusion bed or for the insertion of

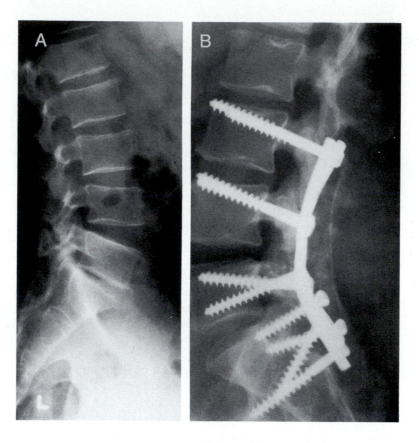

FIG 33–15.
A, this 42-year-old man underwent an L4–S1 intertransverse fusion without instrumentation 2 years previously. A pseudoarthrosis at L4–5 was believed to account for the persistent pain. **B,** a fusion at L3–S1 was performed using AO plates. Preoperatively a discogram also revealed problems at L3–4. Pseudoarthroses were found at L4–5 and L5–S1. The patient had good posterior bone stock and has gone on to solid fusion.

posterior fixation devices. The stumps of the pedicles, if they remain, are a possible site for insertion of a pedicle screw.

Frequently, extensive scarring and devascularization make the posterior fusion alone unlikely to succeed, and the combined anteroposterior approach is utilized (Figs 33–16, 33–20, 33–21, and 33–22).

A second indication is in cases where there is significant loss of lumbar lordosis from previous surgery. The problems of the iatrogenic flat back deformity must be considered here. The anterior procedure is used to mobilize the disc spaces, which are then filled with morselized bone. Internal fixation is contraindicated. A second-stage posterior procedure is performed for the correction of the deformity by posterior osteotomy and instrumentation to re-create the lordosis. If a pseudarthrosis is present, this may be used in lieu of the osteotomy, but this usually requires widening to achieve the necessary correction.

We do not feel that circumferential fusion is indicated for primary, unoperated-on patients with the possible exception of some cases of degenerative spondylolisthesis or in patients requiring four or more levels of fusion to the sacrum, as noted in surgery for adult scoliosis.[61]

Posterior Lumbar Interbody Fusion

The use of posterior lumbar interbody fusion in itself is controversial because of a high risk of neurologic injury, graft extrusion, and the inability to obtain an adequate rate of fusion, even in primary cases. The major problem is the wide exposure necessary to obtain placement of the grafts, which the critics of the procedure believe results in unusual scarring. However, proponents of the procedure believe that this complication is avoidable.[104]

We believe that in previous failed fusion, the role of posterior lumbar interbody fusion is extremely limited because of the technical problems which are encountered as one approaches the dense scar that is often present. If an interbody fusion is necessary, we believe that the anterior route is preferable, but not everybody agrees.

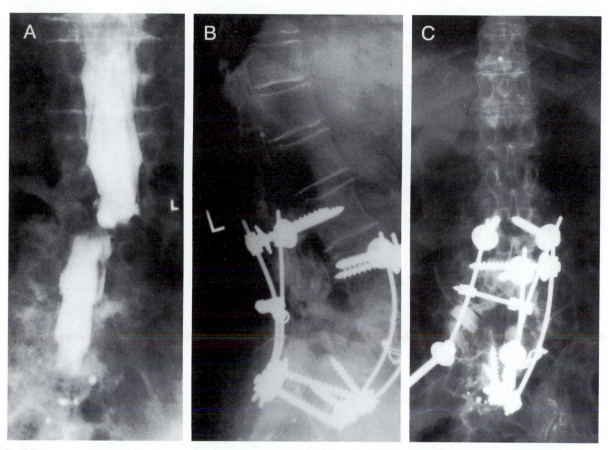

FIG 33–16.
A, a 68-year-old woman. Six previous procedures had been performed including attempts at instrumentation using Harrington rods. Severe sepsis had occurred on one occasion. The patient was paraparetic, in a wheelchair. Note the translation of the dye column on myelography. **B** and **C,** a two-stage procedure was necessary. First, a posterior approach was used to decompress and realign the cauda equina. The stubs of the pedicles were used to provide some fixation because of inadequate area for a fusion as a result of the previous surgery, the laminectomies, and extensive scarring. The second procedure was done via the anterior approach and consisted of interbody grafts. The internal fixation screws (Zielke) were reinforced with methyl methacrylate bone cement for the severe osteoporosis. The patient walks with canes and has regained bowel and bladder control.

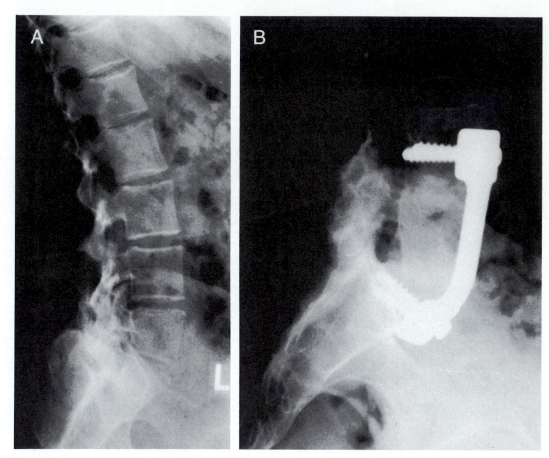

FIG 33–17.
A, this 36-year-old woman underwent two previous attempts at fusions. Pseudoarthroses were located at L4–5 and L5–S1 on plain radiography and tomography. **B,** an anterior interbody fusion of L4–S1 was performed. An I-beam plate was used to enhance fusion. The plate was contoured to the sacral promontory. The patient is pain-free and has returned to work.

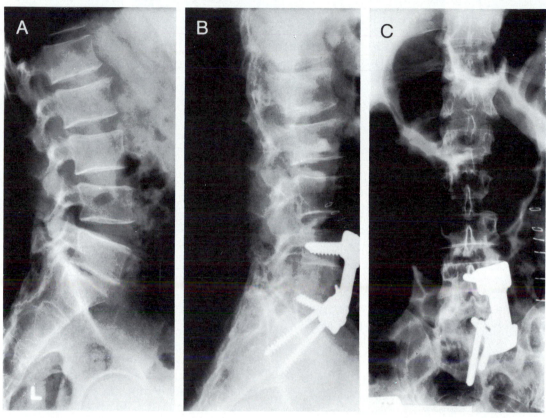

FIG 33–18.

A, this 42-year-old man underwent three previous decompression attempts and fusion plus decompression. Pseudoarthroses were noted at L4–5 and L5–S1. **B** and **C,** an anterior interbody fusion of L4–S1 was successfully done. An I-beam plate was used from L4–5, and two 6.5-mm AO cancellous screws were inserted from L5 into the sacrum. If the promontory (L5–S1 angle) is very prominent, this screw placement is preferred to contouring the plate.

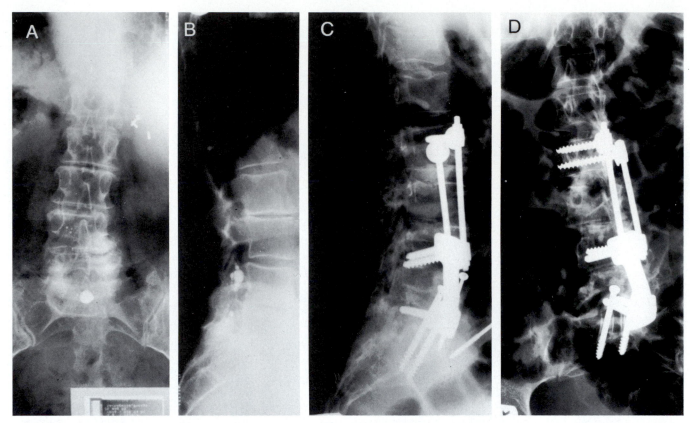

FIG 33–19.

A–D, this 28-year-old woman underwent four previous operations including two decompressions and two posterior attempts at fusion. She had pseudoarthroses at L5–S1, L4–5, and L3–4 and an unstable L2–3 level with little or no posterior elements. **A** and **B,** interbody grafts were used (il- iac crest) for stabilization of L–4, Kostuik-Harrington instrumentation (compression) at L4–5, and an I-plate with 5.5-mm AO cancellous screws at L5–S1. Pain has been considerably lessened and the patient is functional.

Technical Details

Depending on the specific condition being treated, and the history of prior surgery, certain technical details are useful to keep in mind. First, we look at the general issue in posterior repeat fusion.

Posterior Fixation

As noted, we prefer pedicle devices whenever possible, if posterior internal fixation is deemed necessary. In failed prior posterior fusion, the anatomic landmarks of the pedicle may be difficult to define, and radiologic control is essential. If there is a large amount of old bone graft present, the screws may be inserted into the graft without involving the pedicle. More often this is not the case, or osteoporosis is an additional source of concern. Under these circumstances the pedicle should be defined. Time can be saved by estimating the anatomic point of insertion, and making a drill hole. A Kirschner wire is placed

in the hole, and fluoroscopic confirmation obtained. If placement is not acceptable, slight alternations can succeed in achieving the proper entry point, which is then completed with an awl or tap drill.

Once a pedicle fixation system is placed, the linkage must be carefully selected. Plates appear to be more rigid, but are less adaptable. Although they may be contoured for lordosis, it is difficult to adapt them to a rotatory or lateral deviation deformity. Conversely, rods can be easily contoured three-dimensionally, but many of the devices are less rigid than a plate device. Ultimately, the choice of device rests with the surgeon's experience, and the preoperative assessment of which system will deal best with the complexities of the individual patient.

Regardless of the type of device used, it is important to obtain at least two points of fixation, proximal and distal to the pseudarthrosis, such that there are a total of eight points (see Fig 33–15,B). The inclusion of the sacrum also raises a number of

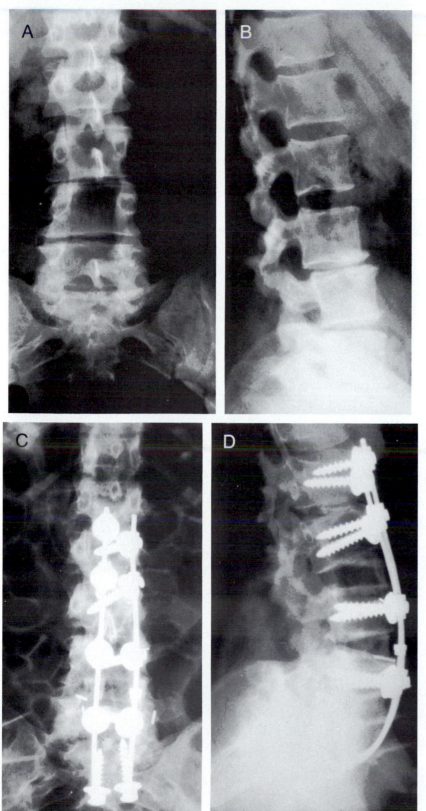

FIG 33–20.
A and **B,** this 51-year-old woman underwent five previous L3–S1 procedures including multiple decompressions and attempts at posterolateral fusion. L2–3 was unstable as well. **C** and **D,** interbody fusion (iliac crest) with double Zielke instrumentation at L2–S1. The patient returned to work as a pharmacist-assistant after being off work for 7 years. Double rods are necessary for rotational control.

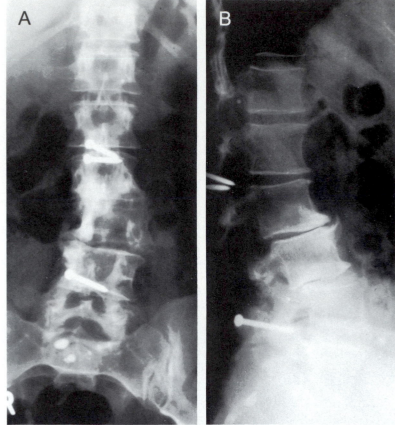

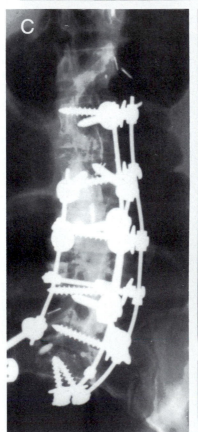

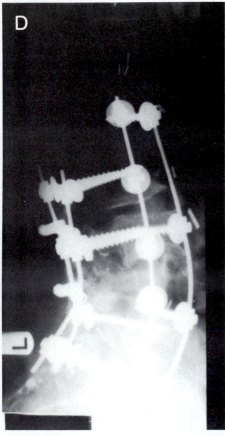

FIG 33–21.
A and **B,** a 62-year-old woman. Six previous procedures had been attempted with resultant severe instability, neurologic pain, and back pain. **C** and **D,** a two-stage procedure was performed including posterior decompression. The pedicle stumps were used for stabilization posteriorly, but because of inadequate bone stock an anterior fusion was done using interbody grafts and double Zielke rods. The patient is remarkably improved 5 years later.

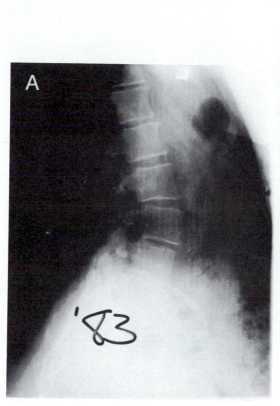

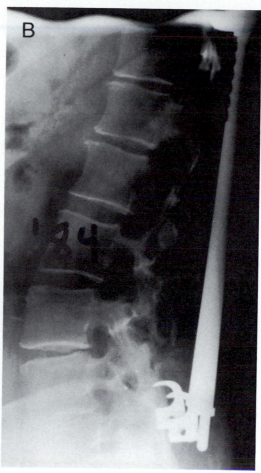

FIG 33–22.

A, this 63-year-old woman underwent a two-level L4–S1 fusion 12 years previously. She developed symptoms of spinal stenosis and segmental instability proximal at L3–4 and L2–3. **B,** the fusion was extended following posterior decompression at L2–3, and L3–4 to T10. One year later the hooks disengaged. The rods were removed but the pseudarthroses were not repaired. **C–E,** the patient's deformity progressed, together with increased instability and pain. The L3 vertebral body appears to be avascular. She developed marked lateral quadriceps weakness and could not stand. A postmyelographic CT showed a residual block. **F,** posterior decompression was performed together with cotrel-dubousset instrumentation and fusion using pedicle screws distally. The L4–S1 fusion was solid, but all other levels had pseudarthroses. Because of the long fusion extending to the fixed sacrum and the poor posterior bone stock **(E)** (small amount, extensive scarring), an anterior fusion was done.

(Continued.)

technical difficulties. The main problems are screw orientation, and the number of screws which can be employed. In our experience, the use of single screws at each side of the sacrum is insufficient, although others have not had that concern (Fig 33–23). In general, we try to introduce four screws, two on each side. The point for entry is usually at the base of the S1 pedicle (Fig 33–24). In the female, access to the sacral promontory from this point of entry is not difficult, but in the narrow male pelvis, the challenge is greater. Thus in males, we have used a similar point of entry but have directed the screw to the thickest part of the ala, aiming distally and laterally at about 30 degrees. A second screw is then introduced into the S2 pedicle, going directly laterally (Fig 33–25). Because of the close proximity of the sacrum to the overlying skin, the use of a bulky fixation device should, if at all possible, be avoided.

More recently, particularly with the Cotrel-Dubousset form of instrumentation, the introduction of two screws, both at the base of the S1 pedicle, has resulted in more easy alignment and introduction of the device rod. The first screw is angled into the promontory and the second is directed laterally into the ala.

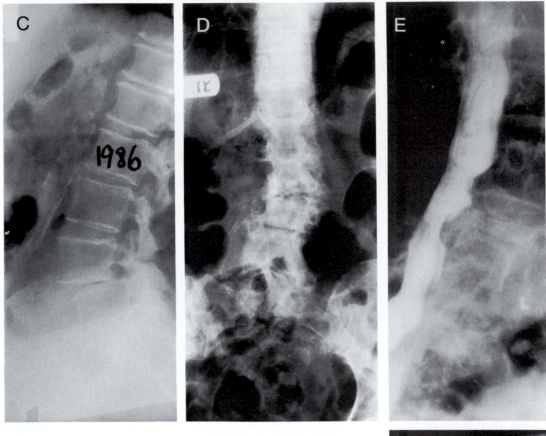

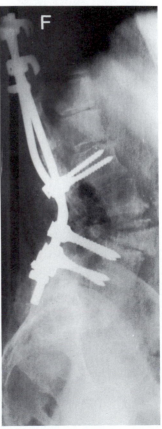

FIG 33-22 (cont.).

Posterior Decortication

In the presence of a preexisting pseudarthrosis, or when a new laminectomy is required which involves the old fusion, a wide exposure is necessary. Although most pseudarthrosis are at right angles to the longitudinal axis of the spine, this is not always the case, and the defect may not be easily identifiable. All too frequently, an exploratory operation fails to identify the pseudarthrosis, even when it was suspected preoperatively. As already noted, one cause is termed a "plate pseudoarthrosis," in which the bone graft has consolidated into a solid plate of bone, which has not adhered to the underlying lamina or transverse processes. Failure to recognize this condition is usually due to inadequate preoperative imaging, including lateral, anteroposterior (AP), and axial tomograms, and also including three-dimensional reconstructions.

Sources of Bone Graft

Although it is tempting to use local bone graft obtained from the old fusion, we believe that in most cases it is important to supplement the fusion with an autogenous graft. Usually sufficient bone can be harvested from one iliac crest, or from both. An alternative is to obtain an anterior iliac crest graft before starting the posterior approach.

When the approach is again anterior, the decision as to the bone graft source is somewhat more debatable. Although autogenous bone is preferable, an allograft may help in this situation.

Management of Osteoporosis

This situation presents a number of major challenges. Firstly, the radiographic determination of fusion after a primary intervention is often difficult. Secondly, fixation devices may be more difficult to apply. As previously noted, we do not advocate the use of methyl methacrylate in the pedicles, with the exception of the S1 pedicle. However, methyl methacrylate can be injected into the vertebral body to enhance fixation, with minimal risk. Let us now consider the technical issues in the anterior approach to repeat fusion.

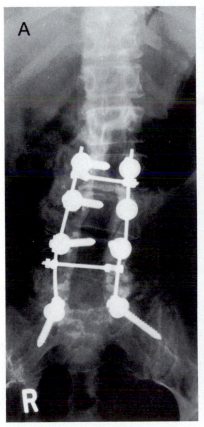
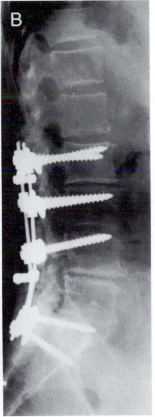

FIG 33–23.

A and **B,** this 63-year-old woman underwent four-level decompression fusion and Zielke instrumentation for severe spinal stenosis 4½ years previously. Only one screw was used on each side of the sacrum at S1 directed into the arch. She developed pseudarthrosis.

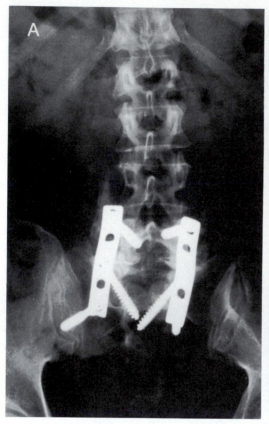
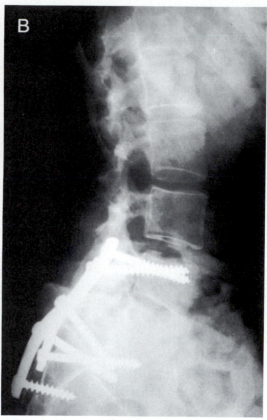

FIG 33–24.
A and **B,** this 42-year-old woman underwent decompression, fusion, and AO plate fixation at L4–S1 for spondylolisthesis. The S1 screws are directed toward the promontory; the S2 screws appear to penetrate too far anteriorly but are really in the ala of the sacrum.

Anterior Fixation Devices

The role of anterior fixation remains more controversial, particularly because of the increased inherent risks of the procedure, and, in general, the less biomechanically favorable devices.

Approaches

For a single simple approach to L5–S1, a transverse suprapubic incision may be used, and is cosmetically more acceptable. A transperitoneal or retroperitoneal approach can then be developed. We prefer the retroperitoneal approach because the bowel contents are well contained, and retraction is easier.

For a two-level approach, a left paramedian incision and retroperitoneal approach are utilized. If fixation devices are affixed to the sacrum and pass beneath the left common iliac system (Fig 33–26) we prefer to lay down a thin sheet of silicone rubber. This prevents direct adherence of the vessels to the scar, and if later surgery is required, the dissection is facilitated.

For approaches to three levels or more, we prefer a flank approach, but when the fusion is to be extended to the sacrum, the bed of the twelfth rib is used. Incision is carried to the rectus sheath, which is then split, and the incision is carried down as a paramedian incision, followed by a retroperitoneal approach.

In all patients rehabilitation of the abdominal musculature is necessary, but in the elderly patient, this may be difficult. Not uncommonly, an incisional hernia is the consequence.

Surgical Results of Repeat Fusion

As noted previously, the results of a second operation are less predictable. In a simple group of patients treated for pseudarthrosis, in whom the previous surgery was simple posterior fusion, a success rate of only 60% was obtained, often despite a subsequent solid arthrodesis.[22] This analytic problem becomes even more difficult when the published series are a mixed population with respect to the orig-

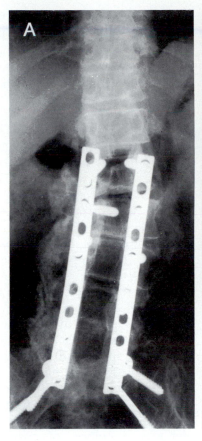
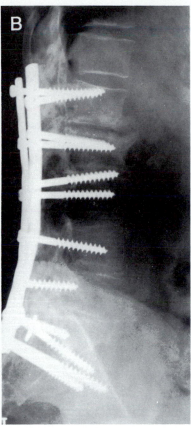

FIG 33–25.
A and **B,** in the male patient the sacral screws are directed laterally into the thickest part of the ala of the sacrum penetrating both cortices. In over 300 cases we (J.P.K) have had

no vascular problems. This patient had two previous procedures and required repeat and proximal decompression to L1, with stabilization. The result was satisfactory.

inal abnormalities, when numerous sources of failures are included, and when a variety of surgical techniques have been used. However, a number of studies are instructive, and give some broad indication of the results which can be achieved.

The first lesson is that patients properly selected can achieve reasonable, but by no means perfect, results, even when the problems are complex. Kostuik and Errico[60] treated 35 patients with fusion and sublaminar wiring. All 35 patients had been off work for an average of 9 years since their last operation. Thirteen returned to work. Satisfactory results were obtained in an additional 9 patients who had a significant decrease in pain, but did not return to work. Pain persisted in 13 patients despite a solid arthrodesis being achieved. A subsequent clinical series was performed between 1984 and 1988,[58, 59] and involved 246 patients treated by a variety of posterior pedicle fixation systems. At 2 years, the pseudarthrosis rate was 8%. During the same period, 51 patients underwent anterior salvage surgery with fu-

sion and instrumentation. The most instructive part of this series were the 38 patients who were treated by anterior salvage surgery for a posterior pseudarthrosis, while an additional group included 6 patients with degenerative disease above or below the previous fusion. The incidence of pseudarthrosis was 9%. Of those who had developed yet another pseudarthrosis following anterior surgery, 50% had pain relief at more than 2 years following the operation. Almost all of the patients were on long-term disability, yet 43% returned to work despite being off for an average of 4 years. Also of interest is that 57% of the patients had significant psychological problems, yet had a satisfactory result. Although these results do not compare with primary spine surgery, they do suggest that there is a group of patients that can benefit. The challenge is how to better the patient selection technique and the surgical approach to improve upon these results.

Other series, in general, give somewhat similar results with respect to the later incidence of

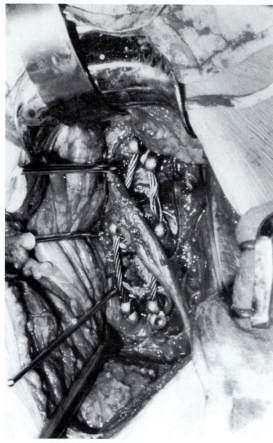

FIG 33–26.
The left common iliac vessels have been dissected out. In this example Dwyer cables go from L4–5 to S1 passing beneath the vessels. The screws pass from anterior to posterior. The vessels have been modified by tying off and sectioning the iliolumbar vessels.

pseudarthrosis following repeat fusion. Fujimaki et al.[34] reported on 38 salvage cases treated by anterior interbody fusion without instrumentation. Only one pseudarthrosis occurred.

Thalgott et al.[112] have reported on the use of AO DCP plates for internal fixation in 31 patients with prior failures of fusion. Of these patients, 17 had failed interbody fusions. Following surgical intervention, a pseudarthrosis rate of 24% was noted. In 14 patients the fusion failure was for a prior posterior operation, where a lower nonunion rate of 14% was obtained.

Zucherman et al.[125] have used the Steffee system, but their failures included a variety of patients who had not been subjected to previous fusion. Of note was their high rate of screw breakage and infection.

Alternative Nonsurgical Treatment

As noted earlier in this chapter, an alternative for many patients is a vigorous rehabilitation program, particularly in the postoperative course, when the fusion is deemed to be solid. Additional therapy which may be considered is the use of electrical stimulation in patients with pseudarthrosis. This technique was first proposed by Dwyer[26] and has been used by Kane[55] in a controlled study of both primary fusion and repair of pseudarthrosis. A large amount of basic research in the peripheral skeleton and some experimental work in animals have also been done. Kahanovitz and Arnoczky[56] suggest that electrical stimulation enhances bone formation. In primary fusion, Kane[55] has observed a rate of fusion of 91.5%. The comparison group achieved success in 81%. In secondary fusion, less certain data are available, but Kane[55] recommends that the procedure be accompanied by bone grafting. In a randomized prospective study of "difficult patients," 15 of 28 controls achieved fusion (54%) compared with 25 of 31 electrically stimulated controls who gained solid arthrodesis (81%) (Chapter 34).

As an alternative, the use of pulsating electromagnetic coils, applied externally, have been advocated by Simmons.[104] In a preliminary study, 13 patients with failures of posterior interbody fusion were analyzed, 10 of whom showed increased bone formation, and 10 (77%) of whom went on to solid arthrodesis. His results have not been replicated by Brodsky,[6] who demonstrated only a 36% success rate in patients with posterior fusion and pseudarthrosis.

REFERENCES

1. Baker AS, Ojemann RG, Swartz MN, et al: Spinal epidural abscess. *N Engl J Med* 1975; 293:463–468.
2. Beals RK, Hickman NW: Industrial injuries of the back and extremities: Comprehensive evaluation— an aid in prognosis and management; a study of one hundred and eighty patients. *J Bone Joint Surg [Am]* 1972; 54:1593–1611.
3. Blasier RD, Munson RC: Acquired spondylolysis after postero-lateral spinal fusion. *J Pediatr Orthop* 1987; 7:215–217.
4. Bosworth DM: Repair of hernia through iliac-crest defects. *J Bone Joint Surg [Am]* 1955; 37:1071.
5. Brodsky AE: Post-laminectomy and post-fusion stenosis of the lumbar spine. *Clin Orthop* 1976; 115: 130.
6. Brodsky AE, Hendricks FL, Khalil MA, et al: Segmental ("floating") lumbar spine fusions. *Spine* 1989; 14:447–450.

7. Brodsky AE, Kahlic MA: Efficacy of electrical bone growth stimulation among 97 patients with pseudo-arthrosis of the lumbar spine. Presented at Pre-Annual North American Spine Society Meeting, Colorado Springs, Colo, June 1988.

8. Brunet JA, Wiley JJ: Acquired spondylolysis after spinal fusion. *J Bone Joint Surg [Br]* 1984; 66:720–724.

9. Burton C: The role of spine fusion: Question 4. *Spine* 1981; 6:291.

10. Burton CV, Kirkaldy-Willis WH, Yong-Hing K, et al: Causes of failure of surgery on the lumbar spine. *Clin Orthop* 1981; 157:191–199.

11. Cleveland M, Bosworth DM, Thompson FR: Pseudo-arthrosis in the lumbosacral spine. *J Bone Joint Surg [Am]* 1948; 30:302–312.

12. Cloward RB: The treatment of ruptured lumbar intervertebral discs by vertebral body fusion: Indications, operative technique, after-care. *J Neurosurg* 1953; 10:154–168.

13. Cochran T, Irstam L, Nachemson A: Long-term anatomic and functional changes in patients with adolescent idiopathic scoliosis treated by Harrington rod fusion. *Spine* 1983; 8:576–584.

14. Collis JS: Total disc replacement: A modified posterior lumbar interbody fusion. Report of 750 cases. *Clin Orthop* 1985; 193:640–667.

15. Cotler JM, Starr AM: Complications of spinal fusions, in Cotler JJ, Cotler HB (eds): *Spinal Fusion, Science and Technique*, New York, Springer-Verlag, 1989.

16. Crock HV: A reappraisal of intervertebral disc lesions. *Med J Aust* 1970; 1:983–989.

17. Crock HV: Observations on the management of failed spinal operations. *J Bone Joint Surg [Br]* 1976; 58:193–199.

18. Crock HV: Internal disc disruption: A challenge to disc prolapse fifty years on. *Spine* 1986; 11:650–653.

19. Dawson EG, Clader TJ, Bassett LW: A comparison of different methods used to diagnose pseudoarthrosis following posterior spinal fusion for scoliosis. *J Bone Joint Surg [Am]* 1985; 67:1153–1159.

20. DePalma A, Rotherman R: The nature of pseudoarthrosis. *Clin Orthop* 1968; 59:113–118.

21. Deyo RA: Reducing work absenteeism and diagnostic costs for backache, in Hadler NM (ed): *Clinical Concepts in Regional Musculoskeletal Illness*. Orlando, Fla, Grune & Stratton, Inc, 1987, pp 25–50.

22. Deyo RA, Diehl AK, Rosenthal M: How many days of bedrest for acute low back pain? A randomized clinical trial. *N Engl J Med* 1986; 315:1064–1070.

23. Dewar FP: Circumferential fusion for degenerative disc disease, Toronto, Unpublished data, 1963.

24. Drury BJ: Clinical evaluation of back and leg pain due to irritation of the superior cluneal nerve. *J Bone Joint Surg [Am]* 1967; 49:199.

25. Dvorak J, Valach L, Fuhrimann P, et al: The outcome of surgery for lumbar disc herniation. II. A 4–17 year follow-up with emphasis on psychosocial aspects. *Spine* 1988; 13:1423–1427.

26. Dwyer AF: Experience of anterior correction of scoliosis. *Clin Orthop* 1973; 93:191–206.

27. Esses SI, Botsford DJ, Kostuik JP: The role of external spinal skeletal fixation in the assessment of low-back disorders. *Spine* 1989; 14:594–601.

28. Fairbank JC, Park WM, McCall IW, et al: Apophyseal injection of local anaesthetic as a diagnostic aid in primary low-back pain syndromes. *Spine* 1981; 6:598–605.

29. Finnegan W, Fenlin JM, Marvel JP, et al: Results of surgical intervention in the symptomatic multiple-operated back patient. Analysis of 67 cases followed for 3–7 years. *J Bone Joint Surg [Am]* 1979; 61:1077–1082.

30. Fogelberg RB, Zittmann EK, Stinchfield FE: Prophylactic penicillin in orthopaedic surgery. *J Bone Joint Surg [Am]* 1970; 52:95–98.

31. Fraser RD, Osti OL, Vernon-Roberts B: Discitis following chemonucleolysis; An experimental study. *Spine* 1986; 1:679–687.

32. Freebody D, Bendall R, Taylor RD: Anterior transperitoneal lumbar fusion. *J Bone Joint Surg [Br]* 1971; 53:617–627.

33. Frymoyer JW: The role of spine fusion. Question 3. *Spine* 1981; 6:284–290.

34. Frymoyer JW: Back pain and sciatica. *N Engl J Med* 1988; 318:291–300.

35. Frymoyer JW, Hanley E, Howe J, et al: Disc excision and spine fusion in the management of lumbar disc disease; a minimum ten-year follow-up. *Spine* 1978; 3:1–6.

36. Frymoyer JW, Hanley EN, Howe J, et al: A comparison of radiographic findings in fusion and nonfusion patients ten or more years following lumbar disc surgery. *Spine* 1979; 4:435–440.

37. Frymoyer JW, Howe J, Kuhlmann D: The long-term effects of spinal fusion on the sacroiliac joints and ilium. *Clin Orthop* 1978; 134:196.

38. Frymoyer JW, Matteri RE, Hanley EN, et al: Failed lumbar disc surgery requiring second operation. A long term follow-up study. *Spine* 1978; 3:7–11.

39. Fujimaki A, Crock HV, Bedbrook GM: The results of 150 anterior lumbar interbody fusion operations performed by two surgeons in Australia. *Clin Orthop* 1982; 165:164–167.

40. Gurdjian ES, Webster JE, Ostrowski AZ, et al: Herniated lumbar intervertebral discs—An analysis of 1176 operated cases. *J Trauma* 1961; 1:158–176.

41. Guyer DW, Wiltse LL, Eskay ML, et al: The long-range prognosis of archnoiditis. *Spine* 1989; 14:1321–1341.

42. Hadler NM: Regional back pain [editorial]. *N Engl J Med* 1986; 315:1090–1092.

43. Hakelius A: Prognosis in sciatica. A clinical follow-up of surgical and non -surgical treatment. *Acta Orthop Scand Suppl* 1970; 129:1–76.

44. Hanley EN Jr, Shapiro DE: The development of low-back pain after excision of a lumbar disc. *J Bone Joint Surg [Am]* 1989; 71:719–721.

45. Harris RI, Wiley JJ: Acquired spondylosysis as a sequel to spine fusion. *J Bone Joint Surg [Am]* 1963; 45:1159–1170.

46. Hayes MA, Tompkins SF, Herndow WA, et al: Clinical and radiological evaluation of lumbosacral mo-

tion below fusion levels in idiopathic scoliosis. *Spine* 1988; 10:1161–1167.

47. Hirsch C, Nachemson A: The reliability of lumbar disk surgery. *Clin Orthop* 1963; 29:189–194.

48. Howe J, Frymoyer JW: The effects of questionnaire design on the determination of end results in lumbar spinal surgery. *Spine* 1985; 10:804–805.

49. Hoyland JA, Freemont AJ, Denton J, et al: Retained surgical swab debris in post-laminectomy arachnoiditis and peridural fibrosis. *J Bone Joint Surg [Br]* 1988; 70:659–662.

50. Hsu KY, Zucherman J, White A, et al: Deterioration of motion segments adjacent to lumbar fusion. Presented at the North American Spine Society Annual Meeting, Colorado Springs, Colorado, July 1988.

51. Jacobs RR, Montesano PX, Jackson RP: Enhancement of lumbar spine fusion by use of translaminar facet joint screws. *Spine* 1989; 14:12–15.

52. Johnsson KE, Redlund-Johnell I, Uden A, et al: Preoperative and postoperative instability in lumbar spinal stenosis. *Spine* 1989; 14:591–593.

53. Jones JB: The training of orthopaedic surgery residents in lumbar disc surgery. *Clin Orthop* 1971; 81:88–92.

54. Jones AA, Stambough JL, Balderston RA, et al: Long-term results of lumbar spine surgery complicated by unintended incidental durotomy. *Spine* 1989; 14:443–446.

55. Kane WJ: Direct current electrical bone stimulation for spinal fusion. *Spine* 1988; 13:763.

56. Kahanovitz N, Arnoczky SP: The efficacy of direct current electrical stimulation to enhance canine spinal fusions. *Clin Orthop* 1990; 251:295–299.

57. Kornberg M: Discography and magnetic resonance imaging in the diagnosis of lumbar disc disruption. *Spine* 1989; 12:1368–1369.

58. Kostuik JP, Carl A, Ferron S: Anterior interbody fusion and instrumentation for lumbar degenerative disc disease. Unpublished data, 1986.

59. Kostuik JP, Carl A, Ferron S, et al: Results of instrumentation and fusion for salvage surgery in degenerative disc disease. Presented at Meeting of Canadian Orthopaedic Association, Vancouver, March 1990.

60. Kostuik JP, Errico T: Luque instrumentation in degenerative conditions of the lumbar spine. *Spine* 1990; 15:318–321.

61. Kostuik JP, Hall BB: Spinal fusions to the sacrum in adults with scoliosis. *Spine* 1983; 8:489–500.

62. Krempen JF, Smith BS: Nerve root injection; A method for evaluating the etiology of sciatica. *J Bone Joint Surg [Am]* 1974; 56:1435–1444.

63. Kurz LT, Garfin SR, Booth RE: Harvesting autogenous iliac bone grafts. A review of complications and techniques. *Spine* 1989; 14:1324–1331.

64. Laasonen EM, Soini J: Low-back pain after lumbar fusion: Surgical and computed tomographic analysis. *Spine* 1989; 14:210–231.

65. Lee CK, Langrana NA: Lumbosacral spinal fusion: A biomechanical study. *Spine* 1984; 9:574–581.

66. Lehmann TR, Spratt KF, Tozzi JE: Long-term follow-up of lower lumbar fusion patients. *Spine* 1987; 12:97–104.

67. Liang M, Kormaroff AL: Roentgenograms in primary care patients with acute low back pain; A cost-effectiveness analysis. *Arch Intern Med* 1982; 142:1108–1112.

68. Lin PM: PLIF complications and pitfalls. *Clin Orthop* 1985;:193:90–102.

69. Lin PM: Technique and complications of posterior lumbar interbody fusion, in Lin PM, Gill K (eds): *Lumbar Interbody Fusion, Principles and Techniques in Spine Surgery.* Rockville, Md, Aspen Press, 1989.

70. Long DM, Filtzer DL, BenDebba M, et al: Clinical features of the failed-back syndrome. *J Neurosurg* 1988; 69:61–71.

71. Lonstein J, Winter R, Moe J, et al: Wound infection with Harrington instrumentation and spine fusion for scoliosis. *Clin Orthop* 1973; 96:222.

72. Love JG, Rivers MH: Spinal cord tumors simulating protruded intervertebral discs. *JAMA* 1962; 179:878–881.

73. Luk KD, Lee FB, Leong JCY, et al: The effect on the lumbosacral spine of long spinal fusion for idiopathic scoliosis. A minimum 10 year follow-up. *Spine* 1987; 12:996–1000.

74. Macdonald G, Pennel G: Lumbar spine fusion. Presented at Workman's Compensation Course, Toronto, June 1966.

75. McKenzie RA: *The Lumbar Spine, Mechanical Diagnosis and Therapy.*, New Zealand, Spinal Publications, 1981.

76. Macnab I, Dali D: The blood supply of the lumbar spine and its application to the technique of intertransverse lumbar fusion. *J Bone Joint Surg [Br]* 1971; 53:628–638.

77. Macnab I: Negative disc exploration; An analysis of the causes of nerve-root involvement in 68 patients. *J. Bone Joint Surg [Am]* 1971; 53:891–903.

78. Malcolm B, Vaughan PA, Maistrelli G: The results of L4–5 disc excision alone versus disc excision and fusion. *Spine* 1988; 13:690–695.

79. Mayer TG, Gatchel RJ, Kishino N, et al: Objective assessment of spine function following industrial injury; A prospective study with comparison group and one-year follow-up. *Spine* 1985; 10:482–493.

80. Michel CR, LaLain JJ: Late result of Harrington's operation. Long-term evolution of the lumbar spine below the fused segments. *Spine* 1985; 10:414–420.

81. Miller PR, Elder FW Jr: Meningeal pseudocysts (meningococci spurtus) following laminectomy. *J Bone Joint Surg [Am]* 1968; 50P:268–276.

82. Mooney V: The failed back—an orthopaedic view. *Int Disabil Stud* 1988; 10:32–36.

83. Mooney V, Cairns D, Robertson J: A system for evaluating and treating chronic back disability. *West J Med* 1976; 124:370–376.

84. Nachemson A: Editorial comments: Lumbar discography—where are we today? *Spine* 1989; 14:555–557.

85. Nashold BA Jr, Blaine S, Hrubec A: *Lumbar Disc Disease: A Twenty-Year Clinical Follow-up Study.* St Louis, Mosby-Year Book, Inc, 1971.

86. Naylor A: Late results of laminectomy for lumbar disc prolapse: A review after ten to twenty-five years. *J Bone Joint Surg [Br]* 1974; 56:17–29.

87. Naylor A, Shentall RD, Micklethwaite B: An electron microscopic study of the segment long spacing colla-

gen from the intervertebral disc. *Orthop Clin North Am* 1977; 8:217–223.

88. Nerubay J, Marganit B, Bubis JJ, et al: Stimulation of bone formation by electrical current on spinal fusion. *Spine* 1986; 11:167–169.

89. Norton WL: Chemonucleolysis versus surgical discectomy; Comparison of costs and results in workers compensation claimants. *Spine* 1987; 11:440–443.

90. O'Brien JP, Dawson MH, Heard CW, et al: Simultaneous combined anterior and posterior fusion. A solution for failed spinal surgery with a brief review of first 150 patients. *Clin Orthop* 1986; 203:191–195.

91. O'Connell JEA: Protrusions of the lumbar intervertebral discs. A clinical review based on five hundred cases treated by excision of the protrusion. *J Bone Joint Surg [Br]* 1951; 33:8–30.

92. Olerud S, Hamberg M: External fixation as a test for instability after spinal fusion L4–S1. A case report. *Orthopaedics* 1986; 9:547–549.

93. Olerud S, Sjostrom L, Karlstrom G, et al: Spontaneous effect of increased stability of the lower lumbar spine in cases of severe chronic back pain. The answer of an external transpedicular fixation test. *Clin Orthop* 1986; 203:67–74.

94. Phytinen J, Lahde S, Tanska EL, et al: Computed tomography after lumbar myelography in lower back and extremity pain syndromes. *Diagn Imaging* 1983; 52:1922.

95. Pilgaard S: Discitis (closed space infection) following removal of lumbar intervertebral disc. *J Bone Joint Surg [Am]* 1969; 51:713–716.

96. Prothero SR, Parkes JC, Stinchfield EE: Complications of low-back fusion in 1000 patients. *J Bone Joint Surg [Am]* 1966; 48:57–65.

97. Quinnell RC, Stockdale HR: Some experimental observations on the influence of a single lumbar floating fusion on the remaining lumbar spine. *Spine* 1981; 6:263–267.

98. Raugstad TS, Harbo K, Hogberg A, et al: Anterior interbody fusion of the lumbar spine. *Acta Orthop Scand* 1982; 53:561–565.

99. Rolander SD: Motion of the lumbar spine with special reference to the stability effect of posterior fusion. *Acta Orthop Scand Suppl* 1966; 90:1–143.

100. Rombold C: Spondylolysis: A complication of spine fusion. *J Bone Joint Surg [Am]* 1965; 47:1237–1242.

101. Sage FP: Post-operative fracture in the lumbar facets following lumbar disc surgery. *J Bone Joint Surg [Am]* 1975; 57:1173.

102. Schofferman L, Schofferman J, Zucherman J, et al: Occult infections causing persistent low-back pain. *Spine* 1989; 14:417–419.

103. Schonstrom N: The narrow lumbar spinal canal and the size of the cauda equina in man. Sahigren Hospital, Gothenburg, Sweden, Department of Orthopaedics, Gothenburg University.

104. Simmons JW: Treatment of failed posterior lumbar interbody fusion on the spine with pulsing electromagnetic fields. *Clin Orthop* 1985; 193:127–132.

105. Smith SE, DeLee JC, Rammamurthy S: Ilioinguinal neuralgia following iliac bone-grafting. Report of two cases and review of the literature. *J Bone Joint Surg [Am]* 1984; 66:1306–1308.

106. Spangfort EV: The lumbar disc herniation: A computer-aided analysis of 2,504 operations. *Acta Orthop Scand Suppl* 1972; 142:1–95.

107. Spengler DM: Lumbar discectomy: Results with limited disc excision and selective foraminotomy. *Spine* 1982; 7:604–706.

108. Spengler DM, Freeman C, Westbrook R, et al: Low back pain following multiple lumbar spine procedures. Failure of initial selection. *Spine* 1980; 5:356–360.

109. Stokes IA, Counts DF, Frymoyer JW: Experimental instability in the rabbit lumbar spine. *Spine* 1989; 14:68–72.

110. Stokes IAF, Wilder DG, Frymoyer JW, et al: Assessment of patients with low back pain by biplanar radiographic measurement of intervertebral motion. *Spine* 1981; 6:233–239.

111. Terry A, McCall IW, O'Brien JP, et al: Graft impingement following posterolateral fusion, in *Proceedings of the International Society for the Study of the Lumbar Spine*, 1981.

112. Thalgott JS, LaRocca H, Aebi M, et al: Reconstruction of the lumbar spine using AO DCP plate fixation. *Spine* 1989; 14:91–95.

113. Unander-Scharin L: Case of spondylolisthesis lumbalis acquisita. *Acta Orthop Scand* 1950; 19:536–544.

114. van Akkerveeken PF: *Lateral Stenosis of the Lumbar Spine*. Utrecht, The Netherlands, Libertas Drukwerkservice, 1989.

115. Waddell G, McCulloch JA, Kummel E, et al: Nonorganic physical signs in low-back pain. *Spine* 1980; 5:117–125.

116. Walsh TR, Weinstein JN, Spratt KF, et al: Lumbar discography; A controlled prospective study of normal volunteers to determine the false-positive rate. Presented at the International Society for the Study of the Lumbar Spine.

117. Watkins RG: Summary of etiologies of postlaminectomy syndrome, in Watkins RG, Collis JS (eds): *Lumbar Discectomy and Laminectomy*. Rockville, Md, Aspen Press, 1987; pp 267–269.

118. Weatherley CR, Pricken CF, O'Brian JP: Discogenic pain persisting despite solid posterior fusion. *J Bone Joint Surg [Br]* 1986; 38:142.

119. Weikel AM, Habal MB: Meralgia paresthetica: A complication of iliac bone procurement. *Plast Reconstr Surg* 1977; 60:572–574.

120. Weinstein JN, Spratt KF, Spengler D, et al: Spinal pedicle fixation: Reliability and validity of roentgenogram based assessment and surgical factors on successful screw placement. *Spine* 1988; 13:1012–1018.

121. Weber H: Lumbar disc herniation. A controlled, prospective study with ten years of observation. *Spine* 1983; 8:131–140.

122. Wiesel SW: The multiply operated lumbar spine. *Instr Course Lect* 1985; 34:68–77.

123. Wiesel SW, Feffer HL, Borenstein DG: Evaluation and outcome of low-back pain of unknown etiology. *Spine* 1988; 13:679–680.

124. Yang SW, Langrana NA, Lee CK: Biomechanics of lumbosacral spinal fusion in combined compression-torsion loads. *Spine* 1986; 11:937–941.

125. Zuckerman J, Hsu K, White A, et al: Early results of spinal fusion using variable spine plating system. *Spine* 1988; 13:570–579.

34

The Use of Electrical Stimulation in Spinal Fusion

Gunnar B. J. Andersson, M.D., Ph.D.

Thomas W. McNeill, M.D.

The use of electrical stimulation to induce or accelerate osteogenesis began in the 1950s[12] and was applied clinically to spinal fusions in the early 1970s.[3] It is only in the last several years, however, that there has been a more widespread use of electrical stimulation in spinal fusions. It is not the purpose of this chapter to review the influence of electric currents on bone and bone remodeling. Present interest, however, is so widespread that we have felt that a review of the literature on the role of electrical stimulation in spinal fusion would be useful in a book on spinal stenosis. After all, spinal stenosis remains one of the main indications for fusions, although as should be apparent from other chapters, opinions differ as to how often fusion is indeed indicated.

Two main techniques are used to deliver the electric current to the fusion area. One involves the implantation of electrodes at or near the site of stimulation and the application of direct current. The second involves the application of pulsed electromagnetic fields (PEMFs) to the fusion site from electromagnetic coils placed externally.

ANIMAL STUDIES

The earliest animal studies that we have found in which stimulation was specifically applied to spinal fusions date back to 1984. In that year, Kahanovitz et al.[5] published a canine study in which the external method with PEMFs was used in a study of 10 large adult mongrel dogs. The study was not double blind but randomized. Thus, all dogs underwent a three-level lumbar spinal fusion and 5 were treated with electromagnetic pulsing while 5 acted as controls. The evaluation was radiographic and histologic. At 4, 6, and 9 weeks, there appeared to be improved new bone formation and a better organization of the fusion mass in the stimulated specimen. However, at 12 and 15 weeks there were no histologic or radiologic differences between the stimulated and control dogs. The conclusions by Kahanovitz et al. were that electromagnetic pulsing did produce an early accelerated osteogenic response. However, PEMFs did not appear to improve the overall result of primary canine spinal fusions. Kahanovitz and Arnoczky[4] later performed another experimental study using direct current stimulation. In this study, 12 mongrel dogs had posterior facet fusions bilaterally at L1–2 and L4–5. A direct current electrostimulator was placed through each of the fusions. Only half of the electrodes were functional. Evaluation with high-resolution, radiographic, and routine histologic studies showed little difference between fusions in animals with active and inactive devices at 2, 4, and 6 weeks. At 12 weeks, however, all stimulated facet joints showed solid bony fusions while none of the 8 control facet joints demonstrated osseous bridging. Clearly, this provided evidence of a treatment effect.

Nerubay et al.[8] performed a double blind study to evaluate the effect of a constant current stimulator on fusions in 30 young pigs. The animals underwent a spinal fusion at the L5–6 level. Active and inactive "bone growth stimulators" were implanted. Results were evaluated histologically and radiographically. Statistically significant differences were observed at 2 months between animals who had active bone growth stimulators compared with those who had inactive devices. There was a detectable difference between the groups at 1 month.

In another study related to the spine, but not to spinal fusion as such, Carter et al.[1] determined electrical field and current density distributions in vertebral bodies of Sprague-Dawley rats. Several important findings related to the parameter influence on the magnitude of electrical field and current density were determined. Further, it was determined that there was reversal of bone loss in these animals who all displayed castration osteoporosis. Clearly, stimulation does reach and influence bone. The direct application to osteoporosis remains uncertain, however.

CLINICAL STUDIES

From February to September 1972, 12 spinal fusion procedures were performed in Australia using an implanted direct current stimulator.[3] In all, a posterior approach was used to achieve union across the posterior joints of spinal segments. Cathodes were drilled into the articular processes and cancellous bone placed about each cathode, and, in addition, the joints were grafted. Five to 16 weeks after the operation, the patients were readmitted to a hospital for reoperation and removal of the stimulator. At that time, a firm homogeneous mass of fresh vascular bone was found in all but one patient. In that case of nonunion, the anodic electrode lead was radiographically demonstrated to have suffered corrosive failure within a few days of operation, and thus no current was delivered. Dwyer[2] later reported radiographic fusion in 40 of 47 patients who had similar procedures, including 27 patients considered difficult because they required multilevel fusions and had a high incidence of previous surgery.

Dwyer's work stimulated a multicenter clinical trial which was initiated in the United States in 1979. By 1981, data were available on 84 stimulated patients. Eighty-two of these 84 patients, who had been operated on by 23 orthopaedic surgeons in 18 clinical centers, were compared with 159 historical controls from two medical centers.[6] The success rate of fusion was 91.5% in the stimulated group compared with 80.5% in the historical controls. This represented a statistically significant difference and led to a second study in which a randomized prospective control design was used.[6] This study included only patients who had had only one or more previously failed fusions, or had a grade II or worse spondylolisthesis, or a multiple-level fusion or the presence of other risk factors for fusion such as obesity. Clearly, this was a group where problems could be anticipated. It was not a double blind study, but rather the patients were randomized by protocol to either a stimulator or none. The fusion groups were assessed radiographically by the operating surgeon and by an independent radiologist at 12 and 18 months. Success was obtained in 15 of 28 control patients (54%) compared with 25 of 31 stimulation-treated patients (81%). This result was again statistically significant.

At the 1989 North American Spine Society meeting, Simmons et al.[11] presented the results of an open trial study using pulsed electromagnetic fields on lumbar fusions. Two different substudies were reported. One was a study to determine the fusion rates in patients receiving PEMF treatment as an adjunct to lumbar fusion surgery, and the second involved the use of PEMF to treat established pseudarthrosis without concomitant regrafting. The first study included 190 subjects operated on by 26 physicians, while the second involved 126 subjects and 25 surgeons. Success was determined radiographically as the percent of graft assimilation, which was assessed by an independent, blinded radiologist. The data were analyzed with respect to a number of prognostic variables of known influence on the outcome of fusion. The use of the PEMF device could be determined because the device records the time of use. The patients could therefore be divided into consistent and inconsistent users. Consistent users had a success rate of 92% with the active stimulation device compared to 69% with the placebo device which was indistinguishable from the active one (Fig 34–1). Inconsistent users had poor fusion rates, with 65% in the active group compared to 61% in the placebo group. Interestingly, the negative effect of smoking appeared to be eliminated by the use of PEMF (Fig 34–2). The success rate was otherwise independent of sex, age, number of levels, and surgical techniques. Autografts had a higher success rate than allografts.

The pseudarthrosis group was defined by a period of at least 9 months from surgery and a lack of

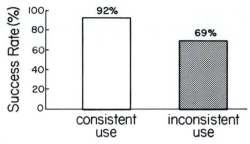

FIG 34–1.
Fusions obtained with consistent and inconsistent use of a brace delivering pulsed electromagnetic stimulation to primary posterolateral lumbar fusions. (Data based on Simmons et al.[11])

healing as documented radiographically for at least 3 months prior to enrollment. A statistically significant higher proportion of those who used the device consistently healed compared with those who were inconsistent in the use of their devices (67% vs. 19%) (Fig 34–3). None of the other variables influenced the success rate in this study where all braces were active. The study confirmed an earlier published study by Simmons[10] in which he had used PEMFs to treat failed posterior lumbar interbody fusions. In that study, which included 13 patients with an average time of 40 months since the last surgical fusion attempt, bone formation was enhanced in 85% and body-to-body fusion through the intervertebral disc space was solid in 77% (10/13).

A subsequent randomized double blind prospective study of the efficacy of pulsed electromagnetic fields for anterior interbody fusions was published by Mooney in 1990.[7] In that study, 98 subjects were randomized to an active device group and 97 to a placebo device group. A brace containing identical equipment was used by both groups (Fig 34–4). The

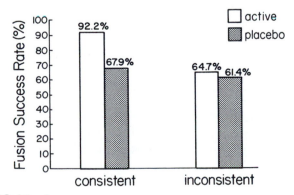

FIG 34–3.
Treatment of pseudoarthroses with PEMF. The success rate was significantly higher in that group of patients who used the stimulator consistently. No regrafting was performed. (Data based on Simmons et al.[11])

success rate of fusion was 92% in the active group compared to 65% in the control group. The negative effect of smoking was again found to be eliminated by the use of pulsed electromagnetic fields.

In the same year, Rosenthal and Edwards[9] presented a paper at the North American Spine Society meeting in which they had used compression instrumentation and an implantable electrical stimulator to treat lumbosacral nonunions. The success rate was 41% in that 11 of 27 nonunions healed. A historical control group where the same operative procedure had been performed, but without stimulation, had a success rate of 86%. This difference was statistically significant and led the investigators to believe that "adult patients with lumbosacral nonunions are best treated with dynamic compression instrumentation and cancellous grafting alone. The addition of an implantable direct current electrical stimulator may actually lessen the chances of a successful fusion."[9]

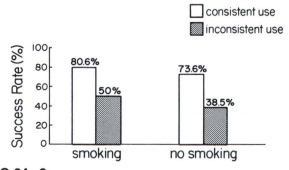

FIG 34–2.
The success rate of fusions in smokers and nonsmokers, with and without consistent use of a pulsed electromagnetic field (PEMF) device. (Data based on Simmons et al.[11])

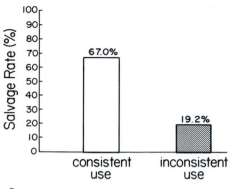

FIG 34–4.
Results of a randomized clinical trial using PEMF on anterior lumbar interbody fusions. (Data based on Mooney[7])

DISCUSSION

Historically, if lumbosacral fusions in adults had had a consistent rate of success, then electrical stimulation post fusion would not be an issue of great interest. However, the failure rate in lumbar spinal fusions has remained at a dismal 20% or worse.[6]

Not all lumbar fusion procedures carry the same risk of failure. Evidence has been accumulating that floating fusions, fusions in smokers, multilevel fusions, fusions in the elderly, obesity, and failed previous fusions carry a greater risk of failure than fusions performed in patients in whom these risk factors are not present. Conversely, the greatest chance for success in an attempted lumbar fusion is in a younger patient with a one-level lumbosacral fusion for a spondylolisthesis of grade I or less or other pathologic condition involving only the lumbosacral joint. Clearly, the indications are stronger in patients with risk factors. Since the evidence appears to support the efficacy of spinal stimulation in lumbar fusions and especially in those with increased risk factors for failure, we have incorporated this treatment modality into our practice.

Once the decision to use electrical stimulation has been made, a number of difficult choices must still be made. First, should the stimulator be implanted or worn externally? Implanted electrodes and battery direct current stimulators have the advantage of convenience, guaranteed patient compliance, and application of the current directly to the area of need. The disadvantage is the need for a second anesthesia and surgical procedure for removal. Further, in the unlikely chance of failure, repair of the device is not possible. External stimulators have the disadvantage of being cumbersome, heavy, inconvenient, and require compulsive patient compliance. They have the advantage of being easily checked and easily repaired and, of course, do not require further surgery. Secondly, should the stimulator be prescribed for all patients or only those at special risk of failure? This factor will become more and more important, as both choices are expensive and becoming more so. The question of the cost-benefit ratio in the low-risk patient is yet to be answered.

In patients with a pseudarthrosis, we believe that it is worthwhile to try an external stimulator before resorting to another surgical procedure. A more conservative approach is attractive in these patients. The prerequisite is that there be bone remaining that can respond to the stimulation.

In summary, we are of the opinion (without being dogmatic) that electrical stimulation has a definite place in lumbar fusions in patients who have increased risk factors for failure, as well as in patients with failed spinal fusions.

REFERENCES

1. Carter EL, Vresilovic EJ Jr, Pollack SR, et al: Field distributions in vertebral bodies of the rat during electrical stimulation: A parametric study. IEEE *Trans Biomed Eng* 1989; 36:333–345.
2. Dwyer AF: The use of electrical stimulation spinal fusion. *Orthop Clin North Am* 1975; 6:265–279.
3. Dwyer AF, Wickham CG: Direct current stimulation in spinal fusion. *Med J Aust* 1974; 1:73–75.
4. Kahanovitz N, Arnoczky SP: The efficacy of direct current electrical stimulation to enhance canine spinal fusions. *Clin Orthop* 1990; 251:295–299.
5. Kahanovitz N, Arnoczky SP, Hulse D, et al: The effect of postoperative electromagnetic pulsing on canine posterior spinal fusions. *Spine* 1984; 9:273–279.
6. Kane WJ: Direct current electrical bone growth stimulation for spinal fusion. *Spine* 1988; 13:363–365.
7. Mooney V: A randomized double-blind prospective study of the efficacy of pulsed electromagnetic fields for interbody lumbar fusions. *Spine* 1990; 15:708–712.
8. Nerubay J, Margaint B, Bubis JJ, et al: Stimulation of bone formation by electrical current on spinal fusion. *Spine* 1986; 11:167–169.
9. Rosenthal MS, Edwards CC: Treatment of lumbosacral nonunions with compression instrumentation and an implantable electrical stimulator. Presented at the 5th Annual Meeting of the North American Spine Society. Monterey, Aug 8–11, 1990.
10. Simmons JW: Treatment of failed posterior lumbar interbody fusion (PLIF) of the spine with pulsing electromagnetic field. *Clin Orthop* 1985; 193:127–132.
11. Simmons JW, Hayes MA, Christensen KD, et al: The effect of post-operative pulsing electromagnetic fields on lumbar fusion: Open trial study. Presented at the Fourth Annual Meeting of the North American Spine Society, Quebec, Canada, June 24–July 2, 1989.
12. Yasuda I, Noguchi K, Sata T: Dynamic callus and electric callus. *J Bone Joint Surg [Am]* 1955; 37:1282.

35

Postoperative Treatment

Thomas W. McNeill, M.D.
Gunnar B.J. Andersson, M.D., Ph.D.

Spinal stenosis is not one entity, and no two patients require exactly the same treatment either surgically or in the postoperative period. The principles of postoperative care presented in this chapter represent one of several approaches, essentially our approach. The suggested management has proved to be rewarding, safe, and generally acceptable to the patient, as well as being easy to implement. The chapter is not intended to be an exhaustive treatise on the care of postoperative patients in general.

Postoperative care begins preoperatively. A postoperative management plan is formulated which takes into account the many factors that are unique to the individual, and is therefore always, in part, custom-made for each patient. Each plan should address six areas of concern: (1) the age and general medical condition of the patient; (2) the nature of the surgery; (3) prevention of complications from the surgery; (4) social and vocational aspects; (5) rehabilitation; and (6) follow-up care with the surgeon and other health care providers.

PREOPERATIVE PLANNING

Age and General Condition

The nucleus of the postoperative plan is the patient's preoperative physical condition. Of first importance is the identification of preexisting medical conditions that require stabilization before surgery and careful follow-up in the immediate postoperative period.[2] For example, a patient with chronic,

stable liver disease may have a bleeding tendency which requires control with fresh frozen plasma before, during, and after surgery. Recent stroke and myocardial infarction are absolute contraindications to surgery, while more remote strokes or myocardial infarctions will require preoperative clearance and close attention following surgery. If protection from stroke or myocardial infarction requires anticoagulation after surgery, we believe that often the most prudent choice is delay of the surgery rather than submitting the patient to the risk of anticoagulation therapy in the immediate postoperative period.

Occasionally, one encounters preoperative coagulopathies in these (usually elderly) patients. In most such instances, surgery should be deferred indefinitely or at least until the defect can be controlled. Preoperative, intraoperative, and postoperative fresh frozen plasma or other blood products must be available for prevention of bleeding (and secondary significant neurologic injury from the pressure of a hematoma on neural elements) when surgery is finally attempted.

Patients with signs and symptoms of peripheral neuropathy along with those of stenosis present a special problem in surgical planning as well as in postoperative care. Peripheral neuropathy from any cause will compromise the quality of the surgical result since many of the preoperative leg and foot symptoms will remain unchanged. The patient and his family need to be informed that the result of the surgery may not include complete relief of radicular symptoms, such as numbness and burning in the feet. The extent and severity of the neuropathy should be documented prior to surgery, as a baseline reference. Postoperatively, careful control of diabetes and alcohol ingestion is required to achieve the best possible result.

Orthopaedic disabilities, when present, may also require careful consideration. When a stenosis patient also has hip or knee disease we often suggest correction of these problems before stenosis surgery. Limping due to hip or knee arthritis puts a severe lateral and rotational stress on the spine which may exaggerate the stenosis symptoms, and hip flexion contracture causes secondary lumbar extension when walking, thus effectively making the stenosis more severe. Further, the hip or knee disease will make rehabilitation more difficult and less effective. The differential diagnosis of what causes the pain is sometimes difficult in these patients, and may require neurodiagnostics as well as joint, nerve, and epidural blocks.

Social and Vocational Issues

Social and vocational issues are important in spinal stenosis as in many other spinal problems. Because many patients are elderly, their home situation becomes critical. Arrangements to support the patients postoperatively should be made preoperatively and the family should be aware of what is required, and what can be expected.

Vocational issues are sometimes also important, and may actually be what forces the patient to a surgical decision. Expectations in this respect must be realistic. Patients in whom a "simple" one-level laminectomy is performed can often return to even a physically demanding job, particularly when the facet joints are minimally excised. Often, however, some accommodation regarding walking, lifting, bending, and twisting is necessary, and in patients with a fusion, return to work may not be possible until well after a fusion has healed, i.e., perhaps 6 months to a year. Patients with sedentary occupations, on the other hand, can return to work after 3 to 4 weeks.

Autologous Blood and Medication

Preoperative preparation for anticipated blood replacement needs is now routine in most hospitals. There is almost always enough time before surgery to obtain blood from the patient or one of the patient's relatives and to store it fresh or frozen. This becomes important if one of the larger reconstructive procedures is planned. Autologous blood should ideally be available in all cases requiring fusion, in-

strumentation, or revision of a previous spinal operation. We do not routinely reinfuse predeposit blood, but use the blood only as needed. A healthy patient can safely be phlebotomized of 450 mL of blood as often as three to four times in the 6 weeks preceding surgery. Oral iron therapy should always be provided.

A special concern in these patients is the frequent use of nonsteroidal antiinflammatory drugs (NSAIDs), which increase the risk of bleeding. They need to be replaced preoperatively with pain medication of another type. The time at which these drugs should be stopped preoperatively varies depending on their half-lives. Salicylates and piroxicam need to be stopped a few days before the operation.[3]

Preoperative Teaching and Rehabilitation

Discussion of the proposed procedure is part of the informed consent process. Informed consent is a mandatory part of clinical practice in United States and, of course, is practiced elsewhere as well. The elements of an informed consent include explaining:

1. The nature and purpose of the proposed procedure
2. Risks, complications, and problems in recuperation
3. Alternative forms of treatment

Preoperative teaching, which, of course, must be in lay language, helps prepare the patient emotionally, ensures cooperation, and makes disappointments less likely. Realistic expectations are the key to satisfied patients. Risks should not be hidden, but, of course, the ways in which these risks will be minimized should be explained as well. In spinal stenosis there are often several alternative approaches to treatment, which need to be discussed. Not infrequently a failure of a more conservative treatment alternative precedes a discussion of an operative treatment. Discussion of why the previous treatment failed should then always be included.

Rehabilitation efforts should ideally begin before surgery. The stationary bicycle is an important tool in the rehabilitation of stenosis patients, and we like the patients to start using the bicycle before surgery to improve their general condition, and prepare them for the later rehabilitation. Bicycling is preferred since patients who cannot walk can usually use the bicycle on which they can lean forward, thus relieving some of the effects of the stenosis on the cauda equina.

POSTOPERATIVE CARE

Blood Replacement

Most patients who undergo the common one- or two-level-wide decompression do not require transfusion. Healthy patients will tolerate a postoperative drop in hemoglobin to 9 or 10 g/dL without replacement. However, the elderly and those with cardiopulmonary disease should not be subjected to the stress of a severely reduced oxygen-carrying capacity even briefly. As indicated previously, our preference is to use autologous blood, which can be stored fresh up to 35 days, and fresh frozen plasma much longer. Autologous blood reduces the hazards of the standard blood transfusion, including the risk of acquired immunodeficiency syndrome (AIDS) and hepatitis. Techniques for reclamation and transfusion of blood lost during surgery have proved useful in some very large spinal reconstructive procedures. However, this is seldom a consideration in stenosis surgery.[7]

Antibiotics and Anticoagulants

Surgical wound infection rates are increased in patients older than 70 years, particularly if obese. Diabetes is another risk factor, as are operative procedures lasting more than 2 hours. All these factors are present in many spinal stenosis procedures. For these reasons, prophylactic antibiotic therapy given as an intravenous (IV) medication (usually a cephalosporin), intraoperatively and postoperatively, and irrigation during the procedure with an antibiotic solution has been the standard in our unit for the past 15 years. We credit this policy with contributing to a reduction of postoperative sepsis to a manageable 0.02%. Prophylaxis should start 30 to 60 minutes before surgery and last for no more than 24 hours.

Wound closure for the smaller operations without bone grafting can be safely done with a subcuticular suture reinforced with sterile adhesive strips. In the elderly patient, or those with extensive incisions, skin sutures or staples are preferred.

The extent and frequency of postoperative hematoma formation can be reduced by a suction drainage system for 48 hours after surgery. Drains should almost always be considered in cases with intertransverse fusion and iliac crest bone graft. They should be avoided if possible in cases where dural repair was necessary.

In contrast to hip operations, spinal surgery does not carry a particularly high risk of deep venous thrombosis (DVT) and pulmonary embolism. Routine prophylaxis is therefore not indicated. Patients with a previous history of DVT, and patients in whom prolonged bed rest for some reason becomes necessary are at high risk, and prophylaxis should be considered. Warfarin, low-dose heparin, and aspirin should not be used routinely because of the risk of bleeding. This is particularly a concern with warfarin. Physical measures including external pneumatic compression are preferred, but are probably less effective. Compression stockings have a modest effect in reducing venous thrombosis, but are simple and inexpensive, and, of course, have no bleeding complications.

Pain Management

Pain management is important. With adequate pain control, rehabilitation is more rapid and effective and chronic pain complaint is less likely. Yet, it has been found repeatedly that a large proportion of postoperative patients experience insufficient analgesia. Addiction is not a problem when medications are used briefly for relief of pain, but must of course be considered. Three different administration techniques are used: intermittent intramuscular injections, continuous infusion, and patient-controlled analgesia (PCA).[5] Intermittent injections are simple and inexpensive but result in fluctuating levels of anesthetic. Self-administration of IV narcotic drugs, through a pump system, is effective and requires a smaller overall dose than narcotic medication administered "as needed." PCA is not an ideal method for elderly or confused patients, however, since they forget instructions or lose the button in the bed at night. These patients do better for the first 48 hours with a moderate dose of intramuscular (IM) narcotics given at regular intervals, not "as needed." The dose should be sufficient to give persistent pain relief without producing severe central nervous system (CNS) depression. This is often a rather fine line in elderly patients.

The need for systemic narcotic medication can be significantly reduced by the use of 80 mg of methylprednisolone acetate given epidurally at the conclusion of the surgical procedure.[4, 17] Epidural morphine (0.01 mg/kg) as a bolus in 10 mL can also be placed in the epidural space proximal to the area of decompression by catheter prior to closure. This is no more effective than methylprednisolone acetate following laminotomy.[17] In fusion patients, however, it may have some added benefit.[1] The problems with epidural morphine are urinary retention requiring bladder catheterization, itching, nausea, ileus, and respiratory depression. The disadvantages appear to outweigh the advantages except in young healthy adults with large procedures (especially fusions). We have not used epidural morphine administered through a catheter postoperatively[6]; pain control has been satisfactory with the PCA system.

NSAIDs should be avoided in the early postoperative period as they increase the risk of bleeding. In patients with fusion, there is also some concern about the use of NSAIDs, which may interfere with bone healing.

Mobilization and Hospitalization

Stenosis is not a single entity, and the surgical treatment varies from a small one-level central decompression to wide multilevel decompressions and fusions, and even anterior corpectomy with instrumentation. Immediate postoperative care is dictated by the procedure. The guiding principle is to achieve the most rapid mobilization with maintenance of spinal structural integrity, neurologic recovery, and healing of the wound and any fusion that was necessary.

A one- or two-level decompression in which the pars interarticularis and at least 50% of both facets remain intact is perhaps the procedure performed in the majority of surgical stenosis patients. These patients require an average of 5 days in hospital following surgery. We begin bedside "dangling" on the first postoperative day, standing and walking on the first or second postsurgical day, and then progress rapidly to a level of activity sufficient to manage in the home. Ideally, the patient should be independent in self-care, able to walk 50 m independently, or at least with a walker or cane, and be able to climb the stairs in the home, if necessary. The guidance of a physical therapist may be helpful. It is, however, not an absolute requirement.

Patients with multilevel wide decompressive laminectomies, fusions, and those patients who have been instrumented may require a longer hospital stay. Generally, however, we follow the program outlined above, except that these patients may require orthotics as discussed subsequently.

Orthotics

Orthotics are not necessary in all patients operated on for spinal stenosis. Special precautions are necessary, however, in patients who have had wide multilevel decompressions in order to reduce the

risk of late fracture of the pars interarticularis or remaining facet. If the remaining pars interarticularis or facet is obviously severely deficient, that level will properly have been fused. In either case, we fit these patients with a custom-made thoracolumbar orthosis (Fig 35–1). In the patients that have not had a fusion but may be at risk of fracture, the use of the orthosis is continued for 6 to 12 weeks. In those patients in whom a fusion was necessary, the brace treatment is continued until the fusion shows good consolidation by radiograph. In patients in whom instrumentation has been necessary, we still believe that the use of a postoperative orthosis is important. This is particularly the case when the bone is osteoporotic. It should be remembered that the strength of osteoporotic bone decreases by the square of the density, and that the modulus increases by the cube of the density. This means that the risk of bony failure at the attachment sites for the instrumentation increases rapidly as the bone becomes more osteoporotic. Strength of all soft tissues decreases with age. Further, the risk of failure above the instrumented level is also great owing to increased stress concentration of the segment adjacent to the rigid instrumented level, and, again, the risk increases with age. Bracing is intended to reduce the risk of screw or hook detachment as well as the stress concentration at the unfused segments while allowing the rehabilitation to progress otherwise.

The need for orthotics after spinal operations is controversial and there are no clean prospective scientific studies. A lumbar orthosis cannot prevent intervertebral motions and can only mildly reduce the load on the spine.[13, 15, 16] By keeping the trunk upright, gross motions and the overall load can be kept at a minimum, however.[12] Micromotion is probably an important factor with respect to the healing of a

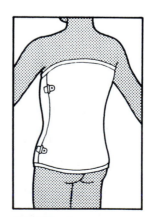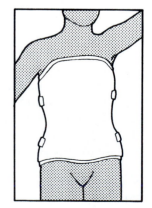

FIG 35–1.
Orthosis used by us postoperatively.

fusion. Recent studies by Johnsson et al.[8, 9] employed internal markers and roentgen stereophotogrammatic analysis (RSA) to determine motions between fused spinal vertebrae postoperatively. It was found that translations begin to decrease 3 to 6 months after a successful noninstrumented posterolateral fusion (Figs 35–2 and 35–3). By 12 months, the fusion was considered rigid. The use of rigid orthoses for 5 months resulted in a significantly higher fusion rate than when the same orthosis was used for 3 months. Apparently the consolidation of a fusion takes as long as 6 months. This observation is in agreement with magnetic resonance (MR) studies of the fusion mass, indicating a decrease in reparative granulation tissue and hyperemia after 6 months.[11] We prefer to treat our fused patients for 6 months postoperatively in a brace.

Electric stimulation is being used increasingly to promote healing of spinal fusions. Direct current stimulation has been demonstrated in nonblinded and nonrandomized clinical studies to enhance fusion,[10] and a randomized double-blind prospective study of pulsed electromagnetic fields for lumbar interbody fusions was found to result in significantly higher fusion rates for active vs. inactive treatment (92% success vs. 65%).[14] We have used pulsed electromagnetic stimulation with excellent results and compliance over the past 5 years for all types of fu-

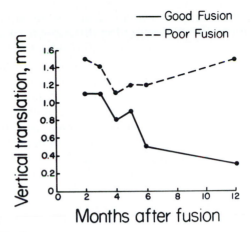

FIG 35–3.
Mean vertical translation between vertebrae in ten fusions with good radiographic results compared with ten with poor fusion. (Adapted from Johnsson R, Strömquist B, Axelsson P, et al: Influence of spinal immobilization on consolidation of posterolateral fusion. Presented to the International Society for the Study of the Lumbar Spine, Heidelberg, Germany, May 13–16, 1991.)

sions, but have not performed a randomized evaluation of its use. Figure 35–4 illustrates the device currently used by us.

Physical Rehabilitation

Physical rehabilitation postoperatively primarily involves reconditioning. Because of their preoperative pain and its relation to activity, most patients with spinal stenosis are deconditioned. In the early

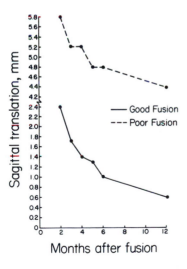

FIG 35–2.
Mean sagittal translation between vertebrae as determined by roentgen stereophotogrammetry. Ten fusions with good radiographic results are compared with ten with poor fusion. (Adapted from Johnsson R, Strömquist B, Axelsson P, et al: Influence of spinal immobilization on consolidation of posterolateral fusion. Presented to the International Society for the Study of the Lumbar Spine, Heidelberg, Germany, May 13–16, 1991.)

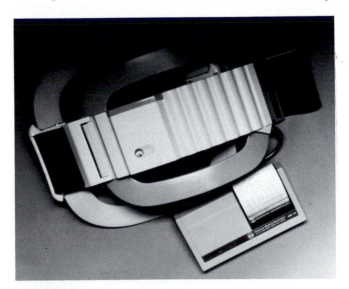

FIG 35–4.
Stimbrace providing pulsed electromagnetic fields to the fused area.

postoperative period we encourage these patients to walk, gradually increasing the distances to at least 1 km after 2 to 3 weeks and then adding distance gradually. Because walking may be uncomfortable at first, the exercise bicycle provides an attractive alternative. This is particularly true in climates where cold, snow, rain, or extreme heat sometimes make outdoor walking a problem. Aquatic exercises or simply walking in water are also excellent alternatives when wound healing is complete.

We do not emphasize muscle strengthening exercises during the first 2 to 3 months after wide laminectomies, and not until healing is complete in spinal fusions. This does not mean that upper or lower extremity exercises are not permitted, but simply that we do not emphasize them. Most of our patients are elderly and need to concentrate on conditioning rather than on muscle strengthening or flexibility.

Home Care

The exceptional patient will require little or no special care at home following stenosis surgery. However, many patients will require several weeks or more of home care with gradually decreasing intensity. This is not so much because of the operation itself as because of the age and general condition of many stenosis patients. The elderly patient with severe intercurrent disease or disability almost certainly will require more care than the average modern family can provide. A patient such as this may require skilled nursing, physical therapy, housekeeping, and "meals on wheels." Where available, an intermediate care facility that provides these services on a temporary basis is ideal. Geriatric and rehabilitation facilities, as well as other long-term care facilities and nursing homes, are examples of such intermediate resources. A plan including these alternatives should be made before the operation, to make certain that they are available. Younger, healthy patients, with able family members at home, will require fewer or none of these services.

The home health care plan includes the patient, the responsible family member, the visiting nurse, physical therapist, and occupational therapist. The patient must take responsibility for his or her care as rapidly as possible. The surgical team must teach the patient the postoperative care plan, short- and long-term goals, and explain the patient's role in the plan. The nurse will provide trained medical eyes and ears. The nurse must be able to appreciate what

is the expected postoperative course and what is unusual so that any significant deviation from the expected can be reported to the surgical team so that timely action can be taken. Additionally, the nurse should be able to remove sutures or clips, teach wound care, explain medications, and in rare instances give IV medications.

The physical therapist needs to provide and supervise a plan of safe aerobic conditioning, and teach use of supports for walking where necessary. Specific physical therapy, including flexibility and muscle strengthening, is a later issue. The occupational therapist (OT) can provide valuable help with simple assistive devices and training in independent living. In our setting, the OT provides the services just prior to discharge from the hospital, but follow-up home visits are often necessary, and sometimes a visit to the patient's home before discharge is needed to evaluate the appropriate assistive needs.

For a postoperative plan to be successful, it must be directed by the surgeon. During the initial 4 weeks after discharge, we try to avoid requiring the patient's attendance at our office or clinic. We place a phone call to the patient during the first week. We also provide written advice in anticipation of the patient's questions and needs and provide phone consultation (when necessary) with the visiting nurse. We ask the visiting nurse to remove sutures or surgical clips at 2 weeks if the wound is well healed and there is no hematoma.

We plan for the first office or clinic visit to take place at 4 to 6 weeks. The purpose of this visit is to assess the patient's progress to date and modify the plan as necessary. The goals should be increased and activity advanced rapidly. In nonfusion patients, the goal should be full function in the home and in the community by 12 to 16 weeks. If this goal is not being achieved, then causes for failure should be sought. Inadequate activation may be the problem. Inpatient rehabilitation should then be considered or a more active physical therapy intervention in an outpatient setting or the patient's home.

CONCLUSIONS

In patients with stenosis, the pre- and postoperative planning and care are as important to the quality of the final result as is surgery itself. Careful attention to the patient's general condition, preoperative planning for blood transfusion and medication, adequate postoperative pain management, and early activity provide for good results. Reasonable expectations and careful preoperative teaching provide for satisfied patients.

REFERENCES

1. Blackman RG, Reynolds J, Shively J: Intrathecal morphine: Dosage and efficacy in younger patients for control of postoperative pain following spinal fusion. *Orthopedics* 1991; 14:555–557.
2. Bolt RJ: *Medical Evaluation of the Surgical Patient*. Mt Kisco, NY, Futura Publishing Co, 1987.
3. Erian RF: Drugs that affect bleeding, in Johnson RG (ed): *Blood Loss in Spinal Surgery*. Philadelphia, Hanley & Belfus, 1991, pp 87–102.
4. Foulkes GD, Robinson JS Jr: Intraoperative dexamethasone irrigation in lumbar microdiscectomy. *Clin Orthop* 1990; 261:224–228.
5. Harmer M, Rosen M, Vickers MD: *Patient-Controlled Analgesia*. Oxford, England, Blackwell Scientific Publishing, 1985.
6. Ibrahim AW, Faraq H, Naguib M: Epidural morphine for pain relief after lumbar laminectomy. *Spine* 1986; 11:1024–1026.
7. Johnson RG: Blood loss in spinal surgery: Is there a problem?, in Johnson RG (ed): *Blood Loss in Spinal Surgery*. Philadelphia, Hanley & Belfus, 1991, pp 1–6.
8. Johnsson R, Selvik G, Strömquist B, et al: Mobility of the lower lumbar spine after posterolateral fusion determined by roentgen stereophotogrammatic analysis. *Spine* 1990; 15:347–350.
9. Johnsson R, Strömquist B, Axelsson P, et al: Influence of spinal immobilization on consolidation of posterolateral fusion. Presented to the International Society for the Study of the Lumbar Spine, Heidelberg, Germany, May 13–16, 1991.
10. Kane WJ: Facilitation of lumbosacral fusions by means of electronic bone growth stimulation. Presented to the Scoliosis Research Society, Seattle, Sept 1979.
11. Lang P, Chafetz N, Genaut HK, et al: Lumbar spinal fusion. Assessment of functional stability with magnetic resonance imaging. *Spine* 1990; 15:581–588.
12. Lantz SA, Schultz AB: Lumbar spine orthosis wearing. I. Restriction of gross body motions. *Spine* 1986; 11:834–837.
13. Lumsden RM, Morris JM: An in vivo study of axial rotation and immobilization of the lumbo sacral joint. *J Bone Joint Surg [Am]* 1968; 50:1591–1602.
14. Mooney V: A randomized double-blind prospective study of the efficacy of pulsed electromagnetic fields for interbody fusions. *Spine* 1991; 15:708–712.
15. Nachemson AL, Andersson GBJ, Schultz AB: Mechanical effectiveness studies of lumbar spine orthoses. *Scand J Rehabil Med Suppl* 1983; 9:193–249.
16. Norton PL, Brown T: The immobilizing efficiency of the back braces: Their effect on the posture and motion of the lumbosacral spine. *J Bone Joint Surg [Am]* 1957; 39:111–139.
17. Schell B, McNeill TW, Andersson GBJ, et al: A comparison of epidural morphine and epidural corticosteroids in controlling postoperative pains for patients undergoing lumbar laminectomy. *Orthop Trans* 1988; 12:112.

Conclusions

36

Putting It All Together: The Stenosis Algorithms

Gunnar B. J. Andersson, M.D., Ph.D.
Thomas W. McNeill, M.D.

To summarize the contents of this book in a single chapter would be presumptuous. As should be clear to the reader, spinal stenosis remains a topic on which there is considerable diversity in thought. This is partly because spinal stenosis is not a single entity, but includes a variety of conditions and presents with greatly variable symptoms. There are many acceptable diagnostic alternatives, and a large number of treatment choices. Clearly, there is a need for unifying concepts, as long as they do not restrict thought and action. Our aim in this final chapter is to provide a frame onto which details and variations can be grafted. To that purpose we have divided stenosis by symptoms and signs, rather than by etiology and morphology. This is how the patient presents to the physician and thus a logical starting point for any investigative and treatment effort.

As discussed in Chapter 17, spinal stenosis presents as four principal symptom complexes: We will refer to those as neurogenic intermittent claudication (NIC), radiculopathy, chronic cauda equina syndrome (CCE), and atypical leg pain (ALP). The main clinical features of the four spinal stenosis subgroups are listed in Table 36–1. Overlap is not uncommon, but most often there are clear distinguishing symptoms and signs. All patients with these presentations do not have spinal stenosis, however.

Table 36–2 lists the main differential diagnoses for each.

The principal diagnostic alternatives to consider for each entity are given in Table 36–3. A minimum evaluation should include a clinical examination and plain film radiographs. When indicated, the next step is spinal imaging. In our opinion, computed tomography (CT) scans have advantages over magnetic resonance imaging (MRI) in that the quality is more uniform, making it easier to distinguish between bone and soft tissue. Further, the cost is less, the time involved shorter, and the availability greater. The rapid advances in technology should be acknowledged, however, and will eventually make MRI even more attractive. Presently, its main advantages lie in its ability to evaluate soft tissue and bone marrow, in its safety, and in the ability to scan the whole of the lumbar spine in one sequence. Myelograms should, we think, only be used when surgery has been decided on as a treatment alternative and only when the information from CT and MRI examinations are incomplete to make appropriate decisions. A CT scan should always follow the myelogram. Neurodiagnostics are complementary as are bone scans. In patients with intermittent spinal claudication, vascular studies may occasionally be required and when a cauda equina syndrome is present, urodynamic studies are often indicated.

TABLE 36–1.

Signs and Symptoms in Patients Presenting With the Four Main Symptom Complexes of Spinal Stenosis.*

Radiculopathy	CCE	NIC	ALP
Sciatica	Urinary/bowel incontinence Urinary urgency/hesitancy	Pseudoclaudication	Leg pain†
Low back pain	Low back pain	Low back pain	Low back pain
Motor deficit	Sciatica	Sciatica	Tingling
Sensory deficit		Motor deficit	
Paresthesias		Sensory deficit	
Weakness			

*NIC = neurogenic intermittent claudication; CCE = chronic cauda equina syndrome; ALP = atypical leg pain. The primary distinguishing symptom is listed at the top of the table.
†Leg pain which is not typical of either radicular or neurogenic claudication. Distribution is often diffuse, bizarre, and is nondermatomal.

The patient with atypical leg symptoms presents a particular diagnostic challenge. A pelvic radiograph should always be obtained to grossly evaluate that area and the hip joints.

Once the diagnosis has been established, appropriate treatment can begin. Not infrequently treatment attempts start on first presentation even before diagnostic tests have been obtained. This treatment usually includes analgesics, nonsteroidal anti-inflammatory agents, and some degree of rest. Conservative treatment is always the first step. Along with medication and rest different types of exercises can be useful, as discussed in Chapter 26. We have been impressed by the results of epidural steroid injections in patients for whom these simple measures are insufficient, but must acknowledge that the results are difficult to predict and sometimes pain relief is short. Failure of conservative therapy, disabling pain, inability to function, and progressive neurologic deficit are the main indications for surgery. Decompressive laminectomy is the required operation for all patients. Fusion should be performed when (1) the spine is preoperatively unstable, or (2) the spine is rendered unstable by the laminectomy. This requires judgment on the part of the surgeon. A fusion should not be performed routinely and should not be taken lightly since secondary effects of fusion on adjacent motion segments cannot be avoided. Also, instrumentation cannot be advised as a routine procedure, as discussed in Chapter 28.

TABLE 36–2.

Differential Diagnoses for the Four Main Symptom Complexes of Spinal Stenosis*

Radiculopathy	NIC	CCE	ALP
Neuropathy	Vascular claudication.	CNS disease	CNS disease
Tumor	Congestive heart failure	Herniated disc	Hip disease
Infection		Cervical myelopathy	Trauma to nerve
Herpes zoster		Primary bladder disease	Pelvic disease
Herniated disc		Pelvic disease	Retroperitoneal disease
Nerve trauma		Multiple sclerosis	Neuropathy
			Herpes zoster
			Polymyalgia rheumatica
			Muscle cramps
			Metabolic
			Postpoliomyelitis syndrome
			Others
			Sympathetic dystrophy

*NIC = neurogenic intermittent claudication; CCE = chronic cauda equina syndrome; ALP = atypical leg pain.

TABLE 36–3.

Diagnostic Tests of Patients With Suspect Spinal Stenosis Presenting as One of the Four Main Symptom Complexes*

Radiculopathy	CCE	NIC	ALP
Imaging	As radiculopathy	As radiculopathy	As radiculopathy
X-ray			
CT	Urinary flow	Stress test	Pelvic radiographs
MRI			
Myelogram	Cystometrogram	Doppler studies	Cervical radiographs
Bone scan			
	Sphincter EMG	Arteriogram	MRI of cervical spine, spinal cord
Electrodiagnostics			
EMG	MRI of cervical spine,		
NCV	spinal cord, brain		Spinal fluid analysis
SSEP			
MEP			MRI of pelvic and retroperitoneal space
Metabolic studies			
Diabetes			
Alcohol			
Laboratory tests			
ESR			
Selective blocks			

*NIC = neurogenic intermittent claudication; CCE = chronic cauda equina syndrome; ALP = atypical leg pain; NCV = nerve conduction velocity.

THE ALGORITHM

The three tables presented in this chapter provide the basis for a spinal stenosis algorithm. (By algorithm we mean a step-by-step plan for arriving at a diagnosis.) These tables, however, do not infer the most direct or elegant means of arriving at the appropriate diagnosis. An experienced physician working with a complaint that he or she sees frequently will institute an appropriate algorithm quickly, easily, and efficiently. It is often called the "plan." Because spinal stenosis is not a single entity and because it may present with a variety of different syndromes (all of which may not be included here) one attempt at a moderately comprehensive series of algorithms seems appropriate (Algorithms 36–1 through 36–4). These algorithms are meant to serve several purposes: (1) as a departure point for a discussion of spinal stenosis; (2) as an overview of this book; and (3) as a guide for teaching young physicians. They are surely not meant to be the only or the definitive algorithms for spinal stenosis. The algorithms represent the stage in the process of accurate anatomic diagnosis that follows an appropriate history and physical examination (see Chapter 17). For purposes of brevity and clarity a key is provided for many of the junction points.

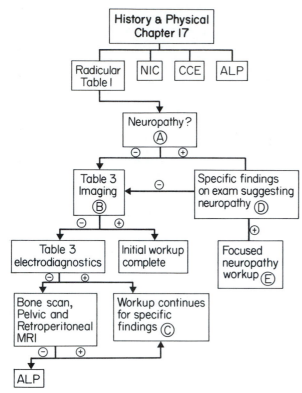

ALGORITHM 36–1.
See Tables 36–3 and 36–3.

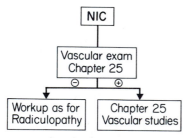

ALGORITHM 36–2.

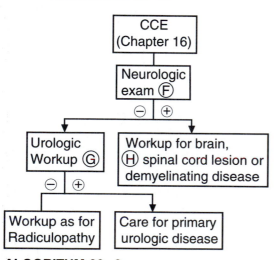

ALGORITHM 36–3.

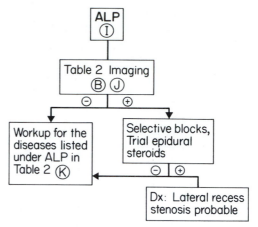

ALGORITHM 36–3.
See Table 36–2.

Key to Algorithms 36–1 to 36–4

Radiculopathy

A. History suggestive of the possibility of peripheral neuropathy: diabetes, alcoholism, tumor, radiation therapy, etc.

B. Imaging should begin with radiographs and either CT or MRI (at the present writing, CT is preferred in the diagnosis of stenosis). Myelography is reserved as a preoperative test.

C. The most likely protocol to be followed at this juncture would be either tumor or infection.

D. Distal findings including absent reflexes, nondermatomal sensory changes, and cutaneous hyperalgesia. Sensory changes are usually greater than motor changes.

E. This should start with a workup for diabetes as it is the most common cause of peripheral neuropathy. If negative, then a complete workup for neuropathy should follow.

Chronic Cauda Equina Syndrome (CCE)

F. Upper motor neuron findings such as hyperreflexia, clonus, positive (+) Babinski or Hoffman reflex, spastic gait.

G. This would include at least a cystometrogram and may include sphincter EMG, urine flow studies, and cystoscopy.

H. If there are cervical complaints or findings, begin the workup directed toward cervical myelopathy.

Atypical Leg Pain (ALP)

I. ALP is diffuse, bizarre, or nondermatomal leg pain often associated with lower back pain.

J. In ALP the most likely spinal cause is lateral recess stenosis.

K. The easiest and quickest examinations should be done first (they were probably already done). These are a hip examination and skin examination for findings of herpes zoster or sympathetic dystrophy. Following this the most serious possible causes should be eliminated, namely occult (pelvic, retroperitoneal, or metastatic to bone) tumor. The other diagnostic categories in Table 36–2 can be worked up without haste.

Index